Replacement Therapies in
Adrenal Insufficiency

Replacement Therapies in
Adrenal Insufficiency

PETER C. HINDMARSH
London, United Kingdom

KATHY GEERTSMA
Dorset, United Kingdom

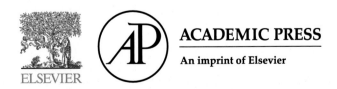

ACADEMIC PRESS
An imprint of Elsevier

Academic Press is an imprint of Elsevier
125 London Wall, London EC2Y 5AS, United Kingdom
525 B Street, Suite 1650, San Diego, CA 92101, United States
50 Hampshire Street, 5th Floor, Cambridge, MA 02139, United States

Notices

Knowledge and best practice in this field are constantly changing. As new research and experience broaden our understanding, changes in research methods, professional practices, or medical treatment may become necessary.

Practitioners and researchers must always rely on their own experience and knowledge in evaluating and using any information, methods, compounds, or experiments described herein. In using such information or methods they should be mindful of their own safety and the safety of others, including parties for whom they have a professional responsibility.

To the fullest extent of the law, neither the Publisher nor the authors, contributors, or editors, assume any liability for any injury and/or damage to persons or property as a matter of products liability, negligence or otherwise, or from any use or operation of any methods, products, instructions, or ideas contained in the material herein.

ISBN: 978-0-12-824548-4

For information on all Academic Press publications visit our website at
https://www.elsevier.com/books-and-journals

Publisher: Stacy Masucci
Acquisitions Editor: Patricia Osborn
Editorial Project Manager: Timothy Bennett
Production Project Manager: Punithavathy Govindaradjane
Cover Designer: Vicky Pearson

Typeset by TNQ Technologies

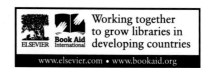

CONTENTS

For additional information on the topics covered in the book, visit the companion
site: https://www.elsevier.com/books-and-journals/book-companion/9780128245484

PREFACE

We have been encouraged by the very positive feedback from people worldwide on our last book 'Congenital Adrenal Hyperplasia: A Comprehensive Guide' and received so many heartfelt messages of gratitude, stating how the information has helped not only with understanding the condition, but also supported many to overcome the problems they were dealing with. These messages largely related not only to the life-threatening aspects as in how and why an adrenal crisis occurs, but as to why both the short and long term side effects caused by taking too little or too much medication, arise. The book was written with cortisol replacement therapy in mind and could be applicable to all with adrenal insufficiency. The responses we received however, pointed to the need for a book more dedicated to those with the various forms of adrenal insufficiency, so with this in mind we set to create a text that would be applicable for all.

Professor Hindmarsh's work in looking at the replacement of the vital life sustaining common factor in adrenal insufficiency, cortisol, is based on his studies of natural cortisol production in individuals without any adrenal problems of all ages, from children and adolescents to the elderly. These studies allowed the development of hydrocortisone pump therapy, which was an idea proposed by Dr Beth Davies, a General Practitioner in Dorset UK, following observations she made in a patient with adrenal insufficiency. Professor Hindmarsh took her observations and combined them with his cortisol studies to devise the first formula to mimic the circadian rhythm of cortisol using continuous subcutaneous hydrocortisone infusion pump therapy. This method using the Peter Hindmarsh formula has been successfully used since 2004 and has resulted in positive life changes in health for many individuals worldwide. The peer reviewed formula requires specific careful testing and determination of an individual's cortisol clearance, which allows rates to be carefully calculated to suit the individual's handling of hydrocortisone. The pump method is particularly helpful in bypassing any problems with the absorption of hydrocortisone, fast clearance and for individuals with gut problems. The benefit of this pioneering work led to the introduction of 24 hour profiling which yielded further experience and knowledge in replacement oral therapy.

Over the years it has become evident that measuring cortisol and other hormones has benefited so many and individualised dosing schedules can make a difference in preventing short and long term side effects. This experience forms the core of Section 3 where simple issues such as the interval between blood samples are very important, as the peak time from the dose can be either 30 minutes, 60 minutes, or 90 minutes so peaks are easily missed when sampling 2 to 3 hourly.

In endocrinology the ethos is to replace the hormone which is missing as close as possible to the way the body naturally produces it. In this case, cortisol is the missing hormone and the circadian rhythm has been well documented with studies showing the same rhythm as the studies Prof Hindmarsh has done. Using the pump to perfectly mimic the circadian rhythm of cortisol, has shown this then leads on to normalise other hormones and although difficult to achieve this with oral dosing, with individualised dosing and using detailed 24 hour profiles, it is possible. There is no doubt the dosing schedules can be challenging to follow. These are explained and suggested to patients, not forced on them.

Getting the cortisol replacement correct, means that the feedback system will respond as it should, so that in Addison's disease and congenital adrenal hyperplasia, ACTH and 17-hydroxyprogesterone (17OHP) respectively, will normalise. Many physicians focus only on supressing ACTH and/or 17OHP often using high doses of hydrocortisone and ensuing side effects. The simple message is that higher doses do not provide better cortisol coverage. This theme runs through this book, as getting replacement right minimises side effects of under and over treatment. We are all individual and nowhere is this more apparent as in the way our bodies handle drugs such as hydrocortisone.

Having adrenal insufficiency does not change the way the physiology of the body works, it just means we have to adapt what we do with our therapies such as hydrocortisone and fludrocortisone, to the metabolism of the patient. There are many causes for adrenal insufficiency and we look at these in Section 1, where we also consider how to identify if the person has adrenal insufficiency and how to determine the cause. Understanding pharmacology is important and we devote a chapter in Section 1 to this as it forms the basis for all our reasoning on dosing and assessing replacement therapy.

Section 2 outlines the problems faced when dosing is either too much or too little, both scenarios can occur within a 24 hour period and we discuss how the common side effects occur. Section 3 uses what we have learnt from pharmacology and hydrocortisone pump therapy to determine the best way to replace cortisol, how to determine cortisol peaks and troughs concentrations and interpret what we have achieved as well as managing day to day events. The circadian rhythm of cortisol is what we want to mimic, so we spend considerable time on this topic, particularly the issue of taking no dose after 6 pm (18:00), why this is not a sensible approach and the possible consequences of using this approach. We have not forgotten the importance of water and sodium balance which is also covered in this section.

One additional piece of information which has also influenced our thinking, are the results of a carefully formulated detailed questionnaire completed by patients and parents, which included questions on dosing, dosing times, and side effects both short and long term. These data, added to the biological information from our extensive repository of 24 hour cortisol profiles from over 100 individuals across all age groups without any adrenal problems, studies of cortisol delivery from hydrocortisone pumps where ideal replacement has been achieved, as well as more than 400 therapeutic cortisol profiles in patients with adrenal insufficiency at different ages receiving hydrocortisone in differing doses and times of the day, has helped refine replacement therapies.

Finally, we should not forget the most common cause of adrenal insufficiency is the use of exogenous glucocorticoids for inflammatory conditions and in organ transplantation. We consider this and how to wean off these treatments in Section 3.

Our aim in writing this book is to improve the knowledge and care for all those with adrenal insufficiency, by providing published peer reviewed data and showing clear examples of how appropriate testing, when undertaken carefully and accurately in conjunction with understanding individual metabolism of hydrocortisone, can improve outcomes. Thank you for taking an interest in this book and we hope the information makes a difference to the wellbeing of all with adrenal insufficiency.

ACKNOWLEDGEMENTS

We would both like to thank Professor Evelina Charmandari who has a wealth of knowledge in adrenal insufficiency, (she previously worked with Professor Hindmarsh in London, as well as at the National Institutes of Health in the United States of America and now in Athens, Greece), for reviewing this and our previous book 'Congenital Adrenal Hyperplasia, A Comprehensive Guide'. Her research has also been very valuable in the effort to improve care for all those with adrenal insufficiency.

Getting a book like this to publication and distribution is a huge task and we thank Stacy Masucci, Patricia Osborn, Timothy Bennett, Punithavathy Govindaradjane and the team at Elsevier for their support.

SECTION 1

Adrenal insufficiency is the term used to describe several conditions that all lead to a reduced or absent production and secretion of the glucocorticoid, cortisol. In some of these conditions the production and secretion of the mineralocorticoid, aldosterone, is also reduced or absent. Adrenal insufficiency can arise when the disease affects the adrenal glands which is termed primary adrenal insufficiency and secondary adrenal insufficiency when the disease affects the pituitary and/or hypothalamus in the brain. The most common cause of secondary adrenal insufficiency is the use of glucocorticoids to treat several conditions such as inflammatory states, for example asthma or rheumatoid arthritis, or when used to manage organ rejection in various organ transplantation programmes. Some patients who have been diagnosed with primary adrenal insufficiency, often refer to their condition as Addison's disease named after a physician who practised in the 19th century, Dr Thomas Addison. In fact Addison described very specific conditions affecting the adrenal glands, mainly tuberculosis.

Thomas Addison (1795-1860) was a physician at Guy's Hospital in London. His original work led to the description of pernicious anaemia which was later shown to be due to a deficiency of vitamin B12. In 1849 Addison came across a constellation of symptoms and signs including weakness, fatigue, anorexia, vomiting, abdominal pain, and weight loss along with skin pigmentation that gave the patient a bronzed sun-tanned appearance. He went on to describe 10 cases in detail and an 11th case as an additional note in 1855 in the publication "On the Constitutional and Local Effects of Disease of the Suprarenal Capsules."

The report described damage to the suprarenal (adrenal) glands caused by tuberculosis and secondary cancer spread. However, two cases are of note. Case 4, a 22 year old man who had died, where examination of the adrenal glands showed they were atrophied with evidence of marked inflammation which are features now recognised as adrenalitis associated with autoimmune adrenal insufficiency.

The second case, Case 10, was a 28 year old woman with tuberculosis found to have normal sized adrenal glands however with obstruction of the adrenal veins. Addison concluded that the manifestation of the adrenal insufficiency arose "upon an interruption of some special function than upon the nature of the organic change." It took another 46 years before the presence of adrenaline was discovered in the adrenal glands of sheep by biochemist Dr Jokichi Takamine in 1901 and it wasn't until 1935 that two biochemists Edward Kendall and Tadeus Reichstein isolated cortisol from bovine adrenal glands. The final discovery of the hypothalamo-pituitary-adrenal system only happened in 1981 with the identification of corticotrophin releasing hormone in the hypothalamus by the scientist Hans Selye. Interestingly, adrenocorticotrophin was identified in 1933 by biochemist James Collip, who in 1922 helped purify insulin along with Drs Frederick Banting, Charles Best and Professor JJ McLeod who were the first to isolate insulin in 1921.

Addison suffered with depression throughout his life and sadly took his own life in 1860 after retiring to Brighton shortly after his 1855 publication.

A collection of the published writings of Thomas Addison. Edited with introductory prefaces to several of the papers by Dr. Wilks and Dr. Daldy. London: New Sydenham Society, 1868. Avaliable from the Wellcome Collection https://wellcomecollection.org/works/s4j8ab8r.

CHAPTER 1

Adrenal Insufficiency

GLOSSARY

Adrenal insufficiency A general term to describe a number of conditions that lead to deficient production or action of cortisol.

Adrenocorticotropin Hormone produced by the pituitary gland that regulates cortisol synthesis and secretion from the adrenal glands.

Corticotropin-releasing hormone A hormone produced by the hypothalamus that regulates adrenocorticotropin synthesis and secretion from the pituitary gland.

False negative result Result from a test that says that a disease is not present when the person does have the condition.

False positive result Result from a test that says that a disease is present when the person does not have the condition.

Glucocorticoid A member of the steroid family similar to cortisol that are particularly involved in carbohydrate, protein and fat metabolism and have anti-inflammatory and immunomodulating properties.

Mineralocorticoid A member of the steroid family similar to aldosterone that is involved in sodium and water balance in the body.

Sensitivity of a test How often a test correctly generates a positive result for people who have the condition being tested for.

Specificity of a test How often a test correctly generates a negative result for people who do not have the condition being tested for.

GENERAL

Adrenal insufficiency is a general term which has been used to describe a number of conditions which lead to deficient production or action of the main glucocorticoid, cortisol. Depending on whether the problem lies in the adrenal glands or is due to impairment of the hypothalamo-pituitary-adrenal axis, there may or may not be alterations in mineralocorticoid and adrenal androgen production.

Adrenal insufficiency is a life-threatening disorder due to the lack of cortisol. This is well recognised in the United Kingdom emergency services call-out pathway. In this pathway an urgent response is triggered when using the phrase 'Adrenal Insufficiency.' Although adrenal insufficiency is commonly used as a description, it is very important to realise it is not in itself, a diagnosis. It merely represents cortisol deficiency of which there are a number of causes.

Broadly, adrenal insufficiency can result from primary adrenal failure, or secondary adrenal failure due to impairment of the hypothalamo-pituitary axis. This is illustrated in Figure 1.1 where the normal cortisol production is demonstrated in panel (a) the left hand side and the effect of primary adrenal disease in panel (b), where no cortisol is produced, but because of the feedback system to the hypothalamus and pituitary gland, adrenocorticotropin hormone (ACTH) from the pituitary gland is raised in an attempt to try to rectify the deficit in cortisol production. Panels (c) and (d) show the situation in secondary adrenal insufficiency where the problem lies in either the generation of corticotropin-releasing hormone (CRH)

Replacement Therapies in Adrenal Insufficiency. https://doi.org/10.1016/B978-0-12-824548-4.00007-3

and arginine vasopressin from the hypothalamus, or ACTH production from the pituitary gland. These are often referred to as secondary adrenal insufficiency if the cause is in the pituitary, or tertiary if the problem lies in the hypothalamus. Occasionally, the secondary and tertiary forms are called central adrenal insufficiency. Deficient ACTH production leads to a reduction in cortisol production from the adrenal glands and a reduction in size of the adrenal glands, because of the loss of the trophic effect of ACTH on adrenal cortical cells.

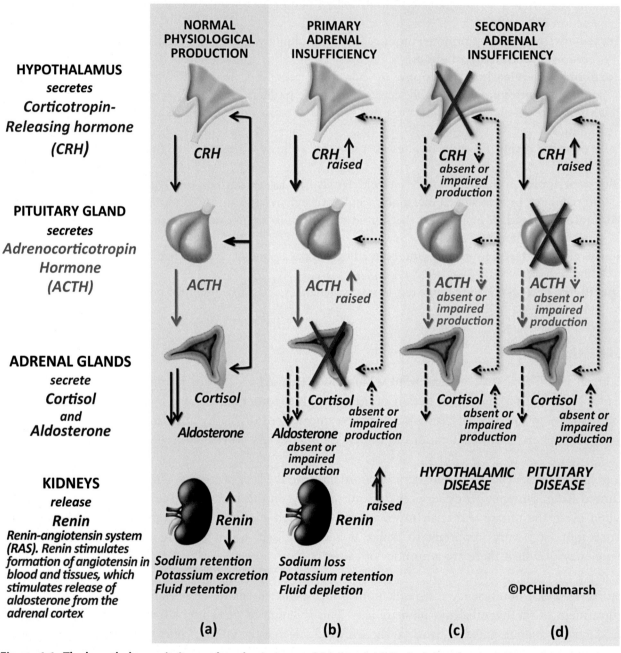

Figure 1.1 *The hypothalamo-pituitary-adrenal axis. In panel (a) the physiological situation is shown with corticotropin-releasing hormone (CRH) produced from the hypothalamus causing release of adrenocorticotropin (ACTH) from the pituitary gland which in turn releases cortisol from the adrenal glands. Cortisol feeds back negatively on CRH and ACTH formation. Sodium and water retention are mediated by the renin-angiotensin system acting to regulate aldosterone production from the adrenal cortex. Primary adrenal insufficiency is shown in panel (b). Cortisol is not produced so CRH and ACTH are raised in an attempt to increase circulating cortisol. Likewise, renin is increased because of the loss of aldosterone production. In secondary adrenal insufficiency (panels (c) and (d)) either CRH or ACTH is not produced leading to absent cortisol production but the renin system is not affected so aldosterone can still be produced.*

We can also introduce a third category of adrenal insufficiency where exogenous glucocorticoids are administered, usually for the treatment of inflammatory conditions. In this situation, there is an increased amount of glucocorticoid which suppresses the endogenous production of corticotropin-releasing hormone and ACTH, leading to reduced cortisol production from the adrenal glands. This situation is only of concern when the glucocorticoid used to control the inflammatory process is weaned down and the individual is left without endogenous cortisol production, because the hypothalamo-pituitary-adrenal axis has been suppressed by the exogenous glucocorticoid. Technically, this is secondary adrenal insufficiency but worth highlighting separately as it is common.

We are not going to discuss every single cause of adrenal insufficiency. There are a number of very good reviews cited in our reading list which can be consulted. To assist the reader, we have tabulated some of the more common causes of primary adrenal insufficiency in Figure 1.2 and for secondary/tertiary adrenal insufficiency, in Figure 1.3.

This book and this chapter are not about the individual conditions in detail, but about the generic use of glucocorticoids and mineralocorticoids although we will provide a brief overview of the more common conditions associated with adrenal insufficiency. We will be looking at replacement of glucocorticoids and mineralocorticoids through the book, across the age ranges and consider how best to monitor replacement therapy. Before progressing to these chapters, a general synopsis of adrenal insufficiency is given.

HOW COMMON IS ADRENAL INSUFFICIENCY?

Looking at primary adrenal insufficiency (predominantly Addison's disease) first, there has been an increase in the number of European cases from 50 per million of the population in the 1960s, to 150 per million at the current time. This gives an estimated incidence of 5 new cases per million of the population per year. In the past, tuberculosis was a common cause for primary adrenal insufficiency but this has been superseded by autoimmune adrenal insufficiency, where the body starts to recognise the cells of the adrenal cortex as foreign and develops antibodies against the enzymes in the adrenal cortical cells, leading to destruction of these cells.

Autoimmune adrenal insufficiency must be rising in incidence because the number of cases of adrenal insufficiency caused by tuberculosis has fallen dramatically during the 20th century. The majority of cases reported by Addison in 1855 were tuberculosis in origin with one case highly suggestive of an inflammatory cause which would be consistent with autoimmune induced atrophy of the adrenal glands. Like most autoimmune conditions, the adrenal form is more common in females than males and can present at any age with a peak age at presentation between 30 and 50 years.

In children, the more common cause of primary adrenal insufficiency is congenital adrenal hyperplasia (CAH). This is most commonly caused by a block at the conversion of 17-hydroxyprogesterone to 11-deoxycortisol due to the absence of the enzyme 21-hydroxylase or CYP21. We have covered this condition extensively in our book Congenital Adrenal Hyperplasia: A Comprehensive Guide and attention is drawn to the further reading list for details of this publication. Congenital adrenal hyperplasia usually presents in the first 2 weeks of life either because of a virilised female with ambiguity of the genitalia, or in males due to a salt-wasting crisis. This is the commonest form of CAH and is known as salt-wasting congenital adrenal hyperplasia (SWCAH). Treatment is with a glucocorticoid and a mineralocorticoid for life.

PRIMARY ADRENAL INSUFFICIENCY

CONDITION	UNDERLYING PROBLEM	OTHER FEATURES
AUTOIMMUNE ADRENALITIS		
Isolated	Associations with HLA system	None
APS 1 (APECED)	*AIRE* gene mutations	Mucocutaneous candidiasis, hypoparathyroidism
APS 2	Associations with HLA system	Hypothyroidism and type 1 diabetes
APS 4	Associations with HLA system	Vitiligo, coeliac and alopecia but not thyroid and type 1 diabetes
GENETIC DISORDERS		
Adrenoleukodystrophy	*ABCD1* and *ABCD2* gene mutations	Neurological involvement
Congenital adrenal hyperplasia		
21-hydroxylase	*CYP21A2* gene mutations	Salt loss and raised androgens
11beta-hydroxylase	*CYP11B1* gene mutations	Hypertension and raised androgens
3beta-hydroxysteroid dehydrogenase type 2	*3beta-HSD2* gene mutations	Ambiguous genitalia in boys
17alpha-hydroxylase	*CYP17A1* gene mutations	Pubertal delay and hypertension
P450 oxidoreductase	*P450 oxidoreductase* gene mutations	Skeletal problems (Antley-Bixler), abnormal genitalia
Side chain cleavage	*CYP11A1* gene mutations	XY sex reversal
Lipoid adrenal hyperplasia	*StAR* gene mutations	XY sex reversal
Adrenal hypoplasia congenita	*NROB1* gene mutations	Hypogonadotropic hypogonadism
IMAGe	*CDKN1C* gene mutations	Intrauterine growth restriction, adrenal hypoplasia, genital and skeletal abnormalities
SF-1 associated	*NR5A1* gene mutations	XY sex reversal
Kerns-Sayre syndrome	Mitochondrial DNA abnormalities	Eye, cardiac and other endocrine problems
Familial glucocorticoid deficiency		
Type 1	*MC2R* gene mutations	
Type 2	*MRAP* gene mutations	
Others	*MCM4* and *NNT* gene mutations	Immune natural killer cell abnormalities
Triple A syndrome	*AAAS* gene mutations	Achalasia, alacrima, deafness
INFECTIONS		
Tuberculosis	Tuberculosis	
AIDS	HIV-1	
Fungal	Histoplasmosis	
DRUG-INDUCED		
Anticoagulants	Haemorrhage	
Trilostane	Inhibition of 3beta-hydroxysteroid dehydrogenase type 2	
Ketoconazole, fluconazole etomidate	Inhibition of CYP11A1 and CYP11B1 enzymes	
Immune checkpoint inhibitors	? autoimmune effect	
OTHERS		
Bilateral adrenal haemorrhage		
Bilateral adrenalectomy		©PCHindmarsh

Figure 1.2 *Causes of primary adrenal insufficiency.*

SECONDARY/TERTIARY ADRENAL INSUFFICIENCY

CONDITION	UNDERLYING PROBLEM	OTHER FEATURES
SPACE-OCCUPYING LESIONS OR TRAUMA		
Pituitary and hypothalamic tumours	Low ACTH and/or CRH secretion	Other pituitary hormone problems
Pituitary stalk trauma following accidents	Low ACTH and/or CRH secretion	Other pituitary hormone problems
Pituitary or hypothalamic surgery	Low ACTH and/or CRH secretion	Other pituitary hormone problems
Pituitary or hypothalamic radiation	Low ACTH and/or CRH secretion	Other pituitary hormone problems
Infections/infiltrates such as Langerhans cell histiocytosis, meningitis, tuberculosis	Low ACTH and/or CRH secretion	Other pituitary hormone problems
Pituitary apoplexy (Sheehan's syndrome in pregnancy)	Low ACTH and/or CRH secretion	Acute severe headache, visual disturbances and other pituitary hormone problems
GENETIC DISORDERS		
HESX homeobox 1	*HESX1* gene mutations	Other pituitary hormone problems, septo-optic dysplasia, developmental problems
LIM Homeobox 4	*LIM homeobox 4* gene mutations	Other pituitary hormone problems
OTX homeobox 2	*OTX homeobox 2* gene mutations	Other pituitary hormone problems
PROP 1	*PROP homeobox 1* gene mutations	Other pituitary hormone problems, can have large pituitary gland
SRY Box 3	*SRY Box 3* gene mutations	Other pituitary hormone problems and developmental delay
T-box 19	*T-box 19* gene mutations	Isolated ACTH deficiency, early presentation
POMC deficiency	*POMC* gene mutation	Obesity, hyperphagia and red hair
DRUG-INDUCED Exogenous glucocorticoids Immune checkpoint inhibitors	? autoimmune effect - hypophysitis	©PCHindmarsh

Figure 1.3 *Causes of central or secondary/tertiary adrenal insufficiency.*

Another condition which illustrates the importance of arriving at a precise diagnosis, is adrenal hypoplasia congenita or AHC. In this condition, there is an abnormality in the gene *NROB1* or *DAX-1* which is a key step in the formation of the adrenal glands from the neuroectodermal ridge close to where the normal kidney forms. The histology of the gland is classic with small cells with dense centres giving an 'owls eye' appearance. The importance in making this diagnosis is that it is also associated with deficiency of luteinising hormone (LH) and follicle-stimulating hormone (FSH), so individuals not only have primary adrenal insufficiency, but also hypothalamic deficiency of the gonadotropin-releasing hormone which normally stimulates luteinising hormone (LH) and follicle-stimulating hormone (FSH) release. Such patients need pubertal induction and testosterone supplementation long term.

Congenital adrenal hyperplasia is more common and is estimated to be present in 1 in 12,000 to 1 in 18,000 live births, whereas adrenal hypoplasia congenita is much less common and because of its inheritance pattern, only affects boys. Secondary adrenal insufficiency is more common than primary adrenal insufficiency. The estimated prevalence is 200 per million and females are affected more than males. The age at which diagnosis can be made, is at any point throughout the life span with a large peak in those aged 50 to 70 years of age, associated predominately with pituitary tumours and primary irradiation for non pituitary tumours. In children, the main cause is congenital disorders of hypothalamo-pituitary development along with cranial irradiation for nonpituitary tumours, as well as pituitary tumours such as craniopharyngiomas.

Adrenal haemorrhage is a heterogeneous condition with several risk factors, underlying adrenal tumour, sepsis, and adrenal vein thrombosis. Even if recognised and treated with glucocorticoids mortality is high. An association with Covid-19 infection or vaccination is recently reported. The most common cause of secondary and tertiary adrenal insufficiency is the use of long term exogenous glucocorticoids which suppress CRH and ACTH production.

CAUSES OF PRIMARY ADRENAL INSUFFICIENCY

Autoimmune adrenalitis

Autoimmune adrenalitis can be isolated (40% of cases) or part of an autoimmune polyendocrinopathy syndrome (APS) (60%) which APS type 2 is the most common. The destruction of the adrenal cortex is mediated by the immune system with antibodies directed at the enzyme 21-hydroxylase in the isolated form. Association with the Human Leukocyte Antigen (HLA) which is the name given to the Major Histocompatibility Complex of man is seen in APS type 2. This complex is a large, fixed position on chromosome 6 of genes that code for proteins that sit on the surface of cells and are essential for regulation of the immune system. The HLA complex is situated on human chromosome 6 quite close to the genes which are involved with salt-wasting congenital adrenal hyperplasia.

The HLA system particularly DR3-DQ2 and DR4-DQ8 haplotypes (a collection of specific DNA sequences in a cluster of tightly linked genes that are inherited together) are strongly associated with APS type 2. APS type 2 is common and includes the constellation of type 1 diabetes mellitus and primary hypothyroidism. APS type 1 is associated with chronic candidiasis (thrush infections particularly of the nail beds) and hypoparathyroidism (underactive parathyroid glands which lead to low plasma calcium). Usually, the manifestations come in the temporal order of candidiasis, low calcium due to the hypoparathyroidism, followed by adrenal insufficiency later in childhood. This is an autosomal recessive inherited condition due to mutations in the *AIRE* gene. Other autoimmune conditions such as hepatitis can develop later in life.

One important point to make is the time course of adrenal insufficiency, particularly due to the autoimmune condition, which can take many years to evolve. This is common in many autoimmune conditions and was first described by Eisenbarth for type 1 diabetes mellitus. The proposal is that there is a genetic predisposition to developing the condition and that an additional precipitating event (such as a viral infection) sets the destructive process in motion. Figure 1.4 illustrates this concept and symptoms and signs only present when a considerable amount of adrenocortical tissue has been lost. The changes in the hypothalamo-pituitary-adrenal and renin-aldosterone axes biochemistry are shown in Figure 1.5. As in insulin dependent diabetes where there is residual insulin production still for several years after diagnosis, there can be some residual cortisol secretion although it is not enough to maintain normal levels of cortisol, so replacement therapy is required. These figures illustrate the difficulty in making an early diagnosis because the clinical features are not manifest until late in the disease process.

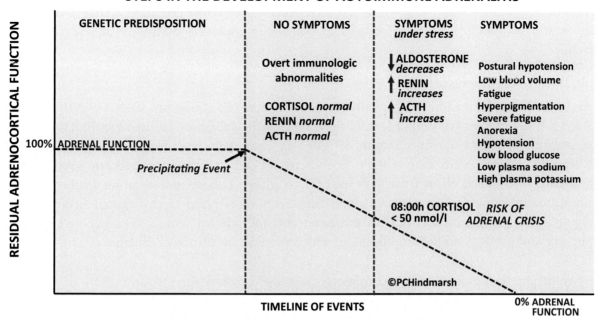

Figure 1.4 *Stages in the development of autoimmune adrenalitis and adrenal insufficiency.*

PROGRESSION OF ADRENAL INSUFFICIENCY

STAGE	ACTH	CORTISOL		PLASMA RENIN ACTIVITY	ALDOSTERONE	SYMPTOMS AND SIGNS
		0 mins	60 mins			
0	N	N	N	N	N	*None*
1	N	N	N	↑	N/↓	*None*
2	N	N	↓	↑	N/↓	*None*
3	N/↑	↓	↓	↑	↓	*Under *stress situations*
4	↑↑	↓↓	↓	↑↑	↓	*Present*

©PCHindmarsh

Figure 1.5 *Stages in the evolution of adrenal insufficiency from Stage 0 (no disease) to Stage 4 (disease present) in terms of adrenocorticotropin (ACTH), cortisol response to synacthen from zero to 60 minutes, plasma renin activity, aldosterone and the presence of symptoms and signs. N is normal response, ↑ increased amount or response compared to normal. ↑↑ very marked increased amount or response compared to normal, ↓ reduced response compared to normal and ↓↓ very reduced amount or response compared to normal. *Stress refers to intercurrent illness, trauma, surgery or intensive exercise.*

Adrenal hypoplasia congenita

Adrenal hypoplasia congenita (AHC) is a X-linked disorder and will affect boys as the gene is situated on the X chromosome. As females have two X chromosomes an affected gene on one of them will not have any affect in the mother, but because the male gets their X chromosome from the mother, if they inherit the affected gene on the X chromosome, they will manifest the condition. So, if one copy of the maternal *NROB1* or *DAX-1* gene is affected, there is 1 in 2 chance that the male offspring will have the condition.

The presentation is usually in an adrenal crisis within the first week of life, although later presentations have been recorded. *NROB1* or *DAX-1* is also important in pituitary gonadotropin and hypothalamic gonadotropin-releasing hormone synthesis, so deficiency leads to absent puberty and infertility.

AHC may also be part of what is known as a contiguous gene deletion syndrome (a clinical picture caused by a chromosomal abnormality that removes several genes lying in close proximity to one another on the chromosome) including the nearby genes for Duchenne muscular dystrophy and glycerol kinase deficiency.

X-linked Adrenoleukodystrophy

Adrenoleukodystrophy is another X-linked recessive disorder. The condition affects 1 in 20,000 men and boys and is caused by mutations in the ATP-binding cassette, subfamily D, member 1 (*ABCD1*) gene. These mutations prevent normal transport of very long chain fatty acids into peroxisomes, preventing their breakdown. Fatty acids have at their core a series of carbon atoms arranged one after another as if on a string. Very long chain fatty acids have 22 or more of these carbon atoms in their structure. Accumulation of abnormal amounts of these fatty acids takes place in the central nervous system, Leydig (testosterone producing) cells of the testes and the adrenal cortex, resulting in neurological impairment and primary adrenal insufficiency, which presents in infancy or childhood.

The two major forms of adrenoleukodystrophy are the cerebral (brain) form (50% of cases; early childhood manifestation with rapid progression) and adrenomyeloneuropathy (35% of cases; onset in early adulthood with slow progression) in which demyelination (loss of the myelin sheath around nerves which is important for transmission of impulse signals along the nerve), is restricted to the nerves running down the spine (spinal cord) and peripheral nerves. Since adrenal insufficiency can be the initial clinical manifestation, the diagnosis should be considered in young male patients with adrenal insufficiency by measurement of plasma concentrations of very long chain fatty acids. Early diagnosis is important as bone marrow transplantation can prevent the onset/worsening of the neurological problems, particularly in the brain.

Congenital adrenal hyperplasia

Congenital adrenal hyperplasia is a group of autosomal recessive disorders resulting from deficiency of one of the enzymes needed for synthesis of cortisol in the adrenal cortex. Figure 1.6 shows the pathway from cholesterol through to cortisol and aldosterone and the adrenal androgens. The most common form is classic 21-hydroxylase (CYP21) deficiency in which there is absence of glucocorticoid (cortisol) and mineralocorticoid (aldosterone) along with adrenal hyperandrogenism. The block is shown as the red line in Figure 1.6 with precursors above the block building up due to the ACTH drive to the adrenal glands to produce cortisol, which it is unable to do. As previously mentioned, the incidence varies between 1 in 12,000 to 18,000 live births and presentation is usually between 10 and 14 days of life with an adrenal crisis, or at birth with virilisation of the external genitalia in females due to the excess adrenal androgens.

The next most common form is 11beta-hydroxylase which is characterised by a lack of cortisol, hyperandrogenism and mineralocorticoid (deoxycorticosterone) excess leading to hypertension. Other enzymatic defects higher in the cortisol biosynthetic chain such as CYP17 deficiency and 3β-hydroxysteroid dehydrogenase, are present in both the adrenal cortex and the gonads leading to under virilisation of males along with signs of adrenal insufficiency.

The gonadal axis is not involved in the two most common forms of CAH, but the other enzyme blocks may lead to gonadal failure in which case LH and FSH may be raised. In untreated CAH or where cortisol replacement is suboptimal in CYP21 deficiency or 11beta-hydroxylase deficiency, LH and FSH may be suppressed due to the high circulating androgen levels. For a full description of these conditions see our companion book Congenital Adrenal Hyperplasia: A Comprehensive Guide by Peter Hindmarsh and Kathy Geertsma and published by Elsevier (2017).

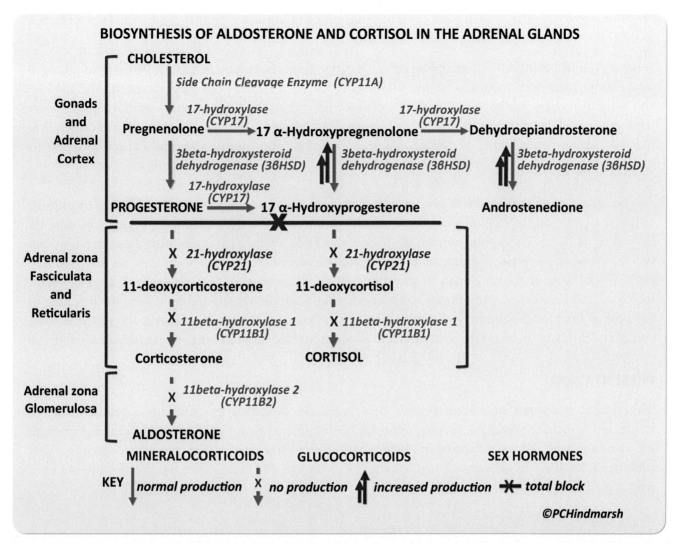

Figure 1.6 *Pathway for cortisol, aldosterone and adrenal androgen formation. Block at CYP21 (solid red line) leads to lack of formation of cortisol and aldosterone and an increase (red arrows) in 17-hydroxyprogesterone and androstenedione in the situation where there is 21 hydroxylase deficiency.*

CAUSES OF SECONDARY ADRENAL INSUFFICIENCY

Secondary adrenal insufficiency results from any process which involves the pituitary gland and interferes with ACTH secretion. ACTH deficiency can be isolated or can occur in association with deficiencies of other pituitary hormones. Genetic causes of ACTH deficiency include loss-of-function mutations in the genes encoding proopiomelanocortin gene and propeptide convertase, which result in early-onset severe obesity, as well as mutations in *TPIT*, a T-box factor (a family of proteins involved in the formation of the limbs and heart at an early stage of development) that controls reading of the proopiomelanocortin gene. These are rare causes which have an early onset manifest as cortisol deficiency. In addition to these causes of isolated ACTH deficiency, ACTH may be lost as part of hypopituitarism resulting from a number of pituitary developmental gene disorders, as well as trauma or tumours of the region.

Tertiary adrenal insufficiency describes loss of the hypothalamic peptides which regulate ACTH, corticotropin-releasing hormone and/or arginine vasopressin. Many clinicians combine tertiary into secondary insufficiency.

Two important drug families impact on the hypothalamo-pituitary-adrenal axis. Firstly, suppression of the hypothalamic-pituitary-adrenal axis by long term administration of high doses of glucocorticoids used for their anti-inflammatory effect, is the most common cause for adrenal insufficiency. These exogenous glucocorticoids switch off corticotropin-releasing hormone production by the hypothalamus and ACTH production by the pituitary. This is considered further in Chapter 15.

Secondly, advances in our understanding of the immune response to cancer and mechanisms of immune modulation, have been translated to immunotherapy for the treatment of many advanced solid tumour and haematological malignancies such as melanomas, renal, liver and lung carcinomas. Immune regulatory modulators are a family of monoclonal antibodies (laboratory produced molecules that serve as substitute antibodies to restore, enhance or mimic the immune system and are targeted to specific proteins within the body) to proteins known as immune checkpoint regulators.

The typical function of these checkpoint regulator proteins is to diminish the immune response to antigen, acting as a brake on the immune system. Monoclonal antibodies to these checkpoint regulator proteins, known as immune checkpoint inhibitors, release the brake which has been placed on the immune system, allowing the patients' immune system to attack cancer cells. Not only do they do this, but they can also lead to an attack on certain healthy tissues. This is known as an immune-related 'adverse event' which is an inflammatory autoimmune response, affecting multiple systems resulting from the blocking of the normal immune regulatory pathways. Hormone deficiencies can result from damage to the adrenal cortex and pituitary gland as well as thyroid and pancreas leading to insulin dependent diabetes mellitus.

PRESENTATION

The clinical symptoms of adrenal insufficiency originally described by Addison in primary adrenal insufficiency include weakness, fatigue, anorexia, abdominal pain, weight loss and low blood pressure on standing and failure to thrive in babies who often have associated projectile vomiting and prolonged jaundice. In primary adrenal insufficiency, salt loss also takes place and the first presentation may actually be a salt-wasting crisis.

Figure 1.7 illustrates the components of an adrenal crisis seen in primary adrenal insufficiency and is characterised by low plasma sodium and raised plasma potassium concentrations along with low blood glucose and blood pressure. In older individuals or patients on established therapy, a crisis may be precipitated by a stress such as surgery, trauma or an intercurrent infection. By stress we do not mean a sudden surprise or watching a scary movie!! What is meant is the effects of infection where the high temperature alters the binding of cortisol to its transport protein in the blood, cortisol binding globulin (CBG). As the body temperature rises, the shape of CBG changes and cortisol is not bound as well. This does not matter if you have normal adrenal glands as you simply increase cortisol production to compensate. The problem is when you are on replacement therapy or cortisol production is insufficient, you cannot increase the amount of cortisol in the body except by increasing the dose. This is why we advise double or triple dosing with illness and high temperatures. A similar situation probably operates with trauma and during surgery.

In the congenital forms of adrenal insufficiency presenting in the first few weeks of life, vomiting, diarrhoea, poor feeding, lethargy, poor weight gain (failure to thrive) and prolonged jaundice may be the presenting features.

The other feature which is quite common in primary adrenal insufficiency is hyperpigmentation. This appears as a dark yellow/brown discolouration in the skin creases particularly around the elbows, backs of the knees, knuckles and at the base of the teeth. We discuss this further in Chapter 8, Part 5. This occurs in approximately 30% to 80% of new cases and the prevalence is even higher in those undergoing treatment, because of poorly distributed cortisol replacement. The hyperpigmentation arises because of the raised ACTH or rather, raised levels of its precursor proopiomelanocortin (POMC).

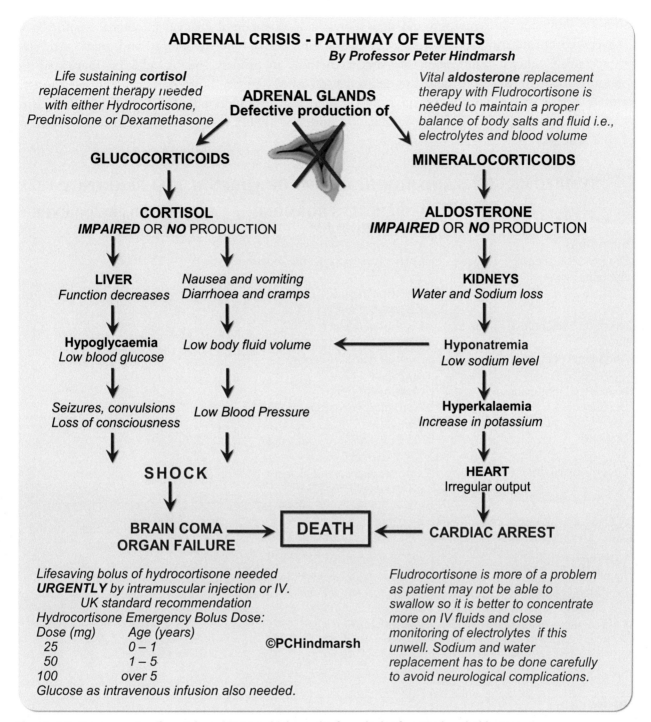

ADRENAL CRISIS - PATHWAY OF EVENTS
By Professor Peter Hindmarsh

*Life sustaining **cortisol** replacement therapy needed with either Hydrocortisone, Prednisolone or Dexamethasone*

ADRENAL GLANDS
Defective production of

*Vital **aldosterone** replacement therapy with Fludrocortisone is needed to maintain a proper balance of body salts and fluid i.e., electrolytes and blood volume*

GLUCOCORTICOIDS

MINERALOCORTICOIDS

CORTISOL
***IMPAIRED* OR *NO* PRODUCTION**

ALDOSTERONE
***IMPAIRED* OR *NO* PRODUCTION**

LIVER
Function decreases

Nausea and vomiting Diarrhoea and cramps

KIDNEYS
Water and Sodium loss

Hypoglycaemia
Low blood glucose

Low body fluid volume ← **Hyponatremia**
Low sodium level

Seizures, convulsions Loss of consciousness

Low Blood Pressure

Hyperkalaemia
Increase in potassium

S H O C K

HEART
Irregular output

BRAIN COMA → **DEATH** ← **CARDIAC ARREST**
ORGAN FAILURE

*Lifesaving bolus of hydrocortisone needed **URGENTLY** by intramuscular injection or IV. UK standard recommendation Hydrocortisone Emergency Bolus Dose:*

Dose (mg)	Age (years)
25	0 – 1
50	1 – 5
100	over 5

©PCHindmarsh

Glucose as intravenous infusion also needed.

Fludrocortisone is more of a problem as patient may not be able to swallow so it is better to concentrate more on IV fluids and close monitoring of electrolytes if this unwell. Sodium and water replacement has to be done carefully to avoid neurological complications.

Figure 1.7 *Components of an Adrenal Crisis which results from lack of cortisol and aldosterone.*

In hypopituitarism in adults, adrenal insufficiency mostly results from treatments to the hypothalamo–pituitary region, these patients will be monitored for the development of hormone deficiencies. One exception to this, is post head trauma where there are still cases of patients developing hypopituitarism several years after the incident. Symptoms and signs include lack of energy, fatigue, loss of sex drive, cold intolerance along with low blood pressure and slow heart rate. The congenital forms such as septo-optic dysplasia or midline developmental syndromes can present in a similar way to those with congenital primary adrenal insufficiency. In addition, hypoglycaemia and prolonged jaundice may reflect cortisol deficiency and thyroxine deficiency is a cause of prolonged jaundice in its own right. A small penis may reflect deficiencies of gonadotropins and/or growth hormone. Growth hormone deficiency does not present with problems with growth until towards the end of the first year of life as the growth hormone receptors are not fully responsive until then.

Figure 1.8 illustrates the symptoms and signs along with biochemical changes in adrenal insufficiency. It covers both primary and secondary adrenal insufficiency. The symptoms and signs associated with secondary adrenal insufficiency are similar to those in primary, but in addition there may be symptoms and signs associated with the deficiency of other pituitary hormones. For example, growth hormone deficiency would be associated with a reduction in childhood growth rate and absence of luteinising hormone (LH) and follicle-stimulating hormone (FSH) would be associated with a lack of pubertal changes.

SYMPTOMS, SIGNS AND BIOCHEMISTRY OF ADRENAL INSUFFICIENCY

	UNDERLYING HORMONE PROBLEM	ESTIMATED PREVALENCE (%)
Symptoms		
Fatigue, lack of energy, reduced strength	*Cortisol and adrenal androgen deficiency* *Thyroxine deficiency* *? Growth Hormone deficiency*	100%
Anorexia, weight loss, failure to thrive	*Cortisol deficiency*	100%
Abdominal pain, nausea, vomiting	*Cortisol and aldosterone deficiency*	90%
Muscle and joint pain	*Cortisol deficiency*	10%
Dizziness	*Mineralocorticoid and cortisol deficiency*	10%
Dry skin	*Adrenal androgen deficiency* *Thyroxine deficiency*	
Loss of sexual drive	*Adrenal androgen deficiency* *Gonadotropin deficiency*	
Signs		
Skin hyperpigmentation	*Cortisol deficiency*	30% at presentation higher during treatment
Pale skin	*ACTH deficiency*	
Jaundice	*Cortisol and thyroxine deficiency*	
Low blood pressure	*Mineralocorticoid and cortisol deficiency*	80%
Loss of pubic and axillary hair	*Adrenal androgen deficiency in females* *Testosterone deficiency in males*	
Small penis	*Testosterone and growth hormone deficiency*	
Biochemistry		
Hyponatraemia	*Mineralocorticoid and cortisol deficiency*	80%
Hyperkalaemia	*Mineralocorticoid deficiency*	65%
Anaemia and eosinophilia	*Cortisol deficiency*	
Increased TSH	*Cortisol deficiency*	
Low TSH	*Thyrotropin-stimulating hormone deficiency*	
Hypercalcaemia	*Cortisol deficiency*	
Hypoglycaemia	*Cortisol and growth hormone deficiency*	**©PCHindmarsh**

Figure 1.8 *Symptoms, signs and biochemical measures in adrenal insufficiency seen only in primary adrenal insufficiency (blue), only in secondary adrenal insufficiency (red) and in both (purple).*

Understanding the causes of secondary adrenal insufficiency and the associated pituitary hormone deficits that go with it is important when we consider glucocorticoid replacement. In older adults with hypopituitarism (secondary adrenal insufficiency) there may be a deficiency of thyroxine and cortisol. In this situation glucocorticoid replacement with hydrocortisone needs to be commenced first before the thyroxine is introduced.

This careful approach is needed because treating with thyroxine first can:

- Produce problems with heart rate, particularly atrial fibrillation and potentially heart failure if there is no cortisol in the circulation.

- Increase the clearance of cortisol and can also increase the basal metabolic rate of the body. This leads to an increased requirement for cortisol which cannot be met as there is no endogenous cortisol and as yet no hydrocortisone treatment, this can precipitate an adrenal crisis.

Introducing growth hormone treatment in an individual already on hydrocortisone replacement, can alter the metabolism of hydrocortisone leading to a reduction in cortisol in the circulation. Similarly, hormone replacement therapy of estrogen in females with hypopituitarism, can alter the availability of cortisol because the estrogen increases cortisol binding globulin (we consider this in Chapters 3 and 13). Finally, cortisol plays an important role in the ability for the kidneys to excrete water and care needs to be taken when changing hydrocortisone dosing in an individual who is receiving treatment for diabetes insipidus (deficiency of, or lack of action of, arginine vasopressin) with synthetic arginine vasopressin (AVP). In addition, hyponatraemia (low plasma sodium concentration) occurs in secondary adrenal insufficiency because of this same problem of cortisol deficiency where the body cannot excrete a water load, leading to water retention and expansion of the blood volume resulting in the low plasma sodium concentration (we cover this in Chapters 13 and 14).

DIAGNOSTIC TESTS FOR ADRENAL INSUFFICIENCY

The principles of diagnosis of adrenal insufficiency are to demonstrate an inappropriately low plasma cortisol concentration, to assess whether the adrenal insufficiency is primary or secondary and to determine the underlying pathological process.

The diagnosis of adrenal insufficiency depends on the demonstration that cortisol secretion is inappropriately low and details of the tests are provided in Chapter 5.

Cortisol secretion follows a circadian rhythm which is illustrated in Figure 1.9.

This figure shows three profiles. Figure 1.9A shows an averaged profile from a number of children who do not have adrenal insufficiency. Figure 1.9B shows the cortisol pattern of an individual child aged 9 years and Figure 1.9C shows an example of the circadian rhythm in a 62 year old individual.

Figure 1.9A shows the high plasma cortisol concentrations between 06:00 (6 am) and 08:00 (8 am) in the morning and trough concentrations between 50 and 100 nmol/l which occur around 22:00 (10 pm) in children. In Chapter 2 we compare the average children normal cortisol production (Figure 1.9A) to a carefully conducted normal cortisol production study in adults (Figure 2.8). Figure 2.8 illustrates similar peak values and timings with a nadir that occurs later approximately 00:00 (midnight) in older adults and 02:00 (2 am) in young adults. We look at the circadian rhythm further in Chapter 9 when we consider the effects of age and gender on the rhythm.

Figure 1.9B shows data from an individual child illustrating that the timing of the peak and nadir are similar to the averaged data set and the rhythm is maintained. This stresses the importance of considering each individual and implies we need personalised dosing for replacement. Note the mini bursts of cortisol in the individual particularly at 16:00 (4 pm) which is a very consistent feature in all individuals. Figure 1.9C illustrates a 24 hour profile in an older person without any adrenal problems and demonstrates again how the timings differ slightly in individuals. These mini bursts of cortisol are only observed with very frequent blood sampling every 15 to 20 minutes and their significance is unclear.

In endocrinology when we anticipate low production of a hormone, we undertake a stimulation test and conversely if we are anticipating excess production of a hormone, we undertake a suppression test. Single measurements of cortisol are not particularly helpful although a 08:00 (8 am) cortisol of 100 nmol/l or less would strongly suggest cortisol deficiency.

It is important to always pair the cortisol measurement with a measurement of ACTH. This is extremely helpful in primary adrenal insufficiency when the ACTH will be considerably raised whilst the plasma cortisol concentration will be absent, reduced or may even be in the normal range which is still inappropriate given the high circulating concentration of ACTH.

Figure 1.5 illustrates the results that might be found during the stages of developing primary adrenal insufficiency. It is worth noting that an elevated plasma renin activity is often the first finding in the evolution of primary adrenal insufficiency, due to the autoimmune process affecting the zona glomerulosa of the adrenal cortex first.

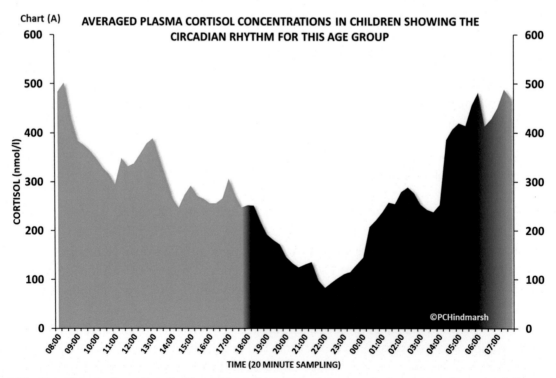

Figure 1.9A *Circadian rhythm of cortisol in children. Averaged plasma cortisol concentrations carefully constructed from a clinical study of 28 children without adrenal problems obtained at 20 minute sampling intervals showing peak values between 06:00 (6 am) and 08:00 (8 am) and the nadir attained around 22:00 (10 pm).*

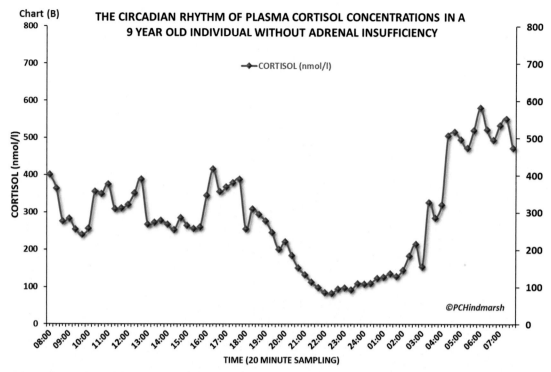

Figure 1.9B *24 hour plasma cortisol profile from an individual aged 9 years without adrenal insufficiency. The profile illustrates that each person has their own particular pattern in terms of peak attained which in this case starts at 06:00 (6 am) and the nadir which occurs at 22:00 (10 pm).*

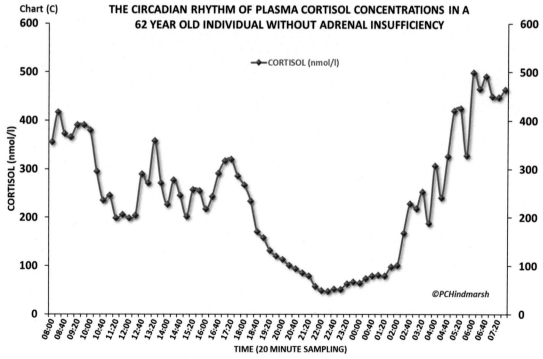

Figure 1.9C *24 hour plasma cortisol profile from an individual aged 62 years without adrenal insufficiency. The profile illustrates that each person has their own particular pattern in terms of peak attained which in this case occurs at 06:00 (6 am) and the nadir at 23:20 (11.20 pm).*

This measurement of cortisol and ACTH should be followed with a synacthen test in which exogenous synthetic ACTH is administered, usually in a dose of 250 mcg and samples measured 30 and 60 minutes after ACTH administration. A normal response should generate a plasma cortisol of over 500 nmol/l. This value is assay dependent which we discuss further below and expand on in Chapter 4. Some patients with adrenal insufficiency show a normal cortisol response to this standard test and lower dose testing may be more sensitive in detecting such cases. This is because the dose of synacthen in the standard synacthen test, leads to an ACTH level that is much higher than encountered during any stress situation including major surgery. Lower dose testing tries to better match the plasma ACTH concentrations encountered during stress.

We also find a 24 hour plasma cortisol profile helpful in determining how good cortisol production is during the day and night. Some people have quite good responses to the synacthen stimulation but have poor cortisol production when we look at it on an hour by hour basis. A modification of this has been proposed with plasma cortisol measured at 07:00 (7 am) or 08:00 (8 am). This can be a helpful guide and can be done at the same time that a synacthen test is undertaken, plasma renin activity and aldosterone should also be measured along with urea and electrolytes.

These cut-off points are based on the traditional cortisol assay in use over the last 15 to 20 years. The newer assay generally underreads on these values so care must be undertaken in assigning a diagnosis. There are various factors which can affect the cortisol measurement, including prior administration of intravenous gamma globulin, estrogens, drugs from the fluconazole family, liver, kidney and gut protein losing states, as well as heterophilic antibodies. The latter are antibodies which the body raises to other proteins that interfere in the assay with the antibodies used to measure cortisol. We cover this in more detail in Chapter 4.

In secondary adrenal insufficiency, ACTH concentrations may be normal or low as may the cortisol concentrations. In secondary adrenal insufficiency in an adult, the insulin induced hypoglycaemia test is helpful as it investigates the integrity of the hypothalamo-pituitary-adrenal axis and is widely regarded as the 'gold standard' (see Chapters 4 and 5). It also has the advantage of assessing growth hormone secretion. It should not be done in patients with cardiovascular diseases or history of seizures and is contraindicated in paediatric practice where the glucagon stimulation test should be utilised. The corticotropin-releasing hormone test assesses pituitary ACTH and is useful in distinguishing secondary (no response of ACTH) from tertiary adrenal insufficiency (delayed rise in ACTH), although this distinction rarely informs treatment.

It is important to realise that none of these dynamic tests, including the insulin induced hypoglycaemia test (IIHT), correctly identify all patients with adrenal insufficiency. There are false positive and false negative results, consequently mild secondary adrenal insufficiency can be missed and healthy individuals can show slightly abnormal responses. The results always need to be interpreted in the light of the clinical symptoms and signs and if these persist the potential diagnosis of adrenal insufficiency should be revisited.

The standard synacthen test has been standardised against the IIHT test of cortisol production which in turn was standardised against the cortisol response to surgical stress in normal patients. One of the difficulties of assessing test performance has been the variety of assays used, the small study patient sizes reported and the heterogeneity of doses used, particularly in the low dose synacthen test.

When we compare how diagnostic tests perform, we assess the sensitivity and specificity of the test. Sensitivity measures how often a test correctly generates a positive result (in this case a low cortisol response) for people who have the condition being tested for. The specificity of a test is the proportion of people without the disease that have a negative (in this case a normal cortisol response) blood test. A test that is 100% specific means all healthy individuals are correctly identified as healthy. Figure 1.10 gives a representation of this in a condition where we use a test to say whether a disease is present or not. In this situation, we say the disease is present or not because there is a way of being sure 100% of the time. We have done this to illustrate these points when applying a test to a condition.

PERFORMANCE OF TESTS

TEST RESULT	DISEASE		TOTAL
	PRESENT	ABSENT	
Test indicates disease **PRESENT**	20 True positive	10 False positive	30
Test indicates disease **ABSENT**	5 False negative	65 True negative	70
©PCHindmarsh TOTAL	25	75	100

Figure 1.10 *Layout of a test carried out in 100 people of whom it is known that 25 have the condition tested for. The test is positive in 20 people who have the condition and positive in 10 who do not have the condition. The test is negative in 65 people who do not have the disease and in 5 who do have the disease. The coloured boxes show the true positives (green), the true negatives (purple), the false positives (orange) and the false negatives (red).*

In this situation our test has been applied to 100 people of whom 25 actually have the condition. Using the layout, the test is positive in 20 people who have the condition and positive in 10 who do not have the condition. The test is negative in 65 people who do not have the disease and in 5 who do have the disease. The sensitivity of the test is the number of times it is positive in those with the condition or 20 out of 25 which is 80%. The specificity is the number of times the test is negative in those that do not have the condition which is 65 out of 75 or 87%. We can also add the false positive percentage which is the number of people that the test says they have the condition who do not, which is 10 out of 75 or 13% and the false negative percentage which is the number of people that the test says do not have the condition when they do, is 5 out of 25 or 20%.

There is often a trade off in deciding the cut-off point defining normality or not. If you make a test very specific where it identifies all that do not have the condition, then the sensitivity falls which means that some people who have adrenal insufficiency might be labelled as having a normal response when they actually have the condition (false negative). Conversely, trying to identify all that have cortisol deficiency runs the risk of saying some people who are actually normal, have a degree of adrenal insufficiency (false positive).

The standard synacthen test when compared to the IIHT and using a cut-off of 600 nmol/l, has an 85% sensitivity and 96% specificity. This means it is really good at excluding adrenal insufficiency as that is what the specificity tells us, but the lower sensitivity means that it will not catch all with adrenal insufficiency. Hence the need for placing the result in the clinical context and being prepared to repeat testing. For the low dose test using a cut-off of 375 nmol/l, reports have placed values close to 86% sensitivity and 88% specificity in defining adrenal insufficiency. When looking at morning cortisol measures, a value over 235 nmol/l has an 84% sensitivity and 71% specificity to exclude cortisol insufficiency and the specificity can be increased to 95% if a cut-off point of 375 nmol/l is used. Note that these cut-off points are based on the traditional assay.

These data tell us that care should be exercised in interpreting results from these tests, in particular the recognition that false positive and false negative results can occur. Any biochemical test result needs to be interpreted in the light of the clinical presentation and history and the clinician should be as certain as is possible that the person has adrenal insufficiency because replacement therapy is life long and once started on therapy it can be very hard to wean off in order to retest or re-evaluate the diagnosis.

Additional testing to establish the diagnosis particularly with primary adrenal insufficiency, should include the measurement of autoantibodies to the adrenal cortex. Autoantibodies (an antibody is a type of protein produced by the immune system, which in this case is directed against one or more of the individual's own proteins) to the adrenal cortex or the enzyme 21-hydroxylase, are present in more than 90% of patients with autoimmune adrenalitis of recent onset. The measurement of plasma 17-hydroxyprogesterone and/or 11-deoxycortisol concentrations in the synacthen test is important when considering a diagnosis of CAH due to 21-hydroxylase and 11beta-hydroxylase deficiencies respectively. A urinary steroid profile 24 hours post synacthen is also useful in determining the type of CAH presenting as primary adrenal insufficiency.

In male patients with isolated Addison's disease and no autoantibodies present, plasma concentrations of very long chain fatty acids (chain length of equal to or greater than 22 carbon atoms; C26, C26/C22, and C24/C22 ratios), should be measured to exclude X-linked adrenoleukodystrophy. Imaging of the adrenals may be useful to identify unusual tumours or tuberculosis. Genetic analysis for *NROB1* or *DAX-1* is also useful in the absence of an explanation for the adrenal insufficiency. Many genetics laboratories offer a panel of genes including *NROB1* or *DAX-1* and those involved in adrenal steroidogenesis.

In secondary adrenal insufficiency, pituitary function should be evaluated to determine whether other pituitary hormones are absent. Imaging of the hypothalamus and pituitary should be undertaken with Magnetic Resonance Imaging. This is important, to identify associated abnormalities in brain development which may warrant further genetic studies as well as excluding pituitary adenomas, craniopharyngiomas, metastases and Langerhans cell histiocytosis or other granulomatous conditions as causes for the secondary insufficiency.

Figure 1.11 illustrates a flow chart for assisting in the diagnosis of the causes of adrenal insufficiency. The orange circles show the tests undertaken at each stage and the results of testing. The key investigations that decide which arm to go down are shown at the very top in the blue box and include plasma ACTH and cortisol, sodium and potassium along with measures of blood glucose and blood acidity in the blood gas measurements. Low plasma sodium, normal plasma potassium with low or normal blood glucose take us down the right arm, whereas low plasma sodium, high plasma potassium, low blood glucose and acidosis on blood gas analysis take us down the left arm. Next step involves interpretation of plasma ACTH and cortisol along with skin colouration which takes us into the categories of primary and secondary adrenal insufficiency. At the primary and secondary level, testing with synacthen helps to confirm cortisol deficiency and additional measures such as 17-hydroxyprogesterone can be added to confirm CAH (CYP21 deficiency). More detailed testing then follows to define autoimmune adrenalitis and adrenoleukodystrophy, as well as tests to identify other hormone deficiencies in secondary adrenal insufficiency.

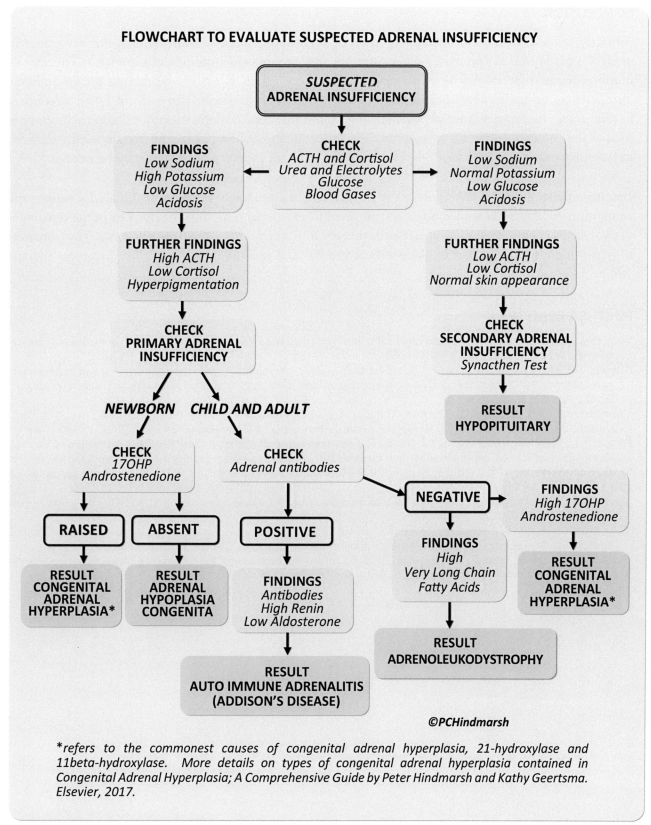

Figure 1.11 *Flow chart from initial presentation to diagnosis based on presenting plasma ACTH and cortisol concentrations, urea and electrolytes, blood glucose and assessment of blood acid status (blood gases). The blue boxes show the tests which should be done next, the orange boxes the results and the purple boxes the diagnosis.*

CONCLUSION

Adrenal insufficiency is a life-threatening series of conditions. Adrenal insufficiency is not a diagnosis in itself, it is merely a description of a glucocorticoid and/or mineralocorticoid deficient state. The adrenal insufficiency may be caused by a disorder of the adrenal glands when it is known as primary adrenal insufficiency or an abnormality of hypothalamo-pituitary function when it is called secondary insufficiency. In primary adrenal insufficiency, additional replacement therapy of adrenal hormones such as the mineralocorticoids is required. This mineralocorticoid replacement therapy is not required in secondary adrenal insufficiency, but replacement of other pituitary hormones may be necessary.

Because adrenal insufficiency is potentially life-threatening, treatment needs to be initiated as soon as the diagnosis is confirmed or sooner if the patient presents in adrenal crisis. It is the purpose of the remainder of this book to consider adrenal replacement therapy in patients with adrenal insufficiency. The principles of replacement therapy, types of glucocorticoid to be used and the monitoring of replacement therapy will be addressed.

FURTHER READING

Banger, V., Clayton, R.N., 1998. How reliable is the short synacthen test for the investigation of the hypothalamic-pituitary-adrenal axis? Eur J Endocrinol 139, 580−583.

Betterle, C., Dal Pra, C., Mantero, F., Zanchetta, R., 2002. Autoimmune adrenal insufficiency and autoimmune polyendocrine syndromes: autoantibodies, autoantigens, and their applicability in diagnosis and disease prediction. Endocr Rev 23, 327−364.

Charmandari, L., Nicolaides, N.C., Chrousos, G.P., 2014. Adrenal insufficiency. Lancet 383, 2152−2167.

Hindmarsh, P.C., Geertsma, K., 2017. Congenital Adrenal Hyperplasia: A Comprehensive Guide. Elsevier, New York.

Perton, F.T., Mijnhout, G.S., Kollen, B.J., Rondeel, J.M., Franken, A.A., Groeneveld, P.H., 2017. Validation of the 1 μg short synacthen test: an assessment of morning cortisol cut-off values and other predictors. Neth J Med 75, 14−20.

Sævik, A.B., Åkerman, A.-K., Methlie, P., et al., 2020. Residual corticosteroid production in autoimmune Addison disease. J Clin Endocrinol Metab 105, 2430−2441.

Sox Jr, H.C., 1986. Probability theory in the use of diagnostic tests. An introduction to critical study of the literature. Ann Intern Med 104, 60−66.

Tan, M.H., Iyengar, R., Mizokami-Stout, K., et al., 2019. Spectrum of immune checkpoint inhibitors induced endocrinopathies in cancer patients: a scoping review of case reports. Clin Diabetes Endocrinol 5, 1.

Yasir, S., Elhassan, Y.S., Iqbal, F., Arlt, W., et al., 2023. COVID-19-related adrenal haemorrhage: multicentre UK experience and systematic review of the literature. Clin Endocrinol 98, 766−778.

CHAPTER 2

Physiology of Cortisol Secretion

GLOSSARY

Adrenocorticotropin Hormone produced by the pituitary gland that regulates cortisol synthesis and secretion from the adrenal glands.

Arginine vasopressin Peptide hormone produced by the posterior pituitary that regulates blood vessel tone and water retention by the kidney.

Backdoor pathway An alternative pathway for the formation of androgen by the fetal adrenal glands.

Catecholamines Hormones which the brain, nerve tissues, and adrenal glands produce with a specific structure — aromatic amines.

Central clock Circadian rhythms are controlled by the central clock of the suprachiasmatic nucleus of the hypothalamus. In the nucleus clock genes respond to the light/dark cycle and through a coupled population of neuronal circadian oscillators, act as a master pacemaker driving rhythms in activity and rest, feeding, body temperature and hormones.

Circadian rhythm Changes in a biological measure in this case cortisol through the 24 hour period where values usually peak in the morning and reach low levels late evening/early hours of the morning.

Corticotropin-releasing hormone Hormone produced by the hypothalamus that regulates adrenocorticotropin synthesis and secretion from the pituitary gland.

Fetal adrenal zone Large structure present in the fetus which mainly produces dehydroepiandrosterone and helps maintain the pregnancy. The fetal adrenal zone disappears by the third month after birth.

Follicle-stimulating hormone Hormone produced by the pituitary gland which is involved in sperm formation from the testes in males. In females, along with luteinising hormone, it is involved in egg selection and production of estradiol.

Growth hormone Hormone produced by the pituitary gland that promotes growth of cartilage growth plates.

Homeostasis The state of steady internal, physical and chemical conditions maintained by the body to optimise function. This includes many variables such as cortisol which need to be regulated despite changes in the environment, diet, or level of activity.

Luteinising hormone Hormone produced by the pituitary gland which generates testosterone from the testes in males. In females, along with follicle-stimulating hormone, it is involved in egg selection and production of estradiol.

Progenitor cells Early descendants of stem cells which can differentiate to form one or more kinds of cells but cannot divide and reproduce indefinitely.

Prolactin Hormone produced by the pituitary gland that is involved in milk production.

Renin-angiotensin system Group of hormones which act together to regulate blood volume and blood pressure.

Stem cells Undifferentiated or partially differentiated cells which can differentiate into various types of cells and proliferate indefinitely.

Thyroid-stimulating hormone Hormone produced by the anterior pituitary that regulates the synthesis and secretion of thyroxine from the thyroid gland.

Replacement Therapies in Adrenal Insufficiency. https://doi.org/10.1016/B978-0-12-824548-4.00003-6

GENERAL

The endocrine system consists of a series of glands distributed through the body. When we are considering cortisol, we are thinking about the hypothalamus and pituitary which are situated at the base of the brain and the adrenal glands situated above both kidneys. In fact, in the adrenal glands we can refine this interest further to the outer portion of the adrenal gland known as the adrenal cortex. The centre of the adrenal gland is made up of the medulla where adrenaline and noradrenaline are made.

ADRENAL GLANDS

The two adrenal glands sit above the kidneys and are made up of two distinct parts: the cortex and the medulla. The adrenal glands are surrounded by a structure known as the capsule. This is an important region because the adrenocortical stem cells and progenitor cells (early descendants of stem cells that can differentiate to form one or more kinds of cells but cannot divide and reproduce indefinitely) which regulate homeostasis (the ability to regulate various physiological processes, e.g. cortisol production, to keep internal states steady and balanced) of the adrenal cortex, reside within the capsule and subcapsular region of the gland. The signalling cues which trigger the movement of a capsular cell to form an adrenocortical cell, remain elusive although we do know that these cells derive from the fetal adrenal zone. How these capsular cells respond in times of stress or following injury to the adrenal glands is unclear.

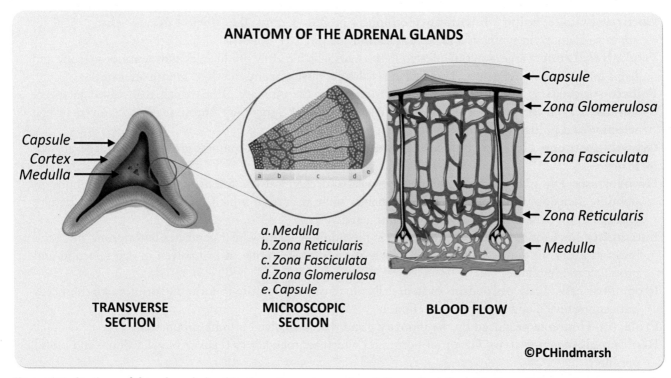

Figure 2.1 *Sections of the adrenal gland to show the cortex and medulla on the left and in the middle a microscopic section of the cortex to show the three cortical zones. On the right is a summary of the blood vessel labyrinth which flows from the capsule through the three zones to the medulla.*

The adrenal cortex is made of three zones (Figure 2.1). The outer zone is the zona glomerulosa where the mineralocorticoid aldosterone is synthesised, the middle zone is the zona fasciculata which synthesises cortisol and then the zona reticularis which synthesises cortisol and the adrenal androgens. In fetal life, these three zones are small compared to the fetal adrenal zone which involutes over the first three months of postnatal life. The blood flow in the adrenal is from the capsule through the cortical zones to the medulla.

In a similar way, the flow of cells from the stem cells in the capsule follows this blood flow pattern, with older cells and dying cells found towards the centre of the gland. This pattern of blood flow is also important because the concentration of cortisol is very high in these blood vessels and this is important for the formation of the catecholamine (hormones that the brain, nerve tissues and adrenal glands produce with a specific structure – aromatic amines), adrenaline from noradrenaline in the medulla by the enzyme phenylethanolamine N–methyltransferase. When cortisol is absent, then formation of adrenaline is reduced and replacement dosing with hydrocortisone is insufficient to restore full activity of the enzyme (Figure 2.2). Aromatic amines are shown in Figure 2.2 as the carbon ring structure attached to an amine group (NH_2).

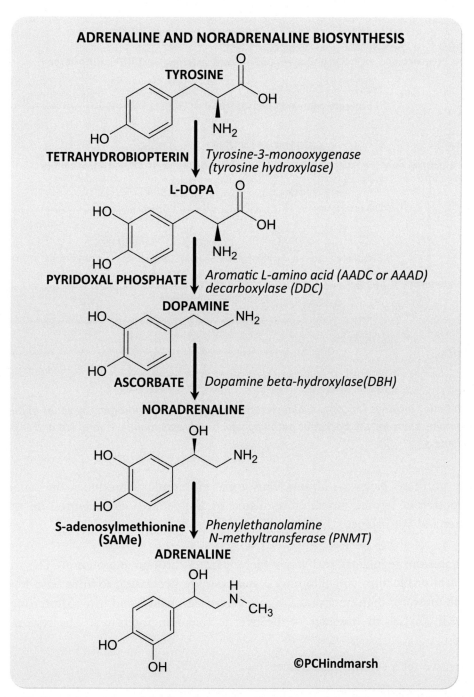

Figure 2.2 *Biosynthetic pathway for adrenaline formation from the amino acid tyrosine. Cortisol influences the activity of the enzyme phenylethanolamine N-methyltransferase which converts noradrenaline to adrenaline.*

It is within the cortex that the three main adrenal steroids are synthesised, cortisol, aldosterone and androstenedione. The products of each of the zones and the synthetic pathways involved are shown in Figure 2.3. All share the common substrate cholesterol and several steps catalysed by enzymes such as 3beta–hydroxysteroid dehydrogenase type 2 (*3β*-HSD) appear in all pathways.

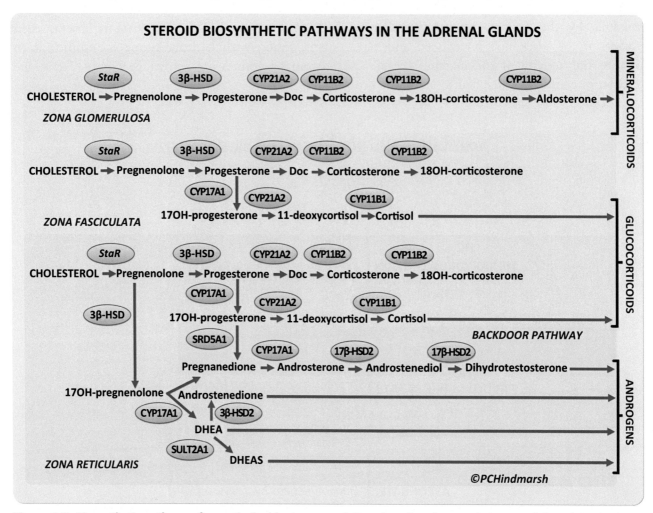

Figure 2.3 *Biosynthetic pathways for cortisol, aldosterone and the adrenal androgens by zones of the adrenal cortex. The green box contains steps for the backdoor pathway which operates mainly in fetal life and is positioned in this figure for completeness.*

The regulation of these pathways differ. The zona glomerulosa produces the mineralocorticoid, aldosterone. Aldosterone is predominantly regulated by the renin system centred on the kidneys and involved in water and salt balance.

Figure 2.4 illustrates this regulatory pathway which operates through angiotensin. The stimuli for renin release, angiotensin production and aldosterone synthesis are decreasing sodium (salt) levels, low blood volume or blood pressure, high potassium, high levels of adrenaline and low aldosterone levels. Renin is a protein which conveys the message to the liver to make angiotensin I. The system functions like an oven thermostat:

- In the oven we set a certain temperature

- The oven then switches on and heats up to that temperature

- Once the set temperature is reached, the heat is switched down

- The thermostat then checks the temperature again increasing or decreasing the oven heat to maintain a constant temperature

In the renin-angiotensin-aldosterone system, if blood volume changes or the amount of sodium varies, renin levels will change.

If the amount of sodium decreases, then the amount of renin increases and similarly if the blood volume decreases, the renin also increases. Angiotensin I is then converted in the lungs to angiotensin II which instructs the adrenal glands to make aldosterone. Aldosterone and angiotensin II constrict the blood vessels and increase cardiac output both of which increase blood pressure. In addition, aldosterone retains sodium in the kidney and aldosterone also retains sodium from the large bowel.

As sodium is retained, then this draws with it water which increases blood volume and blood pressure.

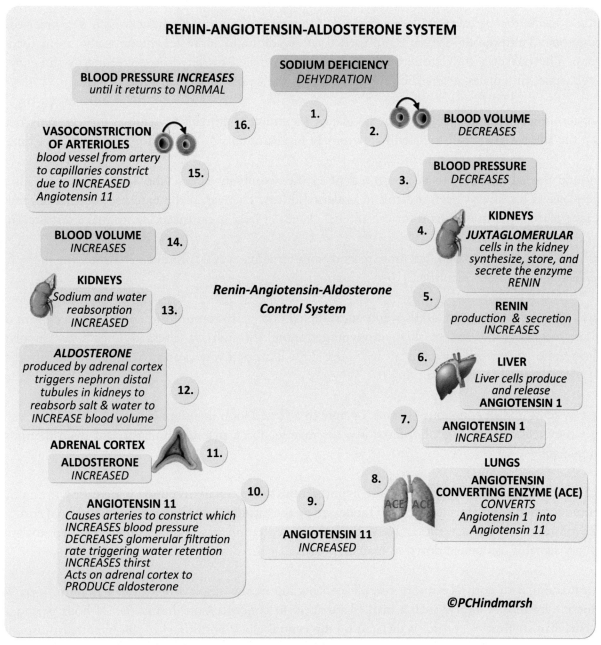

Figure 2.4 *The Renin-Angiotensin-Aldosterone Control System.*

Cortisol is regulated via the hypothalamo-pituitary-adrenal axis which will be described further in this chapter. The adrenal androgens are also regulated by the hypothalamo-pituitary-adrenal axis, although in males the dominant androgen is testosterone produced by the testes. All steroids have cholesterol as the starting point for synthesis. Uptake of cholesterol into the adrenal cortex or the gonads is by the low density lipoprotein receptor.

The cholesterol is then transported by the steroidogenic acute regulatory protein (StAR), which shuttles cholesterol into the mitochondria, where the P450 enzyme CYP11A1 catalyzes the conversion of cholesterol to pregnenolone. These are key steps in biosynthesis of adrenal and gonadal steroids. The pathways diverge after the enzyme 3β-HSD to lead to the formation of cortisol and 18-hydroxycorticosterone in the zona fasciculata and cortisol, dehydroepiandrosterone (DHEA) and androstenedione in the zona reticularis.

Note that DHEAS which is commonly measured in laboratories, is the sulphated form of DHEA and contains very little biological activity.

In the gonads, the pathway is driven towards formation of androstenedione which is converted to testosterone. Testosterone in turn is aromatised to estradiol and androstenedione is also aromatised to estrone. The final step for testosterone is conversion, in males, to dihydrotestosterone by the enzyme 5α-reductase. In females, aromatase activity is high in the ovary and less so in male testes.

Testosterone production from the adrenal glands is extremely difficult to achieve and can only occur when the adrenal gland is stimulated by extremely high amounts of ACTH for long periods of time.

Although this can happen to a certain extent in the womb in babies who have congenital adrenal hyperplasia, it has always been difficult to understand how changes in the external genitalia in females can take place when it is so hard for the adrenal glands, at least in postnatal life, to make testosterone.

This has all seemed rather odd, but more recently an alternative way of producing testosterone in the fetal adrenal glands has been identified.

Rather than going through DHEA and androstenedione, testosterone can also be formed from 17-hydroxypregnenolone and/or 17-hydroxyprogesterone through an alternative pathway involving androsterone (the backdoor pathway in Figure 2.3). This pathway ceases to work after birth as the fetal adrenal zone breaks down.

These systems like all endocrine systems, operate in a closed loop manner. They regulate themselves or rather they regulate the target hormone in a negative feedback manner similar to our oven thermostat example above.

When cortisol concentrations are low, the hypothalamus and pituitary respond by increasing the amount of adrenocorticotropin hormone (ACTH) released by the pituitary, which signals to the adrenal cortex to make more cortisol. Once the ambient cortisol concentration has been attained, the hypothalamo-pituitary signal is dampened down to maintain cortisol at the desired concentration.

The situation with cortisol is more complicated because it also displays a circadian rhythm. Very few endocrine hormones display such a marked variation in concentration during the 24 hour period and the circadian rhythm of cortisol is dictated by the central clock positioned in the hypothalamus which responds to the light/dark cycle. This makes the hypothalamo-pituitary-adrenal axis a very complex feedback system as the cortisol set points are varying throughout the 24 hour period.

THE HYPOTHALAMUS AND PITUITARY GLAND

The regulation of virtually all hormones produced by the body is undertaken by the pituitary gland. The pituitary gland sits at the base of the brain in a bony hollow called the pituitary fossa. This is behind the bridge of the nose and behind the eye socket close to the nerves that come from the eyes.

The anterior pituitary produces six hormones, growth hormone (GH), adrenocorticotropin hormone (ACTH), thyroid-stimulating hormone (TSH), prolactin (PRL), luteinising hormone (LH) and follicle-stimulating hormone (FSH) (Figure 2.5A). The posterior pituitary produces two hormones, arginine vasopressin (AVP) whose effects are shown in Figure 2.5B and oxytocin which is involved in the 'let down reflex' of breast feeding.

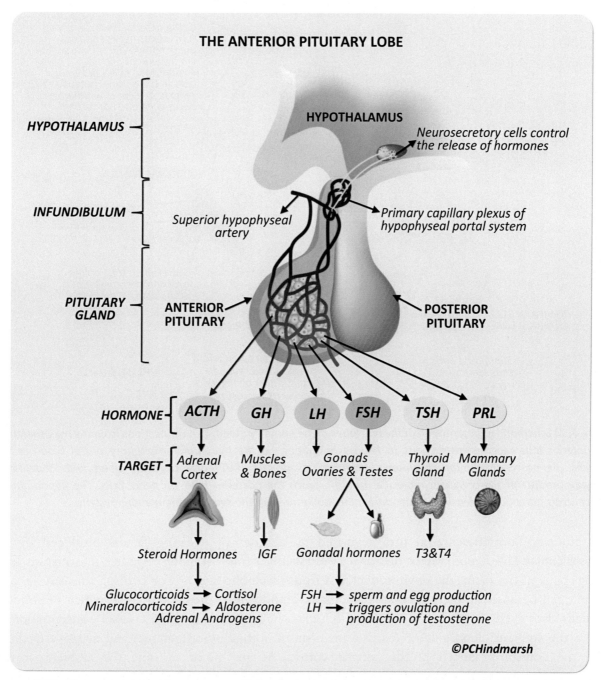

Figure 2.5A *The six major hormones which the anterior pituitary produces: growth hormone (GH), adrenocorticotropin hormone (ACTH), thyroid-stimulating hormone (TSH), prolactin (PRL), luteinising hormone (LH) and follicle-stimulating hormone (FSH).*

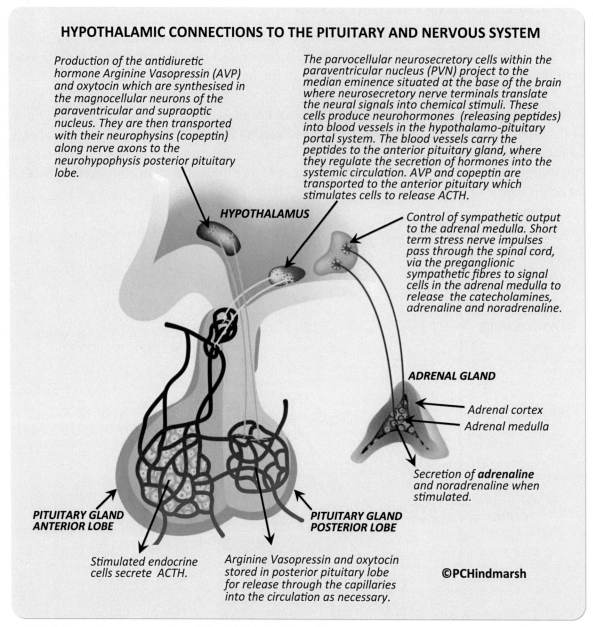

HYPOTHALAMIC CONNECTIONS TO THE PITUITARY AND NERVOUS SYSTEM

Production of the antidiuretic hormone Arginine Vasopressin (AVP) and oxytocin which are synthesised in the magnocellular neurons of the paraventricular and supraoptic nucleus. They are then transported with their neurophysins (copeptin) along nerve axons to the neurohypophysis posterior pituitary lobe.

The parvocellular neurosecretory cells within the paraventricular nucleus (PVN) project to the median eminence situated at the base of the brain where neurosecretory nerve terminals translate the neural signals into chemical stimuli. These cells produce neurohormones (releasing peptides) into blood vessels in the hypothalamo-pituitary portal system. The blood vessels carry the peptides to the anterior pituitary gland, where they regulate the secretion of hormones into the systemic circulation. AVP and copeptin are transported to the anterior pituitary which stimulates cells to release ACTH.

HYPOTHALAMUS

Control of sympathetic output to the adrenal medulla. Short term stress nerve impulses pass through the spinal cord, via the preganglionic sympathetic fibres to signal cells in the adrenal medulla to release the catecholamines, adrenaline and noradrenaline.

ADRENAL GLAND

Adrenal cortex
Adrenal medulla

*Secretion of **adrenaline** and noradrenaline when stimulated.*

PITUITARY GLAND ANTERIOR LOBE

PITUITARY GLAND POSTERIOR LOBE

Stimulated endocrine cells secrete ACTH.

Arginine Vasopressin and oxytocin stored in posterior pituitary lobe for release through the capillaries into the circulation as necessary.

©PCHindmarsh

Figure 2.5B *Schematic representation of the two lobes of the pituitary gland with connections from the hypothalamus. The anterior lobe receives instructions to release hormones via the hypothalamo-pituitary portal blood system whereas the posterior pituitary hormones, arginine vasopressin (AVP) and oxytocin along with copeptin, a cleavage product of the precursor molecule pro-AVP, reach the posterior lobe via nerve cells. The hypothalamus also controls adrenaline release from the adrenal medulla through the sympathetic nervous system.*

The pituitary hormones are in turn regulated by a series of releasing factors produced by the hypothalamus. The hypothalamus acts as a coordinating centre bringing together information from various parts of the brain, the environment and from metabolic agents. For cortisol, this can be quite complicated because the hypothalamus coordinates outputs from the central clock which responds to the light/dark cycle, stressful events such as trauma which raises the blood cortisol concentration, as well as the ambient blood glucose (cortisol maintains a normal blood glucose) and negative feedback from the cortisol produced in the adrenal cortex. At any point in time the ambient cortisol concentration reflects this integrated activity. Finally, the hypothalamus is connected through the nervous system with the adrenal medulla where adrenaline is made and this plays an important role in regulating metabolism.

PITUITARY DEVELOPMENT

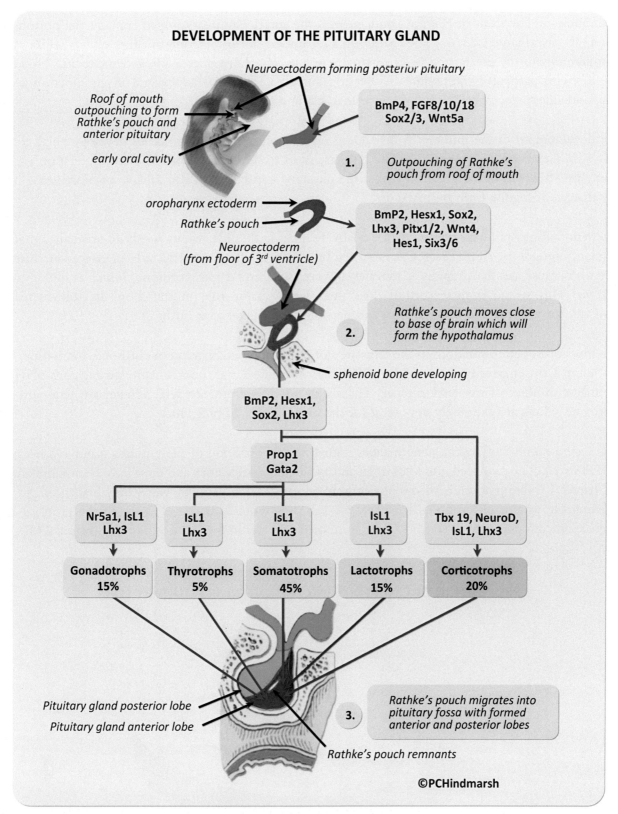

DEVELOPMENT OF THE PITUITARY GLAND

Neuroectoderm forming posterior pituitary

Roof of mouth outpouching to form Rathke's pouch and anterior pituitary

early oral cavity

BmP4, FGF8/10/18 Sox2/3, Wnt5a

1. *Outpouching of Rathke's pouch from roof of mouth*

oropharynx ectoderm

Rathke's pouch

Neuroectoderm (from floor of 3rd ventricle)

BmP2, Hesx1, Sox2, Lhx3, Pitx1/2, Wnt4, Hes1, Six3/6

2. *Rathke's pouch moves close to base of brain which will form the hypothalamus*

sphenoid bone developing

BmP2, Hesx1, Sox2, Lhx3

Prop1 Gata2

| Nr5a1, IsL1 Lhx3 | IsL1 Lhx3 | IsL1 Lhx3 | IsL1 Lhx3 | Tbx 19, NeuroD, IsL1, Lhx3 |

| Gonadotrophs 15% | Thyrotrophs 5% | Somatotrophs 45% | Lactotrophs 15% | Corticotrophs 20% |

Pituitary gland posterior lobe

Pituitary gland anterior lobe

3. *Rathke's pouch migrates into pituitary fossa with formed anterior and posterior lobes*

Rathke's pouch remnants

©PCHindmarsh

Figure 2.6A *Factors involved in the development of the pituitary gland and the cell types involved in hormone synthesis. Within the blue boxes are the transcription factors involved in regulating the steps in development of the different cell types shown in the yellow boxes. Note the corticotrophs (ACTH cells) branch off early in the pathway followed by the gonadotrophs (LH and FSH cells). The percentages show the contribution of the various cell lines to the anterior pituitary cell mass.*

The human pituitary develops as a joint product of the outgrowth of ectodermal tissue from the roof of the mouth which is known as Rathke's pouch and a down growth of neural tissue referred to as the infundibulum. The front of Rathke's pouch forms the anterior pituitary which contains the hormones noted above (Figure 2.5A). The back of the pouch forms an intermediate lobe whilst the infundibulum forms the posterior lobe which contains the hormones AVP and oxytocin. Arginine vasopressin is particularly important in that it retains water in the kidney and in conjunction with renin and aldosterone, plays an important role in salt and water balance.

The development of the pituitary is dependent on the interaction of numerous developmental genes which are illustrated in Figure 2.6A. The pituitary starts to develop around 35 days of gestation and it is only by 18 weeks of the pregnancy, that the pituitary is vascularised and capable of functioning in a way that we recognise from postnatal life.

The hypothalamo-pituitary-adrenal axis is relatively quiet in the first twenty weeks of pregnancy, but as pregnancy progresses, ACTH secretion increases. Interestingly, this is not reflected in a marked increase in cortisol, because the fetus rapidly inactivates any cortisol formed into cortisone, which is biologically inactive. This would suggest cortisol does not play a major role in the fetus. Its role increases however, towards the end of pregnancy and becomes fully active after birth.

The low cortisol concentrations in the fetus are not just due to inactivation to cortisone, but within the fetal adrenal, the enzyme systems which are described in Figure 2.3 are poorly expressed and cortisol is not the major product of the fetal adrenal. The major product from the fetal adrenal are fetal adrenal androgens which are extremely important for the maintenance of pregnancy.

There are a number of genetic abnormalities leading to malformation of the pituitary gland and because ACTH may not be produced, this leads to secondary adrenal insufficiency and these have been summarised in Chapter 1. Note that the corticotrophs are formed early in the pathway when they branch off, so by knowing the pattern of hormone deficiency we can then estimate the level at which the problem has arisen. Corticotrophs form about 20% of the hormonal cell mass in the anterior pituitary (Figure 2.6B).

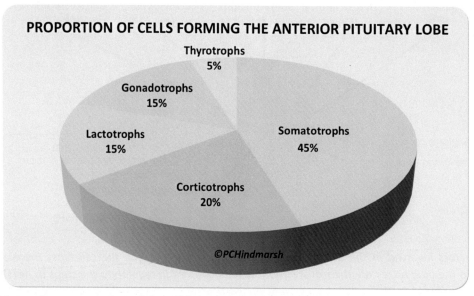

Figure 2.6B *Schematic representation of the cell lines in the anterior pituitary expressed as percentages. The majority of cells in the pituitary are somatotrophs (45%) producing growth hormone.*

Corticotropin-releasing hormone, Arginine vasopressin and Adrenocorticotropin

Corticotropin-releasing hormone (CRH), is a 41-amino acid peptide derived from a 196-amino acid preprohormone secreted by the paraventricular nucleus of the hypothalamus in response to stress and also the circadian clock system. Adrenocorticotropin is a 39-amino acid peptide, which is secreted by the corticotroph cells of the anterior pituitary and is generated from a large precursor called pre proopiomelanocortin, which is broken down to proopiomelanocortin (POMC) which has a molecular weight of 31 kDa. Proopiomelanocortin is broken down into ACTH and other factors such as melanocyte-stimulating hormone and beta-endorphin (see Chapter 8, Part 5, Figure 8.40A).

The feed forward effect of ACTH on the adrenal cortex, operates by rapid short term mechanisms such as the stimulation of cholesterol delivery to the mitochondria and stimulation of CYP11A1 (minutes) and slower long term actions such as stimulation of the genes involved in steroidogenesis, over several hours. Similarly, in the negative feedback loop of cortisol or glucocorticoids on ACTH, cortisol will inhibit CRH secretion by the hypothalamus, which in turn decreases anterior pituitary secretion of ACTH (minutes), whereas a slower effect over hours works through alterations to the rates of POMC gene transcription and peptide synthesis.

Corticotropin-releasing hormone is not the only factor that regulates ACTH release. Arginine vasopressin produced in the hypothalamus and acting on the V_3 receptor on the corticotrophs, also causes ACTH release and is equipotent and synergistic to CRH in causing ACTH release (Figure 2.7). Arginine vasopressin, also known as antidiuretic hormone, is secreted from the posterior pituitary as a result of changes in the osmotic strength of blood. If plasma osmolality rises due to say dehydration, then AVP secretion is increased and via the V_1 and V_2 receptors increases blood pressure by contracting the blood vessels and retaining water from the kidney tubules respectively. Equally, if plasma osmolality falls due to too much water intake, AVP is switched off and blood vessels relax and water is lost from the kidney. This is why the study in Figure 2.7 used hypertonic saline (high osmolality) to stimulate AVP release.

INTERACTION OF CORTICOTROPIN-RELEASING HORMONE AND ARGININE VASOPRESSIN IN MEDIATING RELEASE OF ADRENOCORTICOTROPIN

STIMULUS	CHANGE IN ACTH (pg/ml)	CHANGE IN CORTISOL (nmol/l)
CRH (200 mcg)	30	150
CRH (200 mcg) and hypertonic saline	115	350

Figure 2.7 *Change in adrenocorticotropin and cortisol after intravenous administration of corticotropin-releasing hormone (200 mcg) on its own or during hypertonic saline infusion when plasma vasopressin concentration rose to 9.6 pmol/l. (Data derived from Milsom, S.R., Conaglen, J.V., Donald, R.A., et al., 1985. Augmentation of the response to CRF in man: relative contributions of endogenous angiotensin and vasopressin. Clin Endocrinol 22, 623–628.)*

The precise interaction between these two major ACTH secretagogues is still unclear. Corticotropin-releasing hormone appears to be important in the acute short term stimulation of ACTH release and is probably the prime factor involved in the day to day regulation of cortisol production. Arginine vasopressin on the other hand, appears to play a role in situations where there is more chronic stress to the system. Of note both CRH and AVP are present in large amounts and stimulate high ACTH secretion in untreated primary adrenal insufficiency.

This is extremely important to understand because replacement with cortisol will suppress CRH and AVP which leads to sudden loss of water and a potential dangerous rapid elevation in sodium levels. We will discuss this further when we consider emergency treatment in Chapter 14.

CIRCADIAN RHYTHM AND CIRCADIAN CLOCKS

Several genes which are known as clock genes, are important and are situated in the hypothalamus and their change in activity during the 24 hour period generates what we see when we measure cortisol over a 24 hour period, namely a circadian rhythm (Figure 2.8). Circadian rhythms are endogenously generated rhythms which recur around (circa) 23 to 25 hours examples of which are cortisol, blood pressure and temperature.

This is in contrast to diurnal and nocturnal rhythms which are rhythms around the day or night respectively. Ultradian rhythms are rhythms that occur with a high frequency such as bursts of growth hormone every 3 hours and infradian rhythms are cycles greater than 24 hours (e.g. the human menstrual cycle).

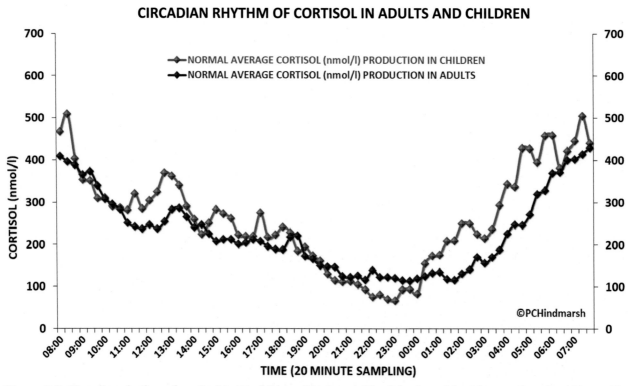

CIRCADIAN RHYTHM OF CORTISOL IN ADULTS AND CHILDREN

Figure 2.8 *Circadian rhythm of cortisol in 28 children (blue) and 80 adults (purple) without adrenal problems. The graphs show the average cortisol levels at each time point. The curves were generated by blood samples obtained every 20 minutes. Peak values of cortisol are attained between 06:00 (6 am) and 08:00 (8 am) in the children and adults and the nadir is attained around 22:00 (10 pm) in children and 00:00 (midnight) in older adults.*

A circadian rhythm is a pattern which changes through a 24 hour period and these clock genes are sensitive to changes in light. It is the light/dark cycle rather than sleep per se which generates the circadian rhythm. This can be seen in experiments where the light/dark cycle has been shifted so day time becomes night time and night time, day time. In these situations, the circadian rhythm changes to fit the light dark cycle rather than the actual clock time. These observations have important implications for night shift workers and probably explain to an extent why jet lag can produce a number of symptoms.

The daily cortisol production is remarkably constant at all ages but the amount of cortisol which can be measured in the blood varies during the 24 hour period. This rhythm of cortisol reflects changes in the amount of CRH and ACTH produced during the 24 hour period. As seen in Figure 2.8, the highest concentrations of cortisol occur in the early hours of the morning, so cortisol can be viewed as the 'get up and go hormone.' During the late afternoon and particularly in the evening, the amounts of cortisol present are very low but there is always some around that can be measured and it rarely goes below 50 nmol/l at its trough value.

It is important to remember this circadian rhythm of cortisol because it determines how we go about replacing cortisol in adrenal insufficiency.

The major objective of endocrinology is to always replace the hormone which is missing as close to the physiological situation as possible. For cortisol replacement this means mimicking this circadian rhythm and our treatment chapters will consider this in depth. This becomes increasingly important as we begin to understand that circadian clocks align behavioural and biochemical processes with the day/night cycle.

Genetic disruption of clock genes in experimental situations, upsets the metabolic functions of tissues at distinct phases of the sleep/wake cycle. Circadian desynchrony or disruption, is a characteristic of shift work and sleep disruption in humans and can lead to metabolic changes similar to those seen in the Metabolic Syndrome, with obesity and diabetes.

Amplification System and Input from Stress and Glucose

The circadian rhythm of cortisol is remarkably reproducible between individuals. For virtually all ages, the peak cortisol concentration is attained between 06:00 (6 am) and 08:00 (8 am). The circadian rhythm of cortisol for males and females is similar in children and adults. The lowest concentration of cortisol in the circadian rhythm is encountered in the late evening. Although the actual amount of cortisol present is remarkably similar and rarely goes below 50 nmol/l, the timing of this nadir varies with age. In children the nadir is around 22:00 (10 pm), in older adults at 00:00 (midnight) and in young adults 02:00 (2 am). Although cortisol concentrations are mainly dictated by the central clock, sleep does probably play some role in the timing of the rise from the nadir and that probably explains why it varies from children through to older adults.

The amount of CRH produced determines the amount of ACTH which is synthesised and released from the corticotroph cells in the anterior pituitary. The amounts of CRH are quite low compared to the amount of ACTH released, which in turn determines the amount of cortisol that can be produced by the adrenal glands. The net effect of this process is that from a small amount of CRH a large amount of cortisol can be produced — roughly a thousandfold increase in concentration compared with the starting point. This amplification system is extremely efficient in terms of the generation of cortisol and it also means that it will be quite sensitive to small changes in cortisol feeding back onto the hypothalamus and pituitary.

The normal circadian rhythm of cortisol dictated by the central clock is extremely important in coordinating the function of the peripheral clocks which are present in every tissue of the body. If this were not to occur, then there would be asynchrony between the tissues for example in terms of energy generation and could lead to some cells over producing, other cells under producing and other cells being exposed to a surfeit or deficit in the particular product that they wish to utilise. The clock system provides a means of coordinating metabolic activity.

The circadian rhythm can be modified throughout the 24 hour period. In addition to metabolic effects, cortisol has a role as a stress hormone and it is released in higher concentrations in situations such as trauma, burns and infection. Cortisol, as we show in Chapter 3, has multiple effects on the body particularly assisting the immune system and maintaining a normal blood glucose. In stress, the hypothalamo-pituitary-adrenal axis increases the production of cortisol. When a person is in intensive care for example, cortisol production is higher than normal and the circadian rhythmicity is often lost. Whether this is part of the overall stress response, or due to the fact that light/dark cues are lost in intensive care because the lights are on all the time, is unclear. What we do know is that cortisol production often doubles and in respiratory infections, can run between 800 and 1200 nmol/l throughout the 24 hour period.

Another situation where the normal cortisol production through the circadian rhythm can be altered, is in hypoglycaemia (low blood glucose), or if blood glucose falls rapidly within the normal range. There is a sequence of events that take place as blood glucose falls. These are shown in Figure 2.9.

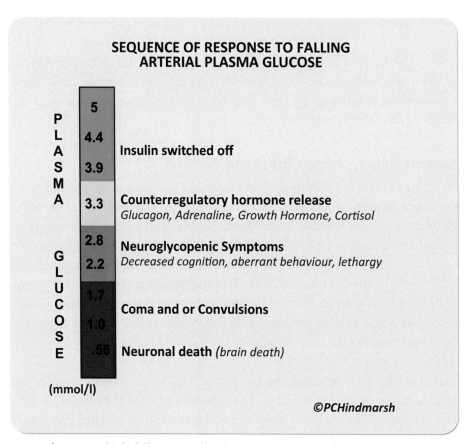

Figure 2.9 *Sequence of events which follow a decline in arterial plasma glucose concentration. To convert blood glucose to mg/dl multiply by 18.*

First of these is that insulin, which is the only hormone that can reduce blood glucose, is switched off at an ambient glucose concentration of 4.4 mmol/l. This is a sensible step as removing the only hormone which can produce hypoglycaemia, would help to alleviate the problem. If that manoeuvre is insufficient, the body mobilises glycogen from the pancreas and adrenaline from the central part of the adrenal glands, both of which in the short term raise blood glucose. In addition, around this trigger point of 3.3 mmol/l (Figure 2.9) the secretion of growth hormone and ACTH (and therefore cortisol) starts to reach a maximum. Both these hormones also raise blood glucose through effects on lipid metabolism predominately, but their effect is slower than glucagon and adrenaline and therefore provide a useful backup to maintain blood glucose within the normal range after the hypoglycaemic episode.

Part of the reason for the circadian rhythm of cortisol, is most likely to prevent nocturnal hypoglycaemia because the individual fasts from the moment of sleep until waking the next morning. In adults with reasonable glycogen stores in the liver, such a period of fasting is not usually a problem, but in children, where glycogen stores in the liver are a lot less than adults, particularly when unwell, the presence of cortisol in the circadian rhythm and the rise overnight will play a protective role against hypoglycaemia.

The stress response with the rise in cortisol is extremely important. In many endocrine systems when there is repeated stimulation of a gland, the amount of hormone which is produced by the gland often declines over time. For example, if we cause growth hormone to be released from the pituitary gland there is an attenuated response to the same stimulus if it is applied within 3 hours of the first. In the case of cortisol and ACTH this is not the case. Repeated stimulation of the adrenal glands with ACTH leads to the same response with no obvious attenuation with time (Figure 2.10). This is an important observation because it means this system is capable of responding repeatedly to stress with the same consistent response.

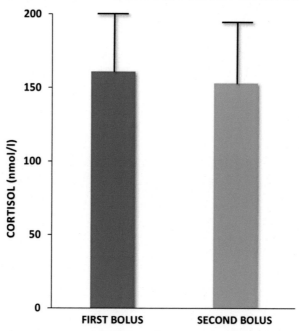

EFFECT OF REPEAT SYNACTHEN STIMULATION OF THE ADRENAL GLANDS ON PLASMA CORTISOL CONCENTRATIONS

Figure 2.10 *The plasma cortisol response to two boluses of synacthen (ACTH 1 - 24) given in a dose of 90 ng/1.73m² body surface area 90 minutes apart. Data are shown as mean and one standard deviation. There was no significant difference between mean values. (Data extracted from Crowley, S., Hindmarsh, P.C., Honour, J.W., Brook, C.G., 1993. Reproducibility of the cortisol response to stimulation with a low dose of ACTH (1-24): the effect of basal cortisol levels and comparison of low-dose with high-dose secretory dynamics. J Endocrinol 136, 167–172.)*

CONCLUSION

The hypothalamo–pituitary–adrenal axis is an integrated system and operates as a closed loop feedback system. This feedback works within a circadian variation of cortisol in the bloodstream which is driven by the central clock via CRH and ACTH. In addition, cortisol is a stress hormone which is increased as a result of increased CRH production in the short term and where more chronic stress is encountered, AVP appears to be an important factor.

Cortisol is one of three steroids produced by the adrenal cortex, the others are aldosterone the mineralocorticoid and the adrenal androgens DHEA and androstenedione. The zonation in the adrenal cortex is associated with each of these steroids. The zona glomerulosa produces aldosterone, the zona fasciculata produces cortisol and the zona reticularis cortisol and the adrenal androgens. There is also an additional pathway present in the fetal adrenal zone that can generate testosterone.

Pituitary development is complex and is closely related to hypothalamic development. The anterior pituitary derives from the ectoderm of the roof of the mouth, whereas the posterior pituitary is of nervous tissue in origin. The anterior pituitary produces six hormones and the posterior two.

FURTHER READING

Allada, R., Bass, J., 2021. Circadian mechanisms in medicine. N Engl J Med 384, 550–561.

Crowley, S., Hindmarsh, P.C., Honour, J.W., Brook, C.G., 1993. Reproducibility of the cortisol response to stimulation with a low dose of ACTH (1-24): the effect of basal cortisol levels and comparison of low-dose with high-dose secretory dynamics. J Endocrinol 136, 167–172.

Kelberman, D., Rizzoti, K., Lovell-Badge, R., Robinson, I.C.A.F., Dattani, M.T., 2009. Genetic regulation of pituitary gland development in human and mouse. Endocr Rev 30, 790–829.

Keil, M.F., Bosmans, C., Van Ryzin, C., Merke, D.P., 2010. Hypoglycemia during acute illness in children with classic congenital adrenal hyperplasia. J Pediatr Nurs 25, 18–24.

Koike, N., Yoo, S.-H., Huang, H.-C., et al., 2012. Transcriptional architecture and chromatin landscape of the core circadian clock in mammals. Science 338, 349–354.

Milsom, S.R., Conaglen, J.V., Donald, R.A., et al., 1985. Augmentation of the response to CRF in man: relative contributions of endogenous angiotensin and vasopressin. Clin Endocrinol 22, 623–628.

Walczak, E.M., Hammer, G.D., 2015. Regulation of the adrenocortical stem cell niche: implications for disease. Nat Rev Endocrinol 11, 14–28.

CHAPTER 3

What are Steroids?

GLOSSARY

Bound Cortisol Cortisol in the circulation attached to binding proteins.

Cholesterol Precursor of all steroids. Characterised by four ring structure with a long carbon chain.

Cortisol binding globulin A protein made by the liver which attaches itself to cortisol and carries it around the bloodstream. This is known as bound cortisol. 90% to 95% of cortisol is bound in this way with 5% in the free state.

Free Cortisol Cortisol in the circulation that is not attached to binding proteins.

Glucocorticoid receptor Docking station for free cortisol within cells. Comprises four components, an immunogenic section, a DNA binding region, a hinge region and a domain where cortisol binds. Steroid receptors are structurally similar but specific for the steroid they bind.

Glucocorticoid resistance A condition where the glucocorticoid receptor does not function correctly leading to high circulating cortisol levels but no features of Cushing's disease.

Low density lipoprotein receptor Receptor which takes up cholesterol attached in the blood to the low density lipoprotein.

Steroidogenesis The process of forming steroids from cholesterol by a series of enzyme mediated steps, leading to the formation of the members of the steroid family in the adrenal glands and gonads.

Steroidogenic acute regulatory protein Protein within steroidogenic cells that transports cholesterol into the mitochondria for steroid synthesis.

Total Cortisol The cortisol which is measured in blood by laboratories which is a combination of free and bound cortisol.

GENERAL

The term 'steroids' has become well embedded in both medical and lay languages. The general view is of an agent that leads to weight gain and acne. In the press, the term steroid is often used synonymously with anabolic steroid use in sport. Neither concept is helpful, nor are terms such as steroid dependent as this tells us nothing about which steroid the person might or might not be dependent on.

CHOLESTEROL

It is far better to think of the term steroid as an overarching description of a family of hormones which all share a similar structure, based on cholesterol. Cholesterol is the precursor of the five major classes of steroid hormones: progestogens, glucocorticoids, mineralocorticoids, androgens, and estrogens. Other branches of this family include the bile salts and vitamin D. Bile salts are synthesized in the liver, stored and concentrated in the gall bladder and then released into the small intestine where they aid digestion. Cholesterol is also the precursor of vitamin D, which plays an essential role in the control of calcium and phosphorus metabolism. Sunlight plays an important role in the formation of vitamin D from cholesterol. The ring structure of cholesterol which defines the steroid family, is broken in the formation of the active form of vitamin D, 1,25-dihydroxycholecalciferol so, although technically not a steroid, vitamin D acts in a similar fashion in binding to a receptor which is structurally similar to the steroid receptors, which together regulate gene expression.

Replacement Therapies in Adrenal Insufficiency. https://doi.org/10.1016/B978-0-12-824548-4.00004-8

The shape of the cholesterol molecule is shown in Figure 3.1A and the numbering system of the carbon atoms that are part of the steroid structure are shown in Figure 3.1B.

STRUCTURE OF CHOLESTEROL

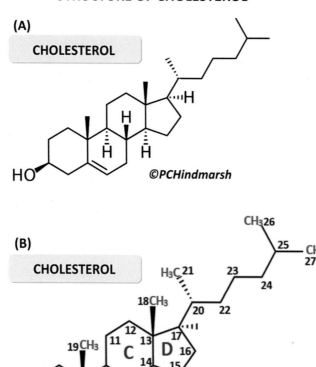

Figure 3.1 *(A) The molecular structure of cholesterol to show the four rings that are the hallmark of the steroid family. Each side links a carbon atom. Carbon double bonds are shown as the double lines. The solid and dashed arrows indicate the orientation of the associated atom (H) or molecule (OH or CH3) around the carbon atom. In the diagram because of the positioning of the oxygen atom around the carbon atom, the OH is written as HO as it is the oxygen which is attaching to the carbon atom, whereas conventionally in a chemical formula and general chemistry texts, it is written as OH. (B) The carbon atoms are numbered in cholesterol from 1 to 27. The rings are labelled A to D.*

We recognise this classification when we use the drug 9-alpha fludrocortisone, which tells us that fluorine has been added to carbon atom number 9 in the alpha orientation. In addition to sharing a similar structure based on cholesterol, the steroid family exerts its individual effect through steroid hormone receptors which are similar in overall structure but employ subtle differences which allow for specific binding to their preferred steroid family member (or ligand).

STEROID BIOSYNTHESIS

Cholesterol forms the basis of steroid biosynthesis in both the adrenal cortex and the gonads (testes or ovaries). There are only two sources of cholesterol, the diet and de novo synthesis predominantly in the liver.

When we look at the various steps involved in steroidogenesis in the adrenal glands or gonads, we can see that hydroxylation reactions play a very important role in the conversion of cholesterol into steroid hormones. You can see that in the name given to some of the enzymes and one that many are familiar with, is 21–hydroxylase which when deficient, is a cause of congenital adrenal hyperplasia. Figure 3.2 shows this reaction where the hydroxyl group (OH) is added to the 17-hydroxyprogesterone molecule to produce 11-deoxycortisol. Hydroxylation requires the activation of oxygen and this is undertaken by a cytochrome P450.

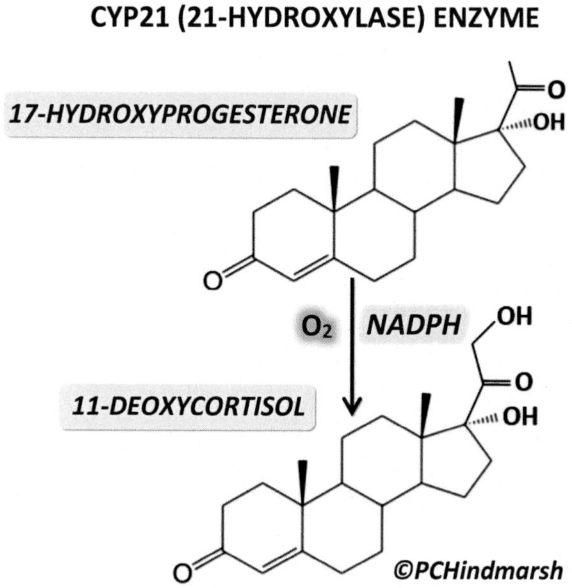

CYP21 (21-HYDROXYLASE) ENZYME

Figure 3.2 *The conversion of 17-hydroxyprogesterone to 11-deoxycortisol by the enzyme CYP21 (21-hydroxylase) which in the presence of oxygen (O_2) and a donor of hydrogen from NADPH (the reduced form of nicotinamide adenine dinucleotide phosphate) places the hydroxyl group (OH) onto the carbon atom at position 21. NADPH is formed as part of the metabolic handling of glucose in cells to form energy.*

The human cytochrome P450 system consists of more than 50 members and its main function is in the liver where it breaks down foreign substances. In fact, some of these liver cytochrome P450s metabolise adrenal steroids. In the adrenal glands and gonads many of the enzyme steps involved in steroidogenesis use these agents.

Figure 3.3 shows the steroid biosynthetic pathway in the adrenal glands and gonads. In the adrenal glands it is the adrenal cortex (outer layer) which is involved in the synthesis of the three main corticosteroids:

1. The mineralocorticoids which are salt retaining hormones, of which aldosterone is the main one.

2. The glucose regulating hormones (glucocorticoids) of which cortisol is the main one.

3. The adrenal androgens which are male like hormones produced by all males and females.

The pathway in the gonads differs in that the gonads do not make cortisol or aldosterone.

The shift of the pathway towards androgen and estradiol formation occurs because the direction of travel, dictated by the enzyme cytochrome P450 17 (CYP17) depends how quickly electrons are provided for the enzyme reaction. If electrons are delivered quickly to the enzyme system, then the reaction moves in favour of androgen generation, whereas slower delivery allows for cortisol development.

In addition, the genes involved in cortisol formation are poorly expressed in the gonads and these structures generate predominately either testosterone or estradiol.

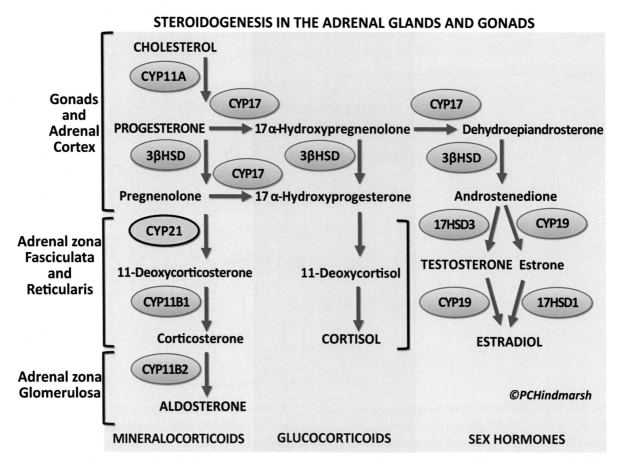

STEROIDOGENESIS IN THE ADRENAL GLANDS AND GONADS

Figure 3.3 *Steps in steroidogenesis in the adrenal glands and gonads. For reference the enzyme defect in salt-wasting congenital adrenal hyperplasia (CYP21) is coloured red. The middle and lower red brackets shows the steps present in the adrenal glands but not in the gonads.*

Aldosterone is regulated mainly by the renin-angiotensin system which we have considered in Chapter 2. The renin-angiotensin system is the main pathway for aldosterone regulation and biosynthesis, although ACTH contributes to a lesser degree. The glucocorticoids and adrenal androgens are regulated by the anterior pituitary gland through the hormone ACTH. This aspect has been considered in Chapter 2. The generation of testosterone and estradiol from the gonads are under the regulation of luteinising hormone (LH) and follicle-stimulating hormone (FSH) also from the anterior pituitary gland.

In order to make cortisol, the adrenal glands need to take up cholesterol from the bloodstream. ACTH signals the cells in the adrenal glands to pick up cholesterol from the blood and it does this by using a series of proteins which help bring cholesterol into the adrenal gland. The first of these is the low density lipoprotein receptor (LDLR) situated on the surface of the adrenocortical cells. The second important protein is called steroidogenic acute regulatory protein (StAR) (Figure 3.4). Cholesterol in the adrenal gland comes via the LDL receptor, de novo synthesis in the cells or from the lipid droplet pool by the action of hormone-sensitive lipase. Steroidogenic acute regulatory protein transports free cholesterol in the cell to the mitochondria for steroid biosynthesis. Steroid hormones contain 21 or fewer carbon atoms, whereas cholesterol contains 27. Thus, the first stage in the synthesis of steroid hormones is the removal of a six-carbon unit from the side chain of cholesterol to form pregnenolone. Each conversion step is brought about by the action of an enzyme. Enzymes are proteins that speed up the process of the chemical reaction, rather similar to the use of baking powder in a cake recipe. Each of the steps requires a special enzyme and each of them have a different name for the different tasks they do. Each enzyme is coded by a separate gene and these are summarised in Figure 3.5.

CHOLESTEROL UPTAKE BY THE ADRENAL GLANDS

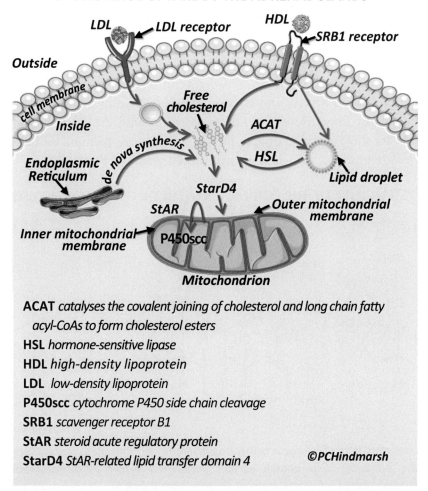

ACAT *catalyses the covalent joining of cholesterol and long chain fatty acyl-CoAs to form cholesterol esters*

HSL *hormone-sensitive lipase*

HDL *high-density lipoprotein*

LDL *low-density lipoprotein*

P450scc *cytochrome P450 side chain cleavage*

SRB1 *scavenger receptor B1*

StAR *steroid acute regulatory protein*

StarD4 *StAR-related lipid transfer domain 4*

©PCHindmarsh

Figure 3.4 *Steps in the incorporation of cholesterol into the adrenal cells via the low density lipoprotein receptor and the steroidogenic acute regulatory protein (StAR). StAR presents cholesterol to the mitochondria in the cell where the side carbon chain of cholesterol is removed.*

STEROIDOGENIC GENE LOCATIONS

ENZYME	GENE	GENE SIZE (Kilobases)	CHROMOSOMAL LOCATION
StAR	*StAR*	8	8p11.2
P450scc	*CYP11A1*	30	15q23-q24
P450c11β	*CYP11B1*	9.5	8q21-22
P450c11AS	*CYP11B2*	9.5	8q21-22
P450c17	*CYP17A1*	6.6	10q24.3
P450c21	*CYP21A2*	3.4	6p 21.1
3βHSD2	*HSD3B2*	8	1p13.1
P450-oxidoreductase	*POR*	69	7q11.2
			©PCHindmarsh

Figure 3.5 *Physical characteristics and location of human genes encoding adrenal steroidogenic enzymes.*

Once the adrenal glands make cortisol, a small amount is stored but the majority is released immediately into the bloodstream. The amounts which are produced at different times of the day vary and generate the circadian rhythm.

BIOCHEMICAL STRUCTURE OF THE STEROIDS

As already noted, steroids share a very similar basic structure. Figure 3.6 shows the structure of the synthetic glucocorticoids (hydrocortisone is synthetic cortisol) with the central ring structure. Double bonds between atoms are shown by the double lines. Chemists can manipulate these double bonds to generate for example, prednisolone which is shown in the middle of Figure 3.6.

STRUCTURE OF THE COMMON SYNTHETIC GLUCOCORTICOIDS

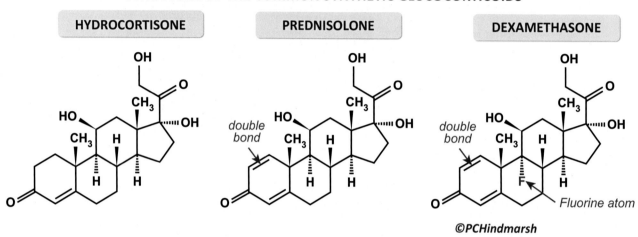

©PCHindmarsh

Figure 3.6 *The chemical structures of hydrocortisone, prednisolone and dexamethasone. Prednisolone differs from hydrocortisone by the presence of a double carbon bond (red arrow) and dexamethasone differs from prednisolone by the introduction of a fluorine atom at carbon atom 9 (red F).*

In this situation, cortisol or hydrocortisone has been modified with an additional double bond shown by the red arrow. The overall effect of this is to increase the potency of the glucocorticoid and to slightly prolong its duration of action as measured by its anti-inflammatory effect. On the right hand side in Figure 3.6, is dexamethasone which again is a synthetic glucocorticoid. It is very similar to both cortisol and prednisolone with a double bond which was introduced into cortisol to generate prednisolone. Dexamethasone has been further modified by the introduction of a fluorine atom at carbon position 9 (as illustrated by the red F for fluorine in Figure 3.6).

This manipulation in all steroids leads to prolongation of the duration of action of the steroid and indirectly increases the potency of the steroid.

In Figure 3.7 you can see some of the differences between aldosterone, cortisol and testosterone and most of the differences between cortisol and aldosterone compared to testosterone, are reflected in the loss of the side chain in the formation of testosterone. These differences lead to the specific effects that these members of the steroid family have on different parts of the body.

The differences between aldosterone and cortisol are not that noticeable and it would be very easy for cortisol to attach itself to the mineralocorticoid receptor (or docking point) in the kidney cells. This would be especially easy as cortisol is present in the circulation in a concentration 1000 times that of aldosterone. If this were to happen, then cortisol would occupy the aldosterone receptor and cause retention of sodium and water leading to hypertension.

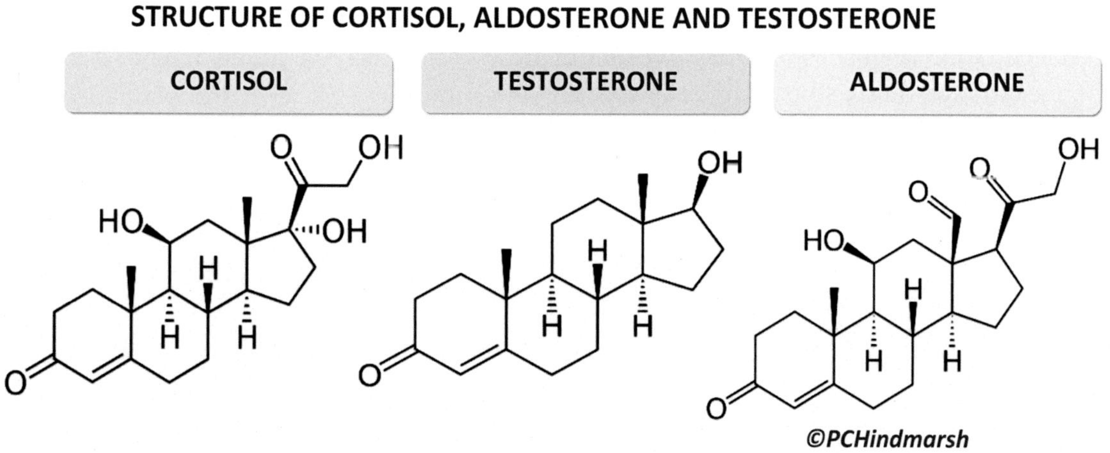

STRUCTURE OF CORTISOL, ALDOSTERONE AND TESTOSTERONE

| CORTISOL | TESTOSTERONE | ALDOSTERONE |

©PCHindmarsh

Figure 3.7 *Structures of cortisol, aldosterone and testosterone. The loss of the side chain in testosterone is very noticeable. The differences between cortisol and aldosterone are less easy to tell with the addition of an oxygen (O) and removal of a hydroxyl group (OH).*

This occurs when the enzyme 11beta-hydroxysteroid dehydrogenase type 2 is missing. This enzyme converts active cortisol to inactive cortisone. The enzyme is found around the target cells for aldosterone, protecting them from the high amounts of cortisol by converting cortisol to cortisone. When missing, this leads to the syndrome of Apparent Mineralocorticoid Excess and very high blood pressure.

A similar effect can be seen with glycyrrhizic acid from liquorice preparations which inhibits the enzyme, leading to hypertension, low potassium, metabolic alkalosis and sometimes fatal heart arrhythmias.

In order for the body to be able to respond to the specific message contained by the steroid in question, the steroids need to get to their target tissues through the bloodstream.

STEROIDAL TRANSPORTATION — CORTISOL AS AN EXAMPLE

Once the adrenal glands make cortisol, a small amount is stored but the majority is released immediately into the bloodstream. The difficulty with the steroid family is they are not very soluble in water — they are hydrophobic. Cortisol in the bloodstream is transported either as cortisol itself which is known as 'free' cortisol, or cortisol bound to proteins in the blood ('bound' cortisol). 'Free' cortisol is cortisol which is ready to act in different cells of the body and is not attached to anything.

A considerable amount of cortisol is attached to different proteins present in the blood, in particular one protein called cortisol binding globulin (CBG) takes up a substantial amount of cortisol and acts almost like a reservoir in the bloodstream. This means that if 'free' cortisol is removed from the circulation, there can be a top up from the cortisol which is attached to the protein reservoir. 'Free' cortisol can be removed by the kidneys and passed out in the urine, but the majority of the cortisol produced is broken down in the liver and passed out of the body in various metabolic forms in the urine.

In addition to CBG, albumin in the blood also carries steroids and will carry cortisol. Both these binding proteins carry cortisol to the various tissues in the body. It is only the unbound ('free' cortisol) that is active. The majority of cortisol, or for that matter steroid that is produced by the endocrine organs in question, is transported attached to the binding proteins so the amount of 'free' cortisol available at any stage is only about 4% to 10%. This means that at any point there is a balance between the amount of cortisol attached to its binding protein, CBG and the amount which is 'free.' This has important implications for the measurement of cortisol in blood samples.

When we do a blood test, we measure both the 'free' and the bound cortisol and this is called the total cortisol concentration (Figure 3.8). In fact, we do not always call it that, we simply refer to it as the plasma cortisol concentration but to be technically correct, we should really call it the plasma total cortisol concentration.

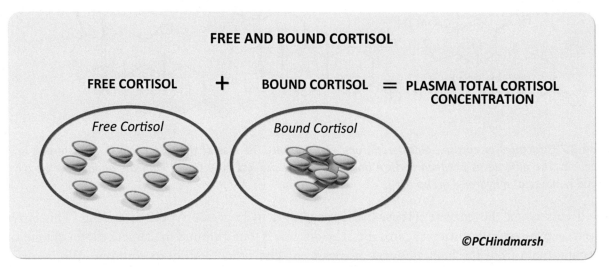

Figure 3.8 *Free cortisol (red discs) circulate unattached to anything in the blood whereas bound cortisol (red discs attached to blue protein) refers to cortisol that circulates attached to various binding proteins such as cortisol binding globulin (CBG).*

This means when we are interpreting cortisol concentrations, we have to remember that some is 'free' and some is bound. Under normal circumstances this does not matter too much, but when CBG concentrations change, for example in people who take the oral contraceptive pill, then the total cortisol concentration we measure will change as well.

Similarly, in conditions where albumin and globulin may be lost in the kidney, in conditions such as nephrotic syndrome, then the plasma total cortisol concentration measured may be lower than expected because the amount of protein available to bind cortisol is reduced because of loss through the kidney. The amount of 'free' cortisol, which is available however, is unchanged, so that unless a large amount of protein is lost through the kidney, the individual will remain well.

Going back to the effect of the oral contraceptive pill, we know if we measure cortisol levels in an individual who is on the pill, then the plasma total cortisol concentration will be high because more CBG is around and that can bind more cortisol, raising the total cortisol concentration. What happens is the free cortisol concentration does not change that much, at least initially.

If, however, you are taking hydrocortisone because you cannot produce cortisol, unless the dose is changed, then more cortisol will be taken up and bound so there will be overall less 'free' cortisol. An example of the effect of the contraceptive pill has on cortisol levels can be seen in Chapter 13 Figure 13.2.

This all adds extra complexity but is extremely important to understand, because it influences many of the things that we do with hydrocortisone replacement. We have seen one example with the oral contraceptive pill. Another example is the whole question of whether you should double, triple or quadruple doses during illness. Standard teaching is to double the cortisol dose.

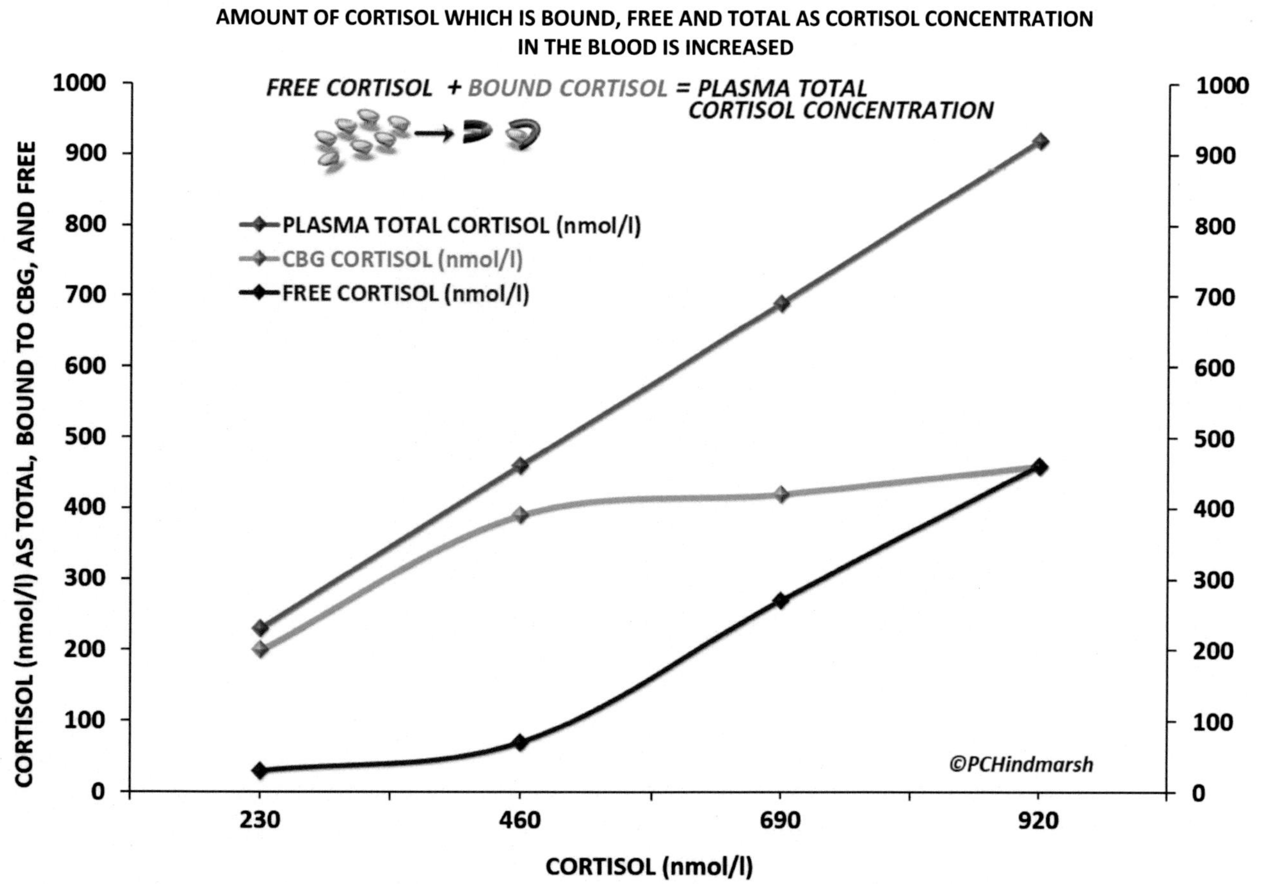

AMOUNT OF CORTISOL WHICH IS BOUND, FREE AND TOTAL AS CORTISOL CONCENTRATION IN THE BLOOD IS INCREASED

Figure 3.9 Changes in the plasma of free (red line) and cortisol binding globulin (CBG) bound cortisol (light blue) that is measured as plasma total cortisol (dark blue) as cortisol concentrations increase.

The question is, what does double the dose do or even tripling or quadrupling the dose?

The answer is perhaps surprising at first. If you double and particularly if you triple the dose, for example go from 10 mg per day of hydrocortisone to 30 mg per day, you do not triple the amount of cortisol in the blood. Although you might triple the dose, cortisol concentrations in the blood, barely double. This happens because of the binding proteins.

When you give more cortisol if you start to exceed plasma cortisol concentrations of 450 to 500 nmol/l, then the proteins (CBG) to which cortisol can attach become saturated.

In other words, there is a limit to how much cortisol can stick onto the protein (Figure 3.9). Once this threshold is reached there will then be an increase in the amount of 'free' cortisol but because this is removed very easily by the liver and the kidney, the amount of total cortisol you actually achieve will not go up proportionately with the amount that you are giving.

This means if you double the dose of hydrocortisone when unwell, then you probably will not double the cortisol concentration.

Although it might be tempting to triple the dose, this will not lead to a triple level of cortisol in the blood, as the threshold will be exceeded and most of the extra cortisol which has been given, will be lost in the urine. Figure 3.10 illustrates this point for a variety of incremental doses of hydrocortisone.

DOUBLE, TRIPLE OR EVEN QUINTUPLING ORAL DOSES OF HYDROCORTISONE DO NOT ACHIEVE DOUBLE, TRIPLE OR QUINTUPLE CORTISOL CONCENTRATIONS DUE TO THE INFLUENCE OF CORTISOL BINDING GLOBULIN

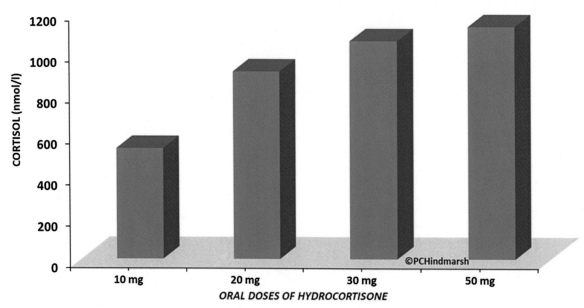

Figure 3.10 *The effect of doubling, tripling and quintupling the oral dose of hydrocortisone from 10 mg on the cortisol level achieved in the blood. Please note, the plasma cortisol levels from the doses should not be used as a guide as the amount achieved in every individual will vary dependent on body size, clearance and other factors, this figure is purely illustrative.*

Figure 3.10 is illustrative of the CBG phenomenon. The doses shown in Figure 3.10 would not necessarily produce similar cortisol levels in everyone, as the peak value obtained from hydrocortisone varies between individuals, due to variations in absorption and clearance which we look at in more detail in Chapter 6. The point to make about Figures 3.9 and 3.10 is when doses are doubled, tripled or even quintupled, the presence and saturation of CBG alters the amount of cortisol you can achieve in the blood, in terms of the plasma total cortisol concentration which is what we measure in the laboratory.

In Figure 3.10 we see that 10 mg of hydrocortisone produces a peak value of 600 nmol/l in this person. If we double the amount to 20 mg of hydrocortisone, we only get to 900 nmol/l. So double dose has not doubled the plasma total cortisol level because as Figure 3.9 shows, we have saturated CBG and all we do is increase the amount of free cortisol which is removed very quickly through the kidneys.

Three times the amount (30 mg) does not triple the plasma total cortisol value and 50 mg hydrocortisone just about doubles the plasma total cortisol value. This is not to say that doubling the dose during illness is not helpful.

In illness, the body has ways to get more cortisol to where it needs it to be as local temperature changes alter how cortisol is attached to CBG. High local temperatures mean more cortisol falls off the CBG molecule delivering a high local amount of cortisol. The point is that CBG plays an important role in determining the amount of cortisol in the circulation preventing the body from getting too much cortisol in the circulation at any one time.

We also see this in cortisol profiles when very high peaks drop quickly as CBG is saturated and the free cortisol is cleared quickly through the kidneys.

These binding proteins act not simply as a buffer and store, but are vital because cortisol does not dissolve very easily in the blood. The way in which cortisol attaches itself to CBG varies considerably between individuals, but even more importantly it is also influenced by body temperature. As body temperature increases, for example during a fever, the amount of cortisol that attaches itself to CBG decreases, so this becomes really important because the 'free' cortisol which now becomes available, particularly to the local tissues, nearly triples. This is a really interesting and important observation, because it is one of the ways in which the body protects itself and gets cortisol out to where it needs to be working in situations of stress and illness.

So, although we do not necessarily double or triple the amount of cortisol in the blood when we double or triple the hydrocortisone dose, what will happen particularly in local tissues, is that 'free' cortisol will increase, so this is an efficient protective way the body has to ensure that during illness the tissues of the body receive exactly the right amount of extra cortisol they need.

As already suggested, the CBG is influenced by several factors. Estrogens, chronic active hepatitis and some anticonvulsant medication will increase CBG whilst cirrhosis, overactive thyroid or protein loss through the kidney in nephrosis or protein loss through the gut in a protein losing enteropathy, will decrease values. Cortisol binding globulin will bind other endogenous steroids. Whilst cortisol strongly associates with CBG, other natural and synthetic steroids also bind to CBG. Amongst these are 17-hydroxyprogesterone (17OHP) and to a certain extent, testosterone. This does not matter as long as the concentration of these particular steroids is low.

However, should 17OHP concentrations be high such as in CAH, then there will be some competition between 17-hydroxyprogesterone and cortisol meaning there will potentially be less cortisol bound to CBG and therefore the total cortisol concentration may appear slightly lower.

STEROID RECEPTORS

What we are now going to consider is how cortisol instructs the cells of the body to carry out all its functions. We will be using cortisol as an example, but the story is similar for the other members of the steroid family. Cortisol has a multitude of effects (Figure 3.11) and nearly two thirds of human genes are regulated by cortisol either by switching them on or off. 'Free' cortisol can cross easily into cells. Within the cell is a special docking station for cortisol — the cortisol or glucocorticoid receptor. There are receptors for other members of the steroid family and the specificity of these receptors for their particular hormone is determined by their shape and size. Steroid hormone receptors are found in the nucleus, cytosol and also on the plasma membrane of target cells. Most of them are generally intracellular receptors (cytoplasmic or nuclear). The glucocorticoid receptor which is a receptor to which cortisol and other glucocorticoids bind is part of the nuclear receptor family.

Interestingly, the glucocorticoid receptor is expressed in almost every cell in the body regulating the genes in the processes outlined in Figure 3.11.

The unbound receptor resides in the cytosol of the cell and after the receptor is bound to cortisol, the cortisol receptor complex then translocates into the nucleus and binds to specific responsive elements on DNA activating gene transcription (Figure 3.12). There are a complex series of interactions that take place at the genetic level which lead to either activation or repression of protein formation. This operates over a time frame of hours to days.

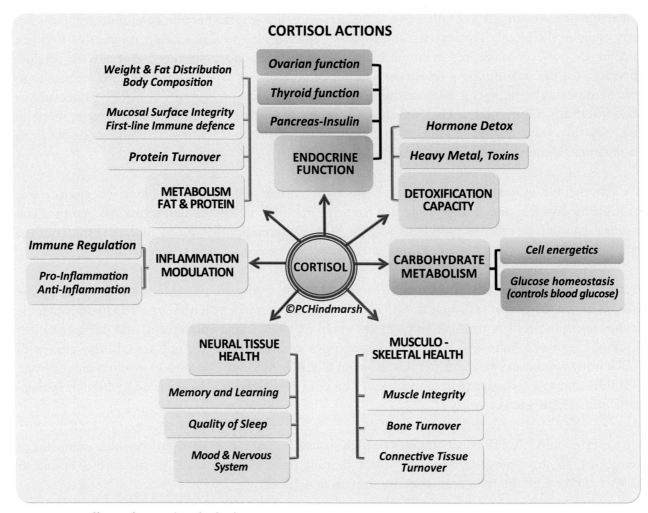

Figure 3.11 *Effects of cortisol in the body.*

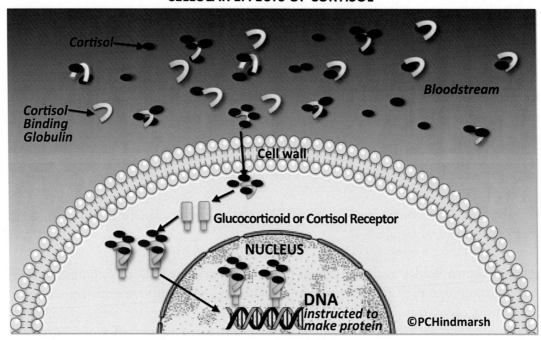

Figure 3.12 *Cortisol enters the cell where it docks with a special glucocorticoid or cortisol receptor. This complex moves into the nucleus of the cell and attaches to a glucocorticoid response element on DNA. This attachment tells the gene to make the mRNA that goes on to form the protein that cortisol regulates.*

The intracellular steroid hormone receptors share a common structure of four units often called 'domains.' The first unit is the variable or immunogenic domain which as its name suggests is the most variable domain between the different receptors. The second domain is the DNA binding domain which is highly conserved and determines which gene will be activated. Between the DNA binding domain and the last domain, the hormone or ligand binding domain, is the hinge region which controls the movement of the receptor to the nucleus. Figure 3.13 shows the various members of the steroid receptor super family with the glucocorticoid receptor at the top and the numbers in the domains expressing percentage identity of each of the domains with the glucocorticoid receptor.

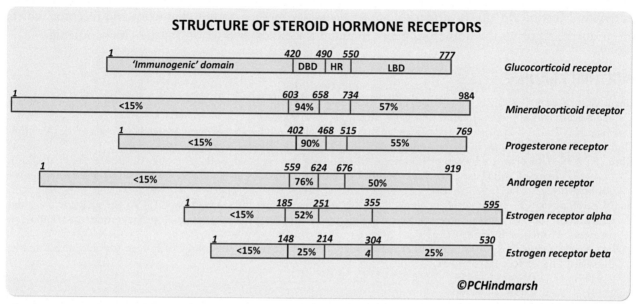

Figure 3.13 *Schematic representation of the six steroid receptors. The percentages compare how similar the domains are to the glucocorticoid receptor shown at the top. As we move down the similarity becomes less. Numbers on top of each receptor indicate the number of amino acids contributing to each domain. DBD - DNA binding domain, HR - hinge region, LBD - ligand binding domain.*

All these effects are mediated through DNA and are known as genome mediated. The steroid family can also mediate effects that do not involve DNA (nongenomic). For example, the cell membrane aldosterone receptor increases the activity of the sodium channels in the kidney tubules and collecting duct as well as in the large bowel and possibly in sweat glands.

Mutations in the glucocorticoid receptor gene result in familial/sporadic generalised glucocorticoid resistance syndrome. The condition is characterized by hypercortisolism without Cushingoid features. To overcome the reduced sensitivity to glucocorticoids in tissues, affected subjects have compensatory elevations in circulating cortisol and ACTH concentrations, which maintain circadian rhythmicity and appropriate responsiveness to stressors. There is loss of or reduced adrenal axis suppression by dexamethasone and no clinical evidence of hypercortisolism. The excess ACTH secretion causes increased production of adrenal steroids with mineralocorticoid and androgen activity. The former leads to hypertension and hypokalaemic alkalosis. The latter accounts for the manifestations of androgen excess, such as ambiguous genitalia and precocious puberty in children, acne, hirsutism and infertility in both sexes, male pattern hair loss, menstrual irregularities and infrequent or absent ovulation in females and adrenal rests in the testes and oligospermia in males. The clinical spectrum of the condition is broad and a large number of subjects may be asymptomatic, displaying biochemical alterations only.

Finally, isoforms (a member of a set of highly similar proteins originating from a single gene) of the glucocorticoid receptor, allows target tissues to differentially respond to the ambient plasma glucocorticoid concentration.

CONCLUSION

Steroidogenesis, the process of forming steroids from cholesterol in the adrenal glands and gonads, requires uptake of cholesterol from the bloodstream and cleavage of the side chain to yield 21 carbon steroids or less. A series of enzymatic steps mainly involving changes in hydroxyl groups yield the principal steroids cortisol, aldosterone and DHEA and androstenedione from the adrenal glands and testosterone and estradiol from the testes and ovaries respectively. Cortisol in the circulation is 90% to 95% bound to cortisol binding globulin and albumin and a complex series of interactions takes place at the local tissue level which is temperature dependent to deliver varying amounts of cortisol in the free state. Most of the effects of cortisol are mediated by binding to the glucocorticoid receptor which up or down, regulates the numerous genes required for the diverse actions of the glucocorticoid.

FURTHER READING

Chan, W.L., Carrell, R.W., Zhou, A., Read, R.J., 2013. How changes in affinity of corticosteroid-binding globulin modulate free cortisol concentration. J Clin Endocrinol Metab 98, 3315–3322.

Charmandari, E., 2011. Primary generalized glucocorticoid resistance and hypersensitivity. Horm Res Paediatr 76, 145–155.

Honour, J.W., 2023. Steroids in the Laboratory and Clinical Practice. Elsevier, Oxford.

Kino, T., 2000. Glucocorticoid receptor [Updated 2017 Aug 15]. In: Feingold, K.R., Anawalt, B., Boyce, A., et al. (Eds.), *Endotext* [Internet]. MDText.com, Inc., South Dartmouth (MA). Available from: https://www.ncbi.nlm.nih.gov/books/NBK279171.

Lu, N.Z., Wardell, S.E., Burnstein, K.L., et al., 2006. International Union of Pharmacology. LXV. The pharmacology and classification of the nuclear receptor superfamily: glucocorticoid, mineralocorticoid, progesterone, and androgen receptors. Pharmacol Rev 58, 782–797.

Miller, W.L., Auchus, R.J., 2011. The molecular biology, biochemistry, and physiology of human steroidogenesis and its disorders. Endocr Rev 32, 81–151.

CHAPTER 4

Biochemical Tests Used in Adrenal Insufficiency

GLOSSARY

21-Hydroxylase Sometimes called CYP21, 21-hydroxylase is the enzyme which converts 17-hydroxyprogesterone to 11-deoxycortisol and also progesterone to deoxycorticosterone. This is the most common enzyme deficiency in congenital adrenal hyperplasia (CAH).

24 hour cortisol profile A test to determine the variation in cortisol as part of the circadian rhythm by drawing blood samples to measure cortisol every hour.

Adrenocorticotropin Hormone produced by the pituitary gland that regulates cortisol synthesis and secretion from the adrenal glands.

Androstenedione Adrenal androgen which is made from dehydroepiandrosterone by the action of the enzyme 3beta-hydroxysteroid dehydrogenase type 2. Level rises in CAH when cortisol replacement is suboptimal.

Fetal adrenal glands Large structures present in the fetus which mainly produce dehydroepiandrosterone and help maintain the pregnancy. The fetal adrenal glands disappear by the third month after birth.

Insulin induced hypoglycaemia test This test uses the stimulus of hypoglycaemia to cause corticotropin-releasing hormone to be released by the hypothalamus which in turn releases ACTH from the pituitary which in turn prompts the adrenal cortex to produce and release cortisol. Growth hormone is also released in response to hypoglycaemia.

Renin–angiotensin system Group of hormones which act together to regulate blood volume and blood pressure.

Sampling interval Time between blood samples in a hormone profile. When measuring natural cortisol production, (i.e. not measuring cortisol replacement from hydrocortisone) blood samples should be drawn at time intervals less than the half-life of the hormone of interest to adequately define peaks and troughs, as well as the frequency and rhythm of the hormone bursts. The average half-life of cortisol is 80 minutes so sampling every 60 minutes will provide a good approximation of the true peaks, troughs, frequency of bursts of cortisol and the circadian rhythm. For measuring cortisol from hydrocortisone replacement therapy, sampling protocols to catch the peak need to be adjusted and individualised to the absorption rate of the dose which means an extra sample needs to be taken 30 minutes after the dose has been given, as well as the usual sample at 60 minutes. Occasionally, the extra sample will need to be taken after the 60 minute sample at 90 minutes if the profile data shows very similar 60 minute and 120 minute cortisol concentrations, indicating the peak may occur at this time.

Synacthen test A means of making the adrenal glands produce and release cortisol. Synacthen is the name given to a synthetic form of ACTH.

Urinary steroid profile Collection of urine over 24 hours and analysed by mass spectroscopy to identify the metabolites of cortisol and other adrenal steroid metabolites.

Urinary free cortisol Measurement of free cortisol in urine obtained over 24 hours. Relies on saturation of cortisol binding globulin by plasma cortisol. Good at detecting high circulating cortisol levels but not discriminatory for low values as it cannot differentiate between low, normal and pathologically low as occurs in adrenal insufficiency.

Replacement Therapies in Adrenal Insufficiency. https://doi.org/10.1016/B978-0-12-824548-4.00023-1

GENERAL

Biochemical tests are used for a number of reasons in patients with adrenal insufficiency. The first and most obvious is to establish the presence or absence of adrenal insufficiency and then to move on to establish the cause. This chapter is focussed on establishing the presence or absence of adrenal insufficiency and Chapter 5 looks at ways of establishing the cause. In addition to diagnostic testing, we can use hormone measurements to help understand the pharmacology of the drugs we use, particularly hydrocortisone. We are interested in two main measures, firstly, how hydrocortisone is absorbed and secondly, how it is cleared from the circulation. We cover how these measurements are achieved in Chapter 6. Finally, we explain how biochemical tests can be used to monitor drug replacement. This in itself is an extremely large topic and one we devote Section 3 of this book.

When we are thinking of testing, whether the body is making too much or too little of a hormone, we use a very broad endocrine principle. If we suspect there is too much of a hormone produced, we look at ways of testing whether we can supress production of the hormone. Conversely, if we are interested in whether a hormone is absent or not, we look at ways of stimulating the release of the hormone of interest. In this book we are clearly interested in documenting whether the adrenal glands are capable of making the glucocorticoid cortisol as well as the mineralocorticoid aldosterone.

In Cushing's syndrome (cortisol excess) we are looking to test whether there is too much cortisol produced throughout the 24 hour period so here we are interested in seeing if we can suppress the cortisol using dexamethasone. We cover this partly in Chapter 5 when we consider dexamethasone suppression tests.

MEASURING CORTISOL

Cortisol is measured in routine chemical pathology laboratories throughout the world. The systems used are increasingly automated and as a result it becomes important to understand factors which may influence the result obtained.

Immunoassays of cortisol

Over the years a number of methods for measuring cortisol predominantly in blood and urine samples have been developed. Common to the majority of these methods is a principle known as immunoassay. In immunoassay, an antibody is raised, usually in an animal or cell line that recognises the protein of interest. An antibody is a large, Y-shaped protein used by the immune system to identify and neutralize foreign objects such as bacteria and viruses. The antibody recognizes a unique molecule of the foreign object, called an antigen. Antibodies are part of a large family known as immunoglobulins.

Unfortunately, steroids are not proteins and generating antibodies to recognise the specific steroids in the circulation can be a very complex process.

In an immunoassay, the antibody which has been generated is usually labelled with a substance we can measure. In the past this was usually a radioactive isotope such as iodine. Iodine is present with different atomic sizes and some are unstable so that when they switch from unstable to stable, they emit radiation which we can measure. Other systems use substances that can be detected using light sensing technology (chemiluminescence), or a substance which then participates in a further enzyme reaction to generate another product or an electric current. The latter, for example, can then be converted into a digital readout.

Historically, the first system to be developed was called a radioimmunoassay. Here a known quantity of an antigen in our case cortisol, was made radioactive by labelling it with an isotope of iodine and mixed with a known amount of antibody raised against the antigen. As a result, the two specifically bound to one another. Then, a sample of plasma from a patient containing an unknown quantity of that same antigen was added.

This causes the unlabelled (or 'cold') antigen from the plasma to compete with the radiolabelled antigen ('hot') for antibody binding sites. As the concentration of 'cold' antigen is increased, more of it binds to the antibody, displacing the radiolabelled variant and reducing the ratio of antibody bound radiolabelled antigen to free radiolabelled antigen.

The bound antigens were then separated and the radioactivity of the free (unbound) antigen remaining is measured (Figure 4.1).

This approach was then refined into an immunometric assay where the antibodies are labelled, not the antigen, so that what you want to measure combines immediately with the labelled antibodies, rather than displacing another antigen by degrees over a period of time. Gradually the radioactive isotopes were replaced with chemicals which could be detected by light sensors. These are known as chemiluminescent assays. They have the advantage of high throughput, but because they use certain light wavelengths for the detection process, they are susceptible to any pigments in the blood such as haemoglobin (red) in haemolysed samples and bilirubin (yellow) in patients with jaundice.

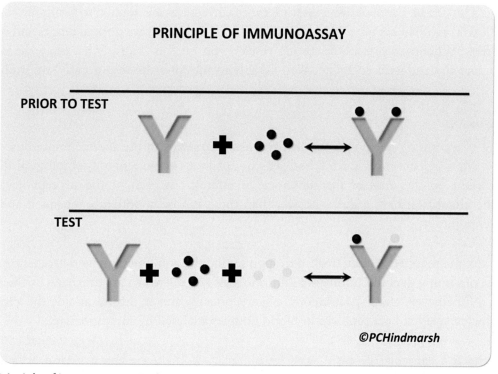

Figure 4.1 *Principle of immunoassay. In the upper panel an antigen (blue circles) say cortisol has been labelled with a chemical or radioactivity that we can measure and combined with an antibody to the antigen. The antibody binds to the blue antigen circles. This complex is then taken and incubated with a blood sample from a patient (yellow circles representing their cortisol which is not labelled). The blue and yellow circles compete to attach to the antibody and the number of yellow circles that can attach will depend on how much cortisol is in the patient's blood.*

This is quite a complex set of biochemical reactions and because it involves many steps, there is potential for error in the measurement of a sample. A single sample measured on several occasions will not necessarily give exactly the same value. For example, if we had a plasma cortisol concentration which was said to be 450 nmol/l repeated measurements might reveal a range between 445 and 455 nmol/l. The error may also vary over the concentration range experienced in physiological and pathophysiological situations.

There are two measures of how the assay performs.

1. First, is the sensitivity of the assay which relates to the lowest concentration of steroid in the blood which the assay can detect. For many cortisol assays this is less than 28 nmol/l.

2. The other measure is the coefficient of variation. The coefficient of variation gives us an estimate of the error attached to each individual measurement. In modern immunoassays this is usually less than 5% and is usually constant across the normal concentration range expected of the steroid of interest.

One problem with these types of assay, is cross-reactivity to endogenous or exogenous compounds other than the target steroid hormone of the assay. Falsely high cortisol measurements can result in some assays in patients with 21-hydroxylase deficiency, due to elevated 21-deoxycortisol (metabolite of 17-hydroxyprogesterone) levels which are picked up in the cortisol assay. An example of exogenous compounds cross-reacting is prednisolone which can have up to 60% cross-reactivity in a cortisol assay.

There has been a move to different assays which are more aligned towards the results obtained by mass spectroscopy. This can be very confusing as sometimes corrections are applied to bring the results which usually read lower, more in keeping with what the clinician has learnt are normal ranges and responses to stimulation tests. Whenever you are discussing results, you need to know what assay the cortisol was measured on and the endocrinologist needs to be able to interpret the results based on studies done in the past.

Mass spectroscopy

Another way of measuring hormones and in particular steroids, is to use the technique known as mass spectroscopy. Mass spectroscopy is a method which separates components of a biological fluid, in this case blood, based on the mass of the substance of interest. As each of the protein hormones and steroids in the circulation have a different size, then these can be confidently separated and identified using this technique.

The sample volume required is quite small, although setting the equipment up and processing the sample is more time consuming than the automated immunoassay systems which are preferred by the majority of laboratories. Nonetheless, mass spectroscopy is very precise, and it mostly avoids the cross-reaction problems which can often be a problem in blood samples analysed by immunoassay.

Cross-reactivity is a particular problem with steroid analysis in the newborn period because the fetal adrenal zone is still active at this time and does not stop working until about 3 months of age. The hormones the fetal adrenal glands produces, look similar to some of the steroid hormones that we wish to measure and because of this we need to use laboratories which can carefully assess the difference between these steroid hormones. There are few laboratories that do this as most laboratories are geared to measuring steroid hormones in adults, who of course do not have the fetal adrenal zone.

As a result, care when interpreting results needs to be exercised. In this situation, the measurement of steroid hormones by the process of liquid chromatography-tandem mass spectroscopy, which is a very specific method for identifying steroid hormones based on their molecular size, comes to the fore. This particular process overcomes the problems associated with the fetal adrenal zone and provides a very specific measure.

TYPES OF SAMPLE

Measuring steroids in blood samples is well established. Obtaining a sample is straightforward and requires nothing more than venepuncture to obtain blood. This is then separated and the steroid of interest, in this case cortisol is measured in the plasma. This direct sampling is extremely useful. Many people collect steroid hormone measurements on filter paper using blood spots (we cover this in Chapter 11). This is a quick method for assessing the level of the steroid hormone but there are considerable problems associated with it, not least the ability to recover all the steroid from the blood spot. This can amount to a 50% difference. There are also collection issues if the actual circle on the filter paper is not filled adequately or is over filled using a series of dabs rather than a free flowing sample.

Virtually all the steroid hormones are metabolised in the liver and excreted in solution in the urine. In the urine there are specific patterns of the metabolites of all the steroid hormones we see in the adrenal pathway. These hormones do not have the same names, but we can easily identify them using chromatography in the same way we can do in blood (Figure 4.2).

EXAMPLE OF A GAS CHROMATOGRAM

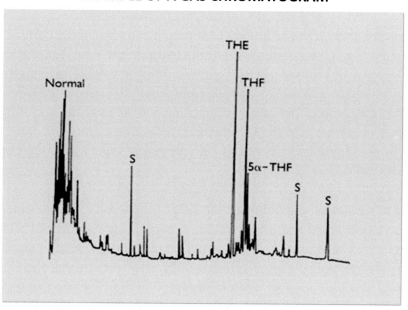

Figure 4.2 *Gas chromatography analysis of a urine steroid profile from a normal subject showing the main metabolites of cortisone − tetrahydrocortisone (THE) and cortisol - tetrahydrocortisol (THF) and 5-alpha tetrahydrocortisol (5α-THF). S are internal standards.*

The advantage of urine testing is the very large volume obtained. In the newborn, we rely very heavily on this technique. From a single processed urine test, we can get an idea of every single steroid hormone above and below a certain block in conditions such as congenital adrenal hyperplasia (CAH). This is a very efficient and effective way of making a diagnosis and it is the one we prefer to use in the initial phases, to blood testing.

Where urine testing becomes less valuable is when we wish to monitor replacement therapy. We will be considering the use of blood profiling later in the book. Suffice to say at this stage, it is very difficult to relate measures in the urine to the delivery of a drug. The reason for this, is there is a temporal gap between ingesting the drug, the drug being absorbed and distributed around the body, the drug acting on tissues of the body, then the drug being metabolised in the liver and distributed around the body again to be excreted in the urine.

The other and perhaps more obvious problem is urine samples cannot be obtained on a regular basis! The best we could possibly obtain samples over, is every 4 to 6 hours which would make correlating drug administration with what subsequently was measured later, extremely difficult. Any time interval greater than this would not be helpful given the duration that hydrocortisone is present in the circulation as cortisol, is only 4 to 6 hours.

Assessment of cortisol and other steroids in saliva has been put forward as a good way of measuring steroid hormones because no blood sample is required. In fact, because what is measured are the free cortisol concentrations, they are not particularly effective. The reason and this applies to the measurement of free cortisol in the urine, is the amount of steroid hormone has to be high in the blood in order to appear in the saliva (and for that matter the urine) and the whole point is that cortisol is likely to be low at times. So, salivary samples are helpful in diagnosing conditions where there are high concentrations of cortisol in the saliva such as in Cushing's disease. However, they should not be used to measure cortisol in conditions where cortisol is being replaced because you cannot adequately measure low cortisol concentrations in saliva.

In particular with cortisol, there is the additional confounding factor that the cortisol measured is highly dependent on the activity of 11beta-hydroxysteroid dehydrogenase type 2 in the salivary glands. This enzyme inactivates cortisol to cortisone. The concentrations of cortisol measured in saliva therefore reflect not just the ambulant circulatory concentration and the impact of factors such as cortisol binding globulin in the blood, but also on the enzymatic activity of 11beta-hydroxysteroid dehydrogenase type 2 in salivary glands. Measurement of salivary cortisone suffers similar problems and is also dependent on 11beta-hydroxysteroid dehydrogenase type 2 activity. This is known as first pass metabolism which we discuss in Chapter 6.

There are also many factors which can influence the saliva sample and cause inaccurate readings, such as too much acid in the mouth, food and drink. In illness, particularly if associated with dehydration, not only could the samples be contaminated, but it would be difficult to obtain enough saliva in which to measure the cortisol concentration. Clearly care has to be also taken when obtaining salivary samples not long after the oral administration of hydrocortisone. The flow of saliva has a circadian variation and flow is also influenced by the ambient temperature. Flow is important for determining what concentration of analyte may be measured and will be susceptible to these effects. Finally, these issues with saliva measurements make the pharmacology of hydrocortisone hard to assess.

VARIATION IN MEASUREMENTS

As previously mentioned, in many of these assay systems there is a variation in the value of cortisol which is obtained even when the same sample is analysed repeatedly. There are other sources of variation, some of which are modifiable and other which are less so. This is important to realise as it adds to the complexity of interpreting the result obtained from testing.

Biological variation

Biological variation refers to differences in cortisol values in a single person and between people. Plasma cortisol concentrations vary as we have already seen throughout the 24 hour period, as part of the circadian rhythm of cortisol (see Chapter 1, Figure 1.9B). This means a value which we obtain at 06:00 (6 am) is quite different to that obtained at 00:00 (midnight) and the normal range which applies at 06:00 (6 am) will be quite different to that at 00:00 (midnight). Consequently, the interpretation of the value will be different. A plasma cortisol concentration of 300 nmol/l at 00:00 (midnight) would be elevated and might indicate Cushing's disease whereas such a value, 6 hours later would be considered normal.

The actual day to day variation in a single person is not that diverse. Any variation largely reflects differences in the light/dark cycle, the latitude where the person dwells, possibly different times of sleep onset, whether the individual is fasting or having regular food intake and the impact of travel particularly across time zones. The majority of these variations we can identify and when we have undertaken 24 hour cortisol profiles in children and adults without adrenal problems (Chapter 2, Figure 2.8), the studies were carried out under strictly controlled conditions including the time of sleep onset, when lights are switched on and off during the evening and night, as well as ensuring meals are taken at standard times.

Variation between people may reflect differences in age and gender. In fact, for cortisol there is very little difference in carefully constructed 24 hour cortisol profiles between young and older individuals, both having similar peak and trough concentrations (Figures 4.3 and 4.4). The only difference which has been observed by us and others in the published literature, is although the timing of the peak is similar at around 06:00 (6 am) to 07:00 (7 am), the timing of the trough concentrations does vary with values of 22:00 (10 pm) in children, 02:00 (2 am) in young adults and 00:00 (midnight) in older individuals.

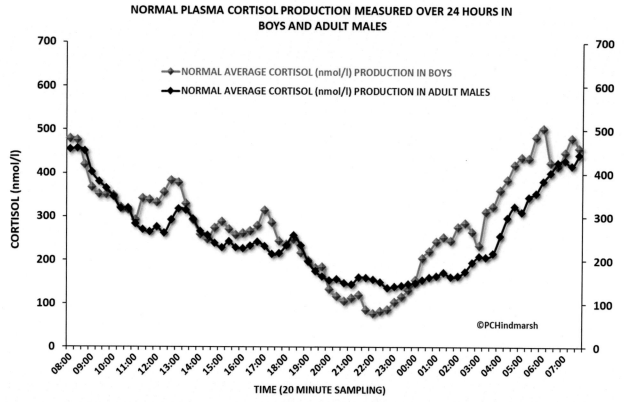

Figure 4.3 *Average 24 hour plasma cortisol concentrations constructed from carefully conducted clinical studies in boys and adult males, by sampling at 20 minute intervals showing differences in timing of the cortisol nadir.*

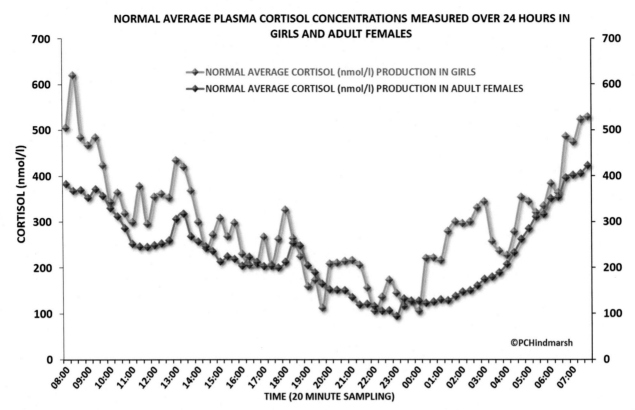

Figure 4.4 *Average 24 hour plasma cortisol concentrations constructed from carefully conducted clinical studies in girls and adult females, by sampling at 20 minute intervals showing differences in timing of the cortisol nadir.*

Other factors which influence the plasma cortisol concentration, largely reflect changes in the amount of cortisol binding globulin (CBG). The cortisol measured in the circulation represents total cortisol, or the plasma total cortisol concentration.

The total concentration is the sum of the cortisol which is bound to the transport proteins particularly CBG and the cortisol which is free in the circulation, not bound to the proteins. There are several diseases which alter CBG, particularly liver disease and the loss of protein through the kidney in conditions such as nephrotic syndrome. Drugs can also alter cortisol binding globulin concentrations, particularly the estrogen component of the oral contraceptive pill which increases CBG concentrations, so the total cortisol concentration measured is higher than might be expected. A similar situation occurs in pregnancy.

Pre-analytic variation

Pre-analytic variation refers to factors influencing cortisol before the sample is received and processed in the laboratory. Pre-analytic variation encompasses biological variation and we tend to use the term to refer to factors which might influence the sample on its way to the laboratory.

As previously mentioned, other medication can impact on the result obtained and it is always important for patients to tell their endocrinologist what medications they are receiving and likewise for the endocrinologist to ask the patient if they are taking any additional medications.

It is not just medications which can alter cortisol concentrations. Liquorice, when taken in large quantities, is known to impair the function of 11beta-hydroxysteroid dehydrogenase type 2, reducing the conversion of cortisol to cortisone and leading to higher circulating amounts of cortisol.

The way in which samples are taken is also important. Many people become anxious and stressed with the idea of an upcoming blood test and if the blood test is difficult and painful, then this can be associated with a rise in cortisol in the circulation. To overcome this problem, we always like to insert a plastic cannula in a vein with as much time as possible before we start to take samples, a minimum period would be 1 to 2 hours, although when we have undertaken our detailed studies which defined normal cortisol production, the cannula was inserted the night before the study commenced. It is not just when we check normal cortisol production but also when we do profiles in patients who have primary adrenal insufficiency. Here, the ACTH stress response is maintained although the patient does not produce extra cortisol. Adrenocorticotropin will rise if cannulation is painful and this rise in ACTH in CAH results in an increase in 17OHP, which is why we do a crossover in time with the samples. We try as diligently as possible to take the sample and give doses at the same time and we can see the amounts of cortisol attained from the hydrocortisone, is very similar and often equal. Figure 4.5 shows this cannulation effect in someone on a continuous subcutaneous hydrocortisone infusion pump using the Peter Hindmarsh formula. Here we know exactly what we are delivering hour by hour, so comparing the first morning with the second morning, shows that the high 17OHP on the first morning reflected stress, as on the second morning it had normalised.

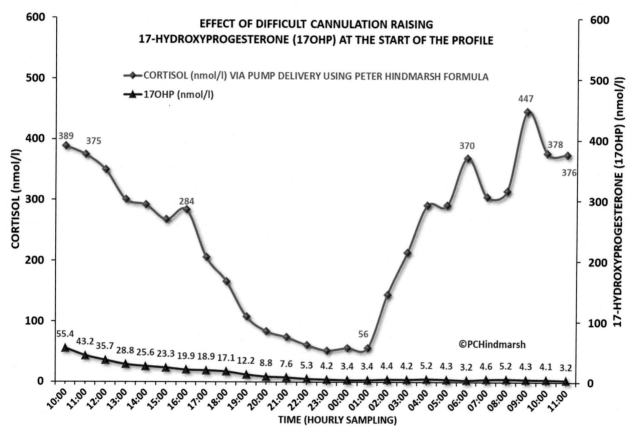

Figure 4.5 *The effect of a difficult cannula insertion on the 17-hydroxyprogesterone (17OHP) level in a patient on a continuous subcutaneous hydrocortisone infusion pump delivering known amounts of hydrocortisone. The pump rates were calculated using the Professor Peter Hindmarsh formula. 17-hydroxyprogesterone is high at the start of the profile and declines compared to the following morning when cortisol is similar, and the 17OHP is within the normal range.*

The time between samples (sampling interval) is also very important. We consider this further in this chapter as well as in Chapters 6, 9 and 10. When measuring natural cortisol production, (i.e. not measuring cortisol replacement from hydrocortisone), the sampling interval should always be less than the half-life of the hormone of interest, so for cortisol with an average half-life of 80 minutes, sampling every hour would ensure that most peak and trough values were properly captured. If the sampling interval is longer than the half-life, then the true peaks and troughs will be underestimated and if the gap is too long, then the rhythm will be lost. Because cortisol is secreted into the bloodstream, half-life or clearance is the most important factor influencing the plasma cortisol concentration, so sampling times within the half-life are important. The situation is different when we come to sample for cortisol during a 24 hour profile to check on oral replacement therapy with hydrocortisone, due to the variance of the half-life of hydrocortisone in individuals (Chapter 6, Figure 6.5). In this situation, half-life or clearance is still important, but now we have to also consider absorption, again absorption is variable (Chapter 6, Figure 6.13). We continue to sample hourly and add in an extra sample 30 minutes after the dose of hydrocortisone has been given. Once we have done a profile in a person, undertaking 30 minute sampling post doses, the results guide us to whether they are a fast, normal or slow absorber. If the data indicates a slow absorption and the peak may occur after the hour sample, we adjust the sampling time and the extra sample should be taken 90 minutes after a dose is taken, (30 minutes after the 60 minute sample). There is an exception with the late night dosing, where we still do a 30 minute sample post dose, but in the majority of patients the peak occurs much later and we then adjust the sampling where necessary.

Blood samples should always be sent to the laboratory as soon as possible after they have been obtained. Cortisol is a relatively robust hormone, unlike ACTH or plasma renin activity which have to be sent on ice to the laboratory immediately they are obtained. All steroids and proteins will degrade if left for long periods of time, particularly over 24 hours and especially if they are left standing in bright sunlight and heat.

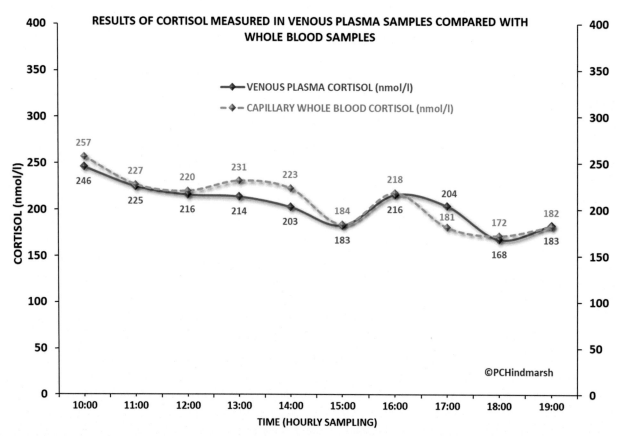

Figure 4.6 *Venous plasma (blue line) and capillary whole blood (light blue dashed line) cortisol concentrations measured at the same time in a short cortisol profile.*

Finally, how the laboratory processes the sample also matters. Cortisol can be measured in blood or serum or plasma and the samples can be drawn from veins or by finger pricks. The differences in concentration between these 3 forms of blood sample will in theory vary slightly. Figure 4.6 shows a short profile of venous plasma and capillary whole blood plasma cortisol measurements. There is actually very little difference between the two and where there are differences it probably reflects the effect of finger squeezing for the capillary sample. This is unlike the situation with glucose for instance, where plasma glucose is about 11% higher than that measured in whole blood.

Analytical variation

We have previously mentioned there is variation in the same sample measured repeatedly. This occurs whether the sample is measured repeatedly in the same assay run, or if the same sample is measured in the same assay but on different days. The former is known as the within assay variation, whereas the latter is known as the between assay variation. This is particularly important when we are assessing 24 hour cortisol profiles. The between assay variation is always slightly greater than the within assay variation. This means when we undertake a 24 hour profile, we have the samples all measured in the same assay run. It does mean if we repeat our profile say one year later, it will clearly not be assayed in the same assay run that the profile was one year previously. We do need to take into account the possible effect of between assay variation in this situation, although the actual variation is usually less than 5%.

Figure 4.7 shows two 24 hour cortisol profiles, (Profile 1 and Profile 2) separated in time by two years from someone on a continuous subcutaneous hydrocortisone infusion pump using the Peter Hindmarsh formula. We know using this system, the amount of cortisol delivered is individually calculated and the infusion rate changes are programmed to deliver these specific amounts of cortisol to mimic the circadian rhythm on an hour to hour basis. This means we know exactly what plasma cortisol concentration will result at any time. We can see the 24 hour cortisol profile is nearly identical over the period of 2 years. In Profile 1 we start at 09:00 (9 am) with a value of 398 nmol/l and the following morning on the second day at 09:00 (9 am), the value is 419 nmol/l. In Profile 2, two years later, we start the sampling slightly later at 10:00 (10 am) with a value of 401 nmol/l and the following morning on the second day at 10:00 (10 am), the value is 406 nmol/l. The rise from the nadir was slightly earlier on the second occasion. All these values are within the 5% variation expected within and between cortisol assays. This would suggest that overall between assay variation matters very little in our interpretation of the data. The actual variation between the assays is probably a lot less than the variation which can take place in 24 hour profiles with respect to food intake, drug administration and sample timing.

There remains for us to consider biochemical problems which can interfere with assay performance. These fall into two broad categories:

1. Interference with the assay.

2. Cross-reactivity with substances which have a similar structure.

In the cortisol assay there are few agents which will interfere with the actual measurement of cortisol. The factors which really influence how the assay works are more related to factors influencing CBG. However, with greater use of immunoglobulin therapies for various medical conditions, upsets to immunoassays can occur. Immunoglobulin therapy upsets these reactions as they are globulins, which is what the antibodies are. They will then participate in the reaction because they are present in high amounts leading to false assay results. In addition, there is the problem of heterophile antibodies. These are antibodies produced against poorly defined antigens or foreign proteins. These are generally weak antibodies and can interfere with immunoassays. The assays for luteinising hormone and follicle-stimulating hormone were particularly prone to this problem.

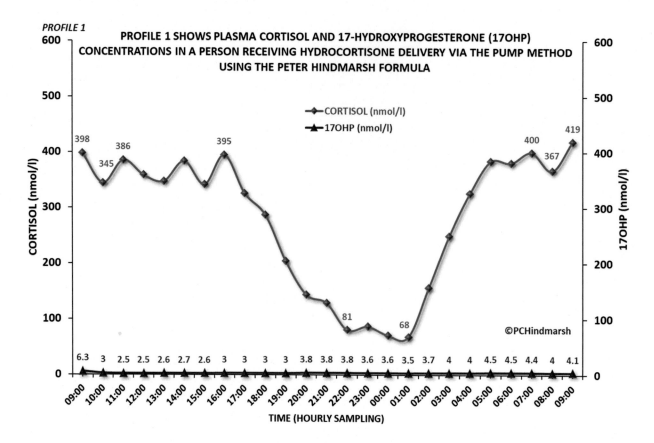

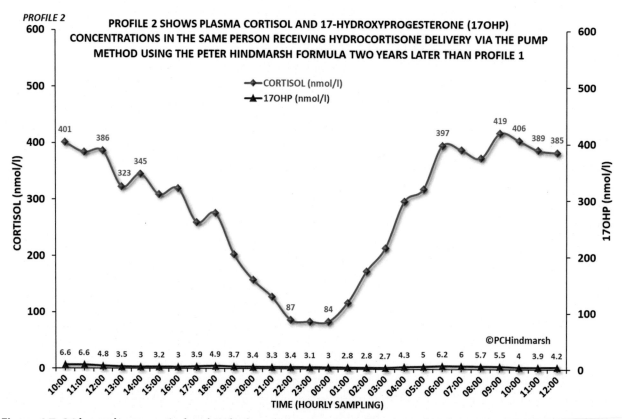

Figure 4.7 *24 hour plasma cortisol and 17-hydroxyprogesterone profiles created with one hourly samples in a patient with congenital adrenal hyperplasia on a continuous subcutaneous hydrocortisone infusion pump using the Peter Hindmarsh formula obtained on two occasions 2 years apart (Profile 1 and 2).*

Cross-reactivity is a problem in all immunoassays and the immunoassays for steroids are particularly prone to this problem. Figure 4.8 shows the structure of cortisol and prednisolone along with 17OHP. If you look at cortisol and prednisolone, there is not much difference structurally between the two. The antibodies which are used in the measurement system for steroids are not quite as specific as those for proteins such as growth hormone. As a result, in the immunoassay system it is quite possible the antibody used will recognise not only what you want it to do in this case, cortisol, but also prednisolone. In fact, in many of the assays there is cross-reactivity in the cortisol assay of prednisolone often up to 60%. This means if a person has no adrenal glands and is taking prednisolone and a blood sample is taken for the measurement of cortisol, it will appear that cortisol is present because the cortisol assay is tricked into believing that cortisol is present because of the look of the prednisolone molecule. This does not mean that these assays measure prednisolone accurately, they don't. Prednisolone needs a specific assay and is not commercially available.

If we now look at the structure of cortisol and 17OHP in Figure 4.8, we might think it would be difficult for 17OHP to cross-react in the cortisol assay. Generally, this is the case. The exception would be if 17OHP concentrations were extremely high (in CAH) when they might alter the cortisol result by this cross-reaction. The problem is not simply with 17OHP but also its metabolite 21-deoxycortisol.

STRUCTURE OF SOME COMMON STEROIDS

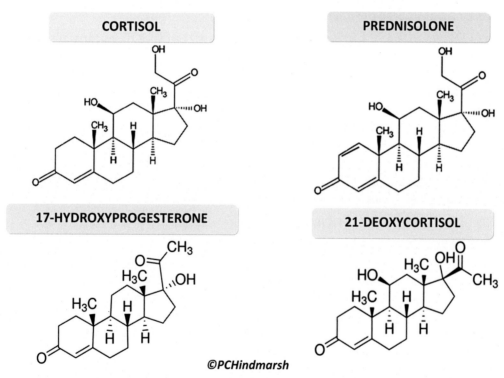

©PCHindmarsh

Figure 4.8 *The chemical structures of cortisol, prednisolone, 17-hydroxyprogesterone and 21-deoxycortisol. 17-hydroxyprogesterone differs from both cortisol and prednisolone whereas its metabolite 21-deoxycortisol is more similar to cortisol.*

Fortunately, cortisol is less susceptible to these cross-reactivities problems than many of the steroids we are interested in for adrenal insufficiency. Standard assays for androstenedione are notoriously unreliable in the newborn because of cross-reactivity with the adrenal androgens produced by the fetal adrenal, which are structurally similar in appearance to androstenedione and will be measurable very easily because of their very high circulating concentration in the newborn baby. Awareness of these assay issues is key for clinicians interpreting all assay results.

TESTS TO ESTABLISH ADRENAL INSUFFICIENCY

The presentation of adrenal insufficiency depends on the degree of adrenal function and the underlying cause. Congenital adrenal hyperplasia most commonly presents in the female at birth with virilisation of the external genitalia. In males with salt-wasting CAH, the diagnosis may not be made until the baby presents with a salt-wasting crisis. In addition, we need to be clear that the presentation with an adrenal crisis due to secondary adrenal insufficiency (ACTH deficiency) is due to lack of glucocorticoids only. This is in contrast to the crisis which results from primary adrenal insufficiency where both cortisol and aldosterone are missing. Secondary adrenal insufficiency generally does not have associated potassium problems. Plasma sodium concentrations may be low, however, because in the presence of cortisol deficiency the kidney is less able to excrete water which leads to a dilution of sodium in the blood and a low plasma sodium concentration.

This is in contrast to primary adrenal insufficiency where the lack of aldosterone leads to sodium loss and water loss through the kidney with dehydration. The loss of sodium in the urine in primary adrenal insufficiency is associated with a rise in the plasma potassium concentration.

BIOCHEMISTRY OF PRIMARY AND SECONDARY ADRENAL INSUFFICIENCY

a). PRIMARY ADRENAL INSUFFICIENCY

1. **High ACTH** due to lack of cortisol feedback and pituitary trying to drive cortisol synthesis.
2. **Low cortisol.**
3. Low blood glucose due to loss of cortisol.
4. Low plasma sodium concentration due to loss of aldosterone production leading to sodium loss in urine and gut.
5. Loss of body water with sodium leading to dehydration with raised plasma urea.
6. High plasma potassium concentration due to loss of aldosterone which exchanges sodium for potassium in the kidney.
7. **Low plasma aldosterone.**
8. **High plasma renin activity** due to lack of aldosterone feedback.

b). SECONDARY ADRENAL INSUFFICIENCY

1. **Low ACTH** due to lack of ACTH production from the pituitary.
2. **Low cortisol** due to lack of ACTH.
3. Low blood glucose due to loss of cortisol and possibly growth hormone.
4. Low plasma sodium concentration due to inability to excrete water, due to cortisol deficiency.
5. Increased body water with low plasma urea.
6. Normal plasma potassium concentration as aldosterone pathway is not affected.
7. **Low Normal plasma aldosterone** due to low normal plasma renin activity.
8. **Low Normal plasma renin activity** due to water retention and increased blood volume.

©PCHindmarsh

Figure 4.9 *Key biochemical features in (a) primary adrenal insufficiency and (b) secondary adrenal insufficiency. Main contrasting features shown in bold.*

Figure 4.9 shows the biochemical characteristics of primary and secondary adrenal insufficiency. A single blood sample may be enough in diagnosing adrenal insufficiency and the time to measure these analytes is at presentation of the individual, usually in Accident and Emergency. If these critical samples are not available, then the conventional approach to assessing adrenal insufficiency is to determine whether the person is able to respond to an appropriate stimulus by increasing cortisol secretion. As the cause of the adrenal insufficiency may be primary or secondary, it may be necessary to test the whole axis.

In this section we are going to consider blood tests which can be used to establish adrenal insufficiency, but before doing so we will consider options for measurements of cortisol in urine and saliva.

URINE AND SALIVARY MEASUREMENTS IN IDENTIFYING ADRENAL INSUFFICIENCY

Virtually all the steroid hormones are metabolised in the liver and excreted in solution in the urine. In the urine there are specific patterns of the metabolites for the steroid hormones which we see in the adrenal pathway. The advantage of doing the test on urine is we can get very large volumes with which to undertake tests. This is extremely useful for determining the cause of adrenal insufficiency such as CAH, but perhaps less so for identifying adrenal insufficiency per se, as the amount of cortisol metabolites will be low and may overlap with the lower end of the normal range. A global reduction in adrenal corticosteroids may be indicative of adrenal insufficiency, but further blood testing will be required.

Another way is to measure the actual amount of cortisol which is present in the urine and this is known as the urinary free cortisol test. This is undertaken by collecting urine over a 24 hour period and measuring the amount of cortisol in the sample. The cortisol that appears in the urine, reflects the plasma free cortisol concentration. Because of the dynamics between cortisol and CBG, the 24 hour urinary free cortisol test is not very helpful when cortisol concentrations are low. For the urinary free cortisol test to be of value, cortisol concentrations have to be high enough to saturate the CBG, so enough cortisol can spill out in the urine to be measured. As a result of this, the 24 hour urinary free cortisol test is very good for detecting high cortisol concentrations in conditions such as Cushing disease (over production of cortisol), but lacks the sensitivity and specificity for establishing whether cortisol production is low or not. The same is true for salivary cortisol/cortisone measurements, which again rely on the amount of free cortisol/cortisone available for processing through the salivary glands.

STIMULATION TESTS MEASURING CORTISOL SYNTHESIS AND RELEASE

The two stimulation tests which are commonly used are the short synacthen test (SST) or the insulin induced hypoglycaemia test of pituitary function (IIHT). In cases of suspected secondary adrenal insufficiency, the full pathway must be tested by the IIHT, along with assessment of the other anterior pituitary hormones by measuring the growth hormone response in the IIHT, as well as the plasma concentrations of luteinising hormone, follicle-stimulating hormone, prolactin and thyroid-stimulating hormone and free thyroxine (see Chapter 5). The reason for this is that isolated ACTH deficiency is rare, unless secondary to exogenous glucocorticoid administration (see Chapter 15). Consideration should also be given to evaluating posterior pituitary function with measurements of paired plasma and urine osmolalities in the first instance.

Synacthen stimulation test

The cortisol response to hypoglycaemia in the IIHT is a good test of adrenal function and is the only test of adrenal function validated against the response to surgical stress. It does test the integrity of the entire hypothalamo-pituitary-adrenal axis.

In contrast, the synacthen test (SST) which uses synthetic ACTH, assesses the response of the adrenal glands to the exogenous ACTH stimulus. It is therefore, a test of adrenal and by inference pituitary function. The premise is that if the adrenal glands are intact and exposed to regular stimulation with ACTH, then normal amounts of cortisol will be synthesised and released. The SST is useful in cases of suspected adrenal insufficiency. It is also useful in CAH, both when the patient is suspected of having the condition and also in determining whether the individual is an unaffected carrier of the gene for CAH. We do the latter test as it helps when we define the carrier status by genetic analysis. Additional adrenal steroids can be measured during the test such as 17OHP.

The test entails stimulation of the adrenal glands by doses of exogenous ACTH (1 − 24) (synacthen), administered either intravenously or intramuscularly which then results in a massive output of cortisol and other adrenal steroids.

The ACTH is made synthetically and is not the full 39 amino acid molecule. Removing the amino acid section 25 − 39, makes the synthetic product less likely to produce an allergic reaction because that section appears to cause the allergic reaction in carefully conducted studies of different sizes of synthetic ACTH.

It is important to realise the dose utilised represents an entire day's output of ACTH and is an excessive stimulus which is only of value in assessing severe adrenal insufficiency. The SST may be insensitive to minor degrees of adrenal suppression, for example, in children with asthma on inhaled steroids. The 30 minute sample obtained after administration of the exogenous ACTH has been standardised against the IIHT.

The dosing schedule is shown in Figure 4.10 along with a comparison of the estimated peak ACTH obtained with various doses of synacthen. Only the lowest synacthen dose of 500 ng/m^2 has an estimated plasma ACTH concentration in adults approaching that encountered at 08:00 (8 am).

The other doses are probably testing more of the stress response of the adrenal cortex and a prolonged stress stimulation at that. After a 500 ng/m^2 dose, normal ACTH levels would be attained 4 - 8 minutes after the injection, whereas with the 250 μg dose normal values would not occur until 40 - 45 minutes later.

SYNACTHEN DOSES

Table A

AGE	DOSE OF SYNACTHEN
< 6 months	62.5 micrograms
6 – 24 months	125 micrograms
> 2 years	250 micrograms

Table B

SYNACTHEN DOSE	PLASMA ACTH (μg/l)	
	NEONATE	ADULT
250μg	1000	50
1μg	4.0	0.2
500ng/m^2	0.6	0.1

©PCHindmarsh

Figure 4.10 *Doses of synacthen used in the standard synacthen test at different ages (Table A) which deliver high estimated plasma ACTH concentrations in both neonates and adults (Table B). For reference 08:00 (8 am) plasma ACTH concentration would be 0.05 μg/l. Only the 500 ng/m^2 synacthen dose approaches this value in adults.*

A cannula is usually inserted at least one hour prior to the test being performed. The test should be performed at 09:00 (9 am) ideally and fasting is not required. In some versions of the low dose synacthen test, the study is undertaken in the early afternoon which brings with it potential problems in what is considered a normal response at that time of day. A point that we will return to further on in this chapter. At time zero, a sample is drawn for the measurement of ACTH and cortisol and if testing for disorders of steroidogenesis, additional samples for the measurement of 17OHP and 11-deoxycortisol can be taken. The synacthen dose is then administered by intravenous or intramuscular bolus injection and a sample obtained at 30 minutes for the measurement of cortisol, 17OHP and 11-deoxycortisol.

It is generally accepted that the peak plasma cortisol concentration following SST should be greater than 500 - 550 nmol/l. This depends on the assay in use by the laboratory and the newer assays read at least 20% below this. An impaired response does not distinguish between adrenal and pituitary failure, since the adrenal glands may be atrophied secondary to ACTH deficiency in the case of the latter. However, measuring ACTH at the same time on the time zero sample, helps distinguish between primary and secondary adrenal insufficiency (Figure 4.11).

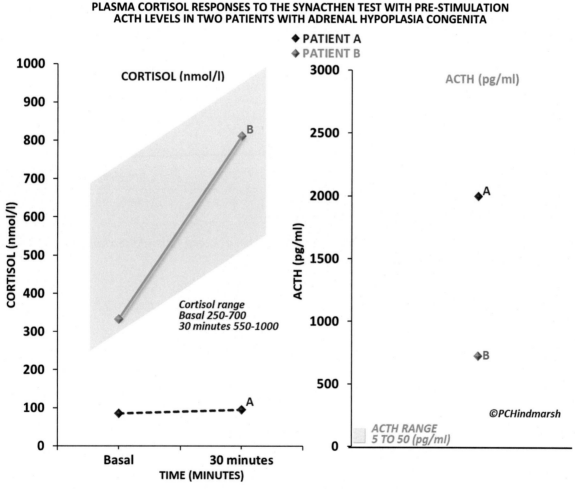

PLASMA CORTISOL RESPONSES TO THE SYNACTHEN TEST WITH PRE-STIMULATION ACTH LEVELS IN TWO PATIENTS WITH ADRENAL HYPOPLASIA CONGENITA

Figure 4.11 *Plasma cortisol response to stimulation with synacthen (left panel) in two patients (A and B) with adrenal insufficiency due to adrenal hypoplasia congenita. Basal plasma ACTH before administration of synacthen is shown in the right panel. The shaded zone indicates the normal range for cortisol during the synacthen test. The yellow panel shows the normal range for ACTH at 08:00 - 09:00 (8 am - 9 am). Patient A (purple) has no cortisol response to synacthen stimulation with a very high basal plasma ACTH concentration. Patient B (green) has a normal cortisol response to synacthen stimulation, but the basal plasma ACTH is also markedly elevated.*

In primary adrenal insufficiency, ACTH concentrations will be high and the time zero plasma cortisol will be low. Note the importance from Figure 4.11 of interpreting the plasma cortisol concentration together with the basal plasma ACTH value.

If only the plasma cortisol response was considered, Patient B would be said to have normal adrenal function but this is at the expense of a high ACTH drive.

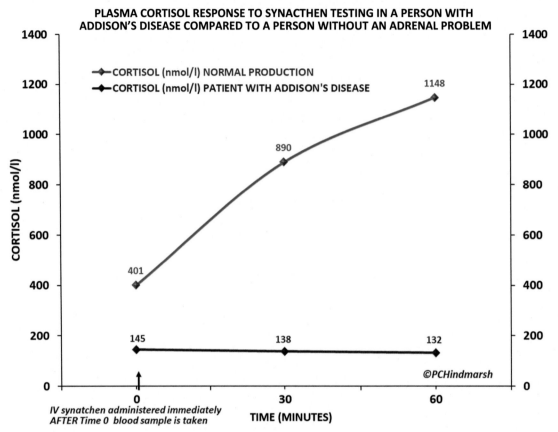

Figure 4.12 *Plasma cortisol response to a standard synacthen test in a patient with Addison's disease (red line) and a person with normal adrenal function (blue line).*

Figure 4.12 shows the responses in a patient with Addison's disease compared to a person with normal adrenal function:

1. Note how the adrenal glands in the individual who has normal adrenal function (blue line) continue to synthesise and release cortisol after 30 minutes in response to the high dose of ACTH administered immediately after the first cortisol measurement (0 minutes) was taken.

2. In contrast, in the individual with secondary adrenal insufficiency due to Addison's disease (red line) the plasma cortisol measurement of 145 nmol/l which was taken immediately before the IV synacthen was administered (0 minutes), was higher than the plasma cortisol concentration taken after 30 minutes (138 nmol/l) and the plasma cortisol concentrations are all lower than in the person with normal adrenal function.

Patients with pituitary dependent cortisol insufficiency will require dynamic testing of the pituitary gland using the IIHT as mentioned in Chapter 5, page 91.

In CAH, the most common cause being 21-hydroxylase deficiency, the plasma cortisol response to stimulation with synacthen may be poor or normal. Figure 4.13 (page 71) illustrates the response to synacthen stimulation in an individual with non-classical CAH (late-onset CAH) (dashed lines) and a person with normal adrenal function (solid lines). Measurements of plasma cortisol (blue lines) and 17-hydroxyprogesterone (purple lines) were taken immediately before IV synacthen was administered (0 minutes) and then again after 30 minutes.

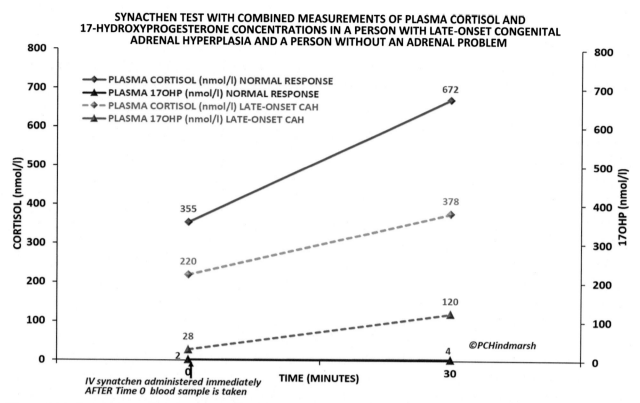

Figure 4.13 *Comparison of response to synacthen in person without adrenal problems (solid lines) and a person with late-onset congenital adrenal hyperplasia (dashed lines). Unstimulated cortisol (blue lines) concentrations are within the normal range but hardly rises in the late-onset patient who also has an elevated 17-hydroxyprogesterone (purple lines) at time zero which becomes exaggerated after synacthen stimulation.*

The synacthen test demonstrates:

1. At time zero the plasma cortisol concentration was greater in the person with normal adrenal function compared to the person with non-classical CAH who also had a raised plasma 17OHP concentration of 28 nmol/l compared to the person with normal adrenal function (2 nmol/l).

2. The magnitude of the plasma cortisol response to synacthen stimulation was greater in the person with normal adrenal function (672 nmol/l) compared to the response in the person with non-classical CAH (378 nmol/l). A normal plasma cortisol response to synacthen stimulation should be over 500 nmol/l.

3. The person with non-classical CAH shows a marked plasma 17OHP response to synacthen stimulation (120 nmol/l) compared to the person with normal adrenal function (4 nmol/l). A normal plasma 17OHP response to synacthen stimulation is characterised by a peak 17OHP response of less than 10 nmol/l whilst in carriers of the 21-hydroxylase gene defect, the peak following synacthen stimulation seen in the plasma 17OHP concentration is between 10 and 20 nmol/l.

Finally, in patients who have been on long term steroid therapy, adrenal function is suppressed and the adrenal glands may not be, or only partially stimulated during the SST.

Modified or physiological synacthen test

It has been argued the SST may not detect subtle degrees of adrenal impairment due to the high dose of synacthen administered. A modified test has been developed by constructing a dose response for ACTH (1 − 24) in terms of the rise in plasma cortisol. A dose of only 500 nanograms of ACTH per 1.73 m^2 body surface area, gave an identical rise in plasma cortisol concentration over the first 20 minutes after intravenous injection, as compared with the standard dose of 250 micrograms. The test needs more frequent cortisol measurements at 5 minute intervals for 45 minutes. Interpretation is similar in that a peak cortisol concentration greater than 500 - 550 nmol/l is considered as adequate. Although a variety of low synacthen doses have been used in the literature as shown in Figure 4.10, the estimated plasma ACTH concentrations achieved even with this lower dose are still high in the newborn, but close to those recorded at 08:00 (8 am) in adults without adrenal problems. One of the difficulties in assessing the performance of these tests has been the variety of cortisol assays used, the small sample sizes often reported and the heterogeneity of doses used, particularly in the low dose test. Further, the results are also altered by anything that alters CBG such as the oral contraceptive pill.

The SST when compared to the IIHT and using a cut-off of 600 nmol/l, had an 85% sensitivity and 96% specificity for the detection of cortisol insufficiency — therefore very similar. For the low dose test using a cut-off of 375 nmol/l, the sensitivity was 100% with a specificity of 20.7% in one study, whereas other reports have placed values closer to 86% sensitivity and 88% specificity in defining cortisol insufficiency.

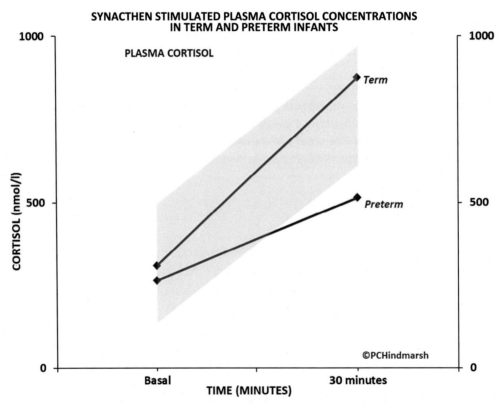

Figure 4.14 *Plasma cortisol responses to synacthen 62.5 micrograms in term (dark blue line) and preterm (red line) infants. Shaded zone shows response in adults and children without adrenal insufficiency.*

One final point is that the adrenal response to synacthen stimulation is lower in the preterm baby compared to term. Term babies have a response to synacthen which is similar to that seen in children and adults. Preterm babies have a lesser response consistent with lower production of cortisol in this group (Figure 4.14).

All these tests need to be undertaken at a certain time of day. This is very important because the cortisol response to stimulation with synacthen varies throughout the 24 hour period. Figure 4.15 shows the effect of stimulation with the same dose of synacthen (100 mcg) administered at 07:00 (7 am), 14:00 (2 pm) and 21:00 (9 pm). The increment in plasma cortisol from the time zero sample, is used to illustrate the differences between the increase in cortisol concentrations after the same dose of synacthen (100 mcg) was administered, at the given time points.

The difference in cortisol concentrations from the same dose at these times is due to the natural circadian rhythm of cortisol.

The greatest increment of 620 nmol/l was seen when the test was undertaken at 07:00 (7 am) which is generally, the time period when ACTH and cortisol are at their highest values. The responses at 14:00 (2 pm) and 21:00 (9 pm) are good and classified as normal at between 500 and 550 nmol/l but are a lot less than observed at 07:00 (7 am).

These observations point to the need for uniformity in the time of undertaking these particular tests, as the response will differ at different times during the day.

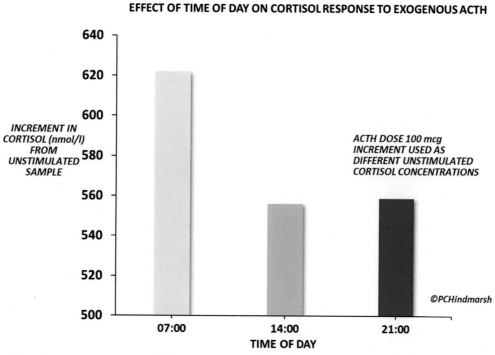

Figure 4.15 *Effect of time of day 07:00 (7 am), 14:00 (2 pm) and 21:00 (9 pm) on the increment in the plasma cortisol response to stimulation with synacthen (100 mcg). The plasma cortisol increment is used in this instance due to the differences in unstimulated plasma cortisol at the start of the test.*

Insulin induced hypoglycaemia test for growth hormone and cortisol secretion

The response to insulin induced hypoglycaemia is widely recognised as the standard test for the assessment of growth hormone and cortisol status. The IIHT consists of the administration of insulin to reduce blood glucose, which in itself acts as a stimulus to the release of growth hormone and cortisol. In Chapter 2, Figure 2.9, we showed that cortisol and growth hormone begin to be secreted as counterregulatory hormones to raise a falling plasma glucose. The threshold for this effect is when the plasma glucose concentration reaches 3.3 mmol/l and is maximal when a plasma glucose concentration of 2.6 mmol/l is attained.

An advantage of using the IIHT is that a known stimulus is applied (a reduction in blood glucose) and a clearly defined response to the stimulus is achieved. From the growth hormone and cortisol responses appropriate conclusions can be drawn.

Measuring growth hormone at all ages is important because in addition to promoting growth in children, it is involved in increasing muscle mass, muscle strength, bone mineral density as well as reducing cholesterol and fat mass in adults.

The test needs to be done over 3 hours and the peak cortisol response is not until 60 – 90 minutes after hypoglycaemia has been achieved (Figure 4.16). This reflects the lag in the system from achieving hypoglycaemia to the brain detecting this level, then acting to release ACTH and ultimately via ACTH, cortisol.

The drawback of the IHHT, is it can be potentially dangerous because we are inducing hypoglycaemia and the test should not be undertaken in individuals with a history of heart problems, epilepsy or in children.

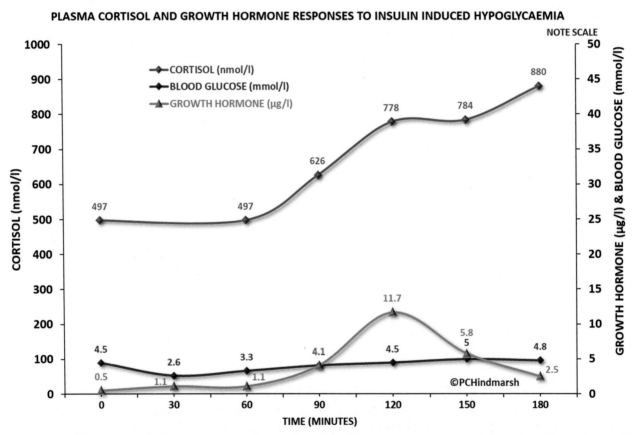

Figure 4.16 *Plasma growth hormone (orange line) and cortisol (blue line) responses to insulin induced hypoglycaemia (red line). Growth hormone displays a normal response greater than 7 µg/l and cortisol has a rise over 500 - 550 nmol/l. Hypoglycaemia at 2.6 mmol/l was attained at 30 minutes with maximum growth hormone and cortisol responses 90 and 150 minutes later respectively.*

Results can only be interpreted if hypoglycaemia has been achieved. The advantage of the test is that information is provided not only on ACTH production (inferred from the measurement of plasma cortisol), but also growth hormone. The test can be combined with assessments of the other pituitary hormones and this is useful in the assessment of secondary adrenal insufficiency where multiple pituitary hormones may be absent. This is reviewed further in Chapter 5.

With respect to cortisol, the plasma cortisol concentration should increase at least twofold from the basal value and a peak of 500 – 550 nmol/l or more should be achieved. This is usually measured in the 90 to 150 minute samples. Further testing of whether the problem lies at the pituitary or hypothalamic level can be undertaken with the corticotropin-releasing hormone test, but this is rarely undertaken in clinical practice.

24 HOUR PLASMA CORTISOL PROFILES

24 hour plasma cortisol profiles present another way of assessing cortisol sufficiency or insufficiency. As a result, the 24 hour mean plasma cortisol concentration can be estimated and the lower limit of the normal range is 180 nmol/l. The 24 hour profile answers a different question to those provided by the synacthen test responses. The synacthen test shows what the adrenal glands can produce when maximumly stimulated, whereas the 24 hour profile provides information on what is happening on a day by day basis in a nonstressed state.

The profile has to be carefully constructed. A cannula needs to be inserted at least 1 to 2 hours before starting, to avoid any stress reaction. Samples then need to be taken hourly. This is essential as the half-life of cortisol is on average 80 to 90 minutes and the rule about sampling interval is it should always be less than the half-life of the drug or hormone that you are interested in measuring. If the length between samples is long or irregular, then inadequate estimation of peak and trough values can happen — a phenomenon known as aliasing. Figure 4.17 shows this in a 24 hour cortisol profile where the timing of samples is hourly or 2 hourly. We should also have sampled every 30 minutes around each dose to give us a better idea of the true peak and how long the previous dose was lasting.

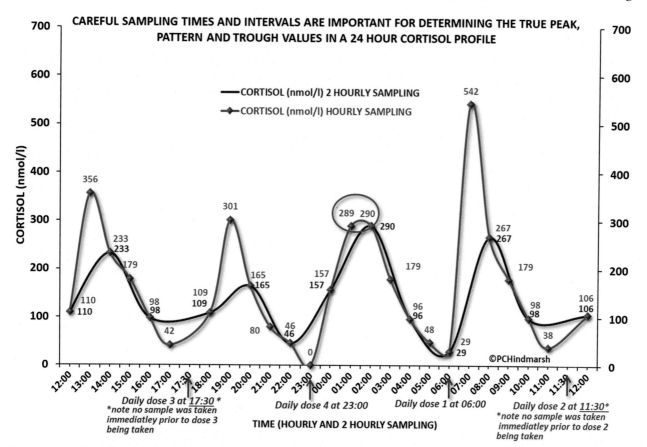

Figure 4.17 *The effect of sampling at irregular intervals on the resulting profile. The red line shows what would result if samples were taken at two hourly and the blue line at one hourly intervals.*

Two hourly sampling:

The two hourly blood sampling misses all the peak and trough values completely. Without the peak values, there is no indication if the dosing schedule is providing too much cortisol and may in fact lead to inaccurate increases in dosing, for example the peak at 07:00 (7 am) is missed. The dose is taken at 06:00 (6 am) with the peak of 542 nmol/l occurring at 07:00 (7 am), in some individuals this peak would occur at 30 minutes, so the difference between the next measurement of 267 nmol/l at 08:00 (8 am) if the peak had occurred at 06:30 (6.30 am), would be even greater. In fact, with two hourly sampling the morning peak value of 267 nmol/l may be considered on the low side and an increase in dose given, when a decrease in the dose may be needed.

The troughs are all missing except for 06:00 (6 am) where the morning dose stacks on the 29 nmol/l remaining from Dose 4. The lowest values are important as these will determine when the optimal time is to stack the next dose on the remaining cortisol and prevent periods without cortisol.

One hourly sampling:

No cortisol measurement was taken immediately prior to Dose 3 which was taken at 17:30 (5.30 pm), the missing pre dose cortisol measurement was probably 0. The 109 nmol/l measurement was taken 30 minutes post dose at 18:00 (6 pm), so the true peak was almost certainly much higher than 301 nmol/l measured after one and half hours post dose at 19:00 (7 pm). These scenarios affect not only the adjustment of doses but also any altering of the dose time which may be needed. To overcome this issue an extra sample should be taken immediately before the 17:30 (5.30 pm) dose is taken, then 30 minutes after at 18:00 (6 pm), followed by an extra sample at 18:30 (6.30 pm). Hourly samples should then resume at 19:00 (7 pm).

At the start of the profile at 12:00 (12 pm) there is already 110 nmol/l of cortisol in the bloodstream and a careful look at the dosing schedule shows Dose 2 was taken at 11:30 (11.30 am) this again leads to the same scenario as seen with the 17:30 (5.30 pm) dose. The cortisol peak from the 11:30 (11.30 am) dose would most likely occur around 12:30 (12.30 pm), so the cortisol peak would be higher than the 356 nmol/l measured at 13:00 (1 pm) which is one and a half hours after the dose is taken. Saying this, it is very important doses are taken at the times they are usually taken at home when undertaking a 24 hour profile, which enables us to get a true picture of what is happening on a daily basis. All medications including the contraceptive pill should also be taken. We discuss this in Chapter 10.

In this example, the profile should be started earlier ensuring samples are taken prior to the dose, with an extra sample at 12:30 (12.30 pm) with hourly sampling resuming at 13:00 (1 pm). Note there is a variation between the amount of time it takes for individuals to reach peak concentrations, some patients will reach the peak concentration around 30 minutes, which is why it is important to take 30 minute sampling after a dose has been given.

In most profiles we see the last dose of the day, dose 4, takes longer to peak and may last longer in the bloodstream. Even with the hourly sampling we can see we have missed the peak value which occurred between 01:00 (1 am) and 02:00 (2 am), (circled in blue) which is evident as the cortisol values are very similar. We cover this in Chapter 9.

Figure 4.18 Charts A & B shows the effect of different sampling times.

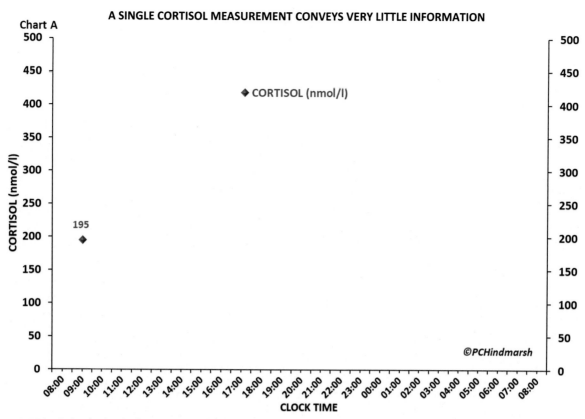

Figure 4.18A *A single cortisol measurement at 09:00 (9 am) leaves little understanding of what has gone previously or what happens for the rest of the day.*

In Chart A we have one plasma cortisol measurement taken at 09:00 (9 am). The value is 195 nmol/l. How do we interpret this? We could look at the normal range at this time quoted by the assay at 09:00 (9 am) as 133 – 537 nmol/l which is quite a variance in range, so this is termed in range!

Is it at the lower end, do we need to increase the dose?

What was the peak value as this measurement is from a dose taken earlier?

When does it run out?

Are there periods during the rest of the day where there is no cortisol?

Are the cortisol levels for the rest of the day optimal?

Is the patient being over or under treated?

What dose needs adjusting?

Lots of questions but essential that we answer them if we are to get the treatment right.

In Chart B we have two measures one at 09:00 (9 am) and the other at 00:00 (midnight) This is often done to diagnose Cushing's syndrome where we are looking at loss of the circadian rhythm. Probably this is acceptable for that diagnosis where the 00:00 (midnight) is high. If it were 100 nmol/l and the 09:00 (9 am) 195 nmol/l, then we might wonder if the person is low throughout the 24 hour period, but we are no closer in defining adrenal insufficiency. This illustrates the importance of sampling at the correct times/intervals which is based in part on the diagnosis being considered.

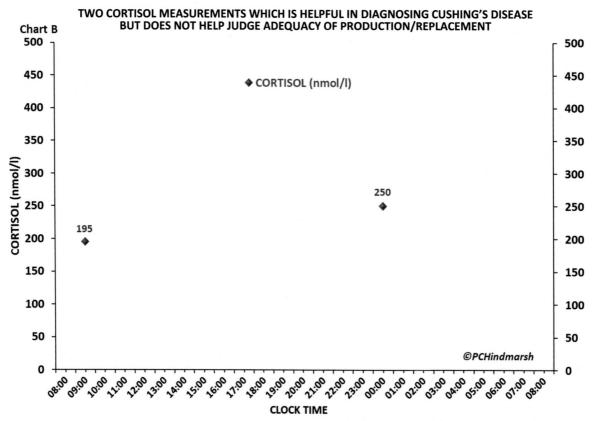

Figure 4.18B *Chart B illustrates two cortisol measurements with a sample taken at 09:00 (9 am) and 00:00 (midnight) which is standard practice to diagnose Cushing's syndrome. This is appropriate for that condition, but these measurements do not add much more information in terms of assessing cortisol production over the 24 hour period.*

Looking at Figure 4.19 we can see the effects of more frequent sampling at 20 minute, 1 and 2 hourly intervals. The 20 minute sampling comes from a research study. The 2 hourly study misses the peaks present in the 20 minute data set, whilst the 1 hourly samples captures more information but still misses the peaks and to overcome this, we do an extra 30 minute sample after each dose as illustrated in Chapter 10. When we look at this over a 24 hour period, then the 2 hourly sampling underestimates the daily cortisol by about 17%. These observations are pertinent not just for diagnostic profiles, but also when we come to assess adequacy of replacement treatment with hydrocortisone.

A suggested modification of the 24 hour profile is to measure plasma cortisol between 07:00 (7 am) and 09:00 (9 am) on the basis that this will capture the peak. This is probably true although in some individuals the peak will occur earlier at 06:00 (6 am). It also does not tell us what happens for the rest of the day. When we look at our normative profiles, the data demonstrate the best time to sample in the morning is between 07:00 (7 am) and 08:40 (8.40 am) when concentrations are very similar and average above 400 nmol/l. In fact, none of the 80 patients studied in this series had a plasma cortisol concentration between 07:00 (7 am) and 08:40 (8.40 am) below 270 nmol/l, so this can be used as a cut-off for this time of the day (Figure 4.20).

This is in a similar range to reported test performance, where a morning plasma cortisol concentration over 235 nmol/l has an 84% sensitivity and 71% specificity to exclude cortisol insufficiency and the specificity can be increased to 95% if a cut-off point of 375 nmol/l is used.

The caveat with all these studies is that the cut-offs may vary depending on the cortisol assay used.

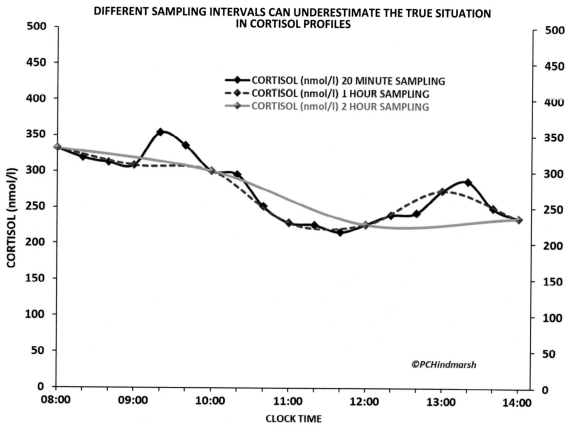

Figure 4.19 *The effect of different sampling intervals on the data obtained. 20 minute sampling (dark blue line) defines actually what is happening. 1 hourly (blue dashed line) sampling approximates this, but 2 hourly (light blue line) sampling leads to less well defined peaks in particular.*

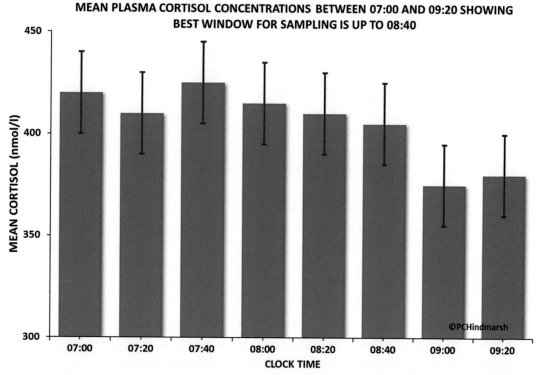

Figure 4.20 *Mean plasma cortisol concentrations at time points between 07:00 (7 am) and 09:20 (9.20 am) in 80 subjects. Bars indicate 1 standard deviation. Note shortened cortisol axis. Mean values are similar between 07:00 (7 am) and 08:40 (8.40 am) with no value recorded less than 270 nmol/l and a working range down to 350 nmol/l.*

TESTING THE MINERALOCORTICOID AXIS

This chapter has focused on the diagnosis of glucocorticoid deficiency associated with adrenal insufficiency. When considering the mineralocorticoid axis, we need to recall the regulatory pathway between the adrenal glands and the kidneys. This is illustrated in Figure 4.21.

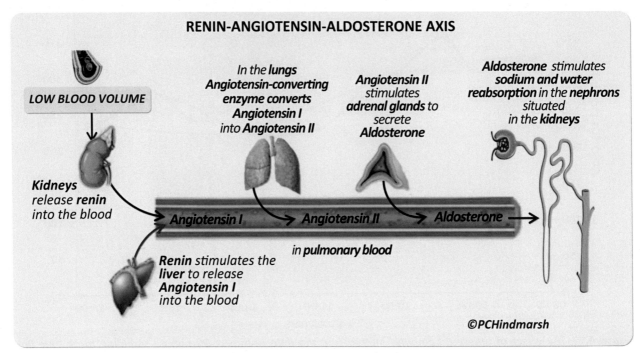

RENIN-ANGIOTENSIN-ALDOSTERONE AXIS

LOW BLOOD VOLUME

In the **lungs** **Angiotensin-converting enzyme converts Angiotensin I** into **Angiotensin II**

Angiotensin II stimulates **adrenal glands to** secrete **Aldosterone**

Aldosterone stimulates **sodium and water reabsorption** in the **nephrons** situated in the **kidneys**

Kidneys release **renin** into the blood

Renin stimulates the **liver** to release **Angiotensin I** into the blood

Angiotensin I   Angiotensin II   Aldosterone

in **pulmonary blood**

©PCHindmarsh

Figure 4.21 *The renin-angiotensin-aldosterone pathway for regulation of salt balance, blood volume and blood pressure.*

The main function of the kidneys is to remove salt and other water soluble waste which the body does not need, by making urine which is then excreted out of the body. The kidneys are also important in maintaining blood volume and blood pressure.

Sodium chloride is the most abundant salt in the body and has many important roles in keeping the body healthy. The hormone which regulates the amount of sodium retained by the body is aldosterone.

Aldosterone is responsible for how much sodium the kidneys retain and how much is passed out in the urine. As sodium retains water, it is very important to have the sodium level correct so the body can retain the correct amount of water and therefore maintain the correct blood volume and blood pressure.

The kidneys are key to the aldosterone feedback system. Any change, particularly in blood pressure, leads to an alteration in renin production which instructs the liver to make angiotensin I from angiotensinogen. Angiotensin I is then converted in the lungs to angiotensin II, which acts on the adrenal glands to regulate the production of aldosterone.

In the diagnosis of adrenal insufficiency, we need to measure the plasma sodium and potassium concentrations along with the plasma renin or renin activity, coupled with the plasma aldosterone concentration. If plasma aldosterone concentrations are low, then plasma renin or renin activity would be very high and this would indicate there is reduced production of aldosterone and the plasma sodium concentration tells us how much sodium loss is occurring.

Another clue the renin-angiotensin-aldosterone system may be involved in adrenal insufficiency is before the sodium plasma concentration starts to fall to low levels, the plasma potassium concentration starts to rise.

In a form of CAH known as simple virilising CAH, the plasma renin or renin activity may be normal, or at least at the top end of the normal range and the plasma sodium concentration normal. In this situation if the individual is placed in an environment which causes increasing sodium loss, for example, a very hot climate where they sweat a lot, or if they are challenged with a very low sodium diet, then the plasma renin or renin activity will rise quite quickly, plasma sodium may fall but more importantly the plasma aldosterone concentration does not rise in response to the increase of the plasma renin or renin activity. If this were to continue unchecked, then a salt-wasting crisis might follow.

When travelling to very hot countries where daily temperatures are 35°C or higher, increased salt intake is recommended.

In primary adrenal insufficiency when an adrenal crisis occurs, the plasma sodium falls and plasma potassium rises due to the lack of aldosterone action on the kidney. The lack of aldosterone results in a whole body potassium surplus. This is exacerbated by low blood glucose which switches off insulin production and this also leads to a higher plasma potassium because insulin plays an important role in driving potassium from the plasma into the cells. This surplus can be accommodated for a while due to the loss of sodium from cells, but a point is reached where this is exceeded and plasma potassium concentrations rise steeply and quickly (Figure 4.22).

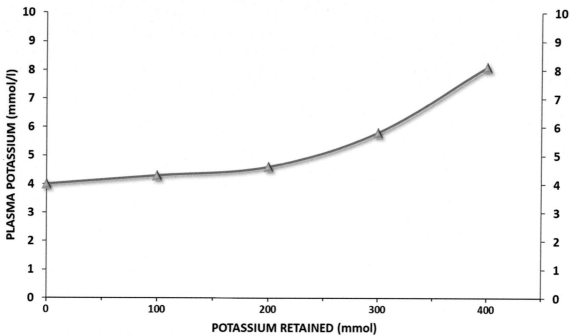

Figure 4.22 *Relationship between potassium retention and plasma potassium concentration showing that once the cellular retention capacity at 250 - 300 mmol is exceeded a rapid increase in plasma potassium takes place. (Redrawn from Lin, S.H., Hsu, Y.J., Chu, J.S., Chu, S.J., Davids, M.R., Halperin M.L., 2003. Osmotic demyelination syndrome: a potentially avoidable disaster. QJM 98, 935—947 with kind permission of the Quarterly Journal of Medicine).*

HYPOTHALAMO-PITUITARY-ADRENAL AXIS

TEST	ROLE	ADVANTAGE	DISADVANTAGE
PLASMA ACTH AND CORTISOL	*Critical samples at presentation to define primary and secondary adrenal insufficiency.*	*Single blood sample before any intervention. Easy to interpret.*	*Needs to be done before any hydrocortisone given. ACTH sample needs to go straight to laboratory.*
24 HOUR URINE STEROID PROFILE	*To show reduced production of cortisol metabolites.*	*Easy to collect. Can use profile to define blocks in steroidogenesis.*	*Low cortisol metabolites can be hard to discern from low normal values.*
24 HOUR URINE FREE CORTISOL	*To show reduced production of cortisol.*	*Easy to collect.*	*Relies on saturation of cortisol binding globulin. Hard to discriminate between low normal and actual pathological low value.*
SALIVARY CORTISOL AND/OR CORTISONE	*To show reduced production of cortisol.*	*Easy to collect.*	*Relies on saturation of cortisol binding globulin. Hard to discriminate between low normal and actual pathological low value. Sample collection needs to be undertaken with care.*
24 HOUR PLASMA CORTISOL PROFILE	*To show reduced production of cortisol.*	*Shows circadian rhythm. Tells what is happening on day by day basis to cortisol production. Well established normal range. Easy to undertake. Can be combined with ACTH measurements.*	*Currently requires 24 hour stay in hospital with hourly blood samples. Does not show what would happen in stress situation.*
07:00-08:40 PLASMA CORTISOL PROFILE	*To show reduced production of cortisol.*	*Well established normal range. Easy to undertake. Can be combined with ACTH measurements.*	*Only provides short time interval and does not describe cortisol for rest of 24 hours. Does not show what would happen in stress situation.*
INSULIN INDUCED HYPOGLYCAEMIA TEST	*Shows contribution of whole axis for cortisol generation so good for primary and secondary adrenal insufficiency.*	*Well established normal range. Can be combined with ACTH measurements. Calibrated against stress of surgery.*	*Needs care to manage the hypoglycaemia and should not be used in children and those with epilepsy or heart problems.*
SYNACTHEN TESTS	*Shows how much cortisol the adrenal can produce.*	*Well established normal range. Can be combined with ACTH measurements. Easy to undertake.*	*Shows how adrenal responds to stress. If measure cortisol alone then does not easily separate primary from secondary adrenal insufficiency. ACTH resulting in the test very high so may not be sensitive to milder degrees of adrenal impairment.*

©PCHindmarsh

RENIN-ANGIOTENSIN-ALDOSTERONE SYSTEM

TEST	ROLE	ADVANTAGE	DISADVANTAGE
PLASMA RENIN ACTIVITY/RENIN	*Test whether mineralocorticoid system is functional.*	*Single blood test.*	*Need to be recumbent for time before test. Sample needs urgent transfer to laboratory. Need to undertake lying and standing samples. Needs to be interpreted in conjunction with plasma aldosterone as well as plasma sodium.*
ALDOSTERONE	*Test whether mineralocorticoid system is intact.*	*Single blood test.*	*Need to be recumbent for time before test. Sample needs urgent transfer to laboratory. Need to undertake lying and standing samples. Needs to be interpreted in conjunction with plasma renin activity/renin as well as plasma sodium.*
PLASMA SODIUM AND POTASSIUM	*Indicates whether problem with mineralocorticoid axis.*	*Single blood test with very rapid result.*	*Care with haemolysed samples which can falsely increase the plasma potassium.*

©PCHindmarsh

Figure 4.23 *Summary of tests used to assess the hypothalamo-pituitary-adrenal and renin-angiotensin-aldosterone axes.*

A further test of the renin-angiotensin-aldosterone axis is to measure blood pressure and plasma renin or renin activity when moving from a lying to a standing position. This leads to a slight decrease in blood pressure and a doubling in plasma renin or renin activity and aldosterone. In a person with adrenal insufficiency in whom aldosterone secretion is compromised, the decrease in blood pressure on standing will be greater than 10 mm Hg and a prominent increase of plasma renin or renin activity will take place, but the aldosterone response will not follow. Incidentally, this is quite a useful test also for determining whether when we replace aldosterone with 9-alpha fludrocortisone, we have attained adequate dosing.

CONCLUSION

When faced with clinical and biochemical features that are suggestive of adrenal insufficiency two steps are required. The first and most obvious is to establish the presence or absence of adrenal insufficiency and then second, to establish the cause. A simple measure of plasma ACTH and cortisol concentrations can be extremely useful in discerning primary from secondary adrenal insufficiency. Because we are trying to identify a deficit in cortisol production, we need to use tests that stimulate production and secretion. The mainstays of this testing are the synacthen test and the IIHT. The IIHT has been standardised against surgical stress and a response of over 500 - 550 nmol/l is considered to indicate normal adrenal cortisol production. The synacthen test performs as well as the IIHT. Lower dose synacthen tests have been devised to better approximate a normal ACTH stimulus.

Following demonstration of cortisol insufficiency, the cause of the primary or secondary failure needs to be established.

In primary adrenal insufficiency, testing of the renin-angiotensin-aldosterone axis is required with measurement of plasma sodium and potassium concentrations along with plasma renin or renin activity and plasma aldosterone concentration. Figure 4.23 brings all these points together into a summary of available tests to demonstrate adrenal insufficiency.

FURTHER READING

Banger, V., Clayton, R.N., 1998. How reliable is the short synacthen test for the investigation of the hypothalamic-pituitary-adrenal axis? Eur J Endocrinol 139, 580—583.

Crowley, S., Hindmarsh, P.C., Holownia, P., Honour, J.W., Brook, C.G., 1991. The use of low doses of ACTH in the investigation of adrenal function in man. J Endocrinol 130, 475—479.

Edwards, R., 1985. Immunoassay: An Introduction. Heinemann, London.

Grassi, G., Morelli, V., Ceriotti, F., et al., 2020. Minding the gap between cortisol levels measured with second-generation assays and current diagnostic thresholds for the diagnosis of adrenal insufficiency: a single-center experience. Hormones 19, 425—431.

Klose, M., Lange, M., Rasmussen, A.K., et al., 2007. Factors influencing the adrenocorticotropin test: role of contemporary cortisol assays, body composition, and oral contraceptive agents. J Clin Endocrinol Metab 92, 1326—1333.

Krasowski, M.D., Drees, D., Morris, C.S., Maakestad, J., Blau, J.L., Ekins, S., 2014. Cross-reactivity of steroid hormone immunoassays: clinical significance and two-dimensional molecular similarity prediction. BMC Clin Pathol 14, 33—46.

Lin, S.H., Hsu, Y.J., Chu, J.S., Chu, S.J., Davids, M.R., Halperin M.L., 2003. Osmotic demyelination syndrome: a potentially avoidable disaster. QJM 98, 935—947.

Perton, F.T., Mijnhout, G.S., Kollen, B.J., Rondeel, J.M., Franken, A.A., Groeneveld, P.H., 2017. Validation of the 1 µg short synacthen test: an assessment of morning cortisol cut-off values and other predictors. Neth J Med 75, 14—20.

Plumpton, F.S., Besser, G.M., 1969. The adrenocortical response to surgery and insulin-induced hypoglycaemia in corticosteroid-treated and normal subjects. Br J Surg 56, 216—219.

Ross, I.L., Lacerda, M., Pillay, T.S., et al., 2016. Salivary cortisol and cortisone do not appear to be useful biomarkers for monitoring hydrocortisone replacement in Addison's disease. Horm Metab Res 48, 814—821. https://doi.org/10.1055/s-0042-118182.

Yo, W.S., Li-Mae, Toh, Brown, S.J., Howe, W.D., Henley, D.E., Lim, E.M., 2014. How good is a morning cortisol in predicting an adequate response to intramuscular synacthen stimulation? Clin Endocrinol 81, 19—24.

CHAPTER 5

Tests to Establish the Cause of Adrenal Insufficiency

GLOSSARY

Adrenal autoantibodies Antibodies raised by the body's immune system against enzymes in the adrenal cortex which the body mistakenly recognises as foreign proteins. The adrenal cortical autoantibodies are raised mainly against the enzyme 21-hydroxylase which means both the cortisol and aldosterone biosynthetic pathways are affected or against CYP17 in which case the aldosterone pathway is preserved.

Adrenal hypoplasia congenita Condition affecting boys where there is a lack of adrenal development and associated gonadotropin deficiency due to a genetic abnormality in the *NROB1* or *DAX-1* gene.

Congenital adrenal hyperplasia A family of enzyme defects in the pathway to cortisol and aldosterone formation in the adrenal cortex which leads to glucocorticoid and mineralocorticoid deficiencies.

Dexamethasone suppression test Test that uses different doses of dexamethasone to determine whether there is autonomous ACTH production or to determine the sensitivity of a person to glucocorticoids.

Diabetes insipidus The passing of large volumes of dilute urine due to either a defect in arginine vasopressin secretion (cranial diabetes insipidus) or loss of action of arginine vasopressin in the kidney (nephrogenic diabetes insipidus).

Hypopituitarism Loss of hormone production from either the anterior or posterior pituitary glands or both.

Insulin induced hypoglycaemia test This test uses the stimulus of hypoglycaemia to cause corticotropin-releasing hormone to be released by the hypothalamus which in turn releases ACTH from the pituitary which in turn prompts the adrenal cortex to produce and release cortisol. Growth hormone is also released in response to hypoglycaemia.

Oxytocin A peptide hormone produced in the hypothalamus and released by the posterior pituitary which is involved in helping the uterus contract after pregnancy and assists in milk delivery from the breast.

X-linked adrenoleukodystrophy This condition affects boys and presentation with adrenal insufficiency may be the first sign of the condition. It is associated with neurological deterioration. The diagnosis can be made by the measurement in the blood of the plasma long chain fatty acids with confirmation by genetic analysis of the *ABCD1* gene.

GENERAL

In Chapter 4, we considered establishing whether the person had adrenal insufficiency using the measurement of adrenocorticotropin (ACTH) and the cortisol response to stimulation tests to confirm the loss of cortisol, as well as to aid in the differentiation of primary from secondary adrenal insufficiency. We also know many of the tests covered in Chapter 4 can be used to establish the impact of exogenous glucocorticoids on the functioning of the hypothalamo-pituitary-adrenal axis. We use the terms endogenous and exogenous to describe the origin of the hormone or drug. In the case of cortisol, endogenous cortisol is cortisol produced by the adrenal glands whereas exogenous glucocorticoids are those which act like cortisol, but are taken in by the person e.g., inhaled glucocorticoids used in asthma. Exogenous glucocorticoids used for their anti-inflammatory effects are the commonest cause of secondary adrenal insufficiency, so understanding their impact on the axis is important.

Replacement Therapies in Adrenal Insufficiency. https://doi.org/10.1016/B978-0-12-824548-4.00021-8

In Chapter 15, we will look in more detail at this area when we consider how to wean down these high exogenous glucocorticoid doses when their anti-inflammatory effect is no longer required. In Chapter 1 we outlined the many causes of primary and secondary adrenal insufficiency and there are a large number of genetic tests which can assist in arriving at the underlying diagnosis. Before we get to that point, we can refine the diagnosis with a number of biochemical tests.

PRIMARY ADRENAL INSUFFICIENCY

In Chapter 1, we outline a number of causes of primary adrenal insufficiency. Some of these such as trauma, adrenal haemorrhage or surgical removal are clear in their causes. Equally, drug therapies which suppress cortisol production or alter adrenal steroidogenesis, come from the clinical history of the patient and the medications they are receiving.

Autoimmune Adrenal Insufficiency

The autoimmune causes of primary adrenal insufficiency may reflect the disease process in which only the adrenal cortex is the target of the generation of antibodies by the body against its own adrenal glands. Alternatively, the autoimmune process may be part of broader polyglandular immune syndromes, Type 1 and 2, as shown in Figure 5.1. These broader syndromes will need to be investigated in their own right, with tests to evaluate other systems such as antibodies raised against the thyroid enzyme thyroid peroxidase in autoimmune hypothyroidism, intrinsic factor in cases of Vitamin B12 deficiency and the enzyme glutamic acid dehydrogenase in type 1 diabetes mellitus. Other associated conditions such as coeliac disease, can be defined by the presence of antibodies to gut cells — anti-endomysial antibodies. Assessment of the *AIRE* gene is helpful to confirm the diagnosis of type 1 polyglandular autoimmune syndrome.

The adrenal cortical autoantibodies are raised mainly against the enzyme 21-hydroxylase which means both the cortisol and aldosterone biosynthetic pathways are affected, or against CYP17 in which case the aldosterone pathway is preserved. Although in the majority of individuals with autoantibodies to 21-hydroxylase both pathways are affected, there are variations in terms of the biochemical changes observed and the deficiency of either the glucocorticoid or mineralocorticoid can precede the other. Autoantibodies to these two enzymes account for 70% of primary adrenal insufficiency cases. These autoantibodies are also involved in the polyglandular syndromes.

TYPES 1 AND 2 POLYGLANDULAR AUTOIMMUNE SYNDROMES

	Type 1	Type 2
INCIDENCE	*Less than 1:100,000/year*	*1 - 2:10,000/year*
INHERITANCE	*AIRE gene*	*Polygenic*
AUTOIMMUNE ENDOCRINE	*Hypoparathyroidism (85%)* *Addison (65%)* *Type 1 Diabetes (20%)* *Hypogonadism (12%)*	*Thyroid (75%)* *Type 1 Diabetes (55%)* *Addison (40%)*
OTHER COMPONENTS	*Mucocutaneous candidiasis (80%)* *Gastritis, hepatitis, pernicious anaemia*	

©PCHindmarsh

Figure 5.1 *Comparison of the autoimmune endocrine components of Types 1 and 2 polyglandular syndromes.*

Imaging of the adrenal glands can be helpful in cases where there have been adrenal haemorrhages or if tuberculosis is suspected. CT scan is the imaging mode of choice. In autoimmune conditions imaging is unhelpful as the gland is often shrunken and hard to visualise.

Adrenal hypoplasia congenita

Adrenal hypoplasia congenita refers to the genetic abnormality in the *NROB1* or *DAX-1* gene that prevents the normal development of the adrenal gland. The fetal adrenal gland makes large quantities of dehydroepiandrosterone (DHEA), which through 16alpha-hydroxylation in the fetal liver and aromatization in the placenta to estriol, allows for maintenance of the pregnancy. Deficiency of *NROB1* or *DAX-1* is associated with a high miscarriage rate. Where pregnancies continue the fetus progresses normally, confirming that the fetus does not need the normal cortisol concentrations which are seen after birth, in children and in adults.

However, once born these babies are at risk of an adrenal crisis.

Diagnosis can be made on a single blood sample because the plasma ACTH concentration is extremely high in the hundreds, cortisol is undetectable, plasma renin activity elevated and aldosterone undetectable. Other causes of adrenal insufficiency such as congenital adrenal hyperplasia (CAH) need to be excluded.

Adrenal hypoplasia congenita is associated with hypogonadotropic hypogonadism due to lack of gonadotropin-releasing hormone (GnRH) in the hypothalamus. This will manifest as a small penis and no entry into puberty. This can be tested for using the GnRH test which we will consider below.

X-linked adrenoleukodystrophy

One metabolic cause for primary adrenal insufficiency important to identify, is X-linked adrenoleukodystrophy. This condition affects boys and presentation with adrenal insufficiency maybe the first sign of the condition. It is associated with neurological deterioration. The importance of making the diagnosis, is that early intervention with bone marrow transplantation before there are progressive signs of neurological problems, holds the disease in check and prevents neurological handicap.

Individuals who have presented with primary adrenal insufficiency and who are adrenal autoantibody negative should be tested for X-linked adrenoleukodystrophy. The diagnosis can be made by the measurement in the blood of the plasma long chain fatty acids with confirmation by genetic analysis of the *ABCD1* gene. There are subdivisions of X-linked adrenoleukodystrophy; adrenomyeloneuropathy, adult cerebral adrenoleukodystrophy, childhood cerebral adrenoleukodystrophy and Addison's only adrenoleukodystrophy. Once raised plasma long chain fatty acids have been documented, then referral should be made to an expert in Inborn Errors of Metabolism.

The *ABCD1* gene contains instructions for creating a protein called X-linked adrenoleukodystrophy protein or ALDP. This is a transporter protein which transports fat in the form of very long chain fatty acids into structures called peroxisomes. Peroxisomes are small membrane bound structures or sacs within the cell and very long chain fatty acids are broken down here. If ALDP is deficient, the transport and breakdown of very long chain fatty acids are disrupted, leading to build up of long chain fatty acids in the tissues of the body. Two specific areas affected are the myelin covering of nerve cells and the adrenal cortex.

Congenital adrenal hyperplasia

This is a large topic which we cover in detail in our book Congenital Adrenal Hyperplasia: A Comprehensive Guide and readers wishing to explore the various enzymatic abnormalities are advised to read the first section of the book. Suffice to say, the commonest form of CAH is due to deficiency of the enzyme 21-hydroxylase, otherwise known as cytochrome P450c21 deficiency. The net effect of the loss of the enzyme function is an inability to generate cortisol and aldosterone. In contrast to other forms of primary adrenal insufficiency, the adrenal glands in CAH are enlarged in the untreated state, whereas in the other forms of adrenal insufficiency the glands are small or absent.

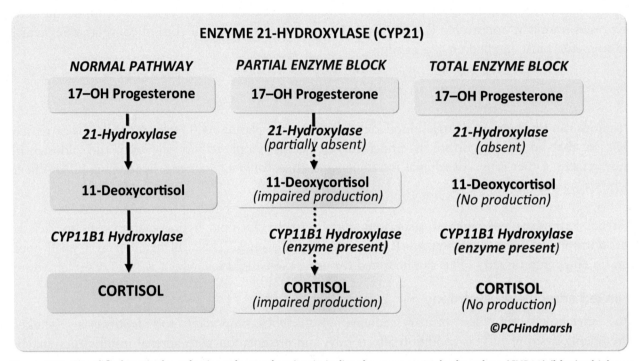

Figure 5.2 *Simplified cortisol synthesis pathway showing in italics the enzyme 21-hydroxylase (CYP21) (blue) which can be completely (on the right) or partially (middle panel) blocked. The enzyme CYP11B1 Hydroxylase is present and functions but because the substrate 11-deoxycortisol is not formed due to the higher block at 21-hydroxylase, little to no cortisol forms.*

Congenital adrenal hyperplasia does provide a useful way of assessing a defect in a metabolic pathway. This uses another endocrine principle that defining a problem in hormone synthesis or action is best done by measuring hormones on either side of where the problem lies. So let's use the example of 21-hydroxylase deficiency. Figure 5.2 shows an abbreviated part of the cortisol biosynthetic pathway based on Chapter 3 Figure 3.3. This shows the steps in converting 17-hydroxyprogesterone (17OHP) to 11-deoxycortisol by the enzyme 21-hydroxylase and the final step converting 11-deoxycortisol to cortisol by the enzyme CYP11B1.

Now we can see what we have to do to fulfil our endocrine principle of measuring before and after an event of interest. In this case, if we want to define a block at 21-hydroxylase, then we measure how much enzyme substrate (17OHP) and enzyme product (11-deoxycortisol) are present. In fact, it is easier to measure cortisol, so in defining the block at 21-hydroxylase we would expect high 17OHP and low cortisol or 11-deoxycortisol.

The easiest way this can be done is by using urine steroid profiles which analyse the steroid metabolites (breakdown products of the various adrenal steroids in the biosynthetic pathway). Again, metabolites of the substrate (in this case 17OHP) and product (11-deoxycortisol or cortisol), are compared and the advantage is that every enzyme we are interested in can be tested in this way. For each of the enzyme blocks, there is a characteristic mass spectroscopy appearance in the urine, of steroids reflecting the accumulation of steroid metabolites before the block and a lack of steroid metabolites beyond the block. It is the ratio of the before and after steroid amounts which are used to define the enzymatic defect.

Another test which is helpful initially if the patient presents with ambiguous genitalia, is fluorescent in situ hybridization of the *SRY* gene. This is a testes determining gene, so if present indicates a male chromosomal make up. The advantage is that it is quicker than conventional chromosomal analysis. Pelvic ultrasound is also helpful because if ovaries and/or a uterus can be identified, it is likely that the patient is female.

Finally, in salt-wasting states, the loss of aldosterone production can be identified as the plasma sodium will be low and the plasma potassium high, indicating loss of aldosterone which can be measured along with plasma renin activity which will be elevated. Once the biochemistry has defined the block, then genetic analysis of the gene encoding the enzyme can be undertaken. This is offered through regional genetics units in the UK for example.

SECONDARY ADRENAL INSUFFICIENCY

Anterior and posterior pituitary hormone testing is essential in cases of secondary adrenal insufficiency. Isolated ACTH deficiency is extremely rare and usually presents in the newborn period or at least in childhood. Isolated ACTH deficiency secondary to exogenous glucocorticoid administration is however, very common and we have reserved a chapter to cover this (Chapter 15).

Congenital causes of secondary adrenal insufficiency usually present in the newborn or early childhood periods. Later onset of secondary adrenal insufficiency may result from pituitary surgery for pituitary tumours, head trauma, meningitis and secondary to radiotherapy to the head for brain tumours. Patients who have had head radiotherapy should be followed for the evolution of anterior pituitary hormone deficiencies.

Figure 5.3 shows the evolution of anterior pituitary hormone deficiencies in adults over time. The effect of irradiation is dose dependent and growth hormone (GH) is the most sensitive hormone to radiotherapy. Doses as low as 10 Gy of radiation are associated with loss of GH production. At doses of 30 Gy as used for brain tumours, growth hormone production is lost in virtually everyone by 5 years following treatment. Adrenocorticotropin and the gonadotropins are next commonly affected with thyroid-stimulating hormone the least.

In contrast to the effects of radiotherapy on pituitary function which increases with time, the post head trauma loss of anterior pituitary hormones becomes less likely with time and is unlikely 10 years after the event.

Posterior pituitary function is generally unaffected by radiotherapy. However, when there is loss of arginine vasopressin secretion at diagnosis, there should be a high index of suspicion of a tumour in the hypothalamo-pituitary region and urgent MRI scan imaging is required in all cases of acquired pituitary hormone deficiency/secondary adrenal insufficiency (Figure 5.4).

Imaging is also useful in the congenital forms of secondary adrenal insufficiency, as the genetic causes of the pituitary problem may also involve other areas of brain development such as the corpus callosum or the optic nerves (Figure 5.5).

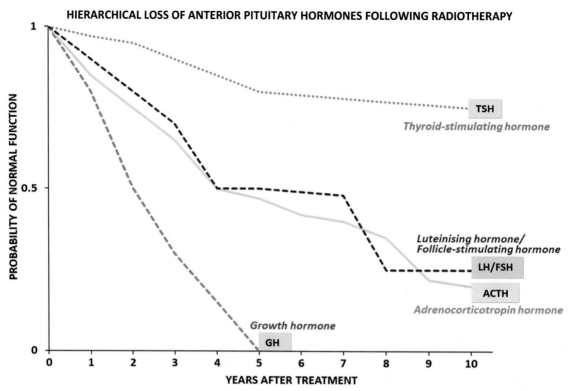

Figure 5.3 *Loss of anterior pituitary hormones following cranial irradiation for brain tumours. Growth hormone is lost first, and the loss is complete 5 years after treatment. Adrenocorticotropin, luteinising and follicle-stimulating hormones are lost next and finally to a lesser extent thyroid-stimulating hormone. (Reproduced with permission from Darzy, K.H., 2009. Radiation-induced hypopituitarism after cancer therapy: who, how and when to test. Nature Clinical Practice Endocrinology & Metabolism 5, 88–99).*

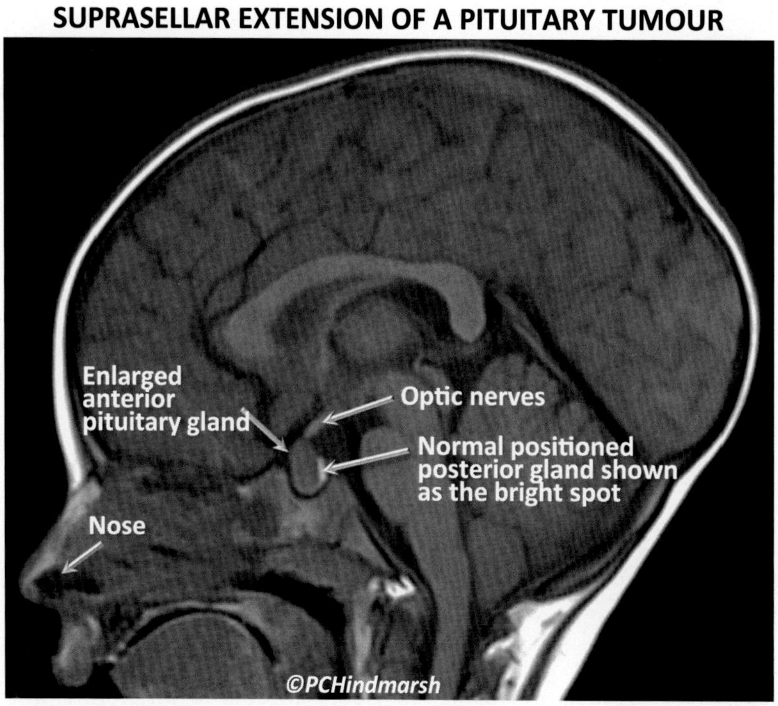

SUPRASELLAR EXTENSION OF A PITUITARY TUMOUR

Figure 5.4 *Enlarged pituitary gland which is encroaching on the optic nerves. Bright posterior pituitary is clearly seen behind the enlarged anterior pituitary in contrast to the loss of this bright spot in this position in Figure 5.5.*

SMALL ANTERIOR PITUITARY GLAND WITH UNDESCENDED POSTERIOR PITUITARY GLAND

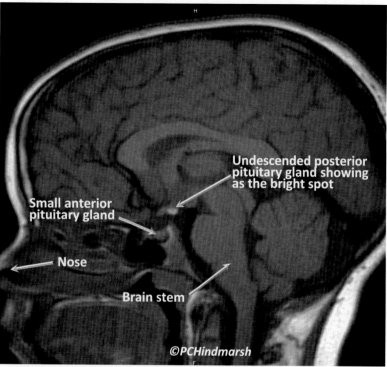

Figure 5.5 *Magnetic resonance scan of the pituitary region showing a small anterior pituitary gland with the normal posterior pituitary bright spot situated at the base of the hypothalamus instead of behind the anterior pituitary. Patient presented with growth hormone and ACTH deficiencies.*

Testing anterior pituitary function

Each of the six anterior pituitary hormones can be measured. Prolactin, which is involved in milk production, can be measured in a single unstimulated sample. Like ACTH, prolactin will rise during stress especially the stress of a painful blood test. High values may reflect pituitary prolactinomas or other lesions affecting the connection between the hypothalamus and pituitary. A number of medications used in psychiatry will also raise prolactin concentrations.

Thyroid-stimulating hormone (TSH) can also be measured in a single sample and is usually measured in conjunction with thyroxine, usually as free thyroxine (FT4). Deficiency of TSH can lead to hypothyroidism (low FT4) or to be more precise, secondary hypothyroidism or central hypothyroidism. Isolated TSH deficiency is rare and more commonly, central hypothyroidism is associated with other anterior pituitary hormone deficiencies.

The remaining hormones, ACTH and growth hormone, are more difficult to interpret from a single measure. Because ACTH has a short half-life of 4 minutes and requires transport immediately to the laboratory on ice, we use cortisol as a marker. As we know, cortisol varies with the circadian rhythm therefore a single measure can be difficult to interpret. Growth hormone has a half-life of 17 minutes so is a bit easier to measure, but during the day levels are low so it is hard to tell what is low normal from low, due to a production problem. In this situation we need a stimulation test, the insulin induced hypoglycaemia test (IIHT) which we reviewed in Chapter 4 when we considered assessing cortisol production. Hypoglycaemia is also a stimulus for growth hormone production, so we can combine cortisol and growth hormone when we undertake this test. During the IIHT, growth hormone and cortisol (driven by a rise in ACTH), are secreted when the blood glucose falls to 3.3 mmol/l and are maximal when the blood glucose reaches 2.6 mmol/l.

Once this maximal stimulus has been reached the hypoglycaemia can be reversed with a glucose drink. Sampling at 30 minute intervals is continued for 3 hours to ensure the peaks for growth hormone and cortisol are detected. In the test, growth hormone should rise over 7 µg/l and cortisol over 500 – 550 nmol/l. Both are dependent on local assays that are used. The IIHT can be combined with tests of the gonadotropin axis (gonadotropin-releasing hormone (GnRH) test) and occasionally the thyrotropin-releasing hormone (TRH) test of TSH release. The latter is usually reserved for situations where there is a concern over isolated TSH deficiency.

Figure 5.6 shows a normal combined IIHT, GnRH and TRH test and the growth hormone, cortisol and blood glucose components are shown graphically in Figure 5.7.

With all tests of growth hormone, care is required to undertake them in the fasting state as fats, proteins and glucose can alter the response obtained. Fats and glucose tend to reduce growth hormone production/release whereas proteins increase release. In this test we look first at the time zero measures of cortisol and thyroxine. Both these hormones along with testosterone and estradiol, facilitate growth hormone synthesis, so deficiencies of any of them can produce a reduced growth hormone response in the test which normalises when the missing hormone e.g., thyroxine is replaced.

This is seen even more clearly in people with delayed puberty, where testosterone or estradiol levels are low and the growth hormone response is blunted. Once puberty is established and testosterone and estradiol levels rise, the growth hormone response normalises. When testing in this age group we always 'prime' the system with sex steroid before we do the test to avoid falsely diagnosing growth hormone deficiency.

RESULTS FROM AN INSULIN INDUCED HYPOGLYCAEMIA TEST

TIME (MINUTES)	-30	0	20	30	60	90	120	150	180
BLOOD GLUCOSE (mmol/l)	4.4	4.5	2.6	3.2	3.8	4.4	5.1	5.0	4.8
GROWTH HORMONE (µg/l)	1.3	1.0	1.2	1.4	12.2	15.7	10.1	8.3	5.6
CORTISOL (nmol/l)	434	389	350	377	452	601	636	583	405
LUTEINISING HORMONE (U/l)		3.1	6.4		5.7				
FOLLICLE-STIMULATING HORMONE (U/l)		2.0	5.0		7.7				
PROLACTIN (mU/l)		225							
THYROTROPIN-STIMULATING HORMONE (mU/l)		1.7	6.8		3.4				
THYROXINE (pmol/l)		15.4							

©PCHindmarsh

Figure 5.6 *Combined anterior pituitary hormone testing using insulin induced hypoglycaemia to stimulate growth hormone and cortisol release, gonadotropin-releasing hormone to stimulate luteinising and follicle-stimulating hormones release and thyrotropin-releasing hormone to generate thyroid-stimulating hormone. Note adequate hypoglycaemic stimulus of 2.6 mmol/l at 20 minutes.*

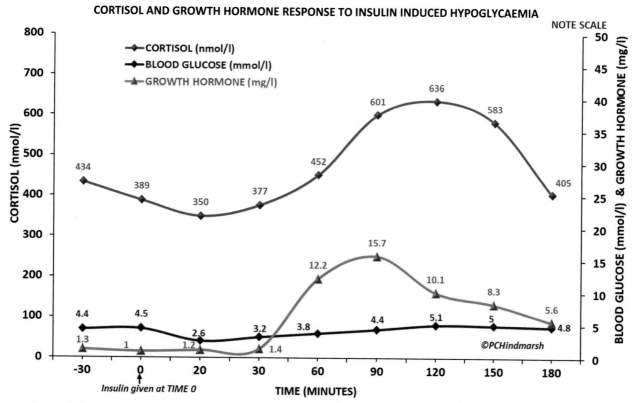

Figure 5.7 *The time course of the growth hormone and cortisol responses to insulin induced hypoglycaemia. A strong stimulus of a blood glucose (red line) of 2.6 mmol/l (at 20 minutes after insulin administration) has been applied (at 20 minutes into the test) and the maximum growth hormone (orange line) and cortisol (blue line) responses are seen at 90 and 120 minutes respectively.*

You will notice that we take a growth hormone measure at –30 minutes. A blood sample to measure growth hormone is taken at –30 minutes before the insulin is administered to determine whether growth hormone levels are rising, falling or unchanged between –30 and zero minutes, as this affects the subsequent growth hormone response.

If the levels are rising, then the response you get is greater than if there was no change or the levels were falling. This is due to the effect of somatostatin which shuts off growth hormone secretion. This occurs after a burst of growth hormone has taken place and we see that with falling or unchanging growth hormone levels, whereas if we catch the upswing of a growth hormone burst, somatostatin is low and the response to the same strength of stimulus is much greater.

This is shown in Figure 5.8 where the same dose of growth hormone-releasing hormone (GHRH) has been given when growth hormone levels are rising, falling or unchanged in the hour before the GHRH is given.

Finally, for completeness, we show the luteinising and follicle-stimulating hormones response to GnRH and the TSH response to exogenous TRH. All show a normal response.

In children and in adults where the IIHT is contraindicated, the glucagon stimulation test can be used. Glucagon will cause the release of growth hormone and less predictably ACTH, so it can be used to test pituitary production of these two hormones with cortisol acting as a surrogate for ACTH.

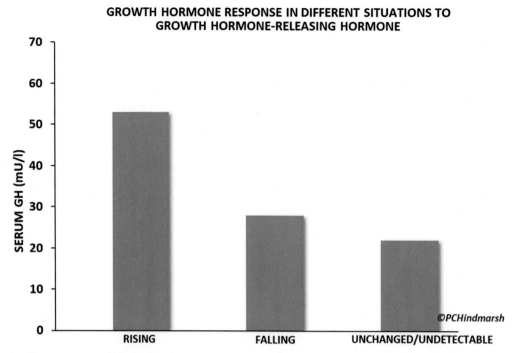

GROWTH HORMONE RESPONSE IN DIFFERENT SITUATIONS TO GROWTH HORMONE-RELEASING HORMONE

Figure 5.8 *Peak serum growth hormone response to an intravenous bolus of 100 μg of growth hormone-releasing hormone depending on whether serum growth hormone concentrations were rising, falling or were unchanged/ undetectable in the hour prior to the administration of the bolus.*

Gonadotropin-releasing hormone tests

'One off' estimations of gonadotropins and sex steroids (testosterone/estradiol see Figure 3.3 for biosynthetic pathway) are fairly unhelpful in the assessment of pubertal delay, with the exception of gonadal failure, when the gonadotropin concentrations are well above the upper limit of the normal adult range. However, in the prepubertal period, the gonadotropin concentrations are low and only increase in the peripubertal phase of development. Gonadotropin secretion is pulsatile in children and adults and its secretion occurs in late prepuberty and early puberty mainly at night whereas in adults it is present throughout the 24 hour period. There is a similar circadian variation of sex steroid secretion. The gonadotropin response to a dose of GnRH (also called LHRH) is low in prepuberty and increases with pubertal progress because of upregulation of the GnRH receptors. More sensitive gonadotropin and sex steroid assays may help diagnostically although there is overlap with the lower values encountered in normal individuals.

The response to stimulation is thus only indicative of the current situation and by no means predicts future development. In gonadal failure, the baseline of LH and FSH is raised and the response to GnRH is accentuated. Testing can be useful in adults to document hypogonadotropic hypogonadism.

The combination of the GnRH test and human Chorionic Gonadotropin (hCG) test is used to distinguish hypothalamo–pituitary problems from gonadal ones in males; these problems may coexist in those who have had radiotherapy and chemotherapy. The hCG component tells us how much testosterone can be generated by direct stimulation of the testes.

Further assessments of gonadal function in males and females can be gained by measuring Anti–Mullerian hormone which is high in males as well as Inhibin B which gives a good measure of testicular and ovarian function on a single blood sample. Figure 5.9 shows the LH and FSH responses to GnRH in a normal individual and in Figure 5.10 a normal LH response and the lack of a response in someone with hypogonadotropic hypogonadism.

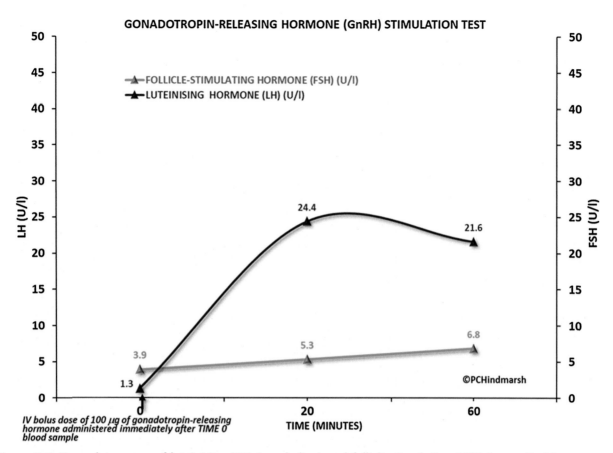

Figure 5.9 *Normal response of luteinising (LH) (purple line) and follicle-stimulating (FSH) (green line) hormones to stimulation with 100 μg gonadotropin-releasing hormone.*

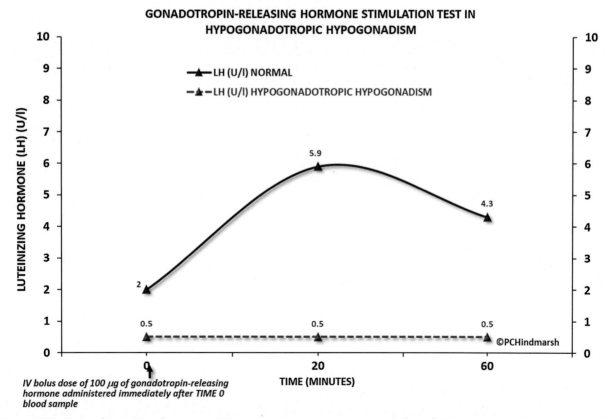

Figure 5.10 *Serum luteinising hormone (LH) response to an intravenous bolus of 100 μg of gonadotropin-releasing hormone in a normal person (purple solid line) and a patient with hypogonadotropic hypogonadism (purple dashed line).*

Thyrotropin-releasing hormone test

With improved sensitivities of the TSH assay, this test is rarely used with perhaps the exception of isolated central hypothyroidism. The test response in various situations is shown in Figure 5.11.

The normal TSH response rises to more than 5 mU/l at 20 minutes, whereas in those where TRH is deficient (hypothalamic problem), the peak is reached at 60 minutes. In TSH deficiency there is no response.

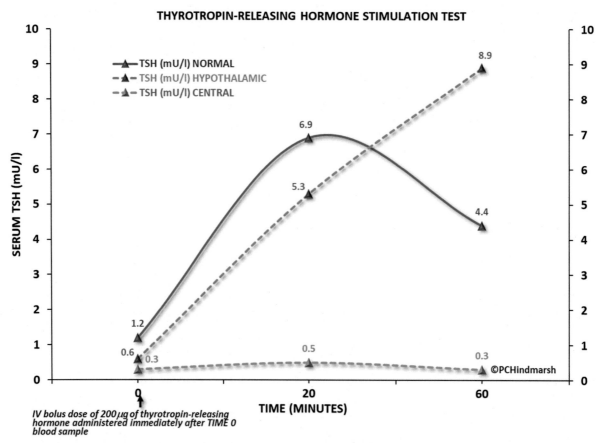

Figure 5.11 *Plasma thyroid-stimulating hormone (TSH) response to an intravenous bolus injection of 200μg of thyrotropin-releasing hormone in a normal subject (blue line) compared to a person with idiopathic central hypothyroidism (green dashed line) and someone with a hypothalamic problem (orange dashed line).*

24 hour profiles

We have looked at 24 hour cortisol profiles already in Chapter 4 and will consider them further in other parts of this book. We can look at any of the pituitary hormones in this way, although we reserve such investigations to growth hormone and cortisol mainly.

We examine growth hormone in a similar way to cortisol and Figure 5.12 shows how growth hormone is produced. Growth hormone technically does not have a circadian rhythm in contrast to cortisol and is more entrained to sleep itself rather than the light/dark cycle. Most of the growth hormone is released in Stage 4 sleep early on at night. The bursts occur on a roughly 3 hour cycle. Growth hormone secretion is regulated by a stimulatory hormone, growth hormone-releasing hormone (GHRH) secreted by the hypothalamus and an inhibitory hormone, somatostatin, also released by the hypothalamus. These two hormones cycle out of phase with each other so that when GHRH is high somatostatin is low and a growth hormone pulse is generated. Somatostatin then starts to rise and GHRH falls switching off growth hormone release from the anterior pituitary.

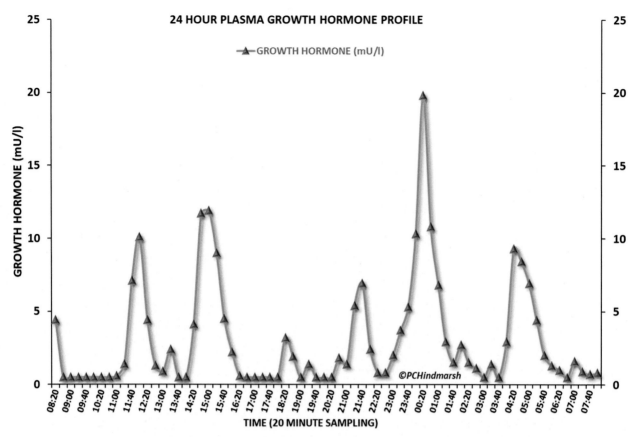

Figure 5.12 *24 hour plasma growth hormone profile with samples drawn at 20 minute intervals showing bursts of growth hormone returning to very low levels between bursts. Bursts occur roughly every 3 hours.*

Testing posterior pituitary function

When we are considering testing posterior pituitary function, we are looking at water balance. Routine measurement of oxytocin, which is involved in milk expression from the breasts, is not undertaken.

Testing for arginine vasopressin (AVP) is largely done in establishing a diagnosis of AVP deficiency (known also as cranial diabetes insipidus), or AVP resistance (nephrogenic diabetes insipidus) where there is lack of action of AVP on the kidney.

Measuring plasma AVP concentrations has proven difficult in terms of processing the sample quickly, a bit like ACTH and like ACTH, it is cleared rapidly from the circulation. More recently measurements of copeptin, a fragment of the AVP prohormone, preprovasopressin, have come to the fore. Preprovasopressin is cleaved into copeptin and AVP inside the posterior pituitary gland and both are released in equimolar amounts into the circulation and cleared by the kidneys. Copeptin is much easier to sample and measure.

Testing AVP production and release is done in two ways. The standard way is to infuse hypertonic saline which increases the plasma osmolality and this stimulates AVP release and reduces urine flow (Figure 5.13). This test is not easy to undertake so many centres use the water deprivation test. In this test the patient is deprived of water intake over a 6 hour period or until 5% of body weight is lost whichever is the sooner.

In diabetes insipidus, water is lost quickly and great care is needed to ensure that the patient does not become very dehydrated. During the test, plasma and urine osmolalities are measured hourly along with body weight.

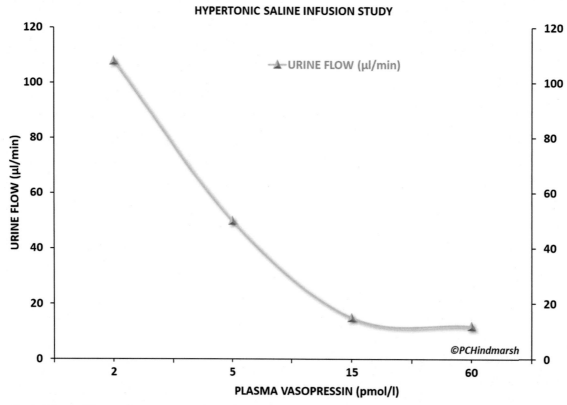

Figure 5.13 *Effect of increasing concentration of vasopressin on reducing urine flow. Hypertonic saline is infused at a rate of 0.05 ml/kg/min into a vein until a plasma osmolality of 300 mOsmol/kg is reached and blood samples drawn at 30 minute intervals from the start of the test to measure arginine vasopressin as well as urine samples to record changes in urine volume. As plasma arginine vasopressin concentrations increase urine volume declines and becomes more concentrated.*

Normally, when deprived of water, the plasma osmolality increases gradually and associated with this is the passage of a more and more concentrated urine (high urine osmolality). When a plasma osmolality of 295 mOsmol/kg is reached, there is a profound desire to drink water. In diabetes insipidus as the plasma osmolality increases, there is no increase in the urine osmolality and the patient continues to pass a large volume of dilute urine (Figure 5.14). Strictly speaking, the water deprivation tests is not as clean as the hypertonic saline study as in the water deprivation test, the stimulus is both an increase in osmolality as well as a reduction in blood volume, whereas the hypertonic saline study only alters osmolality. The sensitivity and specificity of the hypertonic saline study is better than the water deprivation test.

Before undertaking a water deprivation test, fluid intake and urine output should ideally be observed over a 24 hour period: if equal and appropriate for age, then there may be no need to proceed further. Plasma thyroxine and cortisol should be measured before the water deprivation test is undertaken as deficiencies of either or both, will lead to an inability to excrete a water load and may mask the symptoms and signs of diabetes insipidus (false negative result).

In the second part of the water deprivation test, the patient is given DDAVP (desmopressin; synthetic AVP) and urine osmolality recorded. The DDAVP test can help distinguish cranial from nephrogenic diabetes insipidus, because in the former the urine will concentrate in response to DDAVP administration, whereas in the latter it will not, due to a defect in the vasopressin receptors in the kidney. In nephrogenic diabetes insipidus DDAVP will not work even in high doses and a combination of thiazide diuretics, and a non-steroidal anti-inflammatory drug are used to reduce urine production.

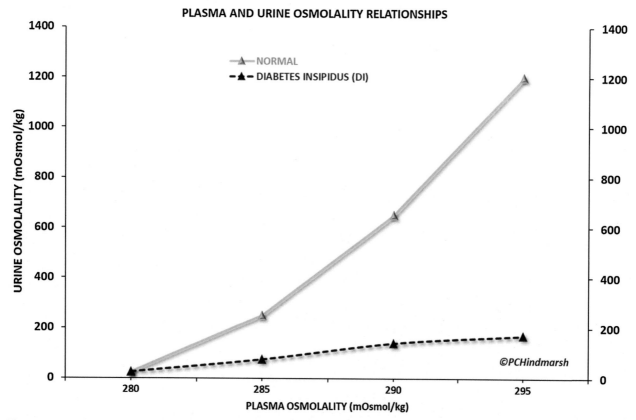

Figure 5.14 *The normal relationship between plasma and urine osmolality (yellow line) showing an increase in urine osmolality (more concentrated urine) as plasma osmolality increases. Maximum urine concentrating ability is attained at a plasma osmolality of 295 mOsmol/kg. In a patient with cranial diabetes insipidus the urine is inappropriately dilute in the face of an increasing plasma osmolality (red dashed line).*

There are two problems to avoid during the water deprivation test. First, the patient must not be allowed to become dehydrated. Fluids must not be limited before the test (no overnight fast) and the test must be terminated as soon as there is a diagnostic result (which may be at the start of the test) or if a weight loss of greater than 5% of total body weight is achieved.

Deprivation of water in a patient with diabetes insipidus is hazardous, due to uncontrolled water loss.

All the measurements must be charted and acted upon promptly. Second, water overload must be avoided following the administration of DDAVP, so water intake must be limited to replacement of losses during the test.

The patient must remain under supervision throughout, and surreptitious drinking must be avoided.

A urine osmolality of greater than 750 mOsmol/kg excludes a diagnosis of diabetes insipidus. If this is at the start of the test there is no need to proceed with water deprivation and the second part of the test, administration of DDAVP, can be undertaken. An elevated plasma sodium of more than 145 mmol/l and/or a plasma osmolality greater than 295 mOsmol/kg in the face of an inappropriately dilute urine (urine osmolality less than 300 mOsmol/kg) also confirms the diagnosis. It is extremely important when interpreting results to have paired samples of plasma and urine osmolality, because how they relate (Figure 5.14) in normal and pathological situations is critical. In terms of duration of the test, if the test is started first thing in the morning and if the urine osmolality at 15:30 (3:30 pm) is less than 450 mOsmol/kg, a diagnosis of diabetes insipidus is likely.

In the range of urine osmolalities between 450 and 750 mOsmol/kg, the diagnosis is probably one of psychogenic polydipsia or compulsive water drinking and gradual fluid restriction under supervision may be indicated, with careful monitoring of plasma and urine osmolalities. The measurement of plasma AVP levels is only helpful if the plasma osmolality is greater than 295 mOsmol/kg. In theory, this could be achieved by the infusion of hypertonic saline, but in practice this is potentially hazardous in children and should not be undertaken. If the patient fails to concentrate urine (greater than 450 mOsmol/kg) in the face of a rising plasma osmolality (greater than 295 mOsmol/kg) and a rising plasma sodium level, the diagnosis of diabetes insipidus is confirmed, and DDAVP is administered in the second part of the test.

Dexamethasone suppression test

The dexamethasone suppression test is usually used to demonstrate high cortisol production that does not suppress in cases of Cushing disease or Syndrome. The doses used are 0.5 mg four times per day for 48 hours followed immediately by 2 mg four times per day for 48 hours. If the condition is caused by an adrenal problem, cortisol will not be suppressed, whereas with a pituitary cause suppression will occur with the higher dose and only partially with the lower one.

In fact, suppression can be achieved at lower doses in people with normal pituitary and adrenal function as shown in Figure 5.15 where a single dose of dexamethasone (0.3 mg/m^2 body surface area) given at 00:00 (midnight) will suppress 08:00 (8 am) plasma cortisol and even 0.1 mg/m^2 will lead to a 50% suppression. We can use these observations for three applications of the dexamethasone suppression test in patients with primary adrenal insufficiency.

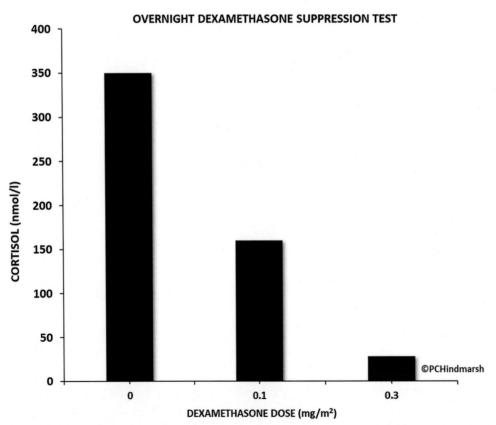

Figure 5.15 *Effect of different doses of dexamethasone given at 00:00 (midnight) on the mean 08:00 (8 am) plasma cortisol concentration measured the following morning. Almost 50% suppression is achieved with a dose of 0.1 mg/m^2 body surface area and full suppression with 0.3 mg/m^2 body surface area in 15 patients with normal pituitary and adrenal function.*

First, if ACTH levels have been high for long periods of time (6 months or more) and do not seem to respond to standard therapy, we would want to know if the ACTH production has become autonomous. In this situation instead of measuring cortisol at 08:00 (8 am) we would measure ACTH as the person cannot produce cortisol anyway. We would use the 0.3mg/m^2 dose given at midnight and see what happens. This might need to proceed to the low and high dose testing above if there is no or only partial suppression but is a good way to start.

Figure 5.16 shows an example where we have used low and high dose dexamethasone suppression to demonstrate that the hypothalamo-pituitary-adrenal system can suppress normally. Of interest is that on Day 4 after the ACTH has been suppressed (undetectable levels), there is still measurable 17OHP (5.2 nmol/l) which probably reflects production of 17OHP from the gonads (in this case the testes).

Incidentally, this shows how much care needs to be exercised in interpreting 17OHP measurements.

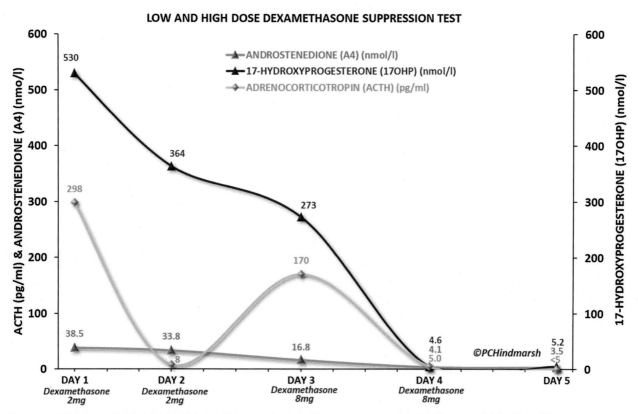

Figure 5.16 *Low and high dose dexamethasone suppression test in a patient with congenital adrenal hyperplasia and persistent high ACTH levels. Low dose dexamethasone 0.5 mg four times per day (2 mg/day) for the first two days reduces the 17OHP (purple line), androstenedione (green line) and ACTH (yellow line). The tests are continued with the high dose of dexamethasone (2 mg four times per day (8 mg/day) for 2 days) which suppresses the ACTH, but not completely the 17OHP and androstenedione which means that the residual 17OHP and androstenedione measured on Day 5 comes from the gonads (testes in this case) and not the adrenal gland as ACTH production has been switched off.*

The second use is to determine how sensitive a person is to glucocorticoids. We talk about tissue responsiveness in Chapter 6 when we consider dose-response curves. In Figure 5.15 the bar chart shows two dexamethasone doses suppressing morning cortisol and we can also use them to determine how responsive a person is to dexamethasone.

A person who was very responsive might suppress completely with a dexamethasone dose of 0.1 mg/m^2, an average person say at 0.3 mg/m^2 and a less responsive person might need 0.5 mg/m^2. This idea is worth researching further as it would help us tailor treatment even further to include how someone might respond to glucocorticoids.

The third use of the dexamethasone suppression test is to determine the source of androgen in CAH. In adults and adolescents both the testes, ovaries and adrenal glands are capable of making androgens (see Chapter 8, Part 4 for further discussion). In CAH and in polycystic ovarian syndrome, it is sometimes useful to understand whether the androgen source is adrenal or gonadal. This is important, because altering the glucocorticoid dosing schedule is unlikely to achieve anything if the gonad is the source of the androgen.

The standard dosing regimen of $0.3mg/m^2$ can be used and if the androgen concentrations (usually androstenedione) are suppressed, this would implicate the adrenal glands as the source of the androstenedione. This can be seen in Figure 5.16 where we have measured 17OHP, as well as ACTH and androstenedione. When the ACTH production is suppressed, there is still some 17OHP and androstenedione measurable on Day 5 and this implies that the gonads are the source of this, (and is normal gonadal production) as any adrenal drive from ACTH has been removed.

GENETIC TESTING

Once the biochemical diagnosis has been made, this can be confirmed by undertaking genetic testing with the gene responsible for the condition. This is becoming more widely available, not just for genes encoding the enzymes involved in CAH, but also for the developmental cascades involved in the formation of the pituitary and adrenal glands. Many of the known genes for pituitary and adrenal disorders are listed in Chapter 1. These tests are available through regional genetics laboratories in the United Kingdom. Genetic testing either uses a series of special probes which are designed to pick up the common mutations, or deletions known in the gene of interest. This is quite an efficient approach to genetic diagnosis.

Another and increasingly used technique is genome sequencing where each of the building blocks of the gene are analysed one by one. This can be quite a task for some of the conditions especially for a large gene such as 21-hydroxylase in CAH, so this technique is reserved for situations where the common mutations/deletions are not identified. As whole genome sequencing becomes cheaper, more easily accessible and quicker to undertake, it is likely this will supersede the other methods of analysis.

CONCLUSION

Making the diagnosis of the cause of adrenal insufficiency requires more detailed biochemical testing with confirmation by genetic analysis. The biochemical tests described are targeted at either defining the biochemical abnormality affected e.g., enzyme deficiencies in CAH or at the causative factor, adrenal antibodies in Addison's disease. In secondary adrenal insufficiency due to hypothalamic and/or pituitary problems, we separate causes into those that are congenital due to a developmental abnormality of the hypothalamus and pituitary, from those which are acquired such as tumours or surgery to the area. As such, MRI scans of the brain and pituitary region play an important role in advancing the diagnosis in secondary adrenal insufficiency.

Testing of the anterior and posterior pituitary gland function in cases of adrenal insufficiency are essential to define the extent of the hormone deficits. In congenital hypopituitarism the loss of anterior pituitary hormones can often indicate the likely genetic defect. For example, growth hormone, TSH, LH and FSH, ACTH and prolactin are missing in abnormalities of the pituitary developmental gene *Prop-1*.

Testing of posterior pituitary function is confined to the assessment of arginine vasopressin production only. This is done indirectly using the water deprivation test which needs to be conducted in a unit that is used to undertaking this test regularly. Water deprivation in a patient with diabetes insipidus can be dangerous and careful monitoring during the test is essential.

FURTHER READING

Borchers, J., Pukkala, E., Mäkitie, O., Laakso, S., 2023. Epidemiology and causes of primary adrenal insufficiency in children: a population-based study. J Clin Endocrinol Metab 108, 2879–2885. https://doi.org/10.1210/clinem/dgad283.

Buonocore, F., Maharaj, A., Qamar, Y., et al., 2021. Genetic analysis of pediatric primary adrenal insufficiency of unknown etiology: 25 years' experience in the UK. J Endocr Soc 11, bvab086. https://doi.org/10.1210/jendso/bvab086.

Darzy, K.H., 2009. Radiation-induced hypopituitarism after cancer therapy: who, how and when to test. Nat Clin Pract Endocrinol Metab 5, 88–99.

Gregory, L.C., Dattani, M.T., 2020. The molecular basis of congenital hypopituitarism and related disorders. J Clin Endocrinol Metab 105, dgz184. https://doi.org/10.1210/clinem/dgz184.

Hindmarsh, P.C., Geertsma, K.H., 2017. Congenital Adrenal Hyperplasia: A Comprehensive Guide. Elsevier, New York.

Refardt, J., Atila C., Chifu, I., et al., 2023. Arginine or hypertonic saline-stimulated copeptin to diagnose AVP deficiency. N Engl J Med 389, 1877–1887. https://doi.org/10.1056/NEJMoa2306263.

CHAPTER 6

Principles of Pharmacology

GLOSSARY

Bioavailability The fraction of the dose administered (usually oral or intramuscular) that reaches the systemic circulation as an intact drug.

Clearance The efficiency of the irreversible elimination of a drug from the body.

Cortisol binding globulin A protein made by the liver which attaches itself to cortisol and carries it around the bloodstream. This is known as bound cortisol. 90% to 95% of cortisol is bound in this way with 5% in the free state.

Duration of action How long a drug produces an effect on the body.

Enteric coated Enteric coatings are polymers that are put on certain tablets (such as prednisolone) to prevent them from dissolving in the acid of the stomach or damaging the lining of the stomach. The coating allows the tablets to survive intact as they pass through the acid in the stomach. Once in the small intestine which is less acidic, they are broken down and absorbed.

Half-life The time taken for the amount of drug in the body, or in the blood, to decrease by fifty percent.

Half-maximal inhibitory concentration A measure of the potency of a substance in inhibiting a specific biological or biochemical function. The amount of an inhibitory substance (e.g. a drug) needed to inhibit a process by fifty percent.

Over stacking The phenomenon which happens if the timing of doses is incorrect. Occurs where the dose is taken too early and builds onto the cortisol remaining from the previous dose, leading to higher levels than expected.

Pharmacokinetics What the body does to the drug.

Pharmacodynamics What the drug does to the body.

Plasma terminal half-life The time required to divide the plasma concentration by 2 after reaching an equilibrium position.

Potency of a drug A measure of drug activity expressed in terms of the amount required to produce a given response. A highly potent drug produces a given response at low levels, while a drug of lower potency produces the same response at higher levels. Note that a higher potency medication does not necessarily mean more side effects. Dose-response curves can be used to compare potency of different drugs. The dose of a drug required to produce 50% of the drug's maximal effect (ED_{50}) is the commonly used measure.

Stacking The addition of a dose upon another dose within a certain time frame, usually the time that the drug is in the circulation.

Under stacking The phenomenon which happens if the timing of doses is incorrect. Occurs where the dose is taken too late and leaves periods of time between doses when there is no drug (cortisol from hydrocortisone) in the circulation.

Volume of Distribution A parameter relating the concentration of a drug in the blood, to the total amount of drug in the body.

GENERAL

Understanding the pharmacology of a drug is essential as it determines the correct dosing regimen to use, which in turn influences the likelihood of side effects either from over or under treatment. Pharmacology

Replacement Therapies in Adrenal Insufficiency. https://doi.org/10.1016/B978-0-12-824548-4.00010-3

also helps us with potential drug interactions which is particularly important in adrenal insufficiency, where multiple drugs may be used for replacement therapy. Medicine has traditionally adopted a 'one size fits all' approach to drug dosing, regardless of the size, gender and ethnicity of the individual. This should no longer be the case because such an approach has led to unwanted side effects and often ineffective treatments. Preferably the treatment regimen used should be individualised. This chapter considers some important pharmacological principles using hydrocortisone as the main example. The reasons for this are twofold.

Firstly, hydrocortisone is the drug of choice for replacing cortisol as it is the synthetic version of the steroid. Prednisolone and dexamethasone were developed not as adrenal replacement therapies, but for their potent anti–inflammatory properties. As such they are not licenced presently in some countries, including the UK, for use in adrenal insufficiency. Secondly, measuring cortisol resulting from hydrocortisone is easy and relates directly to physiological measurements.

The two main concepts in drug pharmacology are pharmacokinetics and pharmacodynamics. The term pharmacokinetics refers to what the body does to the drug, whereas pharmacodynamics is what the drug does to the body. This chapter gives an overview and is not meant to be a detailed appraisal of pharmacology. For that, the reader is directed to the reading list at the end of the chapter.

PHARMACOKINETICS INCLUDING CLEARANCE AND HALF-LIFE

Half-life, Volume of Distribution and Clearance

The two primary pharmacokinetic parameters are clearance and volume of distribution. Clearance and volume of distribution are primary parameters in that they are determined by fundamental physiological processes. The third important pharmacokinetic parameter, half-life, is a composite parameter derived from the clearance and volume of distribution. The three are related by the equation:

$$Half\text{-}life\ (hr) = (0.693\ x\ Volume\ of\ distribution\ in\ litres\ (l))/Clearance\ (l\,/\,hr)$$

This is an important equation as it tells us the half-life will be increased by a rise in the volume of distribution or a decrease in clearance and vice versa.

There are several definitions of clearance, but the most commonly used is that clearance describes the efficiency of the irreversible elimination of a drug from the body or simply quoting the equation above, clearance is the volume of blood cleared of drug per unit time. Volume of distribution is a little more complicated to understand. It is not really a 'volume,' it is actually a parameter relating the concentration of a drug in the blood, to the total amount of drug in the body.

Half-life is a lot easier to understand in that it is the time taken for the amount of drug in the body, or in the blood, to decrease by fifty percent.

Figure 6.1 models the effect of differing maximum peak concentrations (C_{max}) attained after an intravenous bolus injection of hydrocortisone and the subsequent plasma cortisol concentrations attained over the next 240 minutes. In this example for hydrocortisone, we have used the average half-life of 80 minutes. In Figure 6.1 we have started from four different cortisol values 250, 500, 750 and 1000 nmol/l. In each situation the half-life of the drug is the same.

For the 1000 nmol/l C_{max} data, we would expect the plasma cortisol concentration to be 500 nmol/l 80 minutes after the peak, 250 nmol/l 160 minutes after the peak and 125 nmol/l 240 minutes after the peak.

For the 500 nmol/l C_{max} data, we would expect the plasma cortisol concentration to be 250 nmol/l 80 minutes after the peak, 125 nmol/l 160 minutes after the peak and 62.5 nmol/l 240 minutes after the peak.

If we took this out for another 80 minutes to 320 minutes (after four half-lives) we would arrive at 62.5 nmol/l for the 1000 nmol/l peak and 31.25 nmol/l for the 500 nmol/l peak.

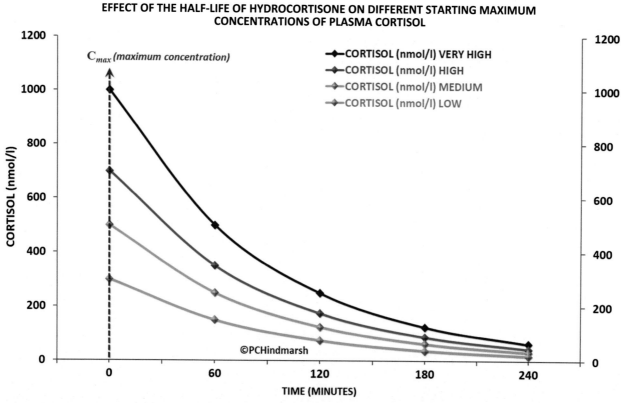

Figure 6.1 *The effect on subsequent plasma cortisol concentrations of starting at different C_{max} (maximum peak concentrations) with the same half-life (80 minutes) in each instance. The overall effect is a minimum difference at 240 minutes despite a fourfold difference in C_{max}.*

This is an important aspect of pharmacology where despite large increments in the starting plasma cortisol concentration, it does not last much longer.

The slightly higher plasma cortisol concentration at 320 minutes, which would have little additional clinical effect, is traded off against a much higher initial plasma cortisol concentration which would carry with it the potential for side effects of over exposure if repeated on a regular basis.

These pharmacologic parameters can be easily determined by administering an intravenous bolus injection of hydrocortisone and measuring the plasma cortisol concentrations achieved over a 3 hour period. Very frequent blood sampling is needed to define the relationship and an example of this is shown in Figure 6.2A (page 108).

From these data, we can determine the three parameters:

- Clearance

- Volume of distribution

- Half-life

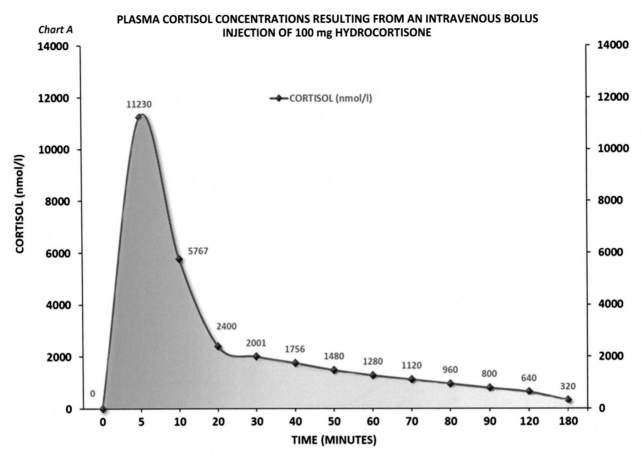

Figure 6.2A *Plasma cortisol concentration following an intravenous bolus injection of 100mg hydrocortisone at time zero. The shaded blue area is the area under the concentration time curve.*

Clearance can be calculated by the following equation using the information in Figure 6.2A. The coloured shaded area represents the area under the curve (AUC) and if we express the plasma cortisol concentration in mg/l instead of nmol/l, then the value obtained will be mg*hour/l.

From this we use the following equation to calculate clearance:

$$Clearance\ (l\,/\,hour) = Dose\ (mg)/AUC\ (mg*hour\,/\,l)$$

Figure 6.2A also illustrates that an intravenous bolus injection of 100mg of hydrocortisone in this individual, produces a very high peak 5 minutes after administration. If the bolus injection was given at 08:00, by 180 minutes the plasma cortisol concentrations are within the range we would expect midmorning in a person without adrenal problems – a large swing! These observations highlight that the dosing regimen we use in emergencies produces very high peak concentrations which do not last very long.

Repeated intravenous bolus injections would lead to oscillations between very high and very low cortisol concentrations which would upset the stability of heart function and blood pressure. This is one reason why a continuous infusion of intravenous hydrocortisone is to be preferred in emergency situations, during surgery and in intensive care.

The peak is very high partly because in adults, dosing is not undertaken on a weight basis so a 65 kg adult will get the same amount as an 85 kg peer. In paediatric practice, the dosing is often 1 mg hydrocortisone per kilogram body weight, so if we used the paediatric weight based dosing these two individuals would get 65 and 85 mg respectively, a thirty percent increase.

The peak comes down quickly partly as a result of mixing of the bolus dose in the circulation, the half-life of hydrocortisone in the individual and also loss of free cortisol into the urine due to saturation of the cortisol binding proteins in the circulation (see Figure 6.3). Incidentally, most laboratory assays do not measure such high plasma cortisol concentrations and in these types of study it is always best to alert the laboratory to the need to undertake dilutional measurements. Because of all these observations, for half-life studies, we now use a standard intravenous bolus dose of hydrocortisone of 30 mg or 0.5 mg/kg body weight to a maximum of 30 mg. This ensures the peak plasma cortisol concentration does not exceed 2000 – 2500 nmol/l which makes dilution by the laboratory easier.

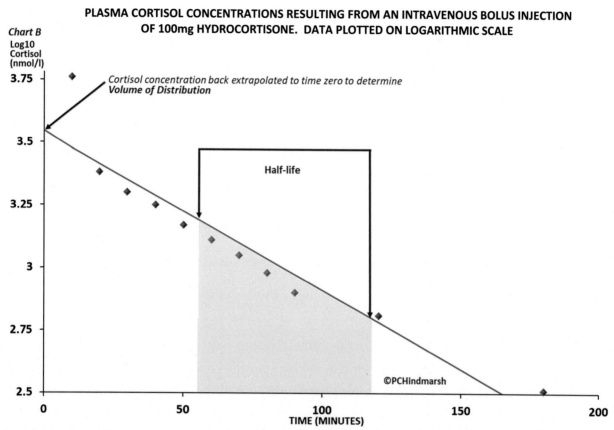

Figure 6.2B *Plot of plasma cortisol concentrations from Figure 6.1A but log$_{10}$ transformed. This yields a straight line which allows easy calculation of the volume of distribution which is the cortisol concentration back extrapolated to time zero and divided into the dose of hydrocortisone administered. Half-life is shown on the same graph in the blue area as the time over which the plasma cortisol concentration resulting from the hydrocortisone administration decreases by half.*

To determine volume of distribution and half-life we need to transform the data in Figure 6.2A. Figure 6.2A is a curvilinear relationship and our mathematics work easier if we have linear relationships. Fortunately, we can achieve this by taking the plasma cortisol concentration data and transforming it which allows us to easily fit a straight line regression as illustrated in Figure 6.2B. This transformation can be either a log$_{10}$ or log$_{e}$ (natural log) transformation. For illustrative purposes we have used log$_{10}$.

The log$_{10}$ system ascribes a value of 1 for the number 10, 2 for 100 and so on. This has the effect of constricting the upper part of the Y axis and stretching out the lower part of the Y axis which allows us to fit a straight line relationship.

We can now calculate volume of distribution by extrapolating the line back to time zero and using the equation:

Volume of distribution (l) = Dose of drug given (mg) / plasma drug concentration at time zero (mg / l)

If we know both the volume of distribution and clearance, we can then work back using the first equation to estimate the half-life, or we can work it from Figure 6.2B which also shows the time taken for the plasma cortisol concentration resulting from the drug administration to fall by 50%.

For example:
If we have worked out that the half-life of cortisol is 120 mins or 2 hours and the volume of distribution is 60 l then:

Clearance = (0.693 x 60) / 2 = 20.79 l/hour

Knowing the clearance is very useful in estimating infusion rates for hydrocortisone in intensive care situations, or for the calculation of the basal rates in a hydrocortisone pump to mimic the circadian rhythm of cortisol (see Chapter 11).

Volume of distribution is also useful as it helps us dose to achieve a steady state quickly. Using the infusion of hydrocortisone in intensive care as an example, if we just start with the infusion rate set to deliver a maintenance dose, it takes some time to get to a steady state. To get to a steady state more quickly, a loading dose can be used and this is where volume of distribution comes in. The loading dose is used to 'fill up' the volume of distribution. This can be written as follows:

Loading dose (mg) = Volume of distribution (l) * target plasma concentration (mg / l)

For example, if we want to get to a steady state of 800 nmol/l quickly:

- 800 nmol/l converts to 0.29 mg/l.

- If the volume of distribution is 60, then the dose we need is 60 x 0.29 which is 17 mg.

Therefore, if we are aiming to get to and maintain a plasma cortisol concentration of 800 nmol/l quickly, we would need to give at the start of the infusion a loading intravenous bolus of 17 mg of hydrocortisone.

Knowledge of the half-life is extremely helpful as well because we can use it to understand how we should dose with hydrocortisone. In endocrine practice when it looks as if there is not enough cortisol in the circulation, clinicians will often simply increase the dose of hydrocortisone in the hope that this will generate more prolonged exposure. A simple rule of thumb is, doubling the dose increases the duration of action by one half-life.

We have looked at this in Figure 6.1 where doubling the dose has not led to more prolonged exposure at a therapeutic concentration. The way to deal with this situation is to dose more frequently and to harness the phenomenon of 'stacking' (see later in this chapter) to improve therapeutic coverage.

The situation is even more complex because of the effect of the binding proteins in the circulation which transport cortisol, namely cortisol binding globulin and albumin. Figure 6.3 (page 111) shows the effect of increasing plasma cortisol concentrations on the amount of cortisol which is bound to the binding proteins and the amount that is unbound or free. Although we have previously looked in detail at the data in Figure 6.3 (Chapter 3, page 45), we are using it again because understanding this effect is so important to our appreciation of the pharmacology of hydrocortisone as well as for clinical practice. The plasma cortisol assay measures total (bound plus free) plasma cortisol.

As the plasma cortisol concentration rises, the cortisol binding globulin becomes saturated and at over 500 nmol/l, the free component increases. The free cortisol is easily filtered by the kidneys and lost in the urine. This can be seen in Figure 6.2A where after the initial high peak from the intravenous bolus injection of hydrocortisone, the values fall quickly as free cortisol is lost and then a much slower decline follows as the body handles the bound cortisol.

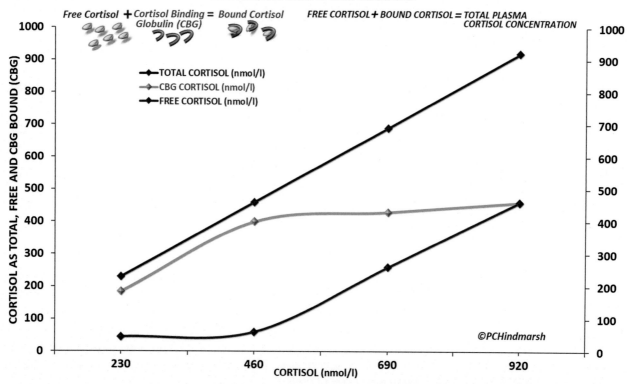

Figure 6.3 *Changes in the amount of free (red line) and cortisol binding globulin bound cortisol (light blue) which is measured as total cortisol (dark blue) as plasma cortisol concentrations increase.*

This phenomenon is important because it means if the hydrocortisone dose is doubled or tripled because of illness, the resulting plasma cortisol concentration will not be doubled or tripled because the cortisol binding globulin will become saturated.

Half-life is also important in determining the following:

- Interval between doses to avoid periods of time when the individual is without cortisol. This occurs when doses are too far apart leaving the patient with insufficient/no cortisol.

- Interval between doses to avoid periods of time when the individual is exposed to too much cortisol. Over exposure can occur when doses are given too close to each other, a phenomenon known as over stacking. This is when a dose is added onto the cortisol from the previous dose.

The converse of over stacking is under stacking. This occurs when the interval between doses is longer than the duration that a drug is at a therapeutic level in the blood stream. For hydrocortisone, this is between 4 and 6 hours. This means that by the time the next dose is due, there is little to no drug available in the bloodstream and this will lead to the effects associated with under exposure. Figure 6.4 (page 112) shows this effect. Two doses of hydrocortisone are given, the first at 07:00 (7 am) and the second at 14:00 (2 pm).

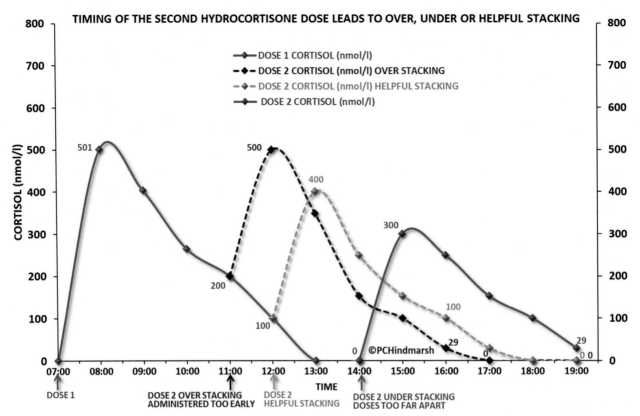

Figure 6.4 *The phenomenon of stacking. Two doses of hydrocortisone (continuous solid blue line) are given, the first at 07:00 (7 am) and the second at 14:00 (2 pm). Before the second dose is taken, cortisol levels fall very low with a period where there is no measurable cortisol in the blood (under stacking as there is no cortisol to stack the next dose on). If the second dose is given earlier at 11:00 (11 am) (dashed red line) then over stacking occurs as the peak attained is much higher (higher than expected). However, if the second dose (light blue dashed line) is given at 12:00 (noon) then helpful stacking takes place attaining a good peak and avoiding the period of low or unmeasurable cortisol between 13:00 (1 pm) and 14:00 (2 pm).*

Before the second dose is due cortisol levels are low (under stacking). If the second dose is given earlier at 11:00 (11 am), then over stacking occurs as the dose is superimposed or stacks on the remaining cortisol from the previous dose, leading to a much higher peak and one higher than expected when compared to the circadian cortisol rhythm at that time. If the second dose is given at 12:00 (noon) then helpful stacking takes place with a good peak and no period of low cortisol at 14:00 (2 pm), as the second dose is given at the point where plasma cortisol concentrations are starting to fall away. This additional dose can summate with what is remaining, to produce a peak cortisol concentration within the favourable circadian range and often a lower dose of hydrocortisone can be used.

It is important to take a cortisol measurement immediately before each dose is taken, as not only will this pre dose measurement give valuable information on how much cortisol is remaining in the bloodstream from the previous dose, it will help guide if the dosing time needs adjustment if over or under stacking is occurring. This measurement will also be valuable in making a decision if any adjustments are required to the dose amount, particularly if the dose is stacking on any remaining cortisol. Considering dose stacking, will help prevent short and long term side effects resulting from over and under dosing.

As previously mentioned, the half-life of cortisol (hydrocortisone) is on average 80 minutes. Figure 6.5 (page 114) shows the variation in cortisol half-life in 75 individuals. The fastest half-life was 40 minutes and this individual needed 6 doses a day of oral hydrocortisone to achieve reasonable concentrations of cortisol in the blood. The individual also needed higher doses to achieve optimal concentrations in the blood.

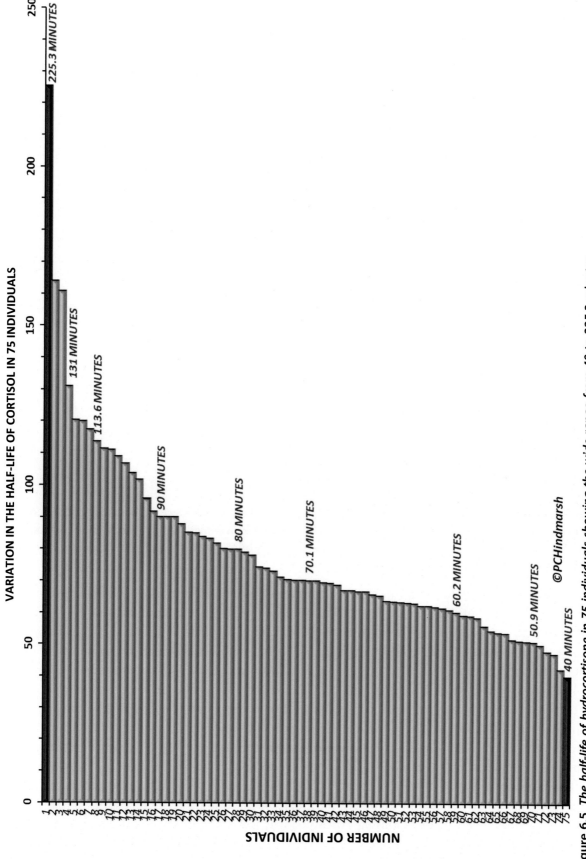

Figure 6.5 *The half-life of hydrocortisone in 75 individuals showing the wide range from 40 to 225.3 minutes.*

Although we often talk about the average half-life this only applies when we are considering populations rather than individuals. This graph illustrates why it is particularly important to individualise the dosing regimen for individuals. The individual with the very fast half-life would need very frequent doses of hydrocortisone, whereas if a similar frequency of dosing was given to the individual with the very slow half-life of 220 minutes, they would become overexposed to cortisol as a result.

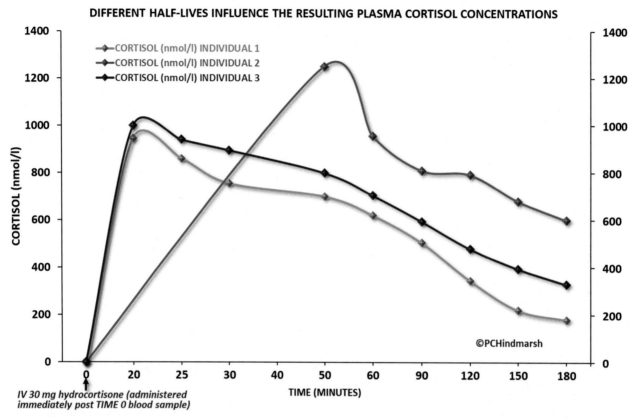

Figure 6.6 *The effect of different half-lives in three individuals given the same intravenous bolus injection of 30 mg hydrocortisone at time zero. A shorter half-life of 75 minutes was observed in Individual 1 (turquoise line), compared to a longer half-life of 150 minutes in Individual 2 (blue line) and a half-life of 85 minutes in Individual 3 (purple line). Note individuals 1 and 3 have similar C_{max}.*

Figure 6.6 illustrates this further with the results from three individuals with similar body mass indices who each received an intravenous bolus of 30 mg of hydrocortisone with measurements taken over 3 hours (180 minutes). In Individual 1 (turquoise line) the plasma cortisol concentration of 945 nmol/l 20 minutes after the bolus was given, declined with a half-life of 75 minutes, leading to a plasma cortisol concentration of 180 nmol/l at the end of the study (180 minutes). In Individual 2 (blue line) a plasma cortisol concentration of 1250 nmol/l was measured 50 minutes into the study. The half-life in this case was slower at 150 minutes, leading to a plasma cortisol concentration of 600 nmol/l at 180 minutes. In Individual 3 (purple line) the plasma cortisol concentration at 20 minutes was similar (1000 nmol/l) to Individual 1, but the half-life was 85 minutes leading to a higher plasma cortisol at 180 minutes (330 nmol/l) compared to Individual 1. A number of factors influence the half-life of hydrocortisone. The main site of cortisol metabolism is the liver. The liver contains many enzymes involved in metabolism and drug metabolism in particular. Three systems are involved in metabolising cortisol. First, the cytochrome P450 enzyme (CYP3A) which with additional sulphation and glucuronidation creates water soluble products for excretion in the urine.

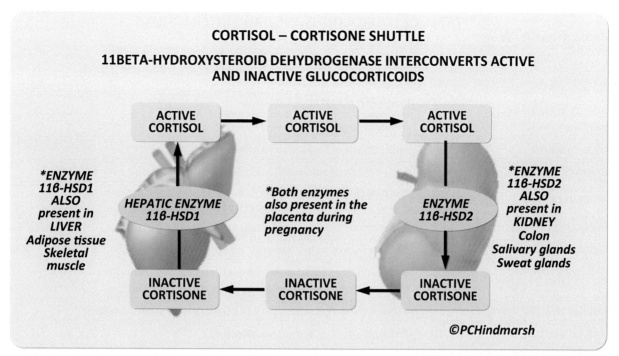

Figure 6.7 *Illustration of the cortisol shuttle where cortisone is converted to cortisol mainly in the liver and adipose tissue by the enzyme 11beta-hydroxysteroid dehydrogenase type 1 (11β-HSD1) and cortisol is converted to cortisone mainly in the kidneys and salivary glands by the enzyme 11beta-hydroxysteroid dehydrogenase type 2 (11β-HSD2).*

The second pathway involves the liver in handling cortisone in conjunction with the kidneys. The hepatic enzyme found mainly in the liver and adipose tissue which is called 11beta-hydroxysteroid dehydrogenase type 1 (11β-HSD1), converts inactive cortisone to cortisol (Figure 6.7). Cortisol is the active form and to ensure there is a balance, 11beta-hydroxysteroid dehydrogenase type 2 in the kidneys, colon and salivary glands converts cortisol to cortisone. This system is known as the cortisol shuttle. Overall, the net effect is that 11β-HSD1 serves to increase local concentrations of biologically active cortisol in a given tissue, whilst 11β-HSD2 serves to decrease local concentrations of biologically active cortisol.

11beta-hydroxysteroid dehydrogenase type 2 is found predominately in the kidneys, so you can measure the effect of this enzyme in urine collections where we look at the ratio of cortisol to cortisone metabolites. Measuring the activity of the type 1 enzyme is not as easy to do as you either need tissue, such as from the liver or to undertake a cortisone acetate loading test. The latter is difficult to carry out now as cortisone acetate is no longer available. In addition to 11β-HSD1 in the liver, there are other enzymes which metabolise cortisol by modifying the main structure, then adding on sulphate or glucuronic acid to facilitate excretion in urine. We can measure these metabolites in the urine.

Thirdly, cortisol is also metabolised into 5alpha-Tetrahydrocortisol (5a-THF) and 5beta-Tetrahydrocortisol (5b-THF), reactions for which 5alpha reductase and 5beta reductase are the rate limiting enzymes, respectively.

As a high percentage of cortisol is metabolised by the liver and because many of the enzymes used in this process are from the Cytochrome P450 (CYP450) enzyme family, the activity of these enzymes is susceptible to modification. Figure 6.8 lists a number of drugs used in common medical practice which are known to impact on hydrocortisone, either increasing or decreasing metabolism and breakdown.

TABLE OF HYDROCORTISONE DRUG INTERACTIONS

Medications A - N

MEDICATION	CONTRAINDICATION
ACE Inhibitors	Antagonism of hypotensive effect
Acetazolamide	Increased risk of hypokalaemia
Adrenergic Neurone Blockers	Antagonism of hypotensive effect
Alpha-blockers	Antagonism of hypotensive effect
Aminoglutethimide	Metabolism of glucocorticoids accelerated (reduced effect)
Amphotericin	**Increased risk of hypokalaemia (avoid concomitant use unless glucocorticoids needed to control reactions)**
Angiotensin-II Receptor Antagonists	Antagonism of hypotensive effect
Antidiabetics	Antagonism of hypoglycaemic effect
Aspirin (also Benorilate)	Increased risk of gastro-intestinal bleeding and ulceration Glucocorticoids reduce plasma-salicylate concentration
Barbiturates and Primidone	**Metabolism of glucocorticoids accelerated (reduced effect)**
Beta-blockers	Antagonism of hypotensive effect
Calcium-channel Blockers	Antagonism of hypotensive effect
Carbamazepine	**Accelerated metabolism of glucocorticoids (reduced effect)**
Carbenoxolone	Increased risk of hypokalaemia
Cardiac Glycosides	Increased risk of hypokalaemia
Clonidine	Antagonism of hypotensive effect
Coumarins	**Anticoagulant effect possibly altered. Check INR**
Diazoxide	Antagonism of hypotensive effect
Diuretics	Antagonism of diuretic effect
Diuretics, Loop	Increased risk of hypokalaemia
Diuretics, Thiazide and related loop diuretics	Increased risk of hypokalaemia
Erythromycin	Erythromycin possibly inhibits metabolism of glucocorticoids
Estrogens	Oral contraceptives increase plasma concentration of glucocorticoids
Hydralazine	Antagonism of hypotensive effect
Ketoconazole	Ketoconazole possibly inhibits metabolism of glucocorticoids
Methotrexate	Increased risk of haematological toxicity
Methyldopa	Antagonism of hypotensive effect
Mifepristone	Effect of glucocorticoids (including inhaled glucocorticoids) may be reduced for 3-4 days after mifepristone
Minoxidil	Antagonism of hypotensive effect
Moxonidine	Antagonism of hypotensive effect
NSAIDs	Increased risk of gastro-intestinal bleeding and ulceration
Nitrates	Antagonism of hypotensive effect
Nitroprusside	Antagonism of hypotensive effect

Medications P - V

Phenytoin	**Metabolism of glucocorticoids accelerated (reduced effect)**
Progestogens	Oral contraceptives increase plasma concentration of corticosteroids
Rifamycins	**Accelerated metabolism of glucocorticoids (reduced effect)**
Ritonavir	Plasma concentration possibly increased by ritonavir
Somatropin	Growth promoting effect may be inhibited
Sympathomimetics, Beta$_2$	Increased risk of hypokalaemia with concomitant use of high doses
Theophylline	Increased risk of hypokalaemia
Vaccines	High doses of glucocorticoids impair immune response; avoid use of live vaccines

Figure 6.8 *Interaction of a number of commonly used drugs with hydrocortisone.*

Estrogen, in the oral contraceptive pill, alters the way in which hydrocortisone is handled in the body and this means the total amount of cortisol present might increase, so dose adjustments might well be needed in order to cope with these changes.

Estrogen produces this effect in part by modifying how the liver enzymes handle cortisol but also by increasing the amount of cortisol binding globulin in the blood (see Chapter 13).

Bioavailability

Bioavailability is the fraction of the dose administered that reaches the systemic circulation as an intact drug. Sometimes, the bioavailability term is used to encompass both the rate and extent of absorption from the site of administration to the systemic circulation. For orally administered drugs, the bioavailability is affected by the amount of drug that is absorbed across the gut wall as well as first pass metabolism through the liver, as the drug crosses the intestine and liver on its way to the systemic circulation.

An increase or decrease in bioavailability directly impacts the total drug exposure.

Bioavailability is determined by comparing the area under the plasma drug concentration curve versus time *(AUC)* for the oral formulation (Figure 6.11) to the *AUC* for the IV formulation (Figure 6.2A).

This is given by the formula:

$$Bioavailability = AUC_{oral} * Dose_{IV} / AUC_{IV} * Dose_{oral}$$
And if the oral and IV doses are the same:
$$Bioavailability = AUC_{oral} / AUC_{IV}$$

You may see the terms absolute and relative bioavailability applied to medications. Absolute bioavailability is measured against an intravenous reference dose, which is 100% by definition. This is what we have described in the equations above. Sometimes the bioavailability of one oral formulation (test formulation) is assessed against a second oral (reference) formulation. This is known as the relative bioavailability of the test versus the reference. This becomes more complicated when we consider different brands of hydrocortisone, where not only may there be a difference in actual tablet content of hydrocortisone, but also in terms of relative bioavailability which can range from 80% to 125%.

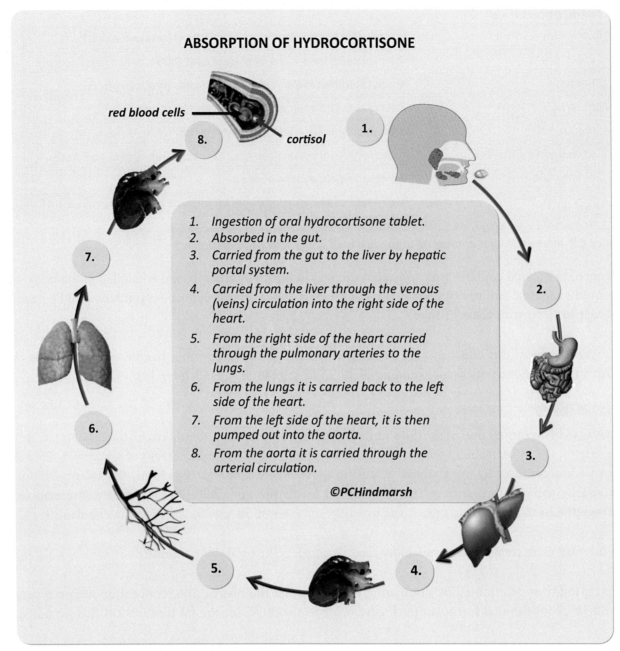

Figure 6.9 *Steps in the absorption and distribution of oral hydrocortisone.*

In Figure 6.9 we see the various steps that take place on taking oral hydrocortisone tablet:

- Ingestion and swallowing of the hydrocortisone tablet deliver the tablet to the stomach and duodenum where the majority of the dose is absorbed. Enteric coated tablets such as some forms of prednisolone or buccal hydrocortisone pass through the stomach and will be absorbed further down the small intestine.

- Taking tablets with food will alter the rate of absorption of a drug and this is the case with hydrocortisone although the difference in T_{max} amounts to only 15 minutes between the fed and fasted states. There is very little effect on C_{max}. This is important because many patients complain of abdominal pain when taking hydrocortisone on an empty stomach. As food impacts little on absorption of hydrocortisone, this means that patients can be advised to take hydrocortisone with food or a milk drink.

- Hydrocortisone is not very soluble in water but very soluble in fat/lipid. The former property means transportation in the circulation as free cortisol is poor but is made possible by the binding protein, CBG, which carries 90% to 95% of cortisol in the circulation. Being lipid soluble means that hydrocortisone is easily absorbed from the stomach and intestines and can access cells of the body very easily due to the lipid content in the cell membranes.

- Passage to the liver through the blood connection between the gut and the liver, known as the portal circulation. Once in the liver, some hydrocortisone will be lost by immediate breakdown, but the majority will then pass through the liver. This is known as first pass metabolism, a phenomenon in which a drug is metabolised at a specific location in the body resulting in a reduced concentration of the active drug when it reaches the circulation and/or its site of action.

  The liver is prominent in this phenomenon as it is a major site of drug metabolism. The lungs, for some medications for example intravenously administered drugs such as propranolol, are another site.

  There is considerable variation between individuals in first pass metabolism particularly due to the expression of the different metabolic enzymes in the liver and variations in plasma protein concentrations. Fortunately, in the case of hydrocortisone, the extraction of hydrocortisone by the liver is low mainly due to hydrocortisone binding to CBG which in turn varies little between individuals.

- Once hydrocortisone has passed through the liver it travels through the heart and lungs and then out into the body where it can alter cell activity.

- A very small amount of hydrocortisone will enter the small intestine where absorption can take place. However, in the small intestine the bacterial flora can metabolise the drug so bioavailability is not as good as higher in the gastrointestinal system and the metabolites can have other actions than a glucocorticoid if absorbed. This is a particular problem for enteric coated preparations and slow release formulations. When drug absorption is dependent on entrance into the small intestine then gut transit time becomes important. Fibre in the diet increases gut transit time while damage to the nerves of the intestinal wall which can occur in diabetes mellitus, slows transit times.

  Thyroid disorders act in both directions. Over activity or over replacement with thyroxine lead to faster gut movement, whereas under activity or under replacement can slow gut movement.

Please note that the rate at which absorption happens is variable. In some patients the peak plasma concentration can be attained within 30 minutes of ingestion whereas in other patients the peak may be 90 minutes or more and the time to peak (T_{max}) also varies within an individual being later during the night than during the day. Careful assessment with cortisol profiling will help individualise the drug profile.

Hydrocortisone is absorbed very quickly from the gut and in particular from the stomach. In fact, the absorption is very efficient and close to 95% – 100% is absorbed although this does vary between individuals. Figure 6.10 shows factors that influence bioavailability. Many of the factors shown in Figure 6.10 are ones that are beyond our control. We can ensure that we do not use enteric coated tablet preparations which will alter the speed of absorption. The gut microbiome is relatively fixed although there are a number of studies underway that are testing how it can be changed to improve health. What is important is that we are aware of all these modifiable and unmodifiable factors, which taken together mean that individuals will have different absorption patterns so careful testing is needed to ensure that the dosing schedules we use match the individual's needs.

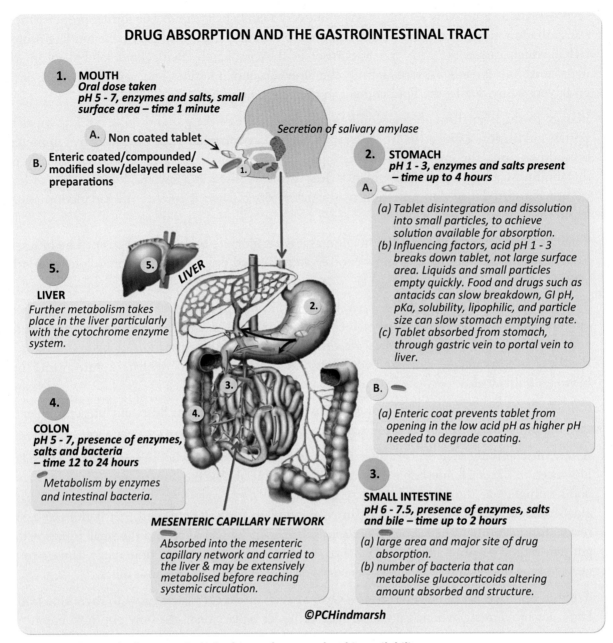

Figure 6.10 *Factors in the gastrointestinal tract that can alter bioavailability.*

Figure 6.11 shows in this individual the peak plasma cortisol concentration is reached 40 minutes after ingestion, but this can vary between individuals from 20 minutes to 3 hours and it can take 4 to 6 hours before the dose is fully out of the system with the values of cortisol achieved decreasing after the peak concentration. For reference, the blue shaded area is the AUC for oral hydrocortisone.

The figure was generated by blood sampling every 20 minutes as part of a research study. This frequent sampling means that the C_{max} and T_{max}, along with the duration that cortisol is present in the bloodstream are accurate representations of the orally administered hydrocortisone. This information tells us that when we are checking what we are delivering from an oral dose of hydrocortisone, we need to take more samples immediately before and 30 and 60 minutes after the dose has been administered. In Figure 6.11 we can see that the 40 minute sample is actually higher than the 60 minute sample.

Please keep in mind due to the pharmacokinetics and pharmacodynamics of hydrocortisone, the value of the cortisol concentrations derived from a dose as illustrated in Figure 6.11, will differ in individuals. The differences include not only the time of the peak, but also the values and duration the cortisol remains in the system.

When hydrocortisone is taken orally (Figure 6.9), the tablet is absorbed very quickly and passes into the liver via the hepatic portal system. It then passes from the liver through the venous circulation to the right side of the heart into the lungs via the pulmonary arteries, then back to the left side of the heart and out into the main circulation.

These observations tell us a lot about how hydrocortisone is absorbed and passed through the liver but not everyone is the same. As previously mentioned, just as there is a variation in half-life of hydrocortisone, the time when the peak is achieved (T_{max}) following oral administration can vary between 20 and 180 minutes, so this individual variation in absorption needs to be factored into the dosing schedule and this can be best evaluated using 24 hour blood cortisol profiles.

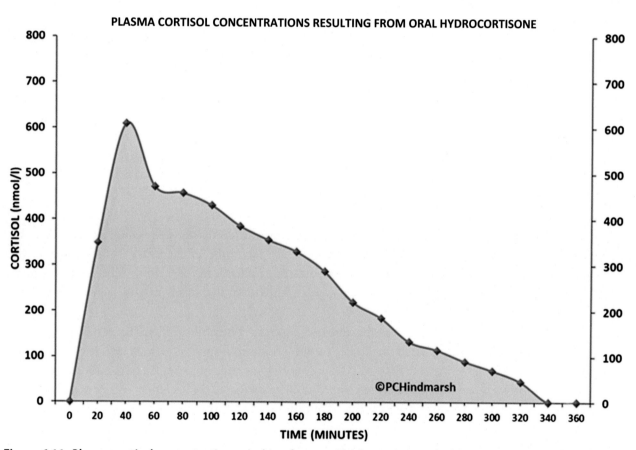

Figure 6.11 *Plasma cortisol concentrations resulting from oral hydrocortisone. The blue shaded area under the curve provides the data needed to calculate the absorption of hydrocortisone and also used to establish bioavailability. Note the cortisol concentrations illustrated are relevant to this person and will differ in other individuals.*

When we are considering oral dosing and undertaking blood sampling to determine how well we are doing with our dosing, we assume that the dose that we are administering is what it says on the prescription. As we will see this may not be the case particularly when we look at different brands. In addition, what happens when we give doses that do not fit exactly to the available tablet size for example doses of 2.5 mg, 5.0 mg, and 7.5mg which are obtained by quartering and halving 10 mg tablets?

Hydrocortisone comes in tablet form and the tablets contain lactose monohydrate, pre gelatinized starch, calcium stearate and hydrocortisone, usually in the acetate form. These additional agents are known as fillers and are used usually to bulk out the tablet.

It is important to note the following:

- Although the packaging may state 10 mg, there is an acceptance that it may vary by ±10%. For a 10 mg tablet this could mean a difference between manufacturer's tablets of between 9 mg and 11 mg. This may also be altered when tablets are halved and quartered.

- We also mentioned the idea of relative bioavailability (page 117) which can have a range between 80% and 125%, therefore heightening potential brand differences.

- This means it is very important that once started on a particular brand, the person does not change the brand otherwise cortisol levels achieved may vary, which over a 24 hour period, every day, may make a difference.

As taking hydrocortisone on an empty stomach can cause problems such as gastritis (inflammation of the stomach wall) and in the long term stomach ulcers, it is best taken after food, or with milk. The rate at which hydrocortisone enters the bloodstream depends on whether the tablets are taken on an empty stomach or not and absorption can be slowed slightly if the tablet is taken with food.

Of importance in terms of absorption, is if hydrocortisone absorption is delayed until it reaches further down the small intestine it may not be absorbed as completely as higher up. This is because the gut bacterial flora changes as we move down the gut and many of the bacteria further down are capable of metabolising steroids and cortisol in particular.

Figure 6.12 illustrates this where cortisol is metabolised into different steroids which do not have the glucocorticoid action cortisol has and have a more salt retaining effect than hydrocortisone (for example 11-hydroxyprogesterone). This has important implications for slow release preparations which may vary in terms of cortisol delivery because of individual variations in gut bacterial flora.

The gut bacterial flora is an area of increasing research interest. The ability of the bacterial flora to alter steroid metabolism was demonstrated in 1957, by an endocrinologist at the Middlesex Hospital in London, John Nabarro. He showed that rectal hydrocortisone suppositories in two patients increased cortisol in the body and in one patient testosterone also increased. This effect on testosterone was reversed when the patient was pretreated with an antibiotic that sterilised the bowel. This approach of measuring steroids before and after administration of antibiotics to the gut, has become the standard approach to defining the importance of the gut microbiome in steroid metabolism.

Interestingly, he also showed the bioavailability of rectal hydrocortisone was markedly reduced compared to the oral route. This is important as it suggests that the rectal route should not be used for the emergency administration of hydrocortisone.

Since then, it has become clear that gut bacterial flora can alter steroid metabolism with evidence for the synthesis by the bacteria of steroids with a mineralocorticoid action which may prove to be an important component in explaining some cases of hypertension.

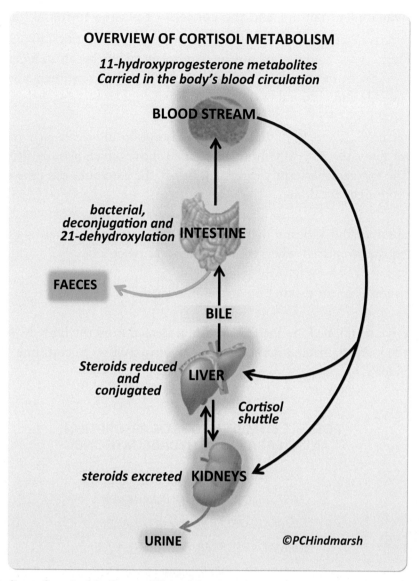

OVERVIEW OF CORTISOL METABOLISM

11-hydroxyprogesterone metabolites
Carried in the body's blood circulation

BLOOD STREAM

bacterial,
deconjugation and
21-dehydroxylation **INTESTINE**

FAECES

BILE

Steroids reduced
and
conjugated **LIVER**

Cortisol
shuttle

steroids excreted **KIDNEYS**

URINE   ©PCHindmarsh

Figure 6.12 *Metabolism of cortisol in the small intestine.*

This variation in absorption is not that high with hydrocortisone but on occasions it can be, particularly if medications or other gut conditions affect bioavailability. If we say that a drug has a mean bioavailability of 50%, or for whatever reason has been reduced to this value, then the drug dose must be doubled to achieve the same concentrations in plasma as achieved using the IV formulation. However, the variability of the bioavailability in the population is more clinically significant than the mean.

To make sure that a person with the poorest absorption is dosed appropriately, the dose must be increased according to the lowest bioavailability, not the mean. For example, if the drug has a mean bioavailability of 50% with a range of 20% to 70%, then to achieve an exposure of 100% for all patients, the dose must be multiplied by 5, not just 2.

However, this will mean that the person with 70% bioavailability will get 3.5 times too much.

This illustrates further the importance of individualising doses and not applying a uniform approach to everyone.

Interaction of bioavailability, half-life and the concept of plasma terminal half-life

We have considered bioavailability and half-life or clearance as separate entities. In practice, they interact very closely generating a very complex picture of cortisol handling by an individual as is shown in Figure 6.13, where we might have people who absorb slowly but clear either quickly or slowly and people who absorb quickly and clear either quickly or slowly.

In addition to influencing C_{max} and T_{max}, these different absorption and clearance rates also influence the duration of time spent above the $50 - 100$ nmol/l threshold above which plasma 17OHP is brought into the normal range. The fast absorbers/fast clearers fell below the threshold the fastest, which would be another reason for more frequent dosing.

This means a quick absorber/quick clearer might need very frequent doses, whereas a slow absorber/slow clearer might be adequately replaced when taking medication twice a day.

Again, the message is replacement therapy has to be individualised.

This is reinforced, as we mentioned, by the fact cortisol is cleared from the body by several mechanisms such as removal by the kidneys, metabolism in the liver and inactivation to cortisone. All these pathways differ between individuals.

POSSIBLE COMBINATIONS OF ABSORPTION AND CLEARANCE OF HYDROCORTISONE

FAST ABSORBER/FAST CLEARANCE

FAST ABSORBER/SLOW CLEARANCE

SLOW ABSORBER/SLOW CLEARANCE

NORMAL ABSORBER/FAST CLEARANCE

NORMAL ABSORBER/SLOW CLEARANCE

VERY FAST ABSORBER/SLOW CLEARANCE

VERY SLOW ABSORBER/FAST CLEARANCE

VERY FAST ABSORBER /VERY SLOW CLEARANCE

NORMAL ABSORBER/ VERY FAST OR VERY SLOW CLEARANCE

VERY FAST OR VERY SLOW ABSORBER/NORMAL CLEARANCE

©PCHindmarsh

Figure 6.13 *List of possible combinations of absorption and clearance for hydrocortisone that could be considered when creating a dosing regimen.*

The data in Figure 6.14 illustrates the variation in how five individuals who have a similar body mass index and are of similar age, metabolise hydrocortisone. The dose each patient took was higher than their usual dose and blood samples to measure cortisol were taken every 20 minutes.

The doses used in Figure 6.14 are from a clinical study undertaken many years ago when higher doses were used but they serve the purpose of defining differences in absorption and metabolism.

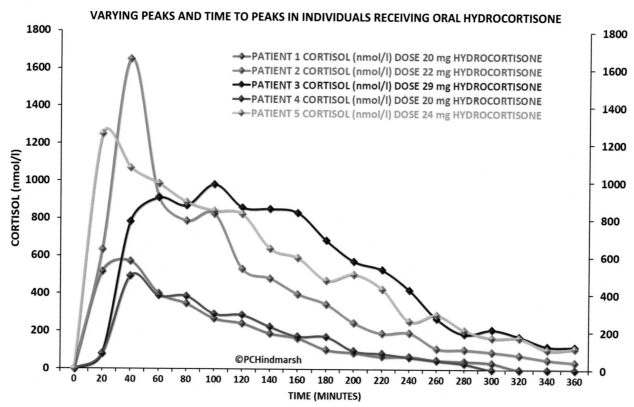

Figure 6.14 *Plasma cortisol concentrations in five individuals showing different peak values and times to peak. Patients 1, 3 and 5 show a clear dose dependent increase in peak values whereas Patients 2, 4 and 5 receive similar doses of hydrocortisone orally but have different peak and time of peaks.*

The following observations clearly show how these 5 patients metabolise cortisol differently:

Patient 1 (orange line) took the lowest dose of 20 mg of hydrocortisone, reached a peak of 571 nmol/l at 40 minutes and reached a situation where cortisol was no longer measurable at 320 minutes. This patient would be classed as a normal absorber and normal clearer.

Patient 2 (green line) took a dose of 22 mg hydrocortisone which attained a peak value of 1600 nmol/l at 40 minutes with a very low cortisol concentration of 40 nmol/l at 360 minutes. This patient would be classed as a fast/normal absorber and normal/slow clearer.

Patient 3 (purple line) took the highest dose of 29 mg of hydrocortisone which reached a high level of 909 nmol/l at 60 minutes with the peak of 981 nmol/l occurring at 100 minutes. The high cortisol values of over 500 nmol/l persisted for 120 minutes and at 360 minutes there was still a value of 123 nmol/l. This patient would be classed as a slow absorber and slow clearer.

Patient 4 (blue line) took 20 mg of hydrocortisone (same dose as Patient 1) which reached a cortisol peak value of 494 nmol/l at 40 minutes, with no measurable cortisol in the blood at 300 minutes. This patient would be classed as a normal absorber and fast clearer.

Patient 5 (yellow line) took 24 mg of hydrocortisone and achieved a peak cortisol of 1250 nmol/l at 20 minutes with a gradual decline to 113 nmol/l at the end of the study which would be classified as a fast absorber and slow clearer.

When we compare the data, we can immediately see these various differences:

- In the time the peak cortisol was attained.
- The peak cortisol concentration attained.
- How differently the cortisol is distributed over the 6 hours.
- How long the dose as cortisol remains in the circulation.

The data unmistakably illustrate the variance in the individual half-life and clearance which we also illustrate in Figure 6.5, as well as the individual absorption/clearance scenarios as described in Figure 6.13. The distribution of the cortisol achieved throughout the 360 minute period, is different for each patient and this has become very evident in the cortisol profiles we have carried out over the last 16 years, on patients with all types of adrenal insufficiency.

These important observations also allow us to determine the following:

- The best time to stack another dose on to avoid levels dropping too low or indeed too early, resulting in a much higher peak than expected (Figure 6.4).
- The most appropriate dose to use.

Blood sampling intervals are important. If Patient 3 (purple line) had a blood sample taken at 60 minutes or even at 120 minutes, they would be unaware of the peak (981 nmol/l) which occurs at 100 minutes and if another dose is added on or before 360 minutes, this would stack on the remaining cortisol (123 mol/l) leading to a higher than expected peak from the next dose. This would lead to weight gain and many other problems associated with long and short term side effects.

If Patient 2 (green line) had a blood sample taken at 60 minutes the result would show a cortisol value of 915 nmol/l, which misses the peak value of 1600 nmol/l which occurred at 40 minutes. Based on this level (915 nmol/l), a dose reduction would be calculated, however due to the substantial difference of 685 nmol/l between the measurements taken at 40 and 60 minutes, this calculated dose reduction may not be sufficient to achieve the required decrease.

We can take this further by considering the fate of the same dose of hydrocortisone when taken by different routes in the same person. In this situation half-life is the same. Figure 6.15 provides this comparison. Note that the time to peak as well as the duration in the circulation differs depending on the route of administration. After 90 minutes, the levels of cortisol are reasonably spread out but as we continue to 240 minutes then because of the effect of half-life, the resulting concentrations start to merge towards each other.

Despite the huge peak from the IV bolus, the value at 240 minutes is the same as the intramuscular injection and not much higher than the oral dose. However, the point here is that the intravenous and intramuscular routes both get cortisol in and to a peak quickly.

These studies were undertaken in an individual with good health. In sickness or where there is a gastrointestinal illness, absorption from the oral route may be compromised hence the recommendation in the sick day rules to administer emergency hydrocortisone by the intramuscular route.

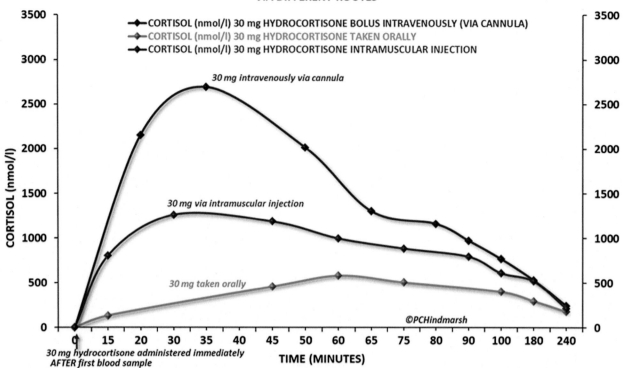

EFFECT OF ADMINISTERING THE SAME DOSE OF HYDROCORTISONE TO THE SAME PERSON BUT VIA DIFFERENT ROUTES

- CORTISOL (nmol/l) 30 mg HYDROCORTISONE BOLUS INTRAVENOUSLY (VIA CANNULA)
- CORTISOL (nmol/l) 30 mg HYDROCORTISONE TAKEN ORALLY
- CORTISOL (nmol/l) 30 mg HYDROCORTISONE INTRAMUSCULAR INJECTION

30 mg intravenously via cannula

30 mg via intramuscular injection

30 mg taken orally

©PCHindmarsh

30 mg hydrocortisone administered immediately AFTER first blood sample

TIME (MINUTES)

Figure 6.15 *The effects of 30mg hydrocortisone given intravenously (red line), intramuscularly (purple line) and orally (green line) over a time course of 240 minutes illustrating the time the peak is attained, the differences in peak values and how after 240 minutes cortisol levels are similar between the three routes.*

Understanding the impact of differences in absorption and clearance is important in interpreting 24 hour cortisol profiles and getting the dosing schedule correct.

What has been suggested as a more useful way to describe the way cortisol is handled in the blood, is something called the terminal plasma half-life. Terminal plasma half-life starts to take into account how the drug is absorbed as this will impact, as we have seen, on the peak level and also how long it takes to reach the peak concentration.

The following information is important:

- Terminal plasma half-life is the time required to divide the plasma concentration by 2 after reaching an equilibrium position.

- It is not the time required to eliminate half the administered dose.

- It is going to become an important aspect of pharmacology as it is especially relevant to multiple dosing regimens as it will influence the degree of drug accumulation.

What is important about these newer techniques of modelling the plasma cortisol curve after oral administration of hydrocortisone, is it will become increasingly simple to individualise therapy very early on. Rather than using a rather rigid dosing schedule, it is going to be possible from the generation of an absorption curve and an estimate of half-life, to model the effect of different frequencies of administration of hydrocortisone to achieve the optimum cortisol profile which can then be verified with a 24 hour plasma cortisol profile.

PHARMACODYNAMICS

We are only just beginning to understand how to measure the effect of cortisol on the body. Cortisol has numerous effects on the body (Figure 6.16 shows a simplified scheme, for more detail see Chapter 3, Figure 3.11) and some of these effects we can start to measure. One of the direct measures we can undertake, is the effect of cortisol on the hypothalamus and pituitary gland and in particular the production of ACTH. Measuring ACTH frequently is a problem because of its unstable nature and the need for very frequent blood sampling.

Whilst we can use ACTH and the hypothalamo-pituitary-adrenal feedback loops to understand cortisol pharmacodynamics, it needs to be remembered that the response of a tissue or organ or biochemical pathway to circulating cortisol may differ between the tissues and organs. For example, plasma 17OHP and androstenedione are unmeasurable when 24 hour mean cortisol concentrations reach 150 nmol/l. This mean concentration is lower than the 24 hour mean cortisol concentration of 350 nmol/l found in the general population implying other pathways may need higher cortisol levels for optimal function.

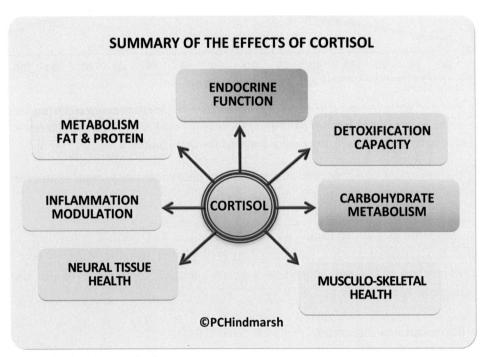

Figure 6.16 *Effects of cortisol in the body.*

In congenital adrenal hyperplasia (CAH), we can use 17-hydroxyprogesterone (17OHP) production as a surrogate marker of the effect of cortisol on ACTH production. Figure 6.17 shows the steroid synthetic pathway in the adrenal glands.

In CAH, due to loss of function of the enzyme CYP21 (P450c21), cortisol production is compromised with a compensatory increase of ACTH released from the pituitary to try to normalise the circulating cortisol concentration which it cannot achieve due to the block in the pathway. This highlights the importance of cortisol to the body as the hypothalamo-pituitary-adrenal axis will work maximally to normalise plasma cortisol concentrations by increasing the ACTH drive to the adrenal glands. As a result, there is an accumulation of 17OHP before the block with a shunting of precursors to the right, as shown in Figure 6.17 and accumulation of increasing amounts of the two adrenal androgens, dehydroepiandrosterone (DHEA) and androstenedione.

Dehydroepiandrosterone is a weak androgen (which some people replace in adrenal insufficiency although the data of its efficacy are equivocal), but when present with androstenedione in increased amounts, this leads to virilisation of the external genitalia of females with CAH and an increase in body hair, odour, height and bone age in those who present with a milder enzyme block.

Measuring the adrenal androgens and 17OHP is an indirect way of assessing the feedback effect of cortisol (or rather hydrocortisone used in treatment) on ACTH production from the pituitary gland.

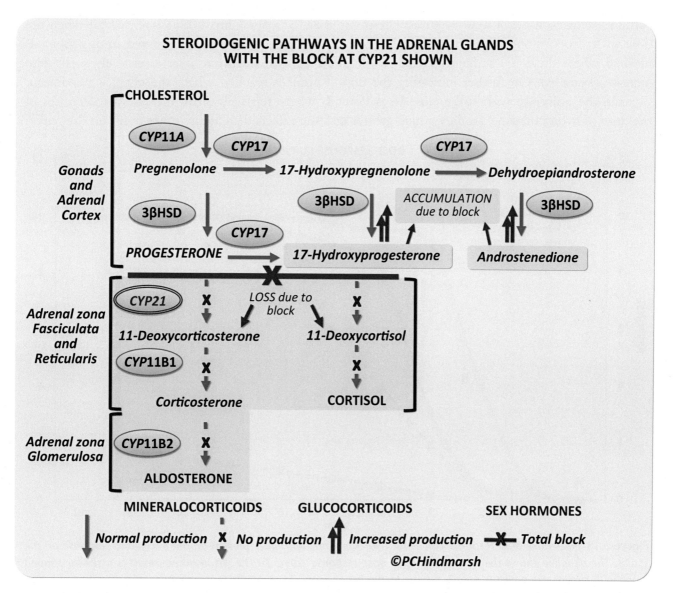

Figure 6.17 *Congenital Adrenal Hyperplasia due to deficiency of the enzyme CYP21 (P450c21). Precursors such as 17-hydroxyprogesterone accumulate before the block and androstenedione also increases as a result. Cortisol and aldosterone formation is lost.*

We can use this situation in patients with CAH to estimate how much cortisol is required to feedback on the system and in this case to reduce the amount of 17OHP. If we undertake this analysis, we come out with a measure known as the half maximal inhibitory concentration (IC_{50}). This value is a measure of the potency of a substance in inhibiting a specific biological or biochemical function. The value indicates how much of an inhibitory substance (e.g. a drug) is needed to inhibit a process by fifty percent. In our case this would be the amount of cortisol you need to have in the circulation to reduce the circulating 17OHP concentration by fifty percent.

Careful studies show the plasma cortisol which needs to be attained is between 50 and 100 nmol/l to produce this effect. This information is extremely important because it means in order to replace cortisol adequately, one component must be to always have plasma cortisol concentrations at or above 50 nmol/l throughout the 24 hour period. This would ensure in CAH the 17OHP concentrations were within the normal range and in Addison's disease the potential for an increased ACTH drive would be switched off.

One of the classic ways of looking at pharmacodynamics is to investigate the dose response curve. In this situation (Figure 6.18), the effect of hydrocortisone is plotted on the Y axis and the dose producing a particular effect, on the X axis. The classic response is an 'S' shaped curve (blue line) so that when the dose of hydrocortisone is increased initially from zero, very little effect is observed until a point is reached where there is a sudden increase in the effect of hydrocortisone over a relatively small dose increase (Point A). On further increasing the dose a point is reached where the effect is maximum. Overall, the point we wish to be close to is Point B where relatively small increases or decreases in the dose of hydrocortisone produce much greater or lesser effects than at any other point on the curve.

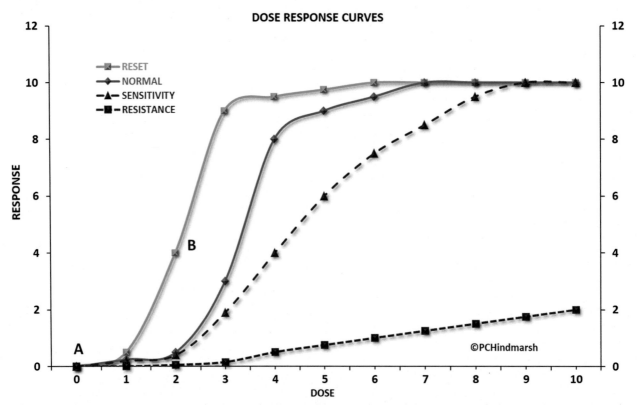

Figure 6.18 *Illustrative dose response curves for hydrocortisone with dose plotted on the X axis and response on the Y axis. The blue line shows the normal S-shaped dose response curve. To the left in green (reset) is a similar shaped curve with similar rise which is merely moved to the left – reset. To the right in purple is a curve (sensitivity) which eventually reaches the full response of 10 but the increase in the response is less per unit increase in the dose. Finally, the red line (resistance) shows a situation where no matter how high the dose the maximal response of 10 is not achieved – resistance. Point A shows the point from which after increasing the dose a response is elicited. Point B is the optimum point to function at where slight changes in dose produce large (amplified) effects in terms of response.*

A number of situations can arise. The purple line shows how changes in the sensitivity of the tissues to hydrocortisone can lead to a greater or in this case, a lesser effect for a given change in the amount of hydrocortisone. This is known as the sensitivity of the body or organ or tissue to the drug. Eventually, if enough drug is given then a maximal effect can be attained. The converse is that a person who is more sensitive will have a greater effect per increment in hydrocortisone dose. These differences in sensitivity also give us further variation in the effect of a drug in a similar way to what we saw with half-life, where there is considerable variation in this measure in many individuals.

Variations in sensitivity to hydrocortisone probably reflect different expression of the glucocorticoid receptor in different tissues. It is important to remember that each tissue or organ may well have a different dose response curve, so what is a reasonable dose and reasonable effect in one organ, may have a completely different effect in another. This is supported by changes to the traditional view that glucocorticoids exert their diverse effects through one receptor protein due to the discovery of multiple isoforms (a member of a set of highly similar proteins originating from a single gene) of the glucocorticoid receptor. It is not just genetic variation in the receptor that may play a part in determining sensitivity to glucocorticoids. Acquired conditions such as immune disorders generate proinflammatory cytokines (substances secreted by cells of the immune system) which reduce sensitivity to glucocorticoids by interfering with local glucocorticoid availability, the glucocorticoid receptor and its signalling pathway and the interaction of the glucocorticoid receptor with target genes. These observations may account for the alterations in tissue sensitivity to glucocorticoids, as well as the variations in response to glucocorticoid treatment documented in clinical practice. This adds an additional layer of complexity when we consider how an individual responds to cortisol or glucocorticoid therapy. We are a long way from understanding how to measure this in the clinical setting other than by the dexamethasone studies mentioned in Chapter 5.

The green line shows a situation where the sensitivity is not changed but the curve is shifted to the left (or it could be to the right) of the normal (blue line). This is known as resetting and means that for any effect, slightly more or less of the drug is needed to get the same effect but increasing the drug will increase the response to the same extent.

The final dose response relationship to consider is shown by the red line where no matter how high the dose of hydrocortisone is raised, little effect is seen in terms of response. This is called resistance and has been described in a number of individuals who are labelled as glucocorticoid resistant. They are not totally resistant as that is probably not compatible with life but need a greater circulating amount of cortisol to achieve effects on the body.

In Figure 6.18 doses of hydrocortisone produce desired responses, but we could also create dose-response curves for adverse effects as well. This means that for any given dose there will be a balance between a desired effect and an adverse effect. This defines a therapeutic window where the dose is chosen to maximise the beneficial effect and minimise any adverse effects. Hydrocortisone has a wide therapeutic window which means it can be used safely although monitoring for side effects is still required.

Comparing the Glucocorticoids

Hydrocortisone is the drug of choice for replacing cortisol as it is the synthetic version of the steroid. Prednisolone and dexamethasone were developed not as adrenal replacement therapies, but for their potent anti-inflammatory properties. As such, they are not licenced in some countries for use in adrenal insufficiency and the use of these agents for cortisol replacement is quite difficult. The only advantages that prednisolone and dexamethasone have is in terms of slightly less frequent administration, but their long duration of action has the potential to cause side effects.

Structure

These glucocorticoids are very closely related to each other. Figure 6.19 shows the structures of hydrocortisone, prednisolone and dexamethasone. The red arrows show where the changes have been made to hydrocortisone to make prednisolone with the introduction of a double carbon bond and in order to make dexamethasone, there is the introduction of a fluorine atom at position 9. The addition of the fluorine atom prolongs the action of dexamethasone, in a similar way to the introduction of the fluorine atom at position 9 in hydrocortisone creates 9 alpha-fludrocortisone which also has a prolonged duration of action.

STRUCTURES OF THE COMMONLY USED SYNTHETIC GLUCOCORTICOIDS

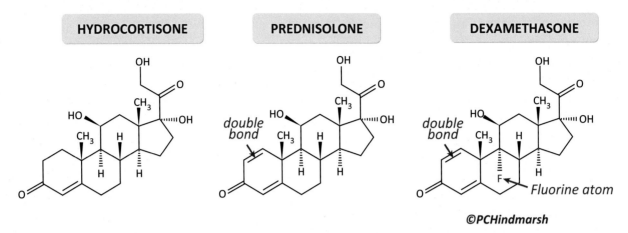

©PCHindmarsh

Figure 6.19 *Comparison of the structures of hydrocortisone on the left, prednisolone in the center with the introduction of a double carbon bond and dexamethasone on the right with the introduction of a fluorine atom and modification of the side chain.*

Potency

Potency is an extremely important concept and can be measured in a number of ways. By definition, potency refers to the dose of a drug required to produce 50% of the drug's maximal effect (ED_{50}). That would be Point B on our dose-response curve shown in Figure 6.18. Here we have the maximum response of 10 so the ED_{50} for the blue line would be 3.5 and for the green and purple lines, 2 and 4.5 respectively.

Potency of a drug should not be confused with drug efficacy, as sometimes the two terms are used interchangeably. We have defined potency above in terms of the drug's ED_{50}. Efficacy (E_{max}) is the maximum effect which can be expected from the drug. In other words when this magnitude of effect is reached, increasing the dose will not produce a greater effect. Using the blue line of our dose response curves in Figure 6.18, that would be at dose 5 as going higher than this does not increase the response greater than 10. A higher potency does not necessarily mean a higher efficacy. Rapid metabolism of a high-potency drug for example, may render it of low efficacy whereas rapid absorption, minimal first-pass metabolism and delayed excretion may create higher efficacy despite much lower potency.

Conventional assessment has been to look at the anti-inflammatory properties of each of the glucocorticoids labelling hydrocortisone with a potency of 1. Based on this approach, prednisolone has potency of 4 despite a very similar blood profile to hydrocortisone, but its duration of action is much longer compared to hydrocortisone. The potency of prednisolone is much greater in terms of growth suppression. This limits its use in pediatric practice and it has proven very difficult to use prednisolone in a way which does not inhibit growth. Equally, dexamethasone is much more potent with a rating of 30 for its anti-inflammatory action and its duration of action also of more than 24 hours leads to problems with side effects. Another way to look at potency in paediatric practice is to look at growth suppression and in Figure 6.20 all these properties are summarised.

As we know more about the half maximal inhibitory concentration (IC_{50}), (the amount of cortisol you need to have in the circulation to reduce the circulating 17OHP concentration by fifty percent), we should in theory be able to construct potencies based on this measure. Measuring drugs such as prednisolone and dexamethasone is not easy and it is difficult to equate the drug measure to plasma cortisol. Nonetheless, this approach is worth considering as the current potency measures have a wide degree of error associated with their ascertainment.

PROPERTIES OF THE COMMONLY USED SYNTHETIC GLUCOCORTICOIDS

Glucocorticoid	Hydrocortisone	Prednisolone	Dexamethasone
Half-Life in Blood (hours)	1.5	2 - 3	3.5 - 4.5
Duration as Glucocorticoid in the Blood (hours)	~6	~8	~12
Duration of Inflammatory Action (hours)	~8	~12	~36
Time to Peak Level (hours)	1 - 2	3 - 4	Rather flat profile
Growth Suppressing Effect	1	5	80
Dosing Effect on Growth Suppression (mg)	30	6	0.35 - 0.45

©PCHindmarsh

Figure 6.20 *Comparison of the half-life, duration of action and anti-inflammatory and growth suppressing potencies of hydrocortisone, prednisolone and dexamethasone. The symbol ~ stands for approximately.*

Duration of Action

We have already talked in this chapter on how long hydrocortisone is in the bloodstream as cortisol. This is shown in Figure 6.20 as the duration of glucocorticoid in the blood (approximately 6 hours for hydrocortisone depending on the individual's half-life of hydrocortisone in the blood). The duration of action of a drug is the length of time that a particular drug is effective. Duration of action is a function of several parameters including plasma terminal half-life, the time to equilibrate from the blood to the cells and how fast/long the drug works in the cell before it is removed. This generates a gap between how long a drug e.g. hydrocortisone as cortisol, lasts in the circulation and its duration of action. This occurs because glucocorticoids act on cells via their receptor. When they do this, there is a time lag between the glucocorticoid attaching itself to the cell and having its effect on the DNA machinery in the cell. This effect on the DNA produces various target proteins which then all have their own individual effects on the cell or maybe locally. This takes time and constitutes what is known as the duration of action.

This means that duration of action includes the time we can actually measure the glucocorticoid in the body (often blood) plus the effect on the target cells. If we look at hydrocortisone, then the duration it can be measured in the blood as the glucocorticoid cortisol is 6 hours, but if we then look at its duration of action as an anti-inflammatory, it is 8 hours. That is not much of a difference, whereas if we look at the same parameters for dexamethasone, then it will be present in the blood for 12 hours, but its anti-inflammatory effect is very much longer at 36 hours. If we look at the glucose raising effect of hydrocortisone as cortisol, this is at a maximum about 4 to 6 hours after the peak cortisol level is achieved (1 to 2 hours) at a time when cortisol levels in the blood are falling from the peak and will be out of the bloodstream by 6 hours.

Whilst there is a clear relationship between many of the side effects of hydrocortisone and the actual dose or concentration achieved in the blood, some of the effects of hydrocortisone and particularly prednisolone and dexamethasone are increased due to the prolonged duration of action of the drugs. Again, it depends on what we are measuring and the classic measurement for the glucocorticoids has been their anti-inflammatory action. This is particularly important for prednisolone and dexamethasone which have measurable times in the circulation of 8 and 12 hours, but their duration of action in anti-inflammatory terms is much longer and measured more in days rather than hours, particularly for dexamethasone. In such situations without understanding the duration of action, inappropriate dosing schedules can be constructed and side effects produced by the additive effects.

Modifying the Glucocorticoids to Minimise Side Effects

Prednisolone is rapidly absorbed by the gastrointestinal tract similar to hydrocortisone and the peak plasma concentration is reached some 1 to 2 hours after oral administration. The half-life in the blood is 180 minutes and the duration of action as an anti-inflammatory agent is a little longer than hydrocortisone at 8 to 12 hours.

As mentioned, one of the main problems with prednisolone, is it cannot be measured accurately in the blood routinely because there are at present no routine commercial assays available, but when they were available, the blood profile looks like that in Figure 6.21. Prednisolone will bind to the plasma proteins such as cortisol binding globulin and albumin, but to a much lesser extent than hydrocortisone. As prednisolone lasts in the blood for approximately 8 hours, this means it needs to be given at least 3 times a day.

What is also seen in Figure 6.21, is the attempt by chemists to avoid some of the stomach side effects by using an enteric coated preparation. By coating the prednisolone, it means the drug is not released until the tablet gets into the small bowel. The profile differs however, with a delayed peak 5 hours after ingestion and a lower peak value. Because of this, the enteric coated preparation is not recommended as a form of cortisol replacement. There could also be further problems with breakdown in the small intestine, because the gut flora itself in the small intestine may have metabolised prednisolone into various inactive components. We review this further in Chapter 9 where we consider various slow release preparations.

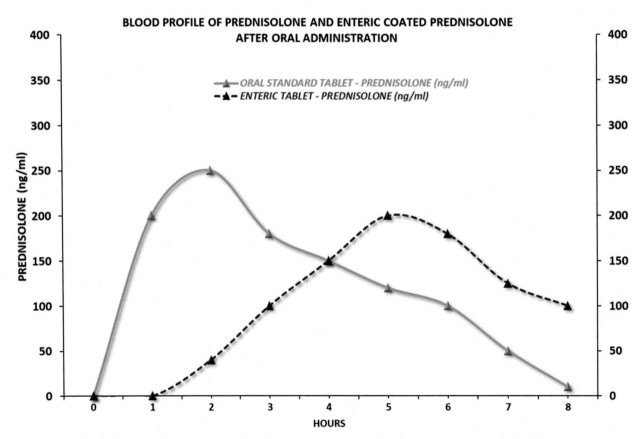

Figure 6.21 *Plasma prednisolone concentrations following oral ingestion of the standard preparation (solid green line) and the enteric coated preparation (dashed dark green line) showing a delay in absorption and peak concentration. It is important to realise the data are from an individual so the actual values will differ between individuals and as with hydrocortisone, people will absorb and clear both forms of prednisolone at different rates. Data taken with permission from Wilson, A.M., Lipworth, B.J., 1999. Short-term dose-response relationships for the relative systemic effects of oral prednisolone and inhaled fluticasone in asthmatic adults. Br J Clin Pharmacol 48, 579–585.*

Whilst on the subject of absorption, prednisone is also available for use, but needs to be metabolised in the liver to its active form, prednisolone. This also slows the presentation of the drug into the circulation.

CONCLUSION

Understanding the pharmacokinetics and pharmacodynamics of a drug are extremely important. With hydrocortisone, there is considerable variation in how the drug is absorbed and how it is removed from the circulation. There are also probably other factors which influence how the drug acts on the body in different organs and tissues.

In considering how we replace cortisol, we use hydrocortisone, as this is the synthetic form of cortisol. The way in which cortisol should be replaced needs to be based on the individual and understanding how the individual absorbs and clears the medication. This is extremely important in determining the amount of hydrocortisone to use, how often it should be given and how the proportion of the dose should be spread across the 24 hour period. Such considerations need to be then tested by measuring the plasma cortisol concentrations which result in the circulation following hydrocortisone administration, using 24 hour plasma cortisol concentration profiles as the gold standard.

Overall, we should always aim to attain plasma cortisol concentrations when replacing missing cortisol, as close to the natural production, the circadian rhythm, as possible to ensure the body can function as it would in any healthy person. As we learn more about circadian clocks and their impact on metabolism, this becomes increasingly important.

FURTHER READING

Birkett, D.J., 1998. *Pharmacokinetics Made Easy*. McGrawHill. Australia.

Charmandari, E., Johnston, A., Brook, C.G., Hindmarsh, P.C., 2001. Bioavailability of oral hydrocortisone in patients with congenital adrenal hyperplasia due to 21-hydroxylase deficiency. J Endocrinol 169, 65—70.

Hindmarsh, P.C., Charmandari, E., 2015. Variation in absorption and half-life of hydrocortisone influence plasma cortisol concentrations. Clin Endocrinol 82, 557—561.

Melin, J., Parra-Guillen, Z.P., Michelet, R., Truong, T., Huisinga, W., Hartung, N., Hindmarsh, P., Kloft, C., 2020. Pharmacokinetic/pharmacodynamic evaluation of hydrocortisone therapy in paediatric patients with congenital adrenal hyperplasia. J Clin Endocrinol Metab 105, e1729—e1740.

Toutain, P.L., Bousquet-Melou, A., 2004. Plasma terminal half-life. J Vet Pharmacol Ther 27, 427—439.

SECTION 2

In Section 2 we consider the side effects which can be encountered with glucocorticoid treatment and how we might monitor this. Monitoring of replacement therapy needs to have clear outcomes and these are summarised in Chapter 7 where we break down follow-up into short, medium and long term aims. To provide a more detailed account of problems which can occur with glucocorticoid use, we have created Chapter 8 and divided it into nine parts each part addressing a specific area such as bone health, effects on glucose handling, fertility, mood and cognitive function as well as growth and development in children. Each part is standalone which allows quick and easy reference to the relative topic. We have kept to the same style that we have used throughout the book for individual chapters. In essence however, it is better to prevent these events happening and that means getting replacement therapies right. We consider this in Section 3.

Of note, please be aware cortisol measurements vary in all individuals not only in those without adrenal problems, but also those on replacement hydrocortisone. An added challenging fact is each individual metabolises the replacement glucocorticoid differently which is influenced by body size, as well as the absorption, clearance and half-life of the drug which makes achieving the optimal dose difficult. Hydrocortisone is the synthetic form of cortisol and is easily measured in the blood, whereas the other more potent glucocorticoids are not. However, this is also not without challenges as the result is also dependent on the cortisol assay used. The vast majority of blood measurements used in this book are using the Immulite assay (including clinical trials), so it is important to know which assay is being used when considering results. When cortisol data is superimposed on the circadian rhythm, these are average values, taken from published, peer reviewed studies and it is the pattern of the circadian rhythm which is important. Solu-Cortef (sodium succinate) which has recently been renamed in the UK to Hydrocortisone Powder for Solution for Injection or Infusion (sodium succinate), has been used for the intravenous and intramuscular studies.

CHAPTER 7

Why It Is Important to Achieve Optimal Glucocorticoid Replacement

GLOSSARY

Adrenal rests The presence of adrenal tissue in the testes. This tissue responds to ACTH stimulation leading to an increase in size. The rests are hard and irregular in shape and can be mistaken for testicular cancers. These can occur wherever there are adrenal cells but mainly in testes and rarely ovaries. These are often referred to as Testicular Adrenal Rest Tissue or TART.

High blood lipids Also known as hyperlipidaemia where cholesterol and triglycerides in the blood are raised. These lipids are known to lead to heart disease if raised for long periods of time.

High blood pressure A blood pressure reading greater than the 90th centile for age. Hypertension is defined as blood pressure reading greater than 95th centile for age.

Hydrocortisone Synthetic form of cortisol.

Hyperpigmentation Areas of yellowy brown skin colour resulting from high ACTH and melanocyte-stimulating hormone levels. Classically observed in skin creases and around the gums.

Metabolic Syndrome The combination of obesity, hyperlipidaemia, hypertension, insulin resistance, type 2 diabetes, which is associated with increased risk of heart disease and stroke.

Polycystic ovaries This is a particular appearance where the ovaries are enlarged and filled with dense stroma in the middle, with lots of small cysts around the periphery of the ovary.

Polycystic ovary syndrome Ovarian appearances on ultrasound in association with increased androgen production, irregular or absent menstrual cycles and often obesity.

Standardised Mortality Rate The death rate of a population adjusted to a standard age distribution.

GENERAL

Monitoring replacement therapy is a critical part of the care of patients with adrenal insufficiency. Both over and under dosing with hydrocortisone or any glucocorticoid leads to many problems and these are illustrated in Figures 7.1 and 7.2.

Some of the effects such as growth acceleration and rapid bone maturation occur in children with congenital adrenal hyperplasia (CAH), but the majority of the remainder in the listing apply to other causes of adrenal insufficiency.

The classification into primary and secondary adrenal insufficiency is very helpful at this stage because some side effects are dependent on whether adrenocorticotropin (ACTH) is present or absent. This is particularly the case with adrenal rests and hyperpigmentation, which are due to high circulating levels of ACTH which can be present in those with primary adrenal insufficiency who are undertreated, but will not occur in those with secondary adrenal insufficiency where ACTH is deficient as part of hypopituitarism, or from suppression by exogenous glucocorticoids.

Replacement Therapies in Adrenal Insufficiency. https://doi.org/10.1016/B978-0-12-824548-4.00016-4

OVER REPLACEMENT WITH GLUCOCORTICOIDS

SIDE EFFECT	PRIMARY ADRENAL INSUFFICIENCY			SECONDARY ADRENAL INSUFFICIENCY
	Primary Adrenal Insufficiency	Salt-wasting Congenital Adrenal Hyperplasia	Simple virilising Congenital Adrenal Hyperplasia	
Gastrointestinal – gastritis and ulcers	Yes	Yes	Yes	Yes
Growth arrest	Yes	Yes	Yes	Yes, less likely as also have GH treatment
Increased appetite	Yes	Yes	Yes	Yes. May be increased anyway due to hypothalamic involvement
High blood glucose	Yes	Yes	Yes	Yes
Weight gain	Yes	Yes	Yes	Yes, and additional hypothalamic component
High blood pressure	Yes, mainly fludrocortisone effect. Incorrect distribution of glucocorticoid	Yes, mainly fludrocortisone effect. Incorrect distribution of glucocorticoid	Less of a problem as aldosterone may not be affected. Incorrect distribution of glucocorticoid	Not common as aldosterone production is intact. Incorrect distribution of glucocorticoid
Bruising and striae	Yes	Yes	Yes	Yes
Osteoporosis	Yes	Yes/No Data unclear	Yes/No Data unclear	Yes, although additional problem because of loss of testosterone/estrogen and growth hormone
Dizziness	Yes	Yes	Yes	Yes, as cortisol acts on blood vessels
Headaches	Yes	Yes	Yes	Yes
Short term memory loss	Yes	Yes	Yes	Yes. May also be related to underlying cause
Low energy	Yes	Yes	Yes	Yes
Diabetes insipidus	No	No	No	Interaction with DDAVP
Poor concentration	Yes	Yes	Yes	Yes. May also be related to underlying cause

Note: Additional Side effects common to adrenal failure only and excess glucocorticoids - stunted growth.

©PCHindmarsh

Figure 7.1 *Side effects of excess glucocorticoids in the various forms of adrenal insufficiency.*

The most important fact about replacement therapy in all forms of adrenal insufficiency, no matter what the cause, is we are replacing the hormone which is missing, namely cortisol with synthetic cortisol (hydrocortisone) and a measure of the replacement should be cortisol in the blood. This is currently not possible when using dexamethasone and only viable in a limited way with prednisolone. It is difficult to equate the prednisolone measurement with what would be an equivalent cortisol measurement and even if we could achieve this, this would not necessarily account for differences in potency.

RESUME OF THE HYPOTHALAMO-PITUITARY-ADRENAL AXIS

The hypothalamo–pituitary–adrenal axis operates as a closed loop negative feedback system. Again, we refer the similarity of this system to being rather like an oven thermostat, in that when the oven is switched on, it will increase the heat until the predetermined temperature is reached and then once that is reached, it will switch down heat production to maintain that level. The thermostat then continues to monitor the temperature making smaller adjustments to the oven to maintain the set temperature required.

UNDER REPLACEMENT WITH GLUCOCORTICOIDS

SIDE EFFECT	PRIMARY ADRENAL INSUFFICIENCY			SECONDARY ADRENAL INSUFFICIENCY
	Primary Adrenal Insufficiency	Salt-wasting Congenital Adrenal Hyperplasia	Simple Virilising Congenital Adrenal Hyperplasia	
Increased body hair	No	Yes	Yes	No
Growth acceleration	No	Yes	Yes	No
Decreased appetite	Yes	Yes	Yes	No as overall masked by hypothalamic involvement
Low blood glucose	Yes (Severity ++ as lose cortisol and adrenaline)	Yes (Severity ++ as lose cortisol and adrenaline)	Yes (Severity ++ as lose cortisol and adrenaline)	Yes (Severity +++ as lose cortisol, growth hormone and adrenaline)
Weight loss	Yes	Yes	Yes	No as overall masked by hypothalamic involvement
Low blood pressure	Yes, mainly fludrocortisone effect	Yes, mainly fludrocortisone effect	Less of a problem as aldosterone may not be affected	No as aldosterone production is intact
Adrenal rests	Yes	Yes	Yes	No
Pigmentation from high ACTH	Yes	Yes	Yes	No

©PCHindmarsh

Figure 7.2 *Side effects of under replacement with glucocorticoids in the various forms of adrenal insufficiency.*

In the closed loop system, the desired output, in this case temperature, depends on the input (gas or electricity that heats the oven). An open loop system means the output of the system is free from the input, which means the oven would continue to get hotter and hotter if the temperature feedback was not present. The hypothalamo-pituitary-adrenal axis with feed 'forward' and feed 'back' paths is shown in Figure 7.3. In the figure we start with the situation where cortisol is low, which leads to increased production of corticotropin-releasing hormone (CRH) from the hypothalamus as well as ACTH from the pituitary. The overall effect is to increase cortisol which feeds back to the hypothalamus and pituitary to reduce CRH and ACTH production.

When cortisol is missing, we say the feedback system is open, so ACTH levels will be high if the problem is primary adrenal insufficiency. In secondary adrenal insufficiency, ACTH will be missing, of course. When we replace cortisol, we close the loop again.

This is extremely important because in this negative feedback loop, if we get the cortisol replacement correct, then the other measures we might use, such as 17-hydroyprogesterone in CAH or ACTH in other forms of primary adrenal insufficiency, should fall into line. We have no such markers in secondary adrenal insufficiency, so the best we can do is match cortisol replacement against the normal circadian rhythm and check parameters such as blood glucose.

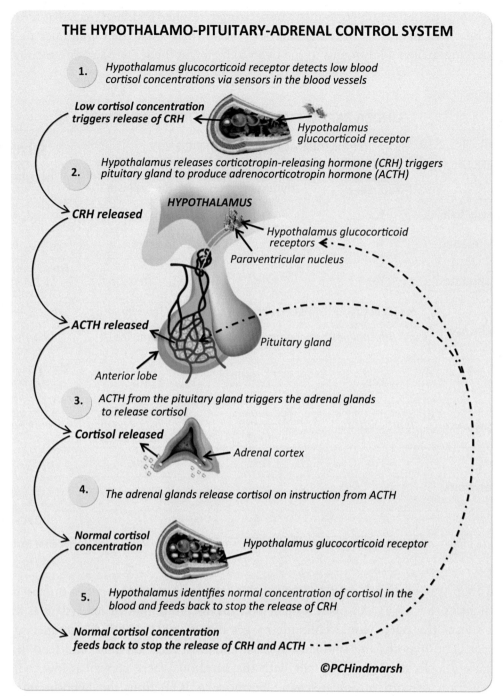

Figure 7.3 *Hypothalamo-pituitary-adrenal axis with feed forward system of corticotropin-releasing hormone (CRH) and adrenocorticotropin (ACTH) shown in red and the feedback system of cortisol in blue.*

MORTALITY AND MORBIDITY

Disorders of adrenal insufficiency due to the replacement regimens used, carry with them many morbidities which we consider in Chapter 8.

These problems may be associated with the underlying condition, such as virilisation in untreated forms of CAH, or with the treatment itself such as osteoporosis when there is overtreatment with glucocorticoids. It can be difficult to separate the condition from the treatment. Under treatment in CAH can lead to an advancement in bone maturation because the condition itself when untreated or under treated, leads to increased adrenal androgen production which matures the growth plates.

It is important to remember however, that adrenal insufficiency is a problem with cortisol production, compounded by any lack of the salt retaining hormone, aldosterone. An adrenal crisis can be severe either at presentation, or during the course of the condition particularly when unwell, which is why we have strict sick day rules. Adrenal crises can be avoided by careful management of sick days, ensuring that emergency intramuscular injections of hydrocortisone are easily accessible and making sure that replacement therapies are all optimised to give full 24 hour coverage with cortisol. Chapter 1 Figure 1.7, illustrates the components of an adrenal crisis which results from lack of cortisol and aldosterone.

Adrenal crises do carry with them a certain mortality. We do not know what that mortality rate is in the undiagnosed situation, although there are data which suggest considerable variation. Adrenal insufficiency following surgery where cortisol deficiency is expected, is associated with 100% survival and where adrenal insufficiency is diagnosed in Accident and Emergency, survival is well over 80% once hydrocortisone is given. That said, there are cases where time from the first symptoms/signs to presentation at Accident and Emergency and death, was 1 to 2 hours. In extremis where there has been adrenal destruction due to sepsis, survival whether hydrocortisone is given or not has been reported as 8% to 9%. This is about the best information there is on acute sudden presentations.

The lifetime risk of an adrenal crisis in a patient with known adrenal insufficiency is about 50% and those with a previous adrenal crisis appear to be at greater risk of subsequent episodes. Another way of looking at this is the estimated risk of an adrenal crisis occurring in a patient with adrenal insufficiency, which is about 6 to 10 cases of adrenal crisis per 100 patient years. There have been reports of increased risk of adrenal crisis in the elderly (older than 60 years old) with no difference between males and females. Better data come from a recent prospective study, which confirmed the rate of 6 to 10 cases per 100 patient years with a mortality rate from crisis of 0.5/100 patient years. To put this in perspective, the prevalence of adrenal insufficiency can be assumed to be 2.18 - 4.20/ 10,000 population and in the UK population of 67 million, adrenal insufficiency would affect between 14,600 to 28,100 people, leading to 730 to 1400 deaths from adrenal crises in a 10 year period.

There are several caveats here such as how well sick days are manged, access to medical attention and the adequacy and monitoring of glucocorticoid replacement, which are all variable factors which could improve these figures. The data can be analysed in more detail with respect to the causes of adrenal insufficiency. This is explored in Figure 7.4 and are expressed as Standardised Mortality Rates or SMRs. As most causes of death vary significantly with people's age and sex, the use of standardised death rates improves comparability over time and between countries or in this case, conditions. The SMR is the death rate of a population adjusted to a standard age distribution.

MORTALITY RATES IN ADRENAL INSUFFICIENCY

CONDITION	STANDARDISED MORTALITY RATE
Congenital Adrenal Hyperplasia	2.8
Adrenal Insufficiency	2.2
Hypopituitarism	1.4
- ACTH Sufficient	0.0
- ACTH Deficient	8.9

©PCHindmarsh

Figure 7.4 *Standardised Mortality Rates for various forms of Adrenal Insufficiency.*

In Figure 7.4 we can see that the SMR for people with CAH is similar to those with adrenal insufficiency which in the report means essentially those with primary adrenal insufficiency. Overall, the rate is about 2 to 3 times the rate expected in an age and sex matched general population, the expected rate given a value of 1 for comparison. This appears to be something to do with needing adrenal replacement therapy, because in the hypopituitary group if ACTH is sufficient and therefore the adrenal glands are working normally, the SMR is zero in other words no different from the general population at any age. However, losing ACTH and therefore needing adrenal replacement therapy increases the rate to 8.9.

Care also needs to be taken in those weaning from or just recently weaned from glucocorticoid treatment, as the rates quoted probably also apply to them.

Common to all the reports is the cause of death, which is mainly from infectious diseases and associated stress to the body. In the adrenal insufficiency population, pneumonia accounted for 66% of the deaths from infectious diseases. This data is all the more important to appreciate as we can vaccinate for pneumococcal pneumonia so this is preventable. We cover this further in our chapter on wellbeing (Chapter 16).

In the CAH study, which included children and young people, salt-wasting crises and infectious diseases were the two commonest causes of death. This was most marked in the 0 to 4 year age group where the SMR was 18.3. This suggests the loss of adrenal function from whatever cause, is an important event and stresses the need for good monitoring of replacement therapy, full immunisation, clear active management of sick days and trauma as well as prevention of hypoglycaemia.

Some of these cases probably also represent a failure to diagnose CAH, particularly in boys who present as infants with a severe salt-wasting crisis.

THE ROLE OF THE ANNUAL REVIEW

When thinking on how to best monitor people with adrenal insufficiency, we need to plot out where we wish to be in the long term and then create a series of intermediate steps, which can guide us to how successful we are in achieving our longer term aims. The long term aims can be broken down into concerns over cardiovascular risk, fertility, bone mineralisation and for paediatric patients, growth.

Cardiovascular risk may be associated with our treatments and a medium term measure might be optimising therapy to avoid high blood pressure and preventing type 2 diabetes mellitus — components of the Metabolic Syndrome.

The Metabolic Syndrome is a constellation of features which arise as a result of a primary defect in the action of insulin on cells. This is known as insulin resistance. To overcome this, the pancreas makes more insulin, which then triggers a series of other responses in other tissues all due to the high insulin levels.

These tissues include fat leading to obesity, the blood vessels leading to high blood pressure and the liver where the balance is shifted towards the production of LDL-cholesterol (bad cholesterol associated with heart disease), from HDL-cholesterol (good cholesterol associated with protection from heart disease). Fat accumulation in the liver leads to non-alcoholic fatty liver disease (NAFLD). When there is associated liver inflammation it is known as non-alcoholic steatohepatitis (NASH) which can cause fibrosis or scarring of the liver, potentially leading to cirrhosis.

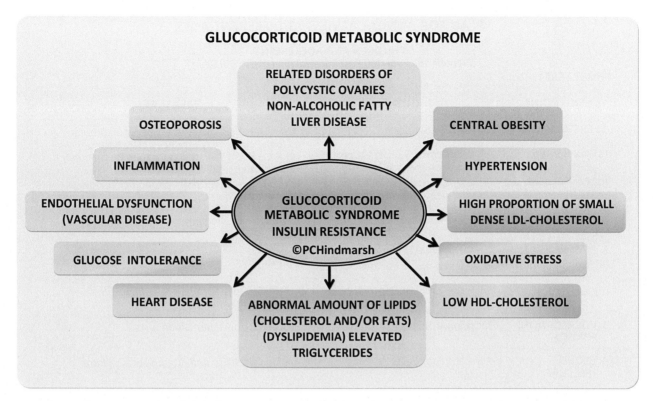

Figure 7.5 *The components of the Glucocorticoid Metabolic Syndrome. Glucocorticoids if present in high amounts, lead to impaired insulin action and insulin resistance which is the central part of the Metabolic Syndrome.*

Glucocorticoids also raise insulin levels in the blood if the cortisol or steroid level is high for long periods of time (see Chapter 8, Part 2). This is why in Figure 7.5, glucocorticoids producing insulin resistance are at the centre of the Syndrome, as these are factors which drive the person to develop this problem.

This cluster of features is not due to adrenal insufficiency itself, but rather from the treatment of the condition with glucocorticoids and fludrocortisone — remembering that fludrocortisone is as potent as dexamethasone. It is not just the dose of glucocorticoid used but also the potency.

The more potent the glucocorticoid is, the more likely there will be problems with this constellation of features.

So, if we are thinking about the Metabolic Syndrome, then our measures might include blood pressure and blood tests for fasting glucose, insulin and cholesterol and the lipid subfractions like LDL-cholesterol, along with body mass index from the obesity standpoint and liver function tests to look at fatty liver development. You can also check this with a liver ultrasound scan, although most clinicians would do liver function tests in the blood first.

If we are looking at bone mineralisation, we would be interested in both short and medium term measures which combine to produce an effect on the skeleton. In the short term, it might be the correct dosing of the steroids we use and in the medium term, in paediatrics for example, if puberty is achieved at the correct time and if it is completed correctly, as this is a key determinant of bone mineralisation.

Figure 7.6 provides a summary of the measures we could undertake at an annual review thinking about short, medium and long term effects.

PLAN FOR ANNUAL REVIEW AT DIFFERENT AGES

CHILDREN AND ADOLESCENT
Prepubertal, Pubertal, Post Pubertal (End of Growth Spurt)

SHORT TERM

END POINT	RATIONALE	MEASURE

1. GROWTH
 	
(a) Acceleration
   CAH
(b) Poor Growth
   CAH
   Addison's Disease
   Hypopituitarism
	1. Assess growth rate
	
	(a) Assess cortisol replacement androgen levels & bone age
	(b) Assess cortisol replacement over treatment & correct distribution
	
	As above include growth hormone
		1. Acceleration - growth acceleration greater than 2cm/year/year needs attention
		(a) Bone age advanced more than 2 years under treatment (CAH)
		(b) Bone age lower than chronological age over treatment
		
		As above including growth hormone replacement

2. WEIGHT **(a) Weight gain** **(b) Weight loss**	2. Assess weight gain/loss (a) Assess amount and distribution of dose (b) Assess amount and distribution of dose	2. Weight gain in excess of 2 kg/year needs attention Weight loss or failure to gain weight needs attention
3. CORRECT DOSE FOR SIZE	3. Optimise Therapy	3. 1 and 2 above and blood tests
4. BLOOD PRESSURE	4. Treatment effects	4. Blood Pressure and plot on centile charts
5. PUBERTY	5. Timing can be altered in CAH & Hypopituitarism	5. Pubertal staging

©PCHindmarsh

CHILDREN AND ADOLESCENT
Prepubertal, Pubertal, Post Pubertal (End of Growth Spurt)

MEDIUM TERM

END POINT	RATIONALE	MEASURE
1. BONE MATURATION	1. Rate of skeletal maturation	1. Yearly Bone age
2. PUBERTAL STATUS	2. Early puberty or rapid progression. Late puberty especially in Hypopituitarism	2. Tanner staging
3. HYDROCORTISONE DOSE	3. Optimise therapy	3. 24 hour profiles measuring cortisol, blood glucose & 17OHP (CAH)
4. FLUDROCORTISONE DOSE	4. Avoid high blood pressure	4. Plasma renin activity & electrolytes Lying/standing blood pressure
5. TESTES AND OVARY HEALTH	5. CAH polycystic ovaries CAH & Addison's Adrenal rests Hypopituitarism function	5. Females: pelvic ultrasound Males: careful examination/sonogram of testes Assessment of sex hormones
6. METABOLIC STATUS	6. Insulin insensitivity and lipids	6. Fasting glucose, insulin and lipids
7. HYPOPITUITARY REPLACEMENT	7. Thyroxine for mental and physical development	7. Free thyroxine measurement
8. VASOPRESSIN REPLACEMENT (DDAVP)	8. Maintain normal sodium to avoid damage to brain tissue from high or low sodium levels	8. Plasma and urine osmolality

©PCHindmarsh

PLAN FOR ANNUAL REVIEW AT DIFFERENT AGES

CHILDREN AND ADOLESCENT
Prepubertal, Pubertal, Post Pubertal (End of Growth Spurt)

LONG TERM

END POINT	RATIONALE	MEASURE
1. GROWTH	1. Outcome	1. Final height within target height of parents
2. BONE MINERALISATION	2. Glucocorticoid effect on bone. Persistent low sodium effect on bone	2. DEXA Scan
3. FERTILITY	3. Effect of CAH/Primary adrenal insufficiency Hypopituitarism	3. Check for regular menstrual cycle in females Polycystic ovaries and syndrome Adrenal rests in males Assessment for fertility treatment. See point 5 for adults below
4. CARDIOVASCULAR RISK	4. Some forms of CAH (11beta-hydroxylase deficiency). Glucocorticoid effect and/or effect of fludrocortisone treatment	4. Fasting glucose and insulin, blood pressure, fasting lipids, body mass index, liver function tests ©PCHindmarsh

ADULTHOOD

END POINT	RATIONALE	MEASURE
1. GENERAL HEALTH	1. Assessing health issues re dosing schedules	1. Blood sampling
2. BLOOD PRESSURE	2. Treatment effects	2. Plasma renin activity & electrolytes Lying/standing blood pressure
3. CARDIOVASCULAR RISK	3. Long term risks from Metabolic Syndrome	3. Fasting glucose and insulin, blood pressure, fasting lipids, body mass index, liver function tests
4. BONE MINERALISATION	4. Glucocorticoid effect on bone. Persistent low sodium effect on bone	4. DEXA Scan Annual or every 2 years
5. FERTILITY	5. Assessing sex hormones	5. Testosterone/Estrogen levels LH and FSH Pelvic ultrasound in females and testicular ultrasound in males
6. CONTRACEPTION	6. Assessing effect of birth control pill on metabolism of hydrocortisone	6. Blood sampling whilst off the pill and blood tests on the pill
7. PREGNANCY	7. Assessing effect of pregnancy hormones on metabolism of hydrocortisone	7. Blood test during pregnancy to ascertain replacement status
8. HORMONE REPLACEMENT IN MALES & FEMALES	8. Assessing testosterone replacement in males Estrogen levels in females	8. Blood tests along with pelvic ultrasound in females and bone mineral density in males and females ©PCHindmarsh

Figure 7.6 *Annual Review plan for patients with various forms of adrenal insufficiency split into age groups.*

CONCLUSION

Cardiovascular disease with or without type 2 Diabetes Mellitus remains the major cause of death in Western society and increasingly around the world. There are many aspects of care, such as glucocorticoid dosing we provide for patients with adrenal insufficiency, which might worsen risks for these conditions. A careful balance between replacement therapy which mimics physiology and wellbeing is essential. Getting as close as possible to the circadian rhythm in terms of replacement dosing will help minimise these risks. This, along with attention to the management of sick day rules will lead to reductions in mortality from illness.

There are also several measures that we can put in place and develop over time. Education of doctors not only those in endocrine training, but also in emergency medicine and anaesthetics around the management of adrenal crises is important. This also includes other health care professionals such as nurses and members of general practices. The conditions we are considering are not common but the associated morbidity and mortality is high. Regular clinic appointments with the same consultant are vital components of the management of chronic health conditions, because consistency is a key component of care delivery and engenders trust between health care practitioners and patients and vice versa.

FURTHER READING

Allolio, B., 2015. Adrenal crisis. Eur J Endocrinol 172, R115–R124.

Auchus, R.J., Witchel, S.F., Leight, K.R., et al., 2010. Guidelines for the development of comprehensive care centers for congenital adrenal hyperplasia: guidance from the CARES Foundation initiative. Int J Pediatr Endocrinol, 2010, Article ID 275213, https://doi.org/10.1155/2010/275213.

Bergthorsdottir, R., Leonsson-Zachrisson, M., Odén, A., Johannsson, G., 2006. Premature mortality in patients with Addison's disease: a population-based study. J Clin Endocrinol Metab 91, 4849–4853.

Burman, P., Mattsson, A.F., Johannsson, G., et al., 2013. Deaths among adult patients with hypopituitarism: hypocortisolism during acute stress, and de novo malignant brain tumors contribute to an increased mortality. J Clin Endocrinol Metab 98, 1466–1475.

Puar, T.H.K., Stikkelbroeck, N.M.M.L., Lisanne, C.C.J., Smans, L.C.C.J., Zelissen, P.M.J., Hermus, R.M.M., 2016. Adrenal crisis: still a deadly event in the 21st century. Am J Med 129, 339.e1–339.e9.

Swerdlow, A.J., Higgins, C., Brook, C.G.D., et al., 1998. Mortality in patients with congenital adrenal hyperplasia: a cohort study. J Pediatr 133, 516–520.

Vella, A., Nippoldt, T.B., Morris, J.C., 2001. Adrenal hemorrhage: a 25 year experience at the Mayo Clinic. Mayo Clin Proc 76, 161–168.

CHAPTER 8

Problems Associated With Adrenal Insufficiency

In Chapter 7, we laid out what a plan for follow up and annual review would look like for people with adrenal insufficiency. In Chapter 8, we look in more detail at some of the common problems associated with glucocorticoid treatment. For mineralocorticoid problems including blood pressure, we cover these in Chapter 14.

We have broken down these common problems into smaller sections so that each part is a standalone mini chapter. We have kept the same format for each of these mini chapters as we have used throughout the book. This means you can delve into each area and get a complete overview which should make access to a wider topic easier.

Replacement Therapies in Adrenal Insufficiency. https://doi.org/10.1016/B978-0-12-824548-4.00024-3

CHAPTER 8.1

Bone Health

GLOSSARY

Avascular necrosis of bone Bone death usually at the head of the femur due to damage to blood vessels supplying the head.

Bone mineral density A measure of how much mineral is present in the bone.

DEXA A scan that measures the bone mineral density.

Fludrocortisone Cortisol modified with a fluorine atom which prolongs action on the mineralocorticoid receptor retaining salt and water.

Glucocorticoids A member of the steroid family similar to cortisol that are particularly involved in carbohydrate, protein and fat metabolism and have anti-inflammatory and immunomodulating properties.

Ligand A substance that binds to a receptor (docking station) to produce an effect on a cell. Ligands can also bind to other substances such as binding proteins. Cortisol (ligand) binding to cortisol binding protein is an example of the latter.

Osteomalacia Softening of the bones in adults. Known as rickets in children.

Osteopenia This is a milder form of reduction in bone mineral density compared to osteoporosis, which is defined on DEXA.

Osteoporosis A marked reduction of mineral in bone which weakens the bone structure thereby increasing the risk of fracture.

RANK(L) Receptor Activator of Nuclear factor—Kappa B (RANK) and its Ligand (L).

Receptor A protein molecule usually in the cell wall to which a ligand can bind to produce an effect inside the cell.

Slipped femoral epiphysis Slippage of the coverings of the head of the femur.

GENERAL

The development of osteoporosis in the general population is a major public health problem. Osteoporosis is the term used to describe the reduction in the amount of mineral in bone. The main mineral is calcium and in osteoporosis there is a loss of calcium deposited in the fine structure of bone. Approximately 1% of all adults and 3% of adults older than 50 years of age receive glucocorticoids for a number of indications such as inflammatory conditions, as well as for adrenal insufficiency.

The reason osteoporosis is of concern is because it is associated with weak bones and increased risk of fracture.

The risk of fracture increases in patients who have adrenal insufficiency with:

- Age as it does in the general population.
- Type of glucocorticoid used - potency and duration of action.
- The dose and distribution of the dose over 24 hours.

Generally speaking, when we are talking about fracture, we are talking about high dose glucocorticoid use such as when used as anti-inflammatory agents. Given that in adrenal insufficiency we are trying to replace cortisol as close as possible to the normal circadian rhythm, to prevent over treatment we still must be aware of the effects of glucocorticoids on bone density. This is particularly the case when glucocorticoids with high potency such as prednisolone and dexamethasone are used.

Before we address this question, we need to look at how the body handles calcium and what is happening in the bones to use calcium to form bone and maintain bone strength.

CALCIUM REGULATION

Like many blood components, calcium is regulated quite tightly and is maintained in the blood with a plasma concentration between 2.2 and 2.6 mmol/l. Low calcium can lead to spasms, seizures and heart rhythm problems, as well as bone pain. High calcium can produce abdominal pain, kidney stones, and confusion and depression (Figure 8.1).

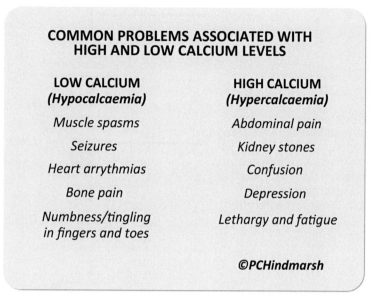

COMMON PROBLEMS ASSOCIATED WITH HIGH AND LOW CALCIUM LEVELS

LOW CALCIUM (Hypocalcaemia)	HIGH CALCIUM (Hypercalcaemia)
Muscle spasms	Abdominal pain
Seizures	Kidney stones
Heart arrythmias	Confusion
Bone pain	Depression
Numbness/tingling in fingers and toes	Lethargy and fatigue

©PCHindmarsh

Figure 8.1 *Common health problems associated with low or high calcium levels in the circulation.*

The level of the calcium in plasma is regulated by the hormones parathyroid hormone (PTH) and calcitonin. PTH is released by the parathyroid glands which are situated immediately behind the thyroid gland in the middle of the neck just below the 'Adam's apple.' Parathyroid hormone is secreted when the plasma calcium level falls below the normal range in order to raise it; calcitonin is released by the parafollicular cells of the thyroid gland when the plasma level of calcium is above the normal range in order to lower it.

Calcium levels are sensed in the parathyroid cells by the calcium sensing receptor. If calcium levels are low, then PTH is released. Parathyroid hormone regulates the last step in the formation of the active form of vitamin D — 1,25-dihydroxycholecalciferol.

The whole pathway starts from cholesterol or rather 7-dehydrocholesterol, which under the effect of ultraviolet radiation from the sun, is converted into cholecalciferol in the skin and is further modified in the liver to calcidiol and then to calcitriol (1,25-dihydroxycholecalciferol) in the kidney (Figure 8.2, page 150). Dietary sources of vitamin D such as ergocalciferol from eggs are also metabolised in the liver to calcidiol.

Vitamin D plays a crucial role in regulating calcium in the body and its absence leads to a softening of the bone which is known as rickets in children. When softening of the bones occurs in adults, it is known as osteomalacia. Osteomalacia occurs when there is a problem with the formation of bone as the condition keeps the bones from mineralizing or hardening as they should.

Osteomalacia should not to be confused with osteoporosis, as although both conditions can cause bones to fracture, osteomalacia is a problem with bone not hardening, whereas osteoporosis is the weakening of bones once they have been formed.

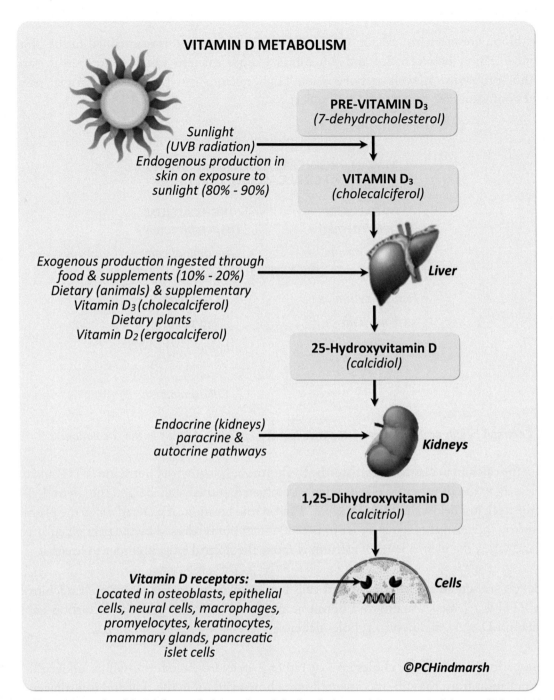

Figure 8.2 *Formation of calcitriol from cholesterol. 7-dehydrocholesterol is converted by sunlight in the skin to cholecalciferol which is metabolised further in the liver to calcidiol. Vitamin D in the diet such as in eggs comes in as ergocalciferol and it too is metabolised by the liver to calcidiol. The final step, the formation of calcitriol takes place in the kidneys.*

This means that vitamin D and calcium supplements are really good as they are involved in bone formation, but less so in preventing bone loss, therefore they are better at preventing osteomalacia rather than osteoporosis. It is important that the endocrinologist is involved in prescribing and monitoring these supplements to avoid over treatment.

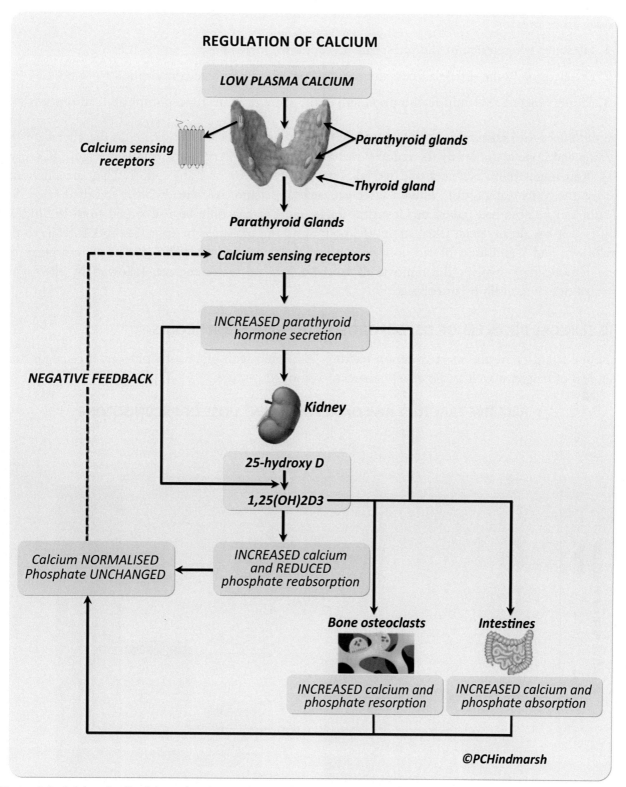

Figure 8.3 *Calcium feedback loop showing activation of parathyroid hormone release as a result of a low plasma calcium level leading to increased calcium resorption from bone and calcium reabsorption from kidneys and increased calcium absorption from the intestine mediated by parathyroid hormone and 1,25-dihydroxycholecalciferol formation in the kidney.*

Now back to our low calcium problem. We now have PTH produced as well as 1,25-dihydroxycholecalciferol which work together to raise calcium concentrations. They do this through three organs:

1. Intestines where calcium and phosphate absorption is increased.

2. Bones through the osteoclast cells increase calcium and phosphate reabsorption from bone.

3. Kidneys increase calcium reabsorption and at the same time decrease phosphate reabsorption.

The net effect is to raise calcium concentrations without any effect on phosphate, as the effects on the intestine and bone are offset by the reduced reabsorption of phosphate by the kidneys (Figure 8.3, page 151). You might think that it is odd we talk about reabsorption and absorption. They are different!! We use the term reabsorption when a substance such as calcium has already been absorbed once. So, calcium can be absorbed (taken up) from the intestines, but can only be reabsorbed from the kidney tubules as it has already been taken up by the body from the intestine. In bone, resorption refers to the breakdown and assimilation of old bone in the cycle of bone growth. The process of resorption (or bone remodelling) involves the removal of hard bone tissue by osteoclasts, followed by the laying down of new bone cells by osteoblasts.

THE CLINICAL PROBLEM OF OSTEOPOROSIS AND GLUCOCORTICOIDS

Vertebral fractures are the most common fractures associated with glucocorticoids and a cause of back pain, loss of height as well as the development of a stooped posture.

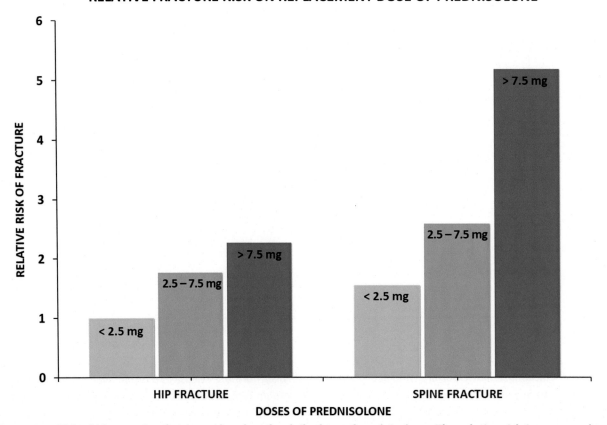

Figure 8.4 *Risk of hip or spine fracture related to the daily dose of prednisolone. The relative risk is compared to a control group of age and gender matched individuals which are allocated a relative risk of one. Reproduced from data in Van Staa, T.P., Leufkens, H.G., Abenhaim, L., Zhang, B., Cooper, C., 2000. Use of oral corticosteroids and risk of fractures. J Bone Miner Res 15, 993–1000.*

The risk of a vertebral fracture increases within 3 months after initiation of treatment and peaks at 12 months. The relative risk of a fracture doubles and the risk of hip fracture increases by 50% among people receiving 2.5 to 7.5 mg of prednisolone daily. Note these doses of prednisolone are not too far away from replacement therapy and probably reflect the greater potency of prednisolone compared to hydrocortisone. Figure 8.4 shows the increased risk of fracture at the spine and hip sites with a clear increase once total daily prednisolone doses exceed 2.5 mg per day. On an equivalent dose for dose basis, prednisolone has a much greater effect on bone mineral density than hydrocortisone.

Figure 8.5 shows risk factors for fractures in patients receiving glucocorticoids.

Many of these are related to the risk of developing osteoporosis in general. In particular, when we are considering secondary adrenal insufficiency due to hypopituitarism, it is important that adequate replacement of estrogens or testosterone when missing, is undertaken to protect the bones long term.

FRACTURE RISK FACTORS
ASSOCIATED WITH GLUCOCORTICOID REPLACEMENT THERAPY

- *Age greater than 55 years*
- *Female*
- *Menopause*
- *Smoking*
- *Caucasian*
- *Long term use of prednisolone at a dose of more than 2.5mg per day*
- *Glucocorticoid associated myopathy*
- *Hypogonadism*
- *Lack of weight-bearing physical activity*
- *Obesity*

©PCHindmarsh

Figure 8.5 *Risk factors for fractures in patients receiving glucocorticoids.*

When secondary adrenal insufficiency is due to treatment of inflammatory conditions with high dose of steroids, then consideration should be given to how easily the glucocorticoid dose schedule can be reduced. Careful monitoring of bone health should be undertaken using DEXA scans. How often these should be undertaken depends on what the results of the initial scan are. If the results show osteoporosis, then intervention is required and that would mean annual scans to check on progress will be required. There is no need for scans more frequently than yearly as density changes are not reflected quickly in the scan results obtained, so yearly is adequate. If the scan is normal then repeat scans every 2 years will be adequate. The difficult area is osteopenia (see definitions in the measuring bone mineral density section) where intervention is mainly with vitamin D therapy and scans probably should be checked on a yearly basis. In fact there is a good argument that anyone on long term glucocorticoid treatments should receive vitamin D and calcium supplements.

Exposure to glucocorticoids should be minimised as much as possible in order to protect bone health.

An additional problem associated with high dose glucocorticoid treatment, is myopathy or weakness of the muscles can occur which can increase the risk of falls and the risk of fracture.

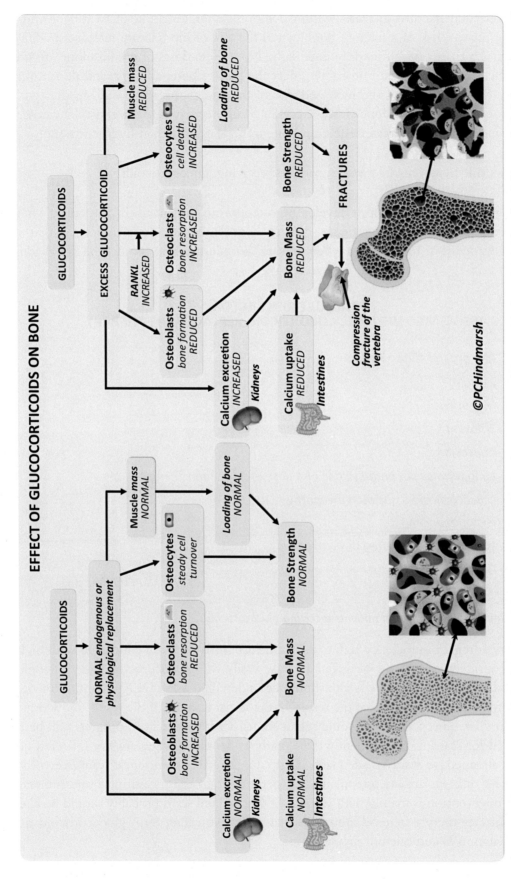

Figure 8.6 *Effect of glucocorticoids in physiological amounts in the left panel compared to excess glucocorticoid in the right panel. Both bone mass and bone strength are impacted upon by glucocorticoids with a switch in favour of osteoclast numbers leading to increased bone resorption.*

GLUCOCORTICOID EFFECTS ON BONE

Glucocorticoids affect bone structure quickly. The effect takes place at multiple levels altering bone mass and bone strength (Figure 8.6, page 154).

We have already mentioned that calcium and vitamin D play an important role in bone formation and glucocorticoids impact on this, by reducing calcium uptake from the intestine and increasing calcium excretion from the kidney into the urine. They also decrease the cells involved in bone formation (osteoblasts), whilst at the same time through the RANKL system (the importance of which we will look at when we consider therapies to improve osteoporosis), increase bone resorption through the osteoclasts.

Normally, the osteoblasts and osteoclasts as well as the osteocytes, are balanced so none predominate over the others. Bone is actively forming and remodelling due to the activity of these cells. In fact, RANKL, which stands for Receptor (docking station for a ligand), Activator of Nuclear factor—Kappa B (RANK) and its Ligand, is involved in both processes. A ligand is a substance (in endocrinology usually a protein or steroid) which binds specifically to a receptor or another substance such as a binding protein. RANKL is released by the osteoblasts and stimulates RANK on the surface of bone stem cells to form osteoclasts.

The same pair of proteins can also signal in reverse from osteoclasts to osteoblasts, so the system is balanced.

1. Glucocorticoids, by decreasing the osteoblast population, tip the balance in favour of the osteoclasts and bone resorption.

2. Bone strength is also impacted upon by glucocorticoids.

3. There is an indirect effect reducing muscle mass which reduces the load carried by bone. This reduced muscle mass also leads to falls and fractures.

4. Osteocytes, which form the architecture of bone and are derived from osteoblasts, undergo programmed cell death (apoptosis) in the presence of high amounts of glucocorticoid, reducing the bone's tensile (resistance of a bone to breaking) strength.

It is important to realise that all the information we have available comes from adult patients who have used high doses of glucocorticoids and we simply do not know at this stage the situation which is going to pertain in patients with adrenal insufficiency.

Glucocorticoid doses in adrenal insufficiency are much lower of course and are only used for replacement and even when high doses are used during periods when the person is sick, they are not used for long periods of time which is when most problems are associated with glucocorticoid induced osteoporosis. This may not be the case however, with the more potent glucocorticoids, prednisolone and dexamethasone, as seen in Figure 8.4. There is no information at present to suggest that fracture risk in people with adrenal insufficiency is likely to be any different to the general population.

It is not only glucocorticoids we need to consider, as fludrocortisone has dexamethasone like effects and needs to be considered when looking at the daily glucocorticoid dose (see Chapter 14). In addition, running a low plasma sodium over long periods of time leads to problems. Much of the sodium in the body is found in bone, cartilage and connective tissue. Longstanding low plasma sodium levels are a more potent cause of osteoporosis/osteopenia than vitamin D deficiency. The activity of the osteoclasts which reabsorb bone is increased when sodium levels are low for periods of time.

Measuring bone mineral density

Bone density is measured using a technique called Dual Photon Absorption (DEXA) scanning. The scan passes a small beam of x-ray through a specific area of the bone. The speed at which the beam goes through the bone is dependent on the density of the bone and this is detected by a series of cameras which pick up the passage of the beam. There follows a series of complex calculations to determine what the likely density of that part of the skeleton is. Figure 8.7 gives an idea of the type of image which can be obtained.

The data can be recorded in a variety of ways such as T–scores, which show the individual's DEXA results compared to the ideal peak bone density of a healthy adult, or as a Z–score which compares the individual's DEXA results to the average reference range which is based on the same age, weight, height and gender of the general population as the individual.

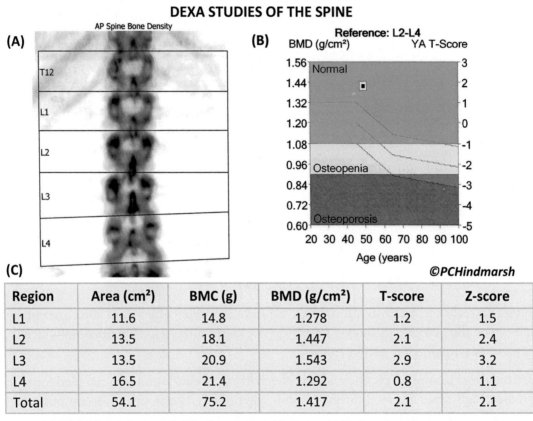

Region	Area (cm²)	BMC (g)	BMD (g/cm²)	T-score	Z-score
L1	11.6	14.8	1.278	1.2	1.5
L2	13.5	18.1	1.447	2.1	2.4
L3	13.5	20.9	1.543	2.9	3.2
L4	16.5	21.4	1.292	0.8	1.1
Total	54.1	75.2	1.417	2.1	2.1

Figure 8.7 *Actual DEXA picture in top left (A) of the spine with the actual value plotted on reference chart on right (B). A table (C) of the data for comparison with reference values is shown below these two pictures for the four lumbar vertebrae individually and as a total. (BMC - bone mineral content); (BMD - bone mineral density).*

A positive Z score means good bone density. A value between 0 and –2 is satisfactory but between –1 and –2 is often referred to as osteopenia or low density. Values below –2 are associated with an increased risk of fractures and this area is termed osteoporosis. A similar set of results can be obtained at the hip (Figure 8.8)

The effects of dexamethasone can be seen in Figure 8.9 in a person who received high doses of dexamethasone for a period of time in an attempt to manage their CAH. The graph and table depict the change in density over a period of time and the effects of the dexamethasone is to flat line the scan data at lower values than expected.

DEXA STUDIES OF THE HIP

(A)

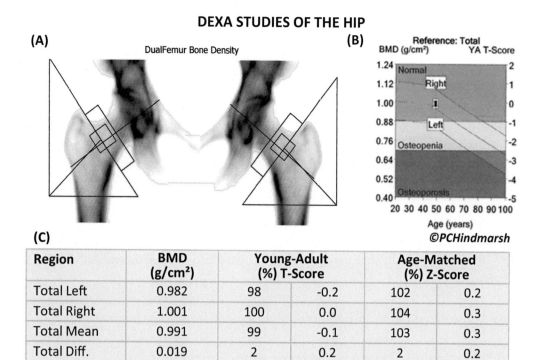

(B)

(C)

Region	BMD (g/cm²)	Young-Adult (%) T-Score		Age-Matched (%) Z-Score	
Total Left	0.982	98	-0.2	102	0.2
Total Right	1.001	100	0.0	104	0.3
Total Mean	0.991	99	-0.1	103	0.3
Total Diff.	0.019	2	0.2	2	0.2

Figure 8.8 Actual DEXA picture in top left (A) of a hip with the actual value plotted on reference chart on right (B). A table (C) of the data for comparison with reference values is shown below these two pictures. (BMC - bone mineral content); (BMD - bone mineral density).

DEXA STUDIES OF THE SPINE FOLLOWING DEXAMETHASONE TREATMENT

(A)   **(B)**

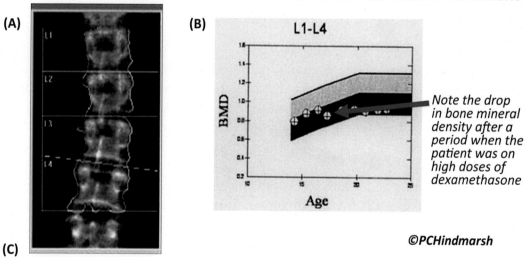

(C)

Region	Area[cm²]	BMC (g)	BMD (g/cm²)	T-Score	PR (Peak reference)	Z-Score	AM (Age matched)
L1	14.32	12.51	0.874	-1.2	87	-1.2	87
L2	14.97	14.03	0.937	-1.4	86	-1.4	86
L3	17.53	16.25	0.927	-1.6	84	-1.6	84
L4	18.87	18.11	0.959	-1.7	84	-1.7	84
Total	65.69	60.90	0.927	-1.5	85	-1.5	85

Figure 8.9 Actual DEXA Scan of the spine (A) of someone who has congenital adrenal hyperplasia and had received a considerable amount of dexamethasone. The actual value is plotted on the reference chart on the right (B) and a table (C) of the data for comparison with reference values is below (BMC - bone mineral content); (BMD - bone mineral density).

WAYS TO IMPROVE BONE MINERAL DENSITY

A variety of non drug interventions can be advised in people on high doses of glucocorticoids and these suggestions probably also apply to those on replacement treatment. The suggestions include undertaking weight bearing exercise, maintenance of normal weight, avoidance of smoking, limited alcohol intake and ongoing assessment of fall risks.

Proton pump inhibitors which are used to reduce gastric acidity may alter absorption of calcium and vitamin D. As these inhibitors are often used in patients receiving glucocorticoid therapy, the continuation of them needs to be considered with the treating endocrinologist.

Calcium and Vitamin D

All people receiving glucocorticoid therapy should receive adequate calcium supplementation of approximately 1200 mg/day in divided doses with added vitamin D supplementation of between 800 and 2000 units per day.

These doses are known to provide an optimum environment for laying down bone.

Studies have shown calcium and vitamin D supplementation prevents a decrease in spinal bone mineral density during long term use of low dose prednisolone (5 mg/day), but did not completely prevent bone loss in those receiving higher doses. We would predict this because vitamin D and calcium are important for bone formation mainly, but if loss exceeds formation the overall effect will be less, but better than no supplementation at all. Another situation which calls for or reinforces the need for assessing whether calcium and vitamin D supplementation is required, is for patients taking proton pump inhibitors for gastritis. Any supplementation should be on the basis of blood testing for calcium and vitamin D.

Treatment for Established Osteoporosis

The treatments to prevent additional fractures should be introduced for any patient with a previous osteoporotic fracture who is receiving glucocorticoids, (prednisolone dose greater than 2.5 mg/day). This is also extended for adults receiving glucocorticoids and have a bone mineral density score of less than 2.5 at either the spine or hip, for men who are 50 years of age or older and for all post-menopausal women.

The mainstay of treatment which helps with glucocorticoid induced osteoporosis is bisphosphonate treatment. This increases bone mineral density. Bisphosphonates have a good safety profile and oral bisphosphonates are the first line agents followed by intravenous bisphosphonates.

Monoclonal antibodies (such as those raised against RANKL) (Denosumab) which inhibit bone reabsorption may actually be superior to bisphosphonates, but there is limited available safety data and in studies there was a higher risk of infection with these agents than with bisphosphonates.

Denosumab blocks RANKL stimulated osteoclast formation (Figure 8.10, page 159).

We still need long term studies to determine the best way to manage bone density for young people with adrenal insufficiency who need long term glucocorticoid treatment.

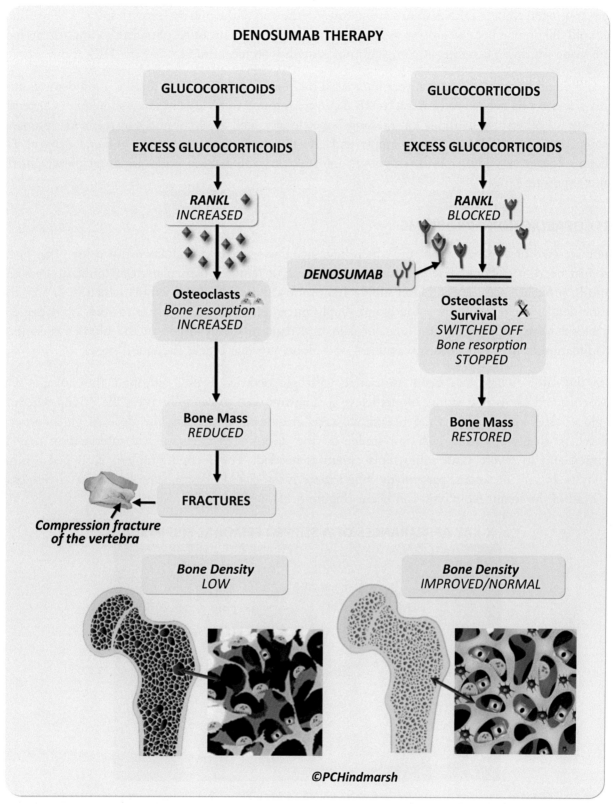

Figure 8.10 *Glucocorticoids increase RANKL which in turn through the osteoclasts increases bone resorption reducing bone mass and leading to fractures. Denosumab is a monoclonal antibody raised against RANKL which binds RANKL and reduces osteoclast survival leading to cessation of bone resorption and restoration of bone mass.*

Monitoring

We recommend routine DEXA scans starting towards the end of the puberty growth spurt. The reason to wait until this point is because growth itself upsets the actual density measures obtained, so adjustments have to be made for this. Therefore, at completion of growth is an ideal time to start the DEXA monitoring.

These should be carried out at two year intervals if the results are normal and there is good density, but a yearly scan may be needed to establish trends if density is found to be lower than it should be. Currently, there are no other easy methods for assessing bone density such as ultrasound and magnetic resonance imaging scanning. DEXA is a very simple and effective way of assessing bone mineral density. The radiation dose is very low, and the important information gained about bone health far outweighs this minor exposure.

ORTHOPAEDIC BONE PROBLEMS

There are two orthopaedic problems which have been associated with glucocorticoid use. The first is avascular necrosis of bone. The head of the thigh bone or femur is particularly susceptible to avascular necrosis, probably because the blood supply has to cross the neck of the femur, which is an area that can be damaged easily, or rather the blood supply interrupted. Possible reasons for this are damage to the blood vessels due to fracture (e.g., broken hip) damage to the inside of the blood vessels (e.g., inflammation of the blood vessels, vasculitis) or a blood clot that blocks the blood vessel.

It is the latter which has been associated with glucocorticoid use, although the linkage with glucocorticoid use is not strong. Nonetheless, it is always wise to carefully assess the dosing schedules of glucocorticoids and this is the reason we take great care in titrating the dose of glucocorticoid exactly, so that we neither over nor under do the dosing schedule. Surgical intervention may be required and in severe cases a hip replacement is needed. The second problem is slipped femoral epiphysis. In rare occasions, particularly when there is associated obesity, slippage of the coverings of the head of the femur (epiphysis) can occur (Figure 8.11).

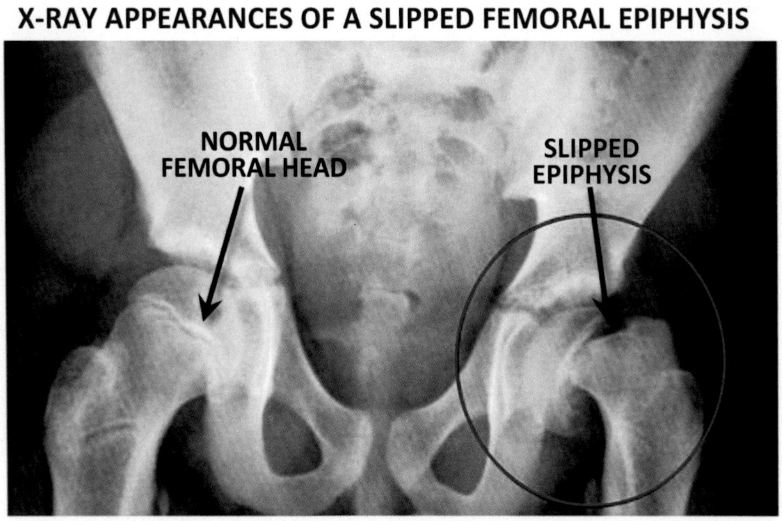

X-RAY APPEARANCES OF A SLIPPED FEMORAL EPIPHYSIS

Figure 8.11 *Hip x-ray showing normal femur fitting into hip socket with epiphysis sitting within the socket on the neck of the femur. On the opposite side (circled) is the head of the femur with a displaced (slipped) epiphysis.*

The femur is the long bone, the thigh bone. The epiphysis can slip quite easily especially in individuals who are overweight and that is why there is a lot of emphasis on monitoring weight and body mass index. Glucocorticoids have not been directly implicated in slipped upper femoral epiphysis and it is probably more a secondary effect of the increase in body weight, rather than an effect of the glucocorticoids on the cartilage. Surgical intervention is needed to stabilise the growth plate and epiphysis.

The final problem that glucocorticoids have on the bone relates to the growth plate and the growth cartilage. This is a problem in children. The growth plate is a complex structure with pre-chondrocytes at the cartilage end, which are selected for multiplication (proliferation) and increase in cell size (hypertrophy) to form chondrocytes by growth hormone and the local generation of insulin-like growth factor-1. The chondrocytes are arranged in columns and kept in this position by the cartilage matrix. The chondrocytes as they progress down the columns, become gradually surrounded by bone forming cells and add onto the bone present causing lengthening of the bone (Figure 8.12).

Glucocorticoids have a direct, inhibitory effect on the growth plate, as demonstrated by in vivo and organ culture studies. Glucocorticoids slow longitudinal bone growth by inhibiting chondrocyte proliferation, hypertrophy, and cartilage matrix synthesis.

ARCHITECTURE OF THE GROWTH PLATE

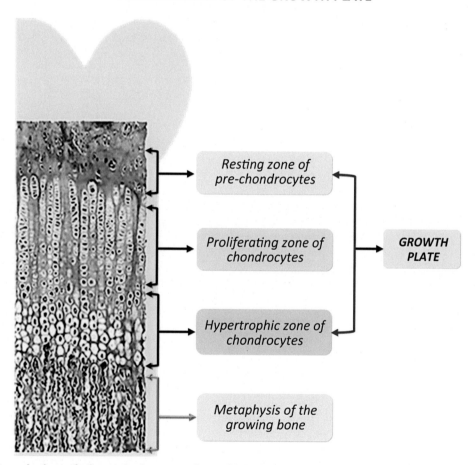

Figure 8.12 *Growth plate of a bone. At the top at the surface of the growth plate cartilage are pre-chondrocytes which develop into chondrocytes which expand in number and size. Note the arrangement of chondrocytes in columns.*

If the exposure to higher than replacement glucocorticoids is over a short period of time (2 to 3 weeks), then growth slows but picks up again and catches up once the high dose is reduced to normal replacement amounts. If the exposure is for longer periods of time or there are repeated exposures, then damage to the growth plate takes place. Unfortunately, we cannot see this on x-rays for bone age that we undertake. The bone age may look fine and the epiphyses look open, but they are damaged and the actual growth which may result may be very compromised and not reversible.

CONCLUSION

Glucocorticoids have effects on bone mineral density directly altering the bone mass and indirectly muscle mass leading to a higher risk of falls and fractures. Osteoporosis is a major public health problem. Supplementation with vitamin D and calcium help in bone formation but are less effective in preventing bone loss. DEXA scanning is a simple and effective way of monitoring bone density and should be undertaken every two years if values are within the normal range and yearly if they are indicative of osteoporosis. Bisphosphonate therapy is proven to improve osteoporosis due to high dose glucocorticoid use. Monoclonal antibody therapy may prove to be even more effective.

FURTHER READING

Hoorn, E.J., Liamis, G., Zietse, R., Zillikens, M.C., 2011. Hyponatremia and bone: an emerging relationship. Nat Rev Endocrinol 8, 33—39.

Koetz, K.R., Ventz, M., Diederich, S., Quinkler, M., 2012. Bone mineral density is not significantly reduced in adult patients on low-dose glucocorticoid replacement therapy. J Clin Endocrinol Metab 97, 85—92.

Liu, J.C., Baron, J., 2011. Effects of glucocorticoids on the growth plate. Endocr Dev 20, 187—193.

Ray, L.B., 2018. RANKL in bone homeostasis. Science 362, 42—43.

Van Staa, T.P., Leufkens, H.G.M., Abenhaim, L., Zhang, B., Cooper, C., 2000. Use of oral corticosteroids and risk of fractures. J Bone Miner Res 15, 993—1000.

Weinstein, R.S., 2011. Clinical practice. Glucocorticoid-induced bone disease. N Engl J Med 365, 62—70.

CHAPTER 8.2

Weight, Glucose and Insulin

GLOSSARY

High blood lipids Also known as hyperlipidaemia where cholesterol and triglycerides in the blood are raised. These lipids are known to lead to heart disease if raised for long periods of time.

Blood pressure In paediatric practice, blood pressure greater than 90th centile for age is regarded as high blood pressure, if greater than 95th centile for age is regarded as hypertension. In adult practice, hypertension is blood pressure greater than 140 mm Hg systolic/90 mm Hg diastolic.

Obesity In paediatric practice overweight is when the body mass index is above the 90th centile and obesity when it is over the 95th centile. In adult practice, a body mass index between 25 and 30 kg/m^2 is within the overweight range, whereas greater than 30 kg/m^2 is defined as obese and is subdivided further into Class 1 between 30 and 34.9 kg/m^2, Class 2 35 and 39.9 kg/m^2 and Class 3 (often referred to as morbidly obese) values greater than 40 kg/m^2.

Type 2 diabetes mellitus Form of diabetes where insulin does not work as well as it should and is associated with high risk of diabetes complications, such as kidney failure, blindness and heart disease.

WEIGHT GAIN

When glucocorticoids were first used in high doses for inflammatory conditions it was clear they had the ability to increase body fat, blood pressure and blood glucose. In fact, the change in the latter was so great that often diabetes was associated with high dose glucocorticoid use. In paediatric practice medicines are dosed on body size and over the years the glucocorticoid doses used has decreased over time from the original hydrocortisone schedule of 25 mg/m^2 body surface area/day in the 1970s and 80s down to the current value of about 10 to 12 mg/m^2 body surface area/day in CAH and 8 to 10 mg/m^2 body surface area/day in other forms of adrenal insufficiency. The original dose of 25 mg/m^2 body surface area/day was derived from urine excretion studies in the 1960s and conversion from the original use of cortisone acetate. Over time as it became apparent the dose was high from a clinical standpoint and with better ways of estimating cortisol production rates the dose gradually declined.

There are two critical doses to note: 30 mg/m^2 body surface area/day, which is associated with poor height gain and excessive weight gain and 18 to 20 mg/m^2 body surface area/day, which has been clearly associated with weight gain but height gain was generally normal. That is not to say that weight gain cannot take place on current dosing schedules because it can, particularly if the distribution of cortisol through the 24 hour period is not correct. Several adult practices tend to use fixed doses irrespective of body size which may potentially lead to problems due to the variance of clearance and absorption of glucocorticoids in individuals (see Chapter 6).

Weight is an easy measure to obtain in both paediatric and adult practice. In paediatrics weight can be plotted on weight charts which are divided into a series of centile lines from 0.4 through to 99.6. Because weight does not change that much year on year in children (only about 2 kilograms/year) it is not as useful as height for monitoring growth but it is quite useful as part of our assessment of the effects of hydrocortisone treatment because if you give too much hydrocortisone then you will put on weight.

Replacement Therapies in Adrenal Insufficiency. https://doi.org/10.1016/B978-0-12-824548-4.00017-6

In adult practice centiles are not available. Here a measurement of weight can be extremely useful if it is combined with a measure of height, as this allows the calculation of body mass index as shown in Figure 8.13. Body mass index (BMI) equals a person's weight in kilograms divided by their height in metres multiplied by their height in metres or:

BMI = Weight (kilograms) / Height (metres) x Height (metres).

WEIGHT AND BODY MASS INDEX

WEIGHT CLASSIFICATIONS	BMI (kg/m²)
Underweight	<18.5
Normal/Healthy Weight	18.5 – 24.9
Overweight	25 – 29.9
Obese	30 – 39.9
Morbidly Obese	>40

Figure 8.13 *Body Mass Index Chart for adults.*

In paediatric practice there are a series of charts for body mass index for females and males (Figure 8.14).

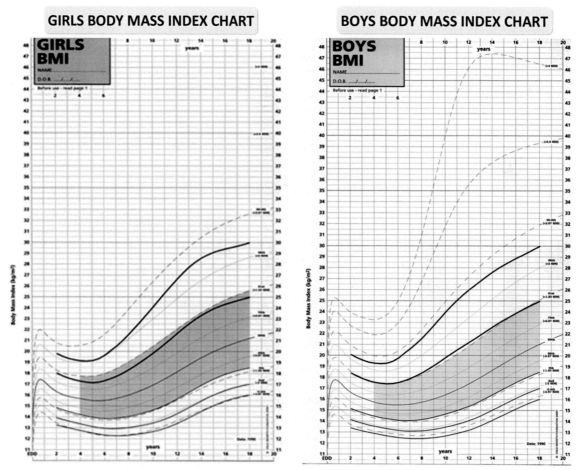

Figure 8.14 *Body Mass Index Charts for boys and girls.* (Charts copyright Child Growth Foundation, reproduced with kind permission).

In paediatric practice overweight is when your BMI is above the 90th centile and obesity when it is over the 95th centile.

In adult practice, a BMI between 25 and 30 kg/m^2 is within the overweight range, whereas a BMI greater than 30 kg/m^2 is defined as obese and can be subdivided further into Class 1 between 30 and 34.9 kg/m^2, Class 2 35 and 39.9 kg/m^2 and Class 3 (often referred to as morbidly obese) values greater than 40 kg/m^2.

In the general population BMI is a useful marker of body fat but it needs to be interpreted with caution because an increase in muscle mass for example, would increase body weight but would not reflect an increase in body fat. The England Rugby Union team are a good example of this.

Weight gain impacts on a number of conditions (Figure 8.15). Some of these effects are direct such as osteoarthritis and episodes when breathing stops (apnoea) particularly at night whereas the effect of obesity on type 2 diabetes is more indirect and mediated through effects on insulin action. Despite the limitations of the study designs, there is consistent evidence that obesity is associated with an increased risk for a number of cancers. Among postmenopausal women, those who are obese have a 20% to 40% increase in risk of developing breast cancer compared with normal weight women.

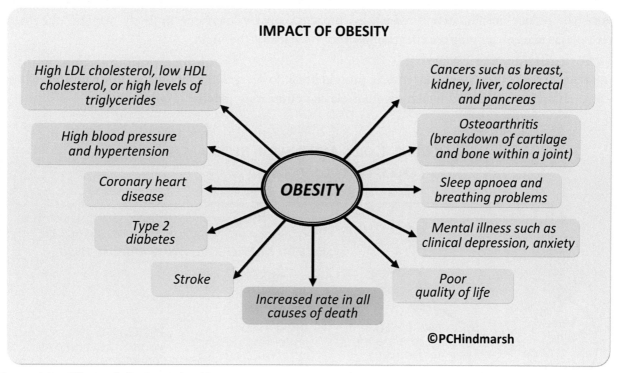

Figure 8.15 *Effects of obesity on health.*

What to Do about Weight Gain

Both overweight and obesity bring with them health problems. Early weight gain is a sign of over treatment and we can resolve the issue by readdressing the amount of glucocorticoid given and the distribution of the glucocorticoid, with carefully constructed 24 hour cortisol profiles. Using this approach along with knowledge of how the individual absorbs and clears hydrocortisone, treatment can be individualised and over treatment avoided. Such an approach can only be used with hydrocortisone as it is not possible to measure dexamethasone and only rarely prednisolone. This is another reason for clinicians not to use the more potent agents, prednisolone or dexamethasone.

Unless the distribution of hydrocortisone is checked and adjusted over the 24 hour period and higher potency glucocorticoids avoided, trying to reduce weight by diet and exercise will not work. It may prevent further increases in weight, but it is unlikely to lead to a reduction. Care can be exercised however, in dietary choices for all on glucocorticoid therapy as we would in any person irrespective of whether they have adrenal insufficiency or not. This includes including grains as the largest portion of food in every meal along with vegetables and fruit and a moderate amount of milk, meat, fish and egg. Intake of foods with high fat, salt and sugar content should be reduced. Above all have regular meal times.

The principles of healthy eating apply to all !!

GLUCOSE AND INSULIN METABOLISM

High Glucose

Glucocorticoids as their name implies are involved in the way the body handles glucose. Their predominant action is to reduce the effect that insulin has on the cells in liver, muscle and fat. This is a complex process and involves many different pathways in muscle and the liver which essentially increase glucose release from the liver or reduce glucose uptake in the muscles.

In fat there are a series of steps that increase glucose uptake and expansion of the fat mass with release of free fatty acids into the circulation which can be used by muscle to release glucose. Free fatty acids themselves reduce insulin action which is impacted on by increases in body weight due to an increased fat mass or by indirect effects of cortisol on parts of the brain.

In muscle, glucocorticoids enhance muscle protein breakdown and in liver glucose formation. At all sites glucose utilization is reduced which together elevate circulating glucose (Figure 8.16).

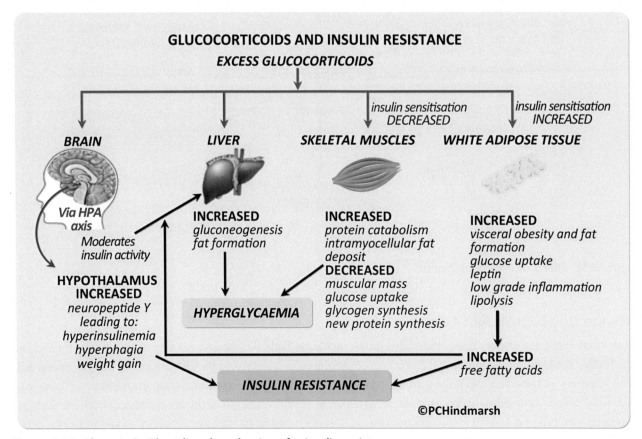

Figure 8.16 *Glucocorticoid mediated mechanisms for insulin resistance.*

This reduction in insulin action is offset by an increase in insulin production to keep the blood glucose levels within the normal range. There is a large capacity in the pancreas to do this but if this increased demand is continued over long periods of time (10 to 30 years), then the cells which make insulin in the pancreas can fail and this can lead to diabetes.

Figure 8.17 shows the relationship between glucose and insulin during fasting and shows although blood glucose concentrations are kept within a very tight range, insulin secretion varies considerably and actually oscillates every 13 minutes to readjust the amount of insulin produced, to meet the needs of the body with respect to the amount of glucose available for energy.

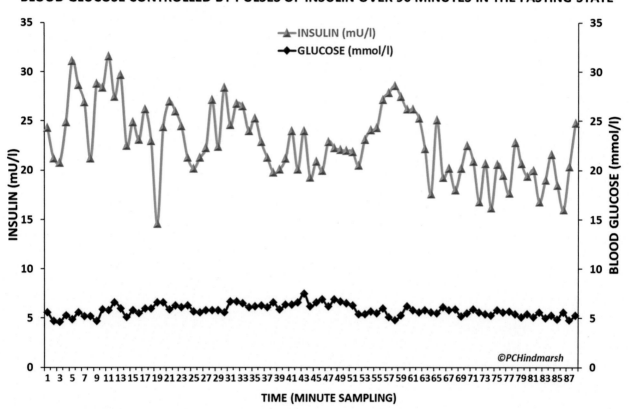

BLOOD GLUCOSE CONTROLLED BY PULSES OF INSULIN OVER 90 MINUTES IN THE FASTING STATE

Figure 8.17 *Insulin levels (green line) oscillate in the fasting state to maintain blood glucose concentrations (red line) constant within a very tight range.*

Although insulin is extremely effective in regulating blood glucose there are problems when insulin concentrations are persistently high.

The first, is insulin resistance of the different organs of the body varies. Initially, the first organ to become less responsive is the liver, followed by muscle and then fat. When the liver becomes less responsive to high levels of insulin, but fat tissue does not, glucose will be diverted into the fat cells where it is converted and stored as fat.

The second problem is, as we have mentioned, although the pancreatic beta cells can compensate for the increased demand this cannot be met over long periods of time. As blood glucose levels start to increase the higher glucose concentrations along with the raised blood fats damage the beta cells. Initially, the insulin pulses are lost which although insulin levels are high, makes insulin less effective and over time the cells are unable to step up their insulin production when required.

High insulin concentrations with insulin resistance are associated with problems developing in the cardiovascular system in the heart, the small blood vessels become narrowed which can lead to heart attacks in the longer term and in the peripheral circulation the high insulin concentrations lead to hypertension.

It is for these reasons we wish to keep the blood glucose levels in the fasting state between 3.5 and 5.6 mmol/l and to ensure that fasting insulin levels do not go any higher than 25 mU/l. Blood glucose is maintained at a very constant level between 4 and 6.5 mmol/l. Occasionally it may dip a little bit lower than this down to 3.5 mmol/l in young children who fast overnight.

We can use the blood glucose measurements in the fasting state and also the glucose measurements obtained when a person drinks a glucose drink. The latter is known as an oral glucose tolerance test and the key glucose measure is at 2 hours after the drink. The test needs to be undertaken after an overnight fast. Laboratory measurements of plasma glucose are made immediately before the glucose drink and again 2 hours later, although some centres sample every 30 minutes over the 2 hours. The test is standardised on the time zero and 120 minute samples. The glucose drink is standardised at 1.75 grams of glucose per kilogram body weight to a maximum of 75 grams.

Figure 8.18 shows the classification of how glucose is handled from normal through to frank diabetes.

GLUCOSE LEVELS AND DEFINITION OF DIABETES

DIAGNOSIS	FASTING GLUCOSE (mmol/l)	2 HOURS AFTER GLUCOSE DRINK (mmol/l)
NORMAL	<5.6	<7.8
IMPAIRED	5.6 – 6.9	7.8 – 11.0
DIABETES	>7.0	>11.1

Figure 8.18 *American Diabetes Association Classification scheme for glucose measurements defining impairment in glucose handling or frank diabetes.*

What to do about high blood glucose concentrations

We can do several things about a high glucose concentration. The first is to look at the amount of glucocorticoid which is given and again, we rely on our profile data to determine if the amounts given are leading to too high cortisol peaks over the 24 hour period.

If they are too high, then we need to take the following steps:

1. Try to normalise cortisol levels by adjusting the hydrocortisone dose in terms of amount, timings and whether stacking is occurring (see Chapters 9 and 10).

2. Think about changes to diet. Quite a few studies show a strict diet and exercise approach can normalise glucose and avoid progression to diabetes.

3. If this step fails, we can then use agents which are used classically in the management of type 2 diabetes. Figure 8.19 shows a step wise approach developed by the American Diabetes Association and the European Association for the Study of Diabetes.

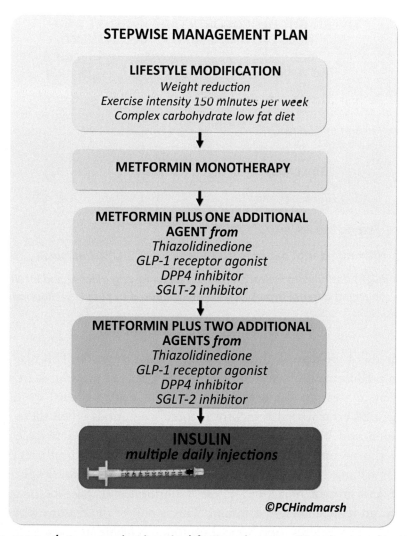

STEPWISE MANAGEMENT PLAN

LIFESTYLE MODIFICATION
Weight reduction
Exercise intensity 150 minutes per week
Complex carbohydrate low fat diet

↓

METFORMIN MONOTHERAPY

↓

METFORMIN PLUS ONE ADDITIONAL AGENT *from*
Thiazolidinedione
GLP-1 receptor agonist
DPP4 inhibitor
SGLT-2 inhibitor

↓

METFORMIN PLUS TWO ADDITIONAL AGENTS *from*
Thiazolidinedione
GLP-1 receptor agonist
DPP4 inhibitor
SGLT-2 inhibitor

↓

INSULIN
multiple daily injections

©PCHindmarsh

Figure 8.19 *Stepwise approach to managing impaired fasting glucose and/or glucose tolerance as well as type 2 diabetes mellitus.*

The mainstay of treatment has been metformin which is a drug that makes the body more sensitive to the effects of insulin. Its predominant effect appears to be on the liver and gut. In the gut it liberates a protein called GD15 which alters the central nervous system response to food intake. Metformin action also tends to oppose the effects of glucocorticoids, so it is a good medication to use in situations where insulin is high as a result of too much exposure to glucocorticoids. The medication is taken once or twice a day and effects on blood glucose and body weight, which it also reduces, can be seen over a 6 to 12 month period.

There are a number of other agents that are highly effective such as the GLP-1 receptor agonist, semaglutide. This drug not only acts synergistically with insulin, but also alters appetite leading to 10% to 15% weight loss. This in itself is sufficient to reduce insulin resistance and improve blood glucose.

It has been suggested that dosing with hydrocortisone later than 6 pm (18:00) leads to glucose problems. This is a misinterpretation of the published paper from a study where the last dose of the day was given at 5pm (17:00) which means that all the glucocorticoid exposure took place during the day when there was also food exposure. Data from our practice shows that taking the correct dose of hydrocortisone after 6 pm (18:00) has no untoward effect on fasting glucose and insulin levels compared to people without adrenal problems (Figure 8.20).

**OVERNIGHT GLUCOCORTICOID EXPOSURE AND
MORNING FASTING GLUCOSE AND INSULIN**

AGE <10 YEARS	NORMAL (N = 56)	CAH (N = 25)
Fasting Glucose (mmol/l)	4.6	4.1
Fasting Insulin (mU/l)	10	5.0
AGE ≥10 YEARS	NORMAL (N = 38)	CAH (N = 32)
Fasting Glucose (mmol/l)	4.6	4.4
Fasting Insulin (mU/l)	11.4	8.9

(N = number of patients studied)   ©PCHindmarsh

Figure 8.20 *Effect of midnight dosing with hydrocortisone on mean fasting glucose and insulin levels taken at 06:00 (6 am) in patients with congenital adrenal hyperplasia (CAH) compared to people without adrenal problems.*

Low Blood Glucose

Low blood glucose is also a problem in those who take glucocorticoids. This may seem odd at first as glucocorticoid action predominantly raises blood glucose or at least prevents it from falling. However, if glucocorticoid levels in the blood are low, for example during illness, or if the distribution of glucocorticoid during a 24 hour period is incorrect, there are periods when there is no glucocorticoid detectable in the blood and blood glucose levels can fall. Low blood glucose levels (often called hypoglycaemia) may also be one of the presenting features of adrenal insufficiency. Cortisol plays an important role in maintaining blood glucose by acting to increase glucose levels in conjunction with glucagon, adrenaline and growth hormone. These 4 hormones all raise blood glucose whereas the only hormone which can reduce glucose is insulin. This is one of the reasons why diabetes occurs and is quite common because there is only one hormone available to bring down blood glucose, compared to the 4 which are available to increase it.

Blood glucose can fall either because there is too much insulin present, or too little of the hormones adrenaline, glucagon, growth hormone or cortisol. Figure 8.21 shows the sequence of events which take place as blood glucose levels fall. As blood glucose decreases from 5 mmol/l to 4 mmol/l, insulin secretion is switched off which is a sensible approach to take as it stops the only hormone which can reduce blood glucose from being produced. If this switch off of insulin does not help the problem, the next step in the process is to switch on the hormones (counterregulatory hormones) which increase blood glucose: glucagon, adrenaline, growth hormone and cortisol.

Glucagon (a hormone made in the pancreas helps regulate blood glucose by releasing glucose from the liver thereby increasing blood glucose levels to prevent them from falling too low) and adrenaline act quite quickly whereas growth hormone and cortisol have a much slower effect on blood glucose. We can see this when we measure blood glucose after hydrocortisone has been administered. It takes some 2 to 3 hours before blood glucose levels increase but they do stay elevated for some 4 to 5 hours after hydrocortisone has been administered. The effect with other glucocorticoids such as prednisolone is even more marked.

The rise occurs some 2 to 3 hours after administration but the persistently high glucose concentrations can last for some 6 to 8 hours.

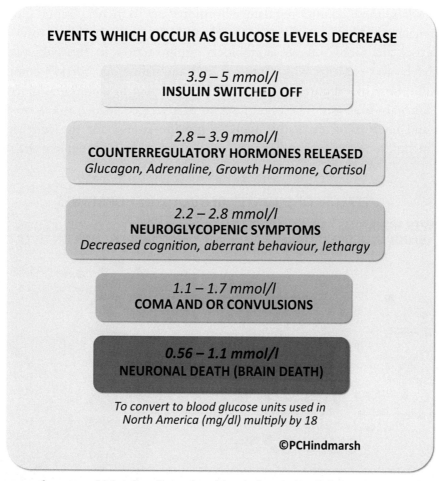

Figure 8.21 *Sequence of events which take place when blood glucose levels fall to the levels as shown.*

As blood glucose drops further to 3.3 mmol/l, a series of additional signs and symptoms become apparent. These are divided into two types:

1. The first, those associated with the effects of low blood glucose on the brain such as poor concentration, behavioural changes, seizure and coma.

2. The second, signs and symptoms due to the activation of various alert systems in the brain and can be seen as an increase in heart rate, blood pressure, sweating and a feeling of hunger.

Role of the counterregulatory hormones

People with adrenal insufficiency, particularly newborn and children before diagnosis is made, are susceptible to hypoglycaemia. Cortisol plays an important role in raising blood glucose, but the most important hormones which raise blood glucose quickly are glucagon and adrenaline. However, in adrenal insufficiency when hypoglycaemia occurs due to the lack of cortisol as well as the compromised synthesis and release of adrenaline from the adrenal medulla, it is not possible for the body to be able to get out of this difficult situation very easily. Growth hormone is also involved in preventing blood glucose from going low. This becomes a problem for those with adrenal insufficiency secondary to hypopituitarism, where the two hormones involved in raising and maintaining a normal blood glucose over the longer term, are missing.

Glucagon will raise blood glucose on its own, but glycogen stores can become depleted quite quickly so glucogen will become less effective at raising blood glucose if hypoglycaemia keeps recurring.

Figure 8.22 shows where these counter regulatory hormones act to increase blood glucose. Notice that glucagon and adrenaline have direct effect to get glucose out from the liver stores whereas growth hormone and cortisol are more indirect and block insulin action in the cells preventing glucose uptake. This probably also explains why glucagon and adrenaline act quickly compared to growth hormone and insulin. Low blood glucose is particularly a problem in children as glucose is an essential source of energy for brain function. The brain reserves of glycogen, which is a way of storing glucose do not last long and reserves of alternative fuels to provide energy for the cells, are limited. Even fasting overnight in children who do not have any adrenal problems, can deplete the stores.

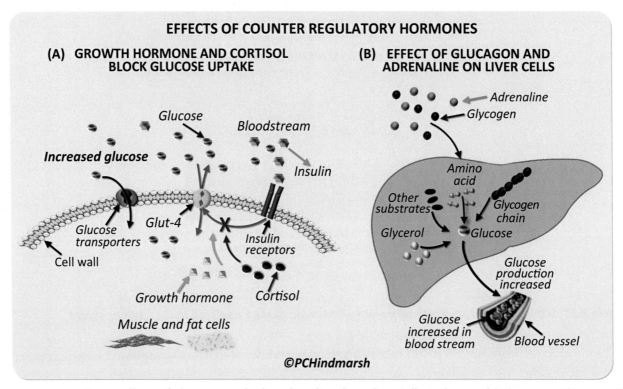

Figure 8.22 *Different effects of glucagon and adrenaline directly on liver cells (right panel (B)) compared to growth hormone and cortisol (left panel (A)) which block glucose uptake by the glucose transporters in muscle and fat cells.*

In adrenal insufficiency and in particular in secondary adrenal insufficiency, additional problems occur. Generally, as long there is a steady input of glucose from food, all will be well. Before diagnosis, however, particularly in the newborn period, a crisis might take place and part of the crisis is a person vomits. Any vomiting which takes place will mean the steady stream of glucose the body needs will be interrupted and because the stores of glycogen particularly in children and the newborn are low, hypoglycaemia will occur quickly.

In adrenal insufficiency and secondary adrenal insufficiency in particular, there is another problem. We mentioned that glucagon, adrenaline and growth hormone will work to raise blood glucose. Is this the case in adrenal insufficiency?

Under normal circumstances adrenaline and glucagon would be present and raise blood glucose if levels were falling. However, because the way the adrenal glands are constructed, the cells which produce adrenaline are in the medulla, which is situated in the middle of the gland and it needs local cortisol production to ensure adequate amounts of adrenaline are made. The blood flow in the adrenal glands goes from the outside right through to the middle where adrenaline is made and means that the middle of the adrenal gland is very rich in cortisol delivered by these blood vessels. We discuss this in Chapter 2. The cortisol producing cells are located on the outside in the cortex and if production cannot take place in the outer cells, then cortisol cannot be released into the small blood vessels which run between the cortex and the centre or medulla, meaning adrenaline production is reduced.

Now not only has the individual lost cortisol, which they could not make anyway, but because of this loss of cortisol the production of adrenaline is also impaired. This double hit leaves the individual with adrenal insufficiency very susceptible to developing hypoglycaemia. There are further problems for all with adrenal insufficiency, because if there are lots of hypoglycaemic episodes the adrenaline response becomes naturally blunted in its own right along with a loss of the symptoms and signs of hypoglycaemia that we described earlier in this section.

The situation is even more concerning in people who have secondary adrenal insufficiency due to hypopituitarism. In this situation they have lost cortisol and probably growth hormone, so if we put these together, they will be deficient in cortisol, growth hormone and adrenaline. This means individuals with hypopituitarism are particularly susceptible to hypoglycaemia and it is extremely important this is recognised and accounted for in the management of their illness.

Treating hypoglycaemia

The most important thing in adrenal insufficiency is to try and prevent the occurrence of hypoglycaemia. This is why it is extremely important to ensure there is good delivery of cortisol, not only by doubling or tripling the dose given when unwell but by giving an extra double dose at 4 am (04:00) (More@4 AM see Chapter 12) when we know the cortisol from the previous night's hydrocortisone dose is likely to be quite low. More@4 AM and double/triple dose during illness or trauma are two ways in which you can prevent hypoglycaemia.

Immediate treatment of hypoglycaemia consists of giving 15 grams of what is known as readily available glucose, in other words neat glucose. This is present in orange drinks and fizzy drinks such as Coca-Cola (not diet or sugar free types). Haribo sweets, jelly babies and dextrose tablets are other sources of readily available glucose (check product packaging for glucose content). Giving 15 grams of glucose will bring the glucose up very quickly and it is useful to have a blood glucose meter available so you can retest to make sure that this has happened. The retest should be done 15 minutes after giving the 15 grams of glucose. If this has not raised the blood glucose, then it is a simple process to repeat with a further 15 grams of glucose and retest 15 minutes later. This is usually sufficient to bring glucose back into the normal range.

Another option, particularly if the person cannot tolerate any oral glucose is to use 'glucogel' and a supply should be kept in your emergency pack. This must be massaged around the gums and into the cheek. Glucose is absorbed very quickly this way and will rectify a low blood glucose very quickly. 'Glucogel' should only be administered if the person is conscious and able to swallow.

The last resort is an emergency injection of hydrocortisone which will also increase the blood glucose, however the best thing to do is to get on top of the low blood glucose problem quickly by giving some easily available glucose. If this is not tolerated then give the emergency injection followed by the glucogel. This order of events ensures normalisation of the blood glucose will take place quickly and be sustained.

To recap, if an emergency hydrocortisone injection is required, for example in situations where the patient is vomiting and cannot keep medication down and the blood glucose is low, the following steps are recommended:

1. Give the injection of hydrocortisone

2. Apply glucogel to gums and cheek if patient able to swallow and is conscious

3. Call an ambulance

If hypoglycaemic episodes are happening on a frequent basis, then it is worth checking the dose and distribution of the glucocorticoid. This can be done by undertaking a 24 hour cortisol profile if they are on hydrocortisone and at the same time, we can measure blood glucose or use continuous glucose monitoring systems, to determine the exact timing and relationship of the amount of cortisol in the blood with the associated blood glucose value. All that may be required is a change in the amount or in the frequency in dosing of the hydrocortisone to avoid that particular period of time during the 24 hour period when blood glucose is low.

CONCLUSION

Glucose is regulated by insulin which is the only hormone that reduces blood glucose. Glucagon, adrenaline, growth hormone and cortisol all increase blood glucose. Hyperglycaemia (Type 2 diabetes mellitus) can occur when glucocorticoid doses are high for long periods of time. However, in the run up to this situation insulin levels are high leading to the development of the Metabolic Syndrome. Careful checking of glucocorticoid dosing and adjusting dose amounts and timing is important to avoid this problem. Hypoglycaemia in adrenal insufficiency is a little more complex than just cortisol deficiency because the production of adrenaline which is one of the hormones the body uses to get out of difficulties with hypoglycaemia very quickly is compromised in its production, so there is a double hit in the way that people with primary adrenal insufficiency respond to hypoglycaemia. The problem is even more pronounced in secondary adrenal insufficiency where in addition the individual may also be deficient in growth hormone.

FURTHER READING

Butler, P.C., Rizza, R.A., 1989. Regulation of carbohydrate metabolism and response to hypoglycemia. Endocrinol Metab Clin North Am 18, 1-25.

Diabetes Prevention Program Research Group, 2002. Reduction in the incidence of type 2 diabetes with lifestyle intervention or metformin. N Engl J Med 346, 393—403.

El Sayed, N.A., Aleppo, G., Aroda, V.R., et al., 2023. American Diabetes Association. 9. Pharmacologic approaches to glycemic treatment: Standards of Care in Diabetes - 2023. Diabetes Care 46 (Suppl. 1), S140—S157.

Green-Golan, L., Yates, C., Drinkard, B., VanRyzin, C., Eisenhofer, G., Weise, M., Merke, D.P., 2007. Patients with classic congenital adrenal hyperplasia have decreased epinephrine reserve and defective glycemic control during prolonged moderate-intensity exercise. J Clin Endocrinol Metab 92, 3019—3024.

Ludwig, D.S., Aronne, L.J., Astrup, A., de Cabo, R., Cantley, L.C., Friedman, M.I., Heymsfield, S.B., Johnson, J.D., King, J.C., Krauss, R.M., Lieberman, D.E., 2021. The carbohydrate-insulin model: a physiological perspective on the obesity pandemic. Am J Clin Nutr 114, 1873—1885.

The GBD 2015 Obesity Collaborators, 2017. Health effects of overweight and obesity in 195 countries over 25 years. N Engl J Med 377, 13—27.

CHAPTER 8.3

Gastrointestinal Problems

GLOSSARY

Enteric formulations A coating applied to a drug to prevent breakdown in the stomach and delivery of the drug at a point further down the gut.

Gastric ulcers and gastritis Breakdown of the normal lining of the stomach. This allows the stomach acid to act on the exposed area leading to pain. If the erosion or ulcer occurs over an underlying blood vessel then gastric bleeding can occur which can be severe. Gastritis refers to a generalised inflammation of the stomach wall.

Proton pump inhibitors Drugs that act by blocking the gastric proton pump of the cells in the stomach. The proton pump is the last stage in gastric acid secretion and is directly responsible for secreting hydrogen ions into the gastric lumen making the contents acidic.

GENERAL

High on the list of side effects of glucocorticoids are effects on the gastrointestinal system. Most common of these is gastritis (an inflammation of the lining of the stomach wall) but there are other effects on gut motility. In addition, there is increasing evidence of an effect of the bacteria which reside in the gut impacting on the glucocorticoids delivered by the oral route.

MOUTH

The effects of glucocorticoids on the mouth vary. There is no doubt local application of hydrocortisone to mouth ulcers leads to increased healing. The data which are available on oral glucocorticoids have tended in the past to focus on changes to the environment in the mouth with respect to how acid/alkaline the salivary secretions are which alter the local environment in the mouth, allowing yeast such as candida to grow and produce a very sore mouth with white patches covering the mouth (Figure 8.23).

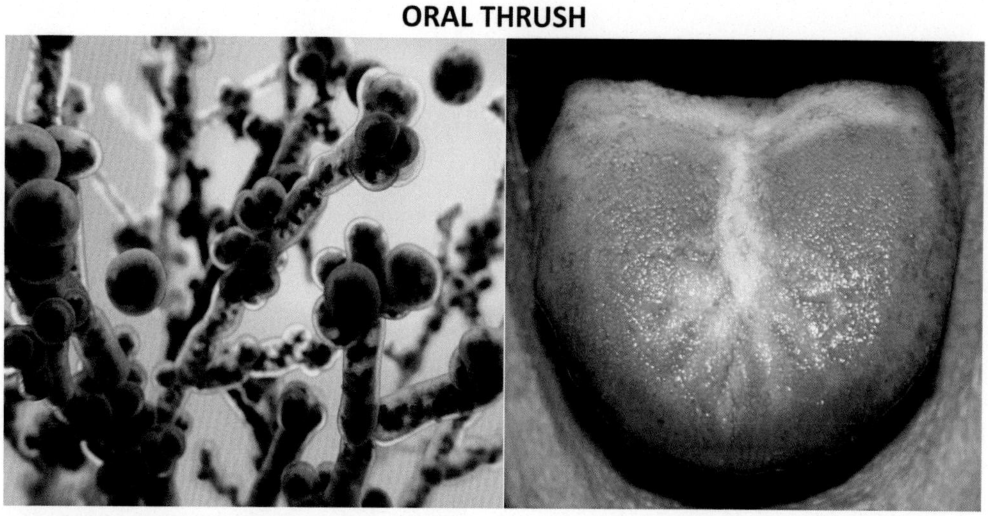

ORAL THRUSH

Figure 8.23 *The causative agent of thrush is candida albicans. The hyphae of the fungus are shown on the left. On the right is thrush infection of the tongue showing the white coating of the fungus.*

Replacement Therapies in Adrenal Insufficiency. https://doi.org/10.1016/B978-0-12-824548-4.00018-8

The problem with candida infections, also known as thrush, of the mouth is the candida can so easily, especially in children, move down into the gut where it can act as a reservoir, so it can be very difficult to eradicate the thrush once it has established itself and recurrent infections are often the norm. Areas which are likely to be affected are the sides of the tongue and further back towards the throat. There are probably two problems associated with glucocorticoids and oral health. The first is the use of extremely high doses of glucocorticoids which are used for anti-inflammatory reasons. The second is the effect of residual glucocorticoids in the mouth following the normal oral intake of replacement therapy. As a guide there are a large number of studies of inhaled glucocorticoids used in asthma treatment which show effects on salivary flow. Saliva is an essential component of the fluid medium of the oral cavity. This contribution of saliva is extremely important and when salivary flow is suppressed, which can happen with glucocorticoids, mouth soreness, alteration in taste and problems with swallowing can ensue. Altering salivary flow along with local immunosuppression due to the residuum of glucocorticoids in the mouth following ingestion, can lead to further damage to the lining of the mouth with ulceration and inflammation of the gums and base of the teeth. A number of studies have also implicated high dose glucocorticoids in causing damage to the teeth and enamel coating of the teeth.

All these observations point to the need to be extremely careful, especially with oral replacement therapy which is for life and means the mouth is constantly exposed potentially to small amounts of glucocorticoid which are locally concentrated in and around the gums and teeth. This would translate into the need to be careful with glucocorticoid administration, to make sure the tablet is swallowed, preferably intact and that any residuum in the mouth should be removed by careful rinsing after the intake of the tablet. The situation might be more pronounced in children where liquid and oral suspensions are used and particularly where particulate (in the form of minute separate particles) methods of delivering hydrocortisone are used, because of potential entrapment of the granules between the teeth.

GASTRITIS AND GASTRIC ULCERS

As already mentioned, many glucocorticoids lead to inflammation of the lining of the stomach known as gastritis. Occasionally, this can be more severe and lead to actual ulceration of the stomach wall. Figure 8.24 shows an example of these conditions.

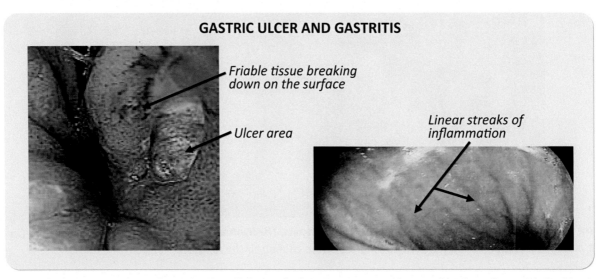

Figure 8.24 *Endoscopic view of gastric ulcer (left panel) showing erosion of normal pink surface with friable tissue surrounding the ulcer. On the right linear streaks of inflammation in patient with gastritis.*

The symptoms which result are upper abdominal pain, particularly after ingestion of food and some people also complain of heartburn. How these symptoms and problems arise are still unclear. Direct application of glucocorticoids onto the stomach wall in experiments show they can produce small ulcers. Several studies have demonstrated there is a dose dependent increased risk of gastric ulcers in patients treated with glucocorticoids, but other studies have not been able to show any relationship. When we look instead at really large studies however, there is overall a 1.8 times higher risk of ulceration for users of steroids than for non users. The risk appears to be greater with steroid doses equivalent to or above 30 mg prednisolone than for the lower doses. In this large review, prednisolone accounted for more than 85% of the systemic steroid used.

More detailed studies have shown that even short term (7 to 28 days) exposure to glucocorticoids, was significantly associated with gastric ulcer bleeding and this risk was dose dependent and higher when aspirin or non steroidal anti-inflammatory drugs were used in conjunction with a glucocorticoid. Although high dose glucocorticoids have been implicated in gastric problems, it is likely that even low dose replacement therapy will be problematic as the exposure is many times a day every day for life. Enteric drugs that delay release beyond the stomach may seem to be a good idea, but the coating alters absorption and we look at this in Chapter 6. Further work on proton pump inhibitors taken to reduce gastric acidity and their interaction with glucocorticoids, is needed.

The exact mechanism of the glucocorticoid induced gastric damage is unclear. In the past it was thought that prostaglandins might be involved, but experimental studies have not been able to confirm. Reflux of gastric acid into the oesophagus which can occur with a hiatus hernia or laxity of the tight junction where the oesophagus joins the stomach, is a problem not simply because of symptoms of heartburn but, if not treated, can lead to Barrett's oesophagus. The cells lining your oesophagus become inflamed and damaged and are replaced by new cells which are more like those lining the stomach. In the meantime, the oesophagus can be damaged by ulcer development as well as scarring, leading to marked narrowing of the oesophagus making it difficult to swallow.

The most important complication of Barrett's oesophagus is that it can develop into cancer, although this is rare. Simple treatments consist of losing any excess weight, stop smoking and eat smaller meals at regular intervals. Proton pump inhibitors are effective. Endoscopic removal of the abnormal cells may be required and very rarely a surgical resection of the area is required.

GASTROPARESIS

Gastroparesis is a condition where the stomach does not contract properly due to impaired nervous innervation of the smooth muscle in the wall of the stomach. A large number of patients do complain of fullness, nausea, vomiting, bloating and abdominal pain and the effect of glucocorticoids can be considered in two ways.

In experimental studies using dexamethasone, enlargement of the stomach was observed and this effect was unrelated to the increased gastric acid secretion seen as a result of the dexamethasone treatment itself. The effect seems to be due to a depletion of arginine in the stomach which impedes the production of nitric oxide which is required for gastric motility.

This is a very important observation because the administration of arginine completely prevented both the enlargement of stomach and the induction of gastroparesis as a result of oral dexamethasone administration.

It is not just exposure to glucocorticoids that produces gastroparesis. There are reports in the literature of people presenting with recurrent episodes of vomiting associated with clear demonstration of gastroparesis in association with cortisol deficiency.

This may explain why babies with adrenal insufficiency present with projectile vomiting. In these cases, hydrocortisone replacement normalised gastric emptying time and relieved the patients of their vomiting. Cortisol deficiency appeared to be the key component of this gastroparesis because it occurred in primary and secondary adrenal insufficiency.

These observations would be consistent with our understanding of the effect of glucocorticoids on smooth muscle. In the body there are three types of muscle. Skeletal muscle, smooth muscle and heart muscle. Smooth muscle is what we find essentially in the tubes of the body such as in the lungs, gut and urinary system.

Cortisol appears to have an important role in maintaining the tone of the smooth muscle. When cortisol is deficient, smooth muscle tone is low and the tubes essentially relax.

That is probably what is happening in gastroparesis when cortisol is deficient. When cortisol is replaced, muscle tone is normalised and the stomach returns to its normal shape. Figure 8.25 summarises some of the features of gastroparesis. It is important to emphasise that the cause of glucocorticoid gastroparesis is different to that observed in patients with poorly controlled diabetes mellitus. In the latter, irreversible damage is done to the nerve cells in the gastric wall by the persistently elevated blood glucose. Whereas, as we have mentioned, in glucocorticoid gastroparesis there is reduced local formation of nitric oxide.

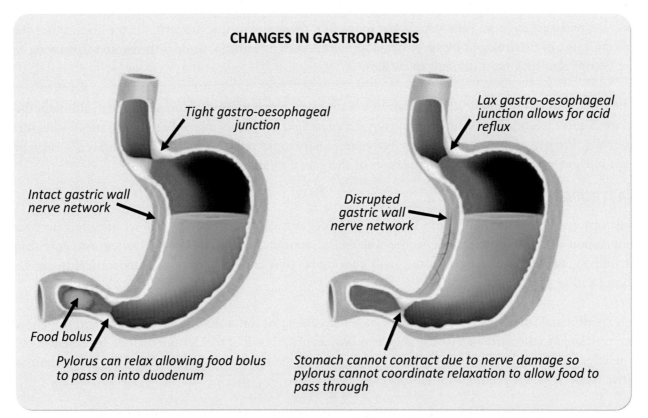

Figure 8.25 Illustration of what happens in gastroparesis. On the left the normal nerve innervation of the stomach is shown in yellow and disrupted in the right panel in gastroparesis. This leads to loss of closure at the gastro-oesophageal junction and narrowing at the pylorus at the other end of the stomach. This leads to fluid accumulation in the stomach and reduced ability to form boluses of food to pass into the duodenum.

SMALL INTESTINE AND MICROBIOME

Glucocorticoids and also bile acids derived from the liver are important to intestinal tract structure and function. Glucocorticoids are particularly important in increasing the enzyme levels which are present in the wall of the intestine which enhance absorption of food. In adrenal insufficiency, there is a reduction in enzyme activity and in the thickness of the lining of the gut, both of which alter absorption of food stuffs.

A new concept which is emerging, is that the bacteria in the gut play an important role in modifying endocrine function and we have explored this in Chapter 6. Breakdown of glucocorticoids by gut bacteria leads to a number of products which are either excreted in the faeces, or some can be absorbed into the bloodstream.

CORTISOL METABOLISM IN THE LIVER AND GASTROINTESTINAL TRACT

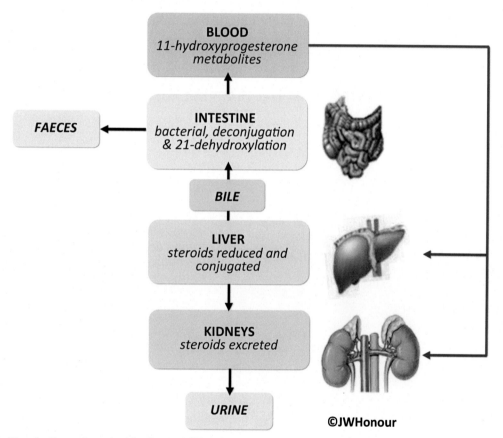

Figure 8.26 *Metabolism of cortisol in the small intestine.*

Generally, cortisol is metabolised in the liver and the breakdown products are either excreted into bile which then goes back into the gut (the enterohepatic circulation), or they are taken to the kidneys and passed out in the urine. How the bacteria in the gut metabolise cortisol varies, depending which part of the gut the steroid is in. As most hydrocortisone is absorbed in the upper gut, the steps detailed in Figure 8.26 apply. As we see shortly, in the lower gut/rectum different steroid conversion products are likely.

The importance of these observations is the gut is not just a passive structure in terms of its interaction which glucocorticoids. The metabolism of cortisol generates a number of products which can go forward to influence hormone functions following absorption in their new state.

In the syndrome of apparent mineralocorticoid excess, patients have congenital mutations leading to nonfunctional 11beta-hydroxysteroid dehydrogenase type 2 in the kidney and as a result, severe hypertension. Normally, 11beta-hydroxysteroid dehydrogenase type 2 protects the mineralocorticoid receptor from excess cortisol, preventing sodium and water retention. Liquorice contains an ingredient called glycyrrhetinic acid which inhibits 11beta-hydroxysteroid dehydrogenase type 2 and can cause hypertension in some individuals.

A series of studies on the gut bacteria have implicated certain types in association with hypertension through the production of glycyrrhetinic acid-like factors (GALFs). This is an important observation because not only might this explain how hypertension occurs in the general population, but this has important implications for the delivery of cortisol, or rather hydrocortisone, as replacement therapy. Most of the hydrocortisone taken in orally, is absorbed in the upper part of the gut where the gut bacteria are completely different to lower down (Figure 8.27). However, if we introduce delayed release or slow release preparations, then hydrocortisone will be released at lower parts of the gut which may lead to the conversion of cortisol into GALFs. Not everything is bad about GALFs because a protective role of GALFs produced by gut bacteria has been implicated in the aetiology of colorectal cancer.

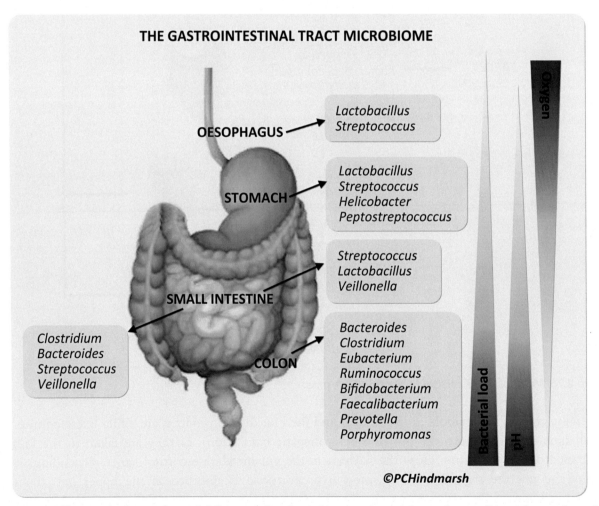

Figure 8.27 *Changes in the gut bacterial flora moving from the oesophagus down the small intestine to the colon. Moving in this direction not only does the bacterial load increase as shown in the side bar but the types change in order to cope with an environment with less oxygen and that is less acidic (pH) (low pH indicates acid, high pH indicate alkali). Note we have used the broad family names such as streptococcus. Some of the members of this family can cause infections but others in the gut are beneficial.*

LARGE INTESTINE

Glucocorticoids along with mineralocorticoid play an important role in water and sodium absorption along with potassium excretion in the large intestine and to a certain degree in the small intestine as well.

Constipation is a particular problem in children and this may relate, in part, to the effect of the mineralocorticoid, fludrocortisone and to some extent hydrocortisone, on the large intestine. We know fludrocortisone acts on the kidney to retain salt, but it also does this in the large bowel. Movement of salt into the body will take with it, water. This means the consistency of the stool formed will have less water in it and become increasingly thicker as it moves through the large bowel. The end result of this would be the generation of stools which are often quite hard and difficult to pass.

As we move through the large intestine down into the rectum, the bacterial flora changes again (Figure 8.27). This is an important step because it also impacts on how we can give hydrocortisone. Hydrocortisone is available in suppository form and has largely been designed for the treatment of inflammatory bowel conditions. It has been suggested the rectal route could be used in an emergency situation rather than resorting to an intramuscular injection.

Part of the problem with this approach is only a very small part of the rectal dose is absorbed which means that for emergency use this preparation is not to be used. One big problem is in many individuals the rectal hydrocortisone is metabolised by the gut bacteria into adrenal androgens and in particular testosterone.

This would mean any hydrocortisone appearing this far down the gut would lead to an increase in the circulating testosterone concentration in both males and females particularly if this were to occur regularly.

WHAT TO DO

Dealing with the upper gastrointestinal problems, particularly gastric ulceration, can only be approached on a more symptomatic basis. A practical solution is to always take glucocorticoids with food and never on an empty stomach. This does slightly alter the absorption of the glucocorticoid but not by very much. A milk drink can be helpful in this situation.

Another approach is to use medicines called antacids which reduce the production of acid in the stomach. There are a variety of these available and the most effective are the proton pump inhibitors (PPI). These reduce acid production and alleviate symptoms. Care needs to be exercised in taking these medications and this should be discussed with your doctor. It has been suggested that proton pump inhibitors may increase the risk of clostridium difficile infection of the colon and that high doses and long term use (1 year or longer) may increase the risk of osteoporosis related fractures of the hip, wrist, or spine.

Long term use of PPIs has also been associated with low levels of magnesium (hypomagnesaemia). Data on the impact of PPIs on heart disease appear contradictory. One retrospective study of patients taking PPIs for long periods of time, showed an increased risk of heart disease but in a large, randomised study of 17,000 patients, no adverse effects such as these were observed over a 3 year period. These differences probably reflect the inclusion of a large number of older patients in the former study who are more likely to have associated heart disease.

A final solution if the stomach problems are severe and in particular if there is gastroparesis, is to bypass the stomach oral route altogether and deliver hydrocortisone using a pump system which is described in Section 3.

We cannot stop the replacement treatment with glucocorticoids to allow the ulcer to heal, more practical solutions are required.

One option is to delay the delivery of glucocorticoid and that is what the enteric coated preparations do. These protect the stomach wall from the effects of the glucocorticoid because they prevent breakdown of the tablet until it reaches the small bowel. Only prednisolone comes in this format and has a number of other problems associated with its potency. It is important to note also that the enteric coat as we have discussed in Chapter 6 affects the absorption and delivery of the glucocorticoid. The same applies to hydrocortisone buccal tablets which are formulated to dissolve slowly in the mouth where they are used to treat mouth ulcers. If used as a source of hydrocortisone for replacement therapy then the absorption will not be as immediate as oral hydrocortisone tablets and similar to enteric coated prednisolone, they will have a delayed delivery of hydrocortisone into the bloodstream.

For constipation, a more pragmatic approach needs to be taken by keeping the diet high in fibre and ensuring good fluid intake. Stool softeners or laxatives can improve the consistency of the stool. Monitoring of both hydrocortisone and fludrocortisone dosing used in blood testing will also allow adjustments to be made to reduce over exposure to either steroid.

CONCLUSION

Gastrointestinal problems are common in people treated with glucocorticoids. The effects whether in producing gastritis or ulceration are dose dependent. Dosing should be evaluated as we describe in Section 3 and medications should be taken with food where possible. 24 hour cortisol profiles can help in defining optimum dosing regimens. Care needs to be exercised with enteric or slow release preparations as they will be susceptible to metabolism by gut bacteria in the small bowel.

Proton pump inhibitors are effective agents to reduce gastric acid production and need to be used in consultation with your endocrinologist.

FURTHER READING

Honour, J.W., 2015. Historical perspective: gut dysbiosis and hypertension. Physiol Genomics 47, 443—446.

Ito, T., Jensen, R.T., 2010. Association of long-term proton pump inhibitor therapy with bone fractures and effects on absorption of calcium, vitamin B12, iron, and magnesium. Curr Gastroenterol Rep 12, 448—457.

Moayyedi, P., Eikelboom, J.W., Bosch, J., ... COMPASS Investigators, 2019. Safety of proton pump inhibitors based on a large, multi-year, randomized trial of patients receiving rivaroxaban or aspirin. Gastroenterology 157, 682—691.

Nakamura, T., Kurihara, I., Kobayashi, S., et al., 2018. Intestinal mineralocorticoid receptor contributes to epithelial sodium channel—mediated intestinal sodium absorption and blood pressure regulation. J Am Heart Assoc 7, e008259. https://doi.org/10.1161/JAHA.117.008259.

Prozialeck, W., Kopf, P., 2019. Gastrointestinal disorders and their treatment. In: Wecker, L., Taylor, D.A., Theobald, R.J. (Eds.), Brody's Human Pharmacology, 6th ed. Elsevier, Philadelphia, PA. chap 71.

Ruiz-Sánchez, J.G., Moreno-Domínguez, O., Herranz de la Morena, L., et al., 2021. Adrenal insufficiency misdiagnosed as diabetic gastroparesis. Hormones 20, 599—601. https://doi-org.libproxy.ucl.ac.uk/10.1007/s42000-021-00284-4

CHAPTER 8.4

Fertility

GLOSSARY

Adrenal rests The presence of adrenal tissue in the testes. This tissue responds to ACTH stimulation leading to an increase in size. The rests are hard and irregular in shape and can be mistaken for testicular cancers. These can occur wherever there are adrenal cells but mainly in testes and rarely ovaries. These are often referred to as Testicular Adrenal Rest Tissue or TART.

Anovulatory A menstrual cycle in which an egg is not generated.

Follicle-stimulating Hormone Hormone produced by the pituitary gland which is involved in sperm formation from the testes in males. In females, along with luteinising hormone, it is involved in egg selection and production of estradiol.

Human Chorionic Gonadotropin Human chorionic gonadotropin (hCG) is a hormone produced by trophoblast cells that form the placenta. It is similar in structure to luteinising hormone and is used in fertility treatments in place of luteinising hormone.

Hypogonadotropic Hypogonadism Condition where there is deficiency of luteinising and follicle-stimulating hormones either due to a pituitary deficiency of the gonadotropin cells that produce these hormones or due to loss of the stimulatory peptide produced in the hypothalamus, gonadotropin-releasing hormone.

Luteinising Hormone Hormone produced by the pituitary gland which generates testosterone from the testes in males. In females, along with follicle-stimulating hormone, it is involved in egg selection and production of estradiol.

Polycystic ovaries This is a particular appearance where the ovaries are enlarged and filled with dense stroma in the middle, with lots of small cysts around the periphery of the ovary.

Polycystic ovary Syndrome Ovarian appearances on ultrasound in association with increased androgen production, irregular or absent menstrual cycles and often obesity.

GENERAL

The effects on fertility of the treatments or the underlying condition varies with the cause of adrenal insufficiency. In primary adrenal insufficiency caused by congenital adrenal hyperplasia (CAH), there are problems with respect to fertility because of side effects associated with under replacement of glucocorticoids. In hypopituitarism, the fertility issues relate directly to the loss of either the gonadotropins and/or the drive to the gonadotropins from the hypothalamus by gonadotropin-releasing hormone. The situation can become even more complex when we consider adrenal hypoplasia congenita. This is a condition which affects boys and is due to a genetic abnormality in the *NROB1* or *DAX-1* gene which leads to a failure to develop the adrenal cortex. The abnormality in this situation is not simply confined to the failure to form an adrenal gland, but there is also associated hypogonadotropic hypogonadism. The situation is probably even more complex in this condition because *NROB1* or *DAX-1* also appears to play a crucial role in testes differentiation by regulating the development of intact testes cores leading to gonadal dysgenesis and infertility although it remains unclear whether this is the situation in humans. Finally, conditions such as autoimmune adrenalitis

Replacement Therapies in Adrenal Insufficiency. https://doi.org/10.1016/B978-0-12-824548-4.00019-X

(Addison's disease) would not be expected to have an abnormality in gonadal function, because the autoantibody which is generated is directed predominantly towards the adrenal glands, but as in other autoimmune conditions, antibodies particularly against the ovary, can be generated leading to primary ovarian failure.

For the purpose of this chapter, we will concentrate on hypogonadotropic hypogonadism and fertility in CAH.

HYPOGONADOTROPIC HYPOGONADISM

In patients with hypogonadotropic hypogonadism there is a lack of gonadotropin secretion throughout life. The first question which arises in these patients is whether long term gonadotropin deficiency causes a deficiency in the gonadal response and in the female in particular, embryo implantation. This concept arose because in the postnatal period (7 days to 6 months of age) in males particularly, there is a surge of gonadotropins and testosterone which might be important in determining the mass of Sertoli sperm producing cells in the testes.

The issue of embryo implantation stems from the observation that in many females, uterine development is less in terms of size, than might be expected when compared to the normal population. How much this reflects old practices in hormone replacement therapy with estrogens and the induction of puberty remains unclear at this stage and this observation may change as time progresses.

The mainstay of treatment is gonadotropin therapy using a combination of human chorionic gonadotropin (hCG) as the source of luteinising hormone (LH) and recombinant follicle-stimulating hormone (FSH). This treatment is well tolerated and effective in inducing testes growth, spermatogenesis and fertility in gonadotropin deficient men. Figure 8.28 (page 185) shows the effect of injections of hCG on LH, FSH and testosterone production. Here the hCG resulted in increased testosterone production and this acted via positive feedback on the hypothalamus and pituitary to improve LH and FSH secretion. In our discussions on the hypothalamo-pituitary axes we have often referred to negative feedback loops which regulate pituitary hormone release. However, it is important to also mention that positive feedback loops also operate, particularly in the hypothalamo-pituitary-ovarian axis leading to the LH surge mid menstrual cycle and subsequent ovulation. The impact on LH pulsatility in particular is shown 3 months later in Figure 8.29 (page 185).

The availability of assisted reproduction (conception) techniques has improved the success rate in the presence of subnormal sperm counts. However, a near normal testicular volume, no history of bilateral undescended testes, normal sexual maturation and no previous testosterone replacement therapy are the most impressive predictors of success with gonadotropin therapy.

These useful predictors, however, are not present in the hypogonadotropic hypogonadal male. The characteristic of these individuals is that testicular volume is small and there is often a history of bilateral undescended testes and delayed or absent puberty. Therefore, careful management of puberty with adequate testosterone replacement coupled probably with the use of recombinant FSH to increase testicular volume, might be the way to improve outcomes.

Certainly, the outcomes of successful fertility in males with hypogonadotropic hypogonadism is less than that observed in females. Whether this represents the loss of the postnatal testosterone and gonadotropin surge is unclear.

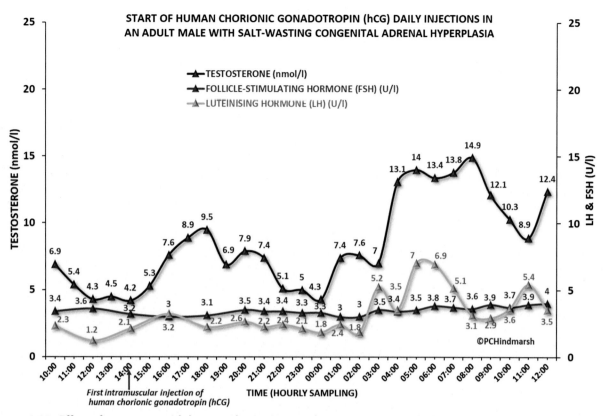

Figure 8.28 *Effect of treatment with human chorionic gonadotropin on overnight luteinising (LH), follicle-stimulating hormone (FSH) and testosterone concentrations prior to the treatment course.*

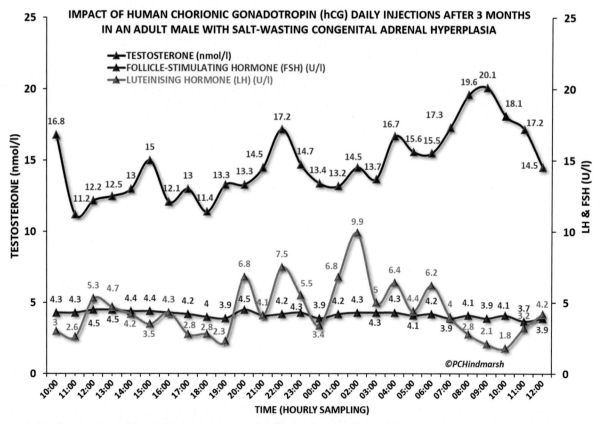

Figure 8.29 *Restoration of luteinising hormone pulsatility and normal testosterone production following treatment with human chorionic gonadotropin. Compared to Figure 8.28 mean LH increased from 3.6 U/l to 5.0 U/l, FSH from 3.5 U/l to 4.1 U/l and testosterone from 9.7 nmol/l to 16.0 nmol/l. The course of human chorionic gonadotropin 'primed' the hypothalamo-pituitary-testicular axis with testosterone leading to improved LH and FSH secretion by positive feedback.*

Currently, pregnancy rates of 50% to 80% can be anticipated during therapy with the combination treatment. Therapy usually takes the form of subcutaneous injections of hCG three times a week until testosterone concentrations are high enough to induce spermatogenesis, followed by the addition of injections of recombinant FSH to support and maintain spermatogenesis. It is important to realise therapy can take 9 to 18 months to be effective, but spermatogenesis can be observed in more than 80% of men using this approach.

In females a similar approach is undertaken. Although patients with hypogonadotropic hypogonadism (HH) have long term estrogen deficiency, their response to controlled ovarian hyperstimulation treatment is similar to normal women. Like in males, the majority of treatment regimens use hCG combined with FSH.

The treatment duration differs between the sexes and is usually approximately 2 weeks in females and 6 to 12 months in males. Usually, the type of treatment used is associated with in vitro fertilisation (IVF) or intracytoplasmic sperm injection (ICSI). It is important to consider different components of the process. In this female population the fertilisation rate is 72% but the actual implantation rate of a fertilised egg is only 36% and from that the live birth rate is 51%. These are not actually significantly different from other infertility cohorts studied. Despite the ovaries being dormant for many years and the need to be stimulated with higher doses of gonadotropins, there is no increased risk of the ovarian hyperstimulation syndrome in the hypogonadotropic hypogonadal group. The ovarian hyperstimulation syndrome occurs when the ovaries overrespond to FSH injections. The symptoms range from mild (swelling and bloated feeling, nausea, heartburn or indigestion), to moderate (abdominal pain and vomiting) and rarely (1% to 1.5% of patients) severe (nausea, vomiting, ovarian enlargement and fluid in the abdomen with a reduction in blood volume and poor circulation). Symptoms usually resolve in 4 to 7 days but observation in hospital is advised.

These observations point to good outcomes for fertility in males and females with hypogonadotropic hypogonadism. Overall, females tend to have better fertility outcomes than males. As with the general population increasing age is associated with reduced fertility and this appears to be exactly the same situation in hypogonadotropic hypogonadism. One important exception to this is the individuals with adrenal hypoplasia congenita where it does appear to be more problematic in stimulating the testes and this may reflect an underlying problem with the testes.

CONGENITAL ADRENAL HYPERPLASIA

In CAH, females have normal ovaries and womb and males form normal testes. Therefore, fertility should not be a problem because the necessary structures are present in both sexes. Females with CAH, if cortisol replacement is optimal and therefore their androgen production is normal, have their first period about 13 years of age which is only slightly later than the average in the general population of 12.4 years. The problems which arise relate to the degree of androgen production from the adrenal glands and can lead to suppression of the hypothalamo-pituitary-gonadal axis. In women with classical CAH on routine replacement therapy, it is estimated that 80% of women with simple virilising and salt-wasting forms are fertile with ovulation rates of 40%. However, woman with classical CAH may have lower pregnancy rates when compared to unaffected individuals. With respect to the non-classical forms, one study stated that 57% of pregnancies occurred naturally without any treatment, 41% were successful with hydrocortisone treatment three times per day and only 2% required ovulation induction agents. Interestingly, the rate of miscarriage was lower in those women with the non-classical form of CAH receiving glucocorticoid treatment compared to those non-classical CAH women that did not.

As already suggested, androgen excess is one of the major factors responsible for poor fertility outcomes in females with CAH. We have already pointed out the suppression of gonadotropin secretion which would lead to lack of egg generation in the ovary. Adrenal androgens may also directly inhibit the formation of the follicles in the ovary by reducing estrogen formation by the aromatase enzyme in ovarian cells. The situation is also complicated because of elevated concentrations of progesterone which occur in the follicular phase of the menstrual cycle and this high level of progesterone can act like a mini contraceptive pill on the lining of the womb (endometrium), leading to lack of egg forming cycles. This is quite a complex situation and even moving towards radical interventions such as adrenalectomy can be successful but carry considerable risks with respect to the adrenal deficiency that results.

Polycystic Ovaries

When we look at the ovary using ultrasound studies (Figure 8.30), we often find an appearance known as a polycystic ovary. The ovary is larger than normal and the follicles which are usually present in the ovary are dotted like a necklace around the edges of the ovary rather than scattered randomly throughout the structure. Contained within the ovary particularly in the centre, there is a dense soft tissue called stroma. This picture is associated with a change in the balance of the hormones so generally speaking, slightly more LH is produced compared to FSH. This appears to be a continuous feature throughout the menstrual cycle and the end result is that periods become irregular and when they do occur, they are often heavy. The development of polycystic ovaries in CAH is unclear but there does appear to be a relationship with suboptimal cortisol replacement. The resulting androgen excess impairs the hypothalamic sensitivity to progesterone, resulting in continuous estrogen production and variable formation of progesterone leading to irregularity in cycle length. During these cycles, the normal ovulatory events do not seem to take place as regularly as in normal cycles and as a result fertility is compromised due to reduced egg production.

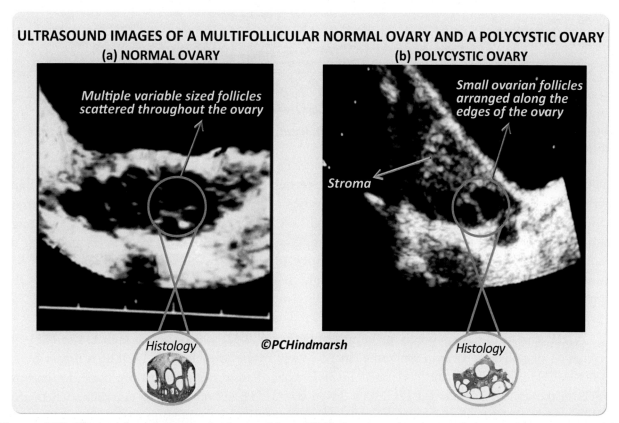

Figure 8.30 *Ultrasound appearances in image (a) multifollicular normal ovary and image (b) polycystic ovary. 1 cm markers are shown in both images, (linear in (a) and dots in (b)) to allow comparison of size. Note the increased stromal tissue in the polycystic ovary with the ovarian follicles about half the size of those in the normal ovary and arranged around the edges of the ovary. Insets show histology of a normal ovary and a polycystic ovary for comparison with the ultrasound pictures.*

This situation is particularly difficult to rectify from the CAH standpoint. The introduction of metformin, in a similar way in which polycystic ovarian syndrome is managed in non adrenal insufficient individuals, certainly assists the situation but does not reverse the condition. Normalising androgen levels is useful in this situation, but as with metformin this does not seem to overcome the inherent problem which has been generated within the ovary and additional in-depth treatment with ovulation induction techniques or in vitro fertilisation might be required.

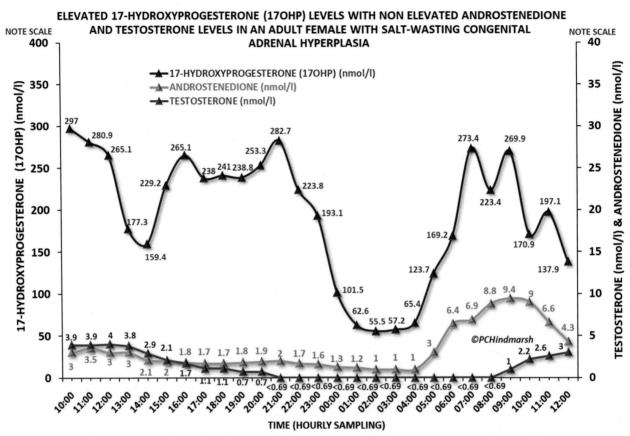

Figure 8.31 *Elevated 17-hydroxyprogesterone (17OHP) levels in the absence of raised androstenedione and testosterone.*

In people with polycystic ovaries 17-hydroxyprogesterone (17OHP) levels are often elevated. Defining whether the source of the 17OHP is from the ovaries or the adrenal glands can be difficult without detailed studies of all the hormones involved. High 17OHP with low androstenedione values might indicate an ovarian source, but usually further testing is required. This is important as increasing the glucocorticoid replacement if the ovary is the source of 17OHP is not going to work. Figure 8.31 illustrates an overnight profile where the midnight hydrocortisone does not suppress the 17OHP despite the androstenedione not being elevated.

The 17OHP appears to relate more to the bursts of LH (Figure 8.32) which show a high LH to FSH ratio characteristic of polycystic ovarian syndrome. In polycystic ovaries the elevated 17OHP is driven by LH and not ACTH. This is different to elevated 17OHP when derived from adrenal rest tissue, for example, TARTs in the gonads as the raised 17OHP is driven by ACTH and not LH. To determine whether the 17OHP arises from the adrenal glands or ovaries, a dexamethasone suppression test (Chapter 5) can be undertaken and ACTH and 17OHP measured pre and post dexamethasone. If ACTH and 17OHP are suppressed, this implicates the adrenal glands as the source of the 17OHP as the dexamethasone has suppressed the ACTH drive to the adrenal glands.

However, if the 17OHP is unchanged or not suppressed by 50% of its pre dexamethasone value this would suggest the source of the 17OHP are the gonads or in this case the ovaries, as the hypothalamo–pituitary–gonadal axis is not suppressed by dexamethasone.

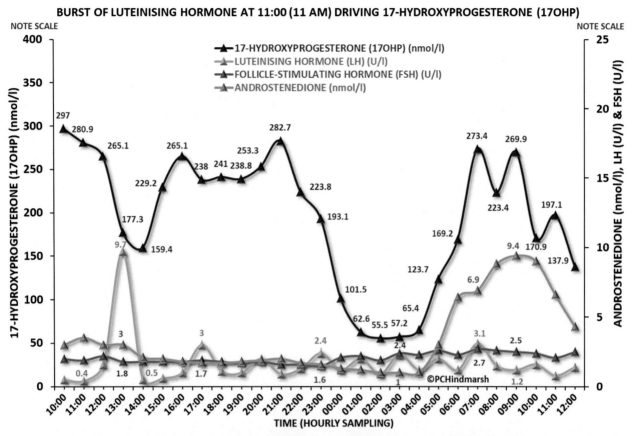

Figure 8.32 *Similar segment of the 24 hour profile shown in Figure 8.31. Hydrocortisone dosing does not lead to suppression of 17-hydroxyprogesterone during the day and night. The androstenedione levels are normal implying that the source is ovarian and the afternoon 17-hydroxyprogesterone rise appears to be more associated with the bursts of luteinising hormone release. In contrast as the hydrocortisone dose wears off by 04:00 (4 am) both androstenedione and 17-hydroxyprogesterone rise together.*

The data in Figure 8.32 illustrate why it is important to consider all hormones when evaluating the reasons for elevated 17OHP concentrations.

For example, as most clinicians make decisions based on 17OHP concentrations derived from blood spots taken pre dose, or even sometimes one hour post dose, the result would show high 17OHP concentrations which would suggest 'poor control' and hydrocortisone doses increased. This would lead to side effects which can often be seen in patients with CAH, particularly weight gain, a repeat series of blood spots would be done with little change in the 17OHP concentrations and this may lead to an incorrect suggestion of noncompliance.

This patient's cortisol was also measured over the 24 hours which needed no adjustment and 3 measurements of ACTH taken over the 24 hours were normal at 08:00 (8 am) 36.5 pg/ml, 04:00 (4 am) 37.7 pg/ml and 22:00 (10 pm) 15 pg/ml.

Finally, we need to consider ovarian adrenal rest tumours which are rare but are similar to those found in males with increased ACTH production.

Adrenal Rests in Females

Ovarian adrenal rest tissue in females with CAH is extremely rare although it is difficult to identify with the commonly used methods of imaging the ovary. This is in contrast to males with CAH, where testicular rests (TARTs) are usually detected by ultrasound are common and thought to be associated with impaired fertility. It remains a question, therefore, whether the presence of ovarian adrenal rest tumours contributes to the reduced fertility outcomes in females with CAH.

Pregnancy in a Person with Congenital Adrenal Hyperplasia

Once pregnancy is achieved new issues regarding management arise. Regular assessment during the pregnancy is required to determine the need for an increase in glucocorticoid or mineralocorticoid therapy. Excessive nausea, vomiting, salt craving and poor weight gain may indicate adrenal insufficiency. Blood glucose needs to be monitored because gestational diabetes might be more frequent in pregnant women with CAH.

Dexamethasone should not be used as replacement therapy because it is not inactivated by the placental 11beta-hydroxysteroid dehydrogenase type 2 enzyme and can cause fetal growth suppression, low birth weight and may lead to developmental problems with the brain (Figure 8.33).

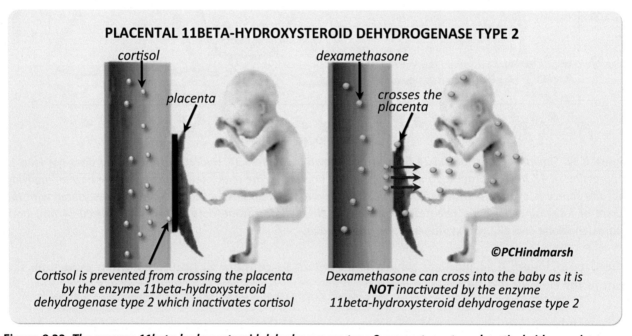

PLACENTAL 11BETA-HYDROXYSTEROID DEHYDROGENASE TYPE 2

cortisol

placenta

Cortisol is prevented from crossing the placenta by the enzyme 11beta-hydroxysteroid dehydrogenase type 2 which inactivates cortisol

dexamethasone

crosses the placenta

©PCHindmarsh

*Dexamethasone can cross into the baby as it is **NOT** inactivated by the enzyme 11beta-hydroxysteroid dehydrogenase type 2*

Figure 8.33 *The enzyme 11beta-hydroxysteroid dehydrogenase type 2 prevents maternal cortisol either endogenous or exogenous from hydrocortisone getting across the placenta into the fetus whereas dexamethasone which is not metabolised by 11beta-hydroxysteroid dehydrogenase type 2 can cross the placenta into the fetus.*

Whilst the baby may not have CAH, if the mother's adrenal androgen levels are high, these can transfer to the baby across the placenta and affect a normal female baby. In fact, this is relatively rare because girls born to mothers with CAH are generally unaffected. The placenta does seem to serve as a barrier and reduces fetal exposure to maternal androgens through placental aromatisation of maternal testosterone and androstenedione. As suggested, changes in the mother particularly the high estradiol and estriol later in pregnancy mean the proteins which carry cortisol around the blood will be increased. It is these carrier proteins such as cortisol binding globulin that are increased and unless the hydrocortisone dose the mother takes is altered, there will be less free cortisol present and adrenal androgens will increase.

As already mentioned, hydrocortisone is the treatment of choice and in pregnancy in particular, this is of immense importance because it does not cross the placenta whereas dexamethasone does. The level of cortisol in the mother's blood is approximately 10 times greater than that of the baby and it will try to equilibrate across the placenta. However, the baby in the womb needs to have a low cortisol level to allow structures to develop and the presence of the enzyme 11beta-hydroxysteroid dehydrogenase type 2 is important, as it inactivates any cortisol coming across from the mother to the placenta, to cortisone. The fetus is not completely cortisol deficient, as very high progesterone concentrations elevate free cortisol concentrations threefold by competing with cortisol for binding to cortisol binding globulin.

The same issues with respect to dosing apply to all on glucocorticoid and mineralocorticoid replacement irrespective of the cause of the adrenal insufficiency, whether primary or secondary.

Thyroxine Dosing During Pregnancy

One further issue is thyroxine dosing during pregnancy in hypopituitarism. In the first 13 weeks of pregnancy, the fetus is dependent on thyroxine from the mother crossing the placenta until the fetal thyroid becomes established around this time. Like cortisol binding globulin, thyroxine binding globulin levels increase during pregnancy so careful monitoring of the thyroxine dose is required throughout the pregnancy.

Fertility in Males with Congenital Adrenal Hyperplasia

Fertility in males with CAH has been less well documented and the influence of the condition on male fertility is not straightforward. As in females, high adrenal androgen concentrations can lead to hypogonadotropic hypogonadism. The high adrenal androgens not only suppress the gonadotropin secretion but because of peripheral aromatisation to estrogens, they also impair Leydig cell function and therefore, testosterone production. From the point of view of the individual, the switching off of the hypothalamo-pituitary-gonadal axis and reduction in gonadal testosterone may not be noticed because it may be compensated by the increased production of adrenal androgens. However, the switching off of the hypothalamo-pituitary-gonadal axis will also reduce the production of FSH and because this hormone is important in sperm formation, infertility will result with a marked reduction of sperm count and size of the testes.

The testes are filled with tiny, coiled tubes called seminiferous tubules. These are lined by Sertoli cells as well as sperm stem cells called spermatogonia. Sertoli cells are stimulated into action by FSH and interact with the spermatogonia to get sperm production underway. The Leydig cells are situated close by and these make testosterone generated by the LH signal. This intratesticular production of testosterone is extremely important because it is involved in the latter stages of sperm maturation, so anything which alters FSH and LH production will lead to impaired sperm formation directly through FSH reduction and indirectly through the loss of the generation of intratesticular testosterone.

This close interaction of the hypothalamo-pituitary-gonadal and adrenal axis is extremely important. What it tells us is that getting cortisol replacement optimal is critical in males with CAH as it is in females. Adrenal androgen excess can be managed by proper cortisol replacement and again stresses the importance of correctly delivering cortisol replacement therapy. This is shown in Figure 8.34 (page 192) where the effects of getting the right balance in hydrocortisone replacement therapy using a continuous hydrocortisone pump infusion, leads to normalisation of LH pulsatility (pulses on average every 90 minutes), with normal testosterone production compared to the reduced LH production due to adrenal androgen suppression and reduced testosterone production which was probably adrenal in origin.

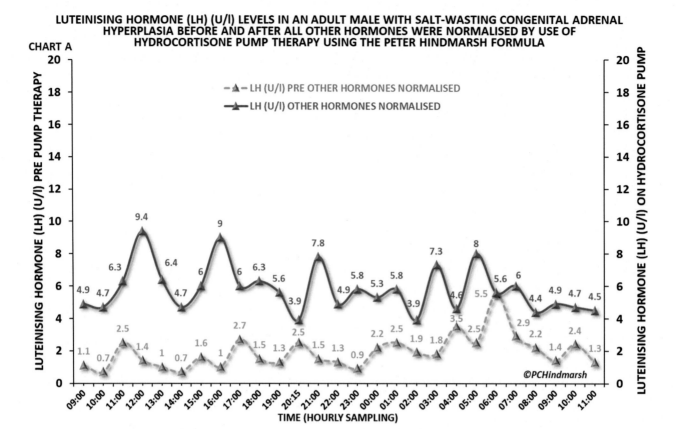

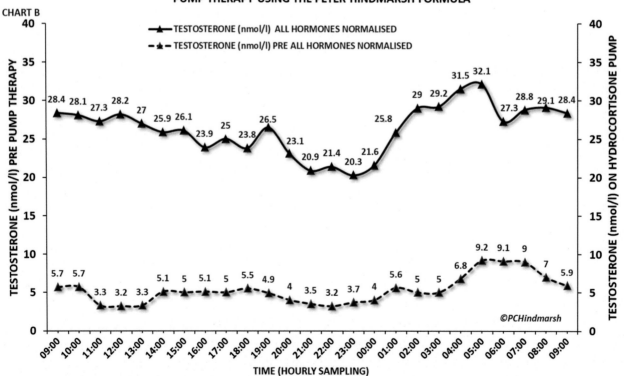

Figure 8.34 *Luteinising hormone secretion (LH) (Chart A) and testosterone production (Chart B) in an adult male with salt-wasting congenital adrenal hyperplasia receiving optimal cortisol replacement via a continuous hydrocortisone infusion pump showing normalisation of LH pulsatility and testosterone production. Excess adrenal androstenedione production dampened LH secretion leading to reduced gonadal testosterone production.*

Adrenal Rests in Males

Adrenal rests, often known as Testicular Adrenal Rest Tissue (TART) have been reported in 27% to 47% of males with classical CAH, as well as in patients with the non-classical form and also individuals with Addison's disease with elevated ACTH concentrations. It is this elevated and prolonged ACTH stimulation which leads to these focal areas of hypertrophic adrenocortical remnants. Adrenal rests are adrenal cells which are present in the testes and these appear in the testes because of the way that the gonads and adrenal glands develop at the very early stage of development. Some have even been found in the liver.

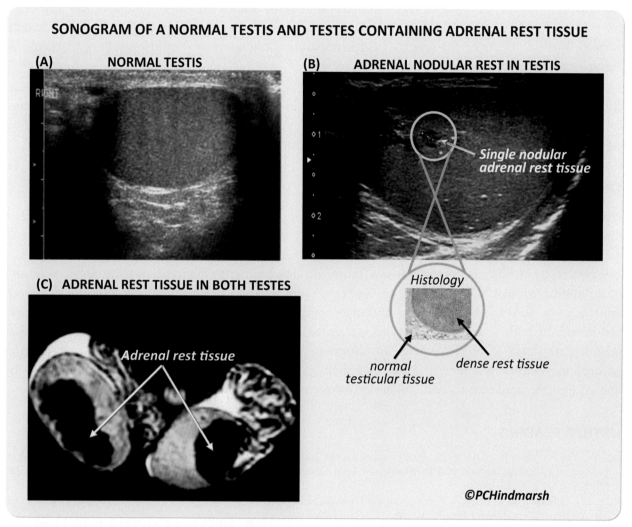

Figure 8.35 *Adrenal rest tissue in the testes. Ultrasound image (A) shows normal testis whereas image (B) shows a single small nodule (small dark area) and (C) shows extensive rest tissue (dark areas) in the testes. Inset shows histology with dense rest tissue surrounded by normal testicular tissue.*

The adrenal glands and gonads form close to each other in the primitive streak so some of the adrenal cells can get into the testes. There is a possibility they will respond to ACTH in the same way that adrenal cells in the adrenal glands do. Normally, this would not matter as long as ACTH concentrations are low. Figure 8.35 shows pictures of testes, one containing a single nodule and the other a dark black irregular shaped adrenal rest. This tissue is hard and irregular and can often be mistaken for a testicular tumour, but these lesions are not malignant although they can increase in size and can cause serious problems with respect to the remaining testicular tissue, which can essentially be squashed and malfunction. The presence of these lesions is associated with a poor outlook for long term fertility.

Not all adrenal rests are palpable, particularly initially. It is important that males have ultrasound studies from puberty onwards.

What can be done in this situation is to optimise cortisol replacement. If adrenal androgens have been suppressing the hypothalamo-pituitary-gonadal axis, spermatogenesis will resume once the axis has become released from the suppressing effect of the adrenal androgens.

The long term outcome for TART is not very good and the likelihood of fertility ensuing in an individual with TART, no matter how optimal the control is after the development of the TART, is very poor indeed. Large doses of dexamethasone can reduce the size of these TARTs but not with complete success. The role for surgery in this situation is unclear and should only be undertaken in consultation with experienced urology teams.

All males with adrenal insufficiency, if they feel a lump in the testes should see their endocrinologist and ask for a sonogram. In situations where there is a TART present, a urologist unfamiliar with the condition may be led to performing an orchidectomy unnecessarily.

CONCLUSION

Fertility needs to be assisted in cases of hypogonadotropic hypogonadism. The outcomes are better in females than males. In primary adrenal insufficiency gonadal function is not impaired apart from in adrenal hypoplasia congenita and when there are gonadal autoantibodies in autoimmune adrenalitis. Persistent high ACTH concentrations can cause the development of adrenal rest tissue in Addison's disease similar to that which occurs in CAH. Careful cortisol replacement can prevent this from happening. In CAH, excess adrenal androgen output can switch off the hypothalamo-pituitary-gonadal axis in both sexes with the additional problem of developing polycystic ovarian syndrome in females. Care needs to be taken with any hormone replacement therapy, particularly in gel form as not only may the person receiving the treatment have effects, but household members also may be exposed directly from skin to skin contact or from contaminated clothing.

FURTHER READING

Gao, Y., Yu, B., Mao, J., et al., 2018. Assisted reproductive techniques with congenital hypogonadotropic hypogonadism patients: a systematic review and meta-analysis. BMC Endocr Disord 18, 85. https://doi.org/10.1186/s12902-018-0313-8.

Otten, B.J., Stikkelbroeck, M.M., Claahsen-van der Grinten, H.L., Hermus, A.R., 2005. Puberty and fertility in congenital adrenal hyperplasia. Endocr Dev 8, 54—66.

Papadakis, G., Kandarakis, E.A., Tseniklidi, E., Papalou, O., Diamanti-Kandarakis, E., 2019. Polycystic ovary syndrome and NC-CAH: distinct characteristics and common findings. A systematic review. Front Endocrinol 10, 388. https://doi.org/10.3389/fendo.2019.00388.

Reichman, D.E., White, P.C., New, M.I., Rosenwaks, Z., 2014. Fertility in patients with congenital adrenal hyperplasia Fertil Steril 101, 301—309.

CHAPTER 8.5

Skin, Muscle and Tendons

GLOSSARY

Melanocyte-stimulating hormone This is a family of peptide hormones consisting of α-melanocyte stimulating hormone, β-melanocyte-stimulating hormone, and γ-melanocyte-stimulating hormone that are cleaved from proopiomelanocortin in the pituitary gland. Alpha-melanocyte-stimulating hormone stimulates the production of melanin by melanocytes in skin and hair which is responsible for skin and hair colour.

Proximal myopathy Weakness of the muscles of the upper leg or arm. Classic effect of excess glucocorticoids. Patients usually cannot raise themselves up from squatting position.

Striae Purple/reddish stretch marks. Glucocorticoids cause thinning of the skin and striae appear when the collagen and elastin fibres in the skin, tear. Where the fibres break, this allows the blood vessels below to show through giving the red or purple colour initially. When the blood vessels eventually shrink the fat below the skin is visible which gives the stretch marks a silvery white colour.

SKIN

Striae

Skin problems occur with glucocorticoid treatment and largely relate to thin skin and bruising, along with the appearance of stretch marks. Stretch marks are also known as striae and result from overtreatment with steroids. These stretch marks are purple/red in colour and are more common when using more potent glucocorticoids, dexamethasone and prednisolone (Figure 8.36). Stretch marks occur because the collagen and elastin fibres in the skin tear. When these fibres break this allows the blood vessels below to show through which is why the stretch marks are red or purple when they first appear. The blood vessels eventually shrink and the pale coloured layer of fat below the skin becomes visible. This then gives the stretch mark a silvery white colour. Stretch marks can also appear when there is a rapid increase in weight which stretches the tissue. In contrast, initially these stretch marks are usually white in colour.

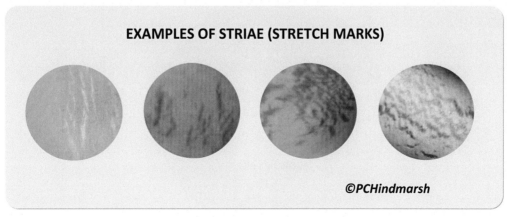

EXAMPLES OF STRIAE (STRETCH MARKS)

©PCHindmarsh

Figure 8.36 *Examples of striae (stretch marks) with red/purple colouration with white colouration shown on the left.*

Replacement Therapies in Adrenal Insufficiency. https://doi.org/10.1016/B978-0-12-824548-4.00020-6

Striae can occur even at low doses and have been noted in 5% of patients taking prednisolone doses as low as 5 mg per day. When glucocorticoids are used in high doses (or even if the total daily dose is delivered over a short time period during the day) steroid acne and hair loss can be seen. Hair loss also occurs in undiagnosed Addison's disease and alopecia areata is an autoimmune condition in its own right where hair follicles are damaged. Excess body hair is a feature of cortisol under replacement in CAH which leads to excess androgen formation. Different areas of the body are affected by the excess androgens so that actual male pattern baldness may result.

Thin Skin and Bruising

Thin skin and bruising have a similar cause to stretch marks. The thin skin itself is a direct effect of the glucocorticoids on the collagen and elastin fibres in the skin. The glucocorticoids break up the tight bonding between these fibres and this means the overlying protection of these fibres for the underlying blood vessels is lost.

These blood vessels which are small capillaries and venules can be easily damaged which explains why the slightest degree of trauma can lead to quite extensive bruising. The most commonly affected sites are the backs of the hands, forearms, sides of the neck, face and lower legs. Figure 8.37 represents the three main groups with adrenal insufficiency showing the percentages of those affected by thin skin, with 51% of the Addison's participants, 33% of the hypopituitarism participants and 16% of the CAH participants having thin skin. The high proportion in the Addison and hypopituitary groups reflected the higher dosing regimens they received, with the total daily dose concentrated between 06:00 (6 am) and 18:00 (6 pm) and a slightly older age group compared to the CAH group.

It is important to remember that skin normally becomes thinner with aging which makes it important to get dosing and distribution correct. Both prednisolone and dexamethasone will affect skin thickness, particularly as they are more potent glucocorticoids. It is also important to remember when using steroid skin creams, particularly those made up with dexamethasone, as continuous use can damage the skin. The key to safe use of steroid skin creams is short term use (3 to 4 weeks) of an appropriate potency steroid (usually 0.5% or 1% hydrocortisone).

SURVEY RESULTS OF THE PERCENTAGE OF PATIENTS WITH ADRENAL INSUFFICIENCY WHO HAVE THIN SKIN

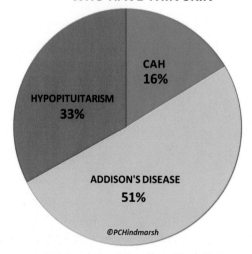

Figure 8.37 *In a questionnaire survey of 226 people with adrenal insufficiency 61 suffered from thin skin and of these 16% had congenital adrenal hyperplasia, 33% hypopituitarism and 51% Addison's disease.*

As we have commented on, glucocorticoids play a key role in thinning of the skin and this gives it a whiter appearance. This has been used in some unbranded skin whitening creams and may lead not only to damage to the skin but also adrenal suppression.

Finally, thinning of the skin and a white appearance should not be confused with vitiligo. This is an autoimmune condition which is often seen in association with Addison's disease. The areas affected are patchy with irregular margins and arise due to damage to the melanocytes in the skin (Figure 8.38).

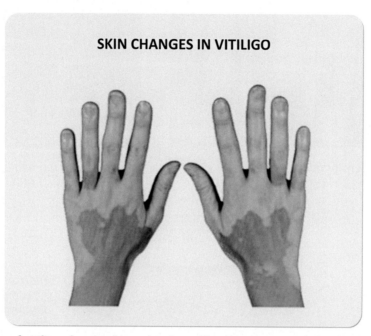

Figure 8.38 *White areas of vitiligo showing large patches of involvement set on the darker normal skin colour.*

Hyperpigmentation

The final skin affect is hyperpigmentation. This is a way inadequate cortisol replacement can show itself in the skin. The effect of this increase in pigmentation is an increase in tanning. This is because ACTH levels rise remarkably high and when they are high the skin tans turning a yellowy brown colour. This is most apparent in skin creases, knuckles (Figure 8.39) as well as the gums. These are often referred to as ACTH patches.

It is sometimes the hyperpigmentation which alerts doctors to the diagnosis of Addison's disease or other causes of primary adrenal insufficiency. Hyperpigmentation can be seen in scars where wounds have healed. Fortunately, the colour disappears when cortisol replacement is optimised and high ACTH levels are normalised. This is unlike the situation with striae which once formed are permanent.

In primary adrenal insufficiency, skin hyperpigmentation is often generalized and involves sun exposed areas, the palmar creases, nail beds, and mucous membranes; isolated tongue discoloration is less common.

The reason why hyperpigmentation occurs is because ACTH is derived from a polypeptide precursor called proopiomelanocortin (POMC). POMC is also the precursor for several other hormones one of these being alpha-melanocyte-stimulating hormone (α-MSH), so making more POMC in order to produce more ACTH, you will also make more α-MSH (Figure 8.40A).

Alpha-melanocyte-stimulating hormone stimulates melanocytes in the skin and the main function of melanocytes is to produce melanin, which is what gives the skin pigment colour so when this level is high, the darker the skin will become.

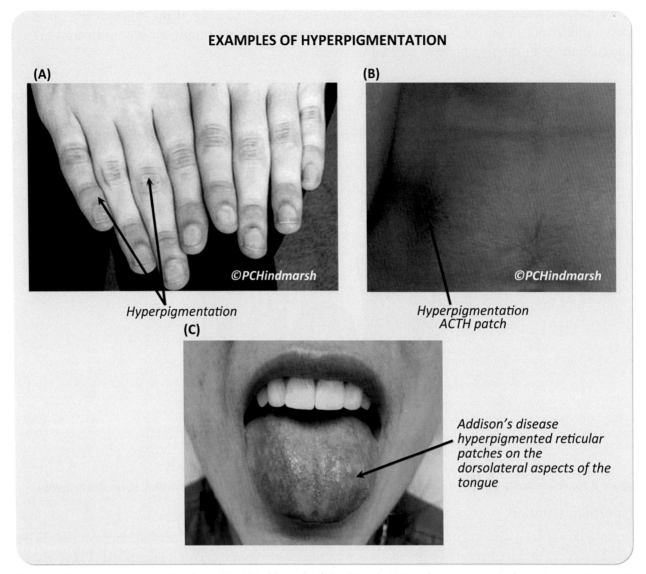

EXAMPLES OF HYPERPIGMENTATION

Figure 8.39 *Hyperpigmentation over the knuckles and finger joints (A) and an ACTH patch (B) in a patient with congenital adrenal hyperplasia who had high ACTH levels. Hyperpigmented reticular patches on the dorsolateral aspects of the tongue (C) in Addison's disease. Photograph C reproduced with kind permission of the Archives of Diseases of Childhood.*

This problem seems to be most common in patients with Addison's disease with 61% of our questionnaire population complaining of it compared to only 3% in the CAH group.

Hyperpigmentation relates to the dosing regimen of glucocorticoid replacement in particular. Leaving long periods of time without cortisol, particularly overnight and into the early morning when the ACTH drive is at its highest, is a major factor in the evolution of hyperpigmentation.

Hyperpigmentation only occurs in primary adrenal insufficiency because in the secondary forms ACTH is not produced. In primary adrenal insufficiency due to adrenal hypoplasia congenita ACTH levels can be extremely high at diagnosis and pigmentation of the newborn scrotum is very common.

Patients with undiagnosed Addison's disease often present with hyperpigmentation and look very tanned despite not having been in the sun and this is due to the persistently high ACTH levels. In contrast, in secondary adrenal insufficiency due to the deficiency of ACTH the skin is very pale, almost like alabaster.

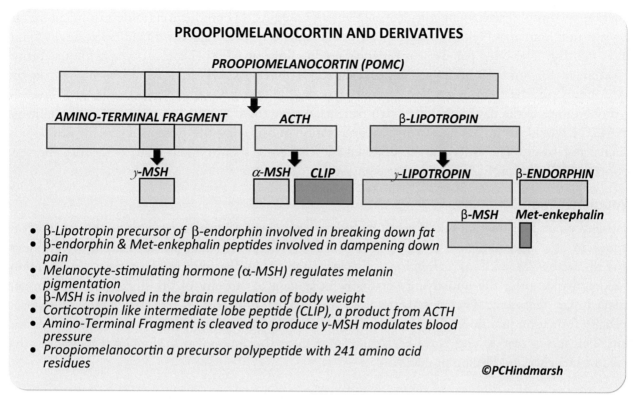

Figure 8.40A *Cleavage of proopiomelanocortin into melanocyte-stimulating hormones (MSH), ACTH and beta-endorphin.*

SURVEY RESULTS OF THE PERCENTAGE OF PATIENTS WITH ADRENAL INSUFFICIENCY WHO HAVE HYPERPIGMENTATION

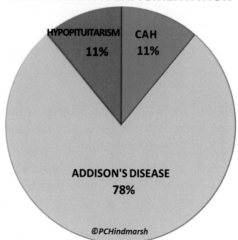

Figure 8.40B *In a questionnaire survey of 226 people with adrenal insufficiency 45 had hyperpigmentation and of these 78% had Addison's disease, 11% had congenital adrenal hyperplasia and 11% hypopituitarism.*

In our survey of 226 participants, 20% (n=45) of the total, suffered from hyperpigmentation (Figure 8.40B). Of the 45, 78% had Addison's disease, 11% CAH (all adults with poor replacement) and interestingly, 11% hypopituitarism. Hyperpigmentation can occur in hypopituitarism when an ACTH secreting tumour is not completely/successfully removed. It can also occur as it did in 3 patients who had undergone adrenalectomy, after failed pituitary surgery for Cushing's disease. In this situation, if cortisol replacement is inadequate then increased ACTH production from the pituitary results in a situation known as Nelson's syndrome. These 3 patients received glucocorticoid replacement 1 to 3 times per day. The once per day patient took prednisolone at 07:00 (7 am), so was without cortisol replacement for some 18 hours per day and especially when ACTH drive would be highest, in the early hours of the morning. This patient also had frequent adrenal crises. The last dose of hydrocortisone of the day in the other two patients, was at 16:00 (4 pm) so again the critical night rise in ACTH would occur, leading to hyperpigmentation and placing the patients at risk of developing adrenal rest tissue. The latter can be detected by frequent testicular ultrasound to identify the rests sooner (see Chapter 8, Part 4 for further discussion).

Wound healing

Impaired wound healing is a side effect of high dose glucocorticoid treatment. This occurs as a result of repression of a series of factors involved in the healing process including pro-inflammatory cytokines, growth factors as well as inhibition of genes important for skin regeneration. In addition, glucocorticoids affect the underlying keratinocytes leading to atrophy of the surface of the skin and delayed skin regrowth. The underlying tissue formed by fibroblast, is also affected with reduced collagen formation in a similar way to the disruption which we see in the formation of striae and thin skin. This means that as long as we keep our replacement therapy similar to the circadian rhythm, we will not incur wound healing problems.

Acne

Skin problems can occur with CAH. These take several forms the most important of which is acne. Acne occurs when sweat glands become blocked with secretions. These glands are very sensitive to the amount of androgen present, so if androgen levels are high then acne spots will appear. Acne spots are of course common in puberty but usually settle. They will also settle in CAH if cortisol replacement it optimised and androgen production is normalised, however occasionally, the acne may not and advice from a dermatologist should be sought. Acne can in fact be a symptom of the condition itself, if it appears in young children who have late-onset CAH as well as a sign of under treatment or inappropriate cortisol replacement.

Acne can also be caused by high steroid doses and this is known as steroid induced acne (Figure 8.41). Steroid acne most often affects adolescent or adult patients who have been taking moderate or high doses of oral steroids such as prednisone or dexamethasone for several weeks. The acne arises probably due to alterations in the types of normal fungi that are on our skin. Once the dose is lowered the acne may clear. If not, advice from a dermatologist might be needed.

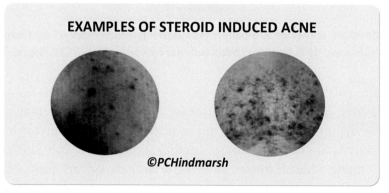

Figure 8.41 *Steroid induced acne.*

MUSCLES AND TENDONS

Glucocorticoids have a direct catabolic effect on skeletal muscle. Glucocorticoids inhibit glucose uptake in skeletal muscle which leads to breakdown of protein in the muscle as well as switching off protein synthesis. These direct effects cause muscle weakness. In addition, there are indirect effects of glucocorticoids such as the inhibition of production of muscle, insulin-like growth factor-1 (IGF-1) which normally stimulates the development of muscle mass by increasing protein synthesis and muscle generation. Insulin-like growth factor-1 is a hormone with a similar molecular structure to insulin and plays an important role in childhood growth and helps build and repair muscle tissue in adults. The production of IGF-1 is regulated by growth hormone so muscle weakness can also be a manifestation of growth hormone deficiency.

Myopathy or muscle weakness usually develops over several weeks to months with the use of glucocorticoids. Most of the observations are based on high dose glucocorticoid use. These effects are usually caused by oral treatment but repeated intramuscular injections can also cause local damage. A single injection as we use in emergency situations will not do any harm but it is important to always try to remember to use a different site if an injection is needed again. The typical clinical features include proximal muscle weakness and atrophy in both the upper and lower extremities. Muscle weakness is classified as either 'proximal' or 'distal' based on the location of the muscles that it affects. Proximal muscle weakness affects muscles closest to the body's midline, while distal muscle weakness affects muscles further out on the limbs.

The quadriceps muscles, which are proximal muscles, are particularly severely affected. The quadriceps are a group of muscles located in the front of the thigh and contain four separate muscles: the vastus lateralis, vastus medialis, vastus intermedius, and the rectus femoris. Each of the vastus muscles originate on the femur and attaches to the patella (kneecap) whereas the rectus femoris originates on the pelvic bone. Incidentally, weakness of these same muscle zones occurs in patients with overactive thyroid glands or in those receiving too much thyroxine replacement. Figure 8.42 shows where these four muscles are located in the thighs.

ANATOMY OF THE QUADRICEPS GROUP OF MUSCLES

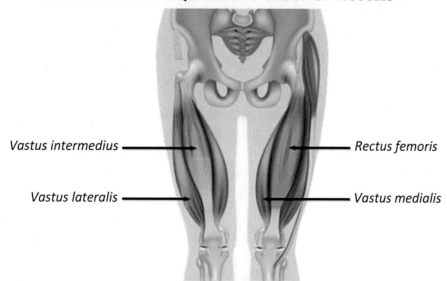

Figure 8.42 *Positions of the four muscles vastus lateralis, intermedius, medialis and rectus femoris that form the quadriceps group. Note on the left of the picture the rectus femoris has been omitted to reveal the vastus intermedius directly beneath it.*

Generally, the higher the dose of glucocorticoid used, the more rapid is the onset and doses of more than 10 mg/day of prednisolone or equivalent, are associated with a much higher incidence of muscle weakness. Unfortunately, there is no definitive diagnostic test to help in determining whether someone is going to develop myopathy associated with glucocorticoids. Readjustment of the dosing schedule can generally improve the myopathy but because it is not possible to withdraw the glucocorticoids, it is better not to get into the position in the first instance and to prevent this occurring. Careful monitoring of cortisol replacement is required.

Interestingly, low or no cortisol leads to muscle weakness as well. The reason for this is not as clear as with exposure to high doses of glucocorticoids. It does appear to be something to do with cortisol action on the muscle fibres and how easily they slide together in their usual mechanism of muscle contraction. Low cortisol concentrations can be accompanied by muscle aches and easy fatigue on exercise which may relate in part to poor glucose availability to the muscle during exercise.

We have already noted the effect of glucocorticoids on collagen and elastin fibres in the skin. Given the high content of collagen in tendons, it is not surprising the glucocorticoids impact on type 1 collagen synthesis in tendons. In addition, they appear to have a direct affect including necrosis of collagen, disruption of the collagen matrix which alters the mechanical properties of the tendons essentially weakening them. However, it should be pointed out that most of the studies of glucocorticoids on tendons, result from glucocorticoid injections administered for the treatment of acutely inflamed tendons and very little is understood of the effect of longer term exposure in individuals receiving glucocorticoid replacement therapy.

Recent studies in patients with congenital adrenal hyperplasia (CAH) have provided another explanation for joint problems. Approximately 10% of patients with CAH carry a deletion of the CAH gene (*CYP21A2*) which extends into the flanking gene for tenascin-X (*TNXB*) causing a contiguous gene deletion syndrome (a syndrome resulting from the loss of multiple neighbouring genes from a particular chromosomal segment) called CAH-X. Tenascin-X is present in connective tissue and *TNXB* mutations cause a severe form of Ehlers–Danlos syndrome (EDS), a connective tissue disorder characterized by hypermobile joints and tissue fragility. Patients with CAH-X suffer from CAH and generalized joint hypermobility, joint subluxations and 25% have cardiac abnormalities mainly of the heart valves.

CONCLUSION

Glucocorticoids have wide ranging effects on skin and connective tissue. The changes due to excess glucocorticoid exposure range from easy bruising to stretch marks and steroid induced acne. Skin pigmentation occurs when ACTH concentrations are high due to increased α-MSH production. Muscle weakness is a particular problem with high dose glucocorticoid use and can lead to falls and fractures as the muscle weakness is often associated with a reduced bone mineral density.

FURTHER READING

Burki, T., 2021. Skin-whitening creams: worth the risk? Lancet 9, 10.

Grose, R., Werner, S., Kessler, D., Tuckermann, J., Huggel, K., Durka, S., Reichardt, H.M., Werner, S., 2002. A role for endogenous glucocorticoids in wound repair. EMBO Rep 3, 575–582.

Miller, W.L., Merke, D.P., 2018. Tenascin-X, congenital adrenal hyperplasia, and the CAH-X syndrome. Horm Res Paediatr 89, 352–61.

Minetto, M.A., Qaisar, R., Agoni, V., Motta, G., Longa, E., Miotti, D., Pellegrino, M.A., Bottinelli, R., 2015. Quantitative and qualitative adaptations of muscle fibers to glucocorticoids. Muscle Nerve 52, 631–639.

CHAPTER 8.6

Eyes

GLOSSARY

Cataracts Opacification of the lens leading to blurred and reduced vision.
Glaucoma Raised pressure within the eye due to a blockage in drainage of water in the eyeball or due to increased volume of the eyeball due to water retention that presses forwards and indirectly blocks the drainage channels.

GENERAL

There are four important ocular side effects of glucocorticoids, steroid induced glaucoma, cataract formation, delayed wound healing and increased susceptibility to infection such as conjunctivitis or after surgery.

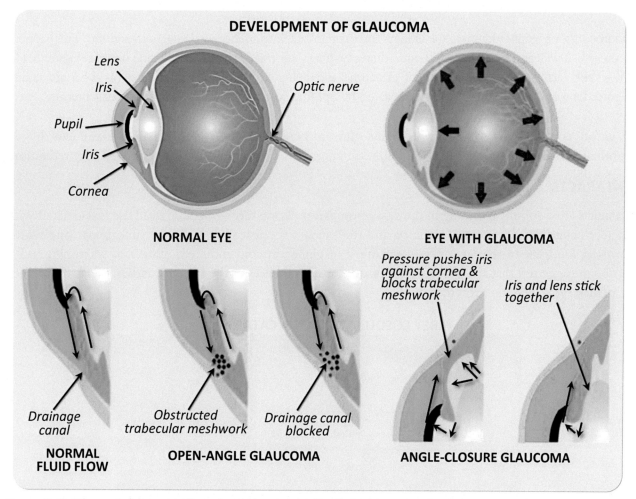

DEVELOPMENT OF GLAUCOMA

Lens
Iris
Pupil
Iris
Cornea
Optic nerve

NORMAL EYE

EYE WITH GLAUCOMA

Pressure pushes iris against cornea & blocks trabecular meshwork

Iris and lens stick together

Drainage canal

NORMAL FLUID FLOW

Obstructed trabecular meshwork

OPEN-ANGLE GLAUCOMA

Drainage canal blocked

ANGLE-CLOSURE GLAUCOMA

Figure 8.43 *Types of glaucoma where the drainage canal is blocked (open angle glaucoma) or where raised pressure in the eye itself pushes the iris of the eye forward blocking the drainage channels.*

Replacement Therapies in Adrenal Insufficiency. https://doi.org/10.1016/B978-0-12-824548-4.00021-8

GLAUCOMA

Glaucoma is a condition in which there is damage to the optic nerve often related to elevated intraocular pressure. The result if not treated quickly, is a progressive permanent vision loss. Glucocorticoids can cause an increase in intraocular pressure by increasing the expression of extracellular matrix proteins which increases the resistance to the outflow of the fluid from the eye (Figure 8.43 — open angle glaucoma).

Glucocorticoids (mainly hydrocortisone) and mineralocorticoids (fludrocortisone) will also retain water which will also contribute to the increase in the aqueous humour or fluid in the eye and produce angle-closure glaucoma (Figure 8.43). The risk of steroid induced glaucoma depends on the duration of use and the potency of the glucocorticoids themselves, as well as the individuals own risk for glaucoma. The exact prevalence of glucocorticoid induced glaucoma is not known. Studies have shown that more than 30% of individuals show a moderate rise of intraocular pressure (6 to 15 mm Hg) after topical hydrocortisone administration to the eye, while about 5% are highly responsive with intraocular pressure elevations of greater than 16 mm Hg). The prevalence is similar in children as in adults. The odds of developing raised intraocular pressure after chronic systemic glucocorticoid treatment ranges from 1.4 to 1.9 times the background rate in the general population. This is dose dependent with a mean increase of 1.4 mm Hg for each 10 mg increase in the daily dose of hydrocortisone.

Fludrocortisone retains sodium in the kidneys and this translates into an increased total body sodium. This happens in the eye as well and the increased sodium draws with it water raising the pressure inside the eye (Figure 8.43). These risk factors are a past history of glaucoma and being very old or young. Patients who are taking steroids long term should be regularly evaluated by ophthalmology for changes in intra-ocular pressure.

If vision is altered in someone receiving glucocorticoids or mineralocorticoids, assessment by an ophthalmologist is required. Glaucoma due to mineralocorticoid use can be reversed by dose reduction.

CATARACTS

Cataracts are a common finding in the aging population. Long term glucocorticoid use is associated with an accelerated development of cataracts and the cataract is classically a posterior subcapsular one which forms at the back of the lens. The mechanism of glucocorticoid induced cataracts is unknown and it has been suggested that the glucocorticoids do not directly act on the lens but rather affect the balance of ocular cytokines and growth factors.

GREY COLOURATION OF A CATARACT

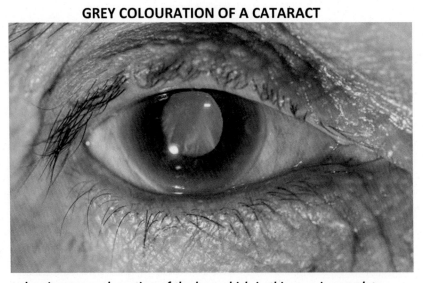

Figure 8.44 *Cataract showing grey colouration of the lens which in this case is complete.*

WOUND HEALING AND INFECTION

Glucocorticoids inhibit growth factors critical in wound healing. It is important to remember that without co-treatment with antibiotics, local ocular infections that are treated with steroids may become worse, especially viral infections.

CONCLUSION

Glucocorticoids play an important role in treating a number of inflammatory conditions. Eye complications can occur and include glaucoma, cataracts, poor wound healing and progressing infections. Careful monitoring is required for patients on high dose glucocorticoid and/or mineralocorticoid therapy and in anyone who notices changes in vision or eye pain. Special care needs to be taken when altering mineralocorticoid doses which should be done in small increments of 25 micrograms and checked with measurement of plasma renin activity. This is because mineralocorticoids can alter the pressure within the eye by changes in sodium levels and also by constricting local blood vessels. As with us all, salt intake should not be excessive and suggested daily intakes are outlined in Chapter 14.

FURTHER READING

Daniel, B.S., Orchard, D., 2015. Ocular side-effects of topical corticosteroids: what a dermatologist needs to know. Australasian J Dermatol 56, 164–169.

Dinning, W.J., 1976. Steroids and the eye – indications and complications. Postgrad Med J 52, 634–638.

Garbe, E., LeLorier, J., Boivin, J.F., Suissa, S., 1997. Risk of ocular hypertension or open-angle glaucoma in elderly patients on oral glucocorticoids. Lancet 350, 979–982.

Kwok, A.K., Lam, D.S., Ng, J.S., et al., 1997. Ocular-hypertensive response to topical steroids in children. Ophthalmology 104, 2112–2116.

Moran Core Opthalmology. University of Utah. From https://morancore.utah.edu/basic-ophthalmology-review/ocular-side-effects-of-corticosteroids/

Sulaiman, R.S., Kadmiel, M., Cidl, J.A., 2018. Glucocorticoid receptor signaling in the eye. Steroids 133, 60–66.

Tripathi, R.C., Kirschner, B.S., Kipp, M., et al., 1992. Corticosteroid treatment for inflammatory bowel disease in pediatric patients increases intraocular pressure. Gastroenterology 102, 1957–1961.

CHAPTER 8.7

Dizziness, Headaches and Dehydration

GLOSSARY

Dehydration Dehydration occurs when more fluid is lost than taken in and the body does not have enough water and other fluids to carry out its normal functions.

Postural hypotension A reduction in blood pressure on standing upright. The person needs to lie for 5 minutes when blood pressure and heart rate are measured then stand upright and the heart rate and blood pressure measures are repeated at 1 and 3 minutes. A drop in systolic blood pressure of more than 20 mm Hg, or in diastolic blood pressure of more than 10 mm Hg, or experiencing light headedness or dizziness is considered abnormal.

DIZZINESS

Dizziness is a common reported side effect. In our questionnaire study of patients with CAH, hypopituitarism and Addison's disease, the percentage reporting dizziness were 12%, 33% and 55% respectively. This also reflected reporting of low blood pressure in 0% of individuals with CAH, 21% of those with hypopituitarism and 79% with Addison's (Figure 8.45). The CAH participants fared better as they take more frequent doses and have the hormone 17OHP as a marker of cortisol replacement therapy. There was a clear increase in the likelihood of reporting dizziness when the gap between glucocorticoid doses was greater than 8 hours (45%) compared to under 8 hours (22%).

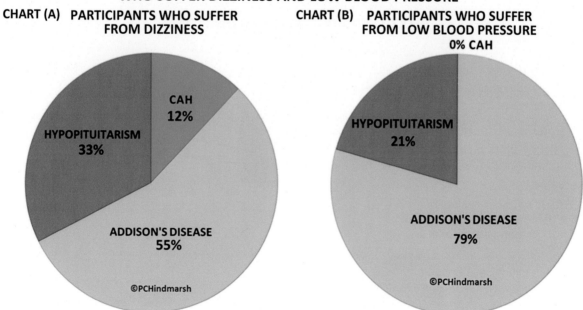

SURVEY RESULTS OF THE PERCENTAGE OF PATIENTS WITH ADRENAL INSUFFICIENCY WHO SUFFER DIZZINESS AND LOW BLOOD PRESSURE

CHART (A) PARTICIPANTS WHO SUFFER FROM DIZZINESS

CHART (B) PARTICIPANTS WHO SUFFER FROM LOW BLOOD PRESSURE

0% CAH

CAH 12%
HYPOPITUITARISM 33%
ADDISON'S DISEASE 55%
©PCHindmarsh

HYPOPITUITARISM 21%
ADDISON'S DISEASE 79%
©PCHindmarsh

Figure 8.45 *Percentages of patients with congenital adrenal hyperplasia, Addison's disease and hypopituitarism who experience dizziness (Chart (A)) and suffer low blood pressure in Chart (B).*

Replacement Therapies in Adrenal Insufficiency. https://doi.org/10.1016/B978-0-12-824548-4.00022-X

In Chapter 14 we look at blood pressure in detail. With respect to low blood pressure in adrenal insufficiency, both glucocorticoids and mineralocorticoids can be involved in the cause of dizziness, usually because of under replacement with either or both corticosteroids. The heart and the large blood vessels play a role in this symptomatology. Mineralocorticoids play an important role in maintaining circulating blood volume through the retention of sodium and water by the kidney. It is quite easy to see therefore, how inadequate mineralocorticoid replacement would lead to a reduction in blood volume which would lead to the experience of dizziness, particularly on standing up from the sitting or recumbent positions. We test for this by measuring blood pressure lying down and then standing up. A drop in systolic blood pressure of more than 20 mm Hg, or in diastolic blood pressure of more than 10 mm Hg is considered abnormal.

A lack of mineralocorticoid will reflect itself in a reduced blood volume which we can detect by measuring the haematocrit, which is the ratio of total red cell volume to total blood volume and by measuring an elevated plasma renin or renin activity (please see Chapter 14 for more detailed discussion).

Glucocorticoids play an important role in the control of vascular smooth muscle tone by their permissive effects in potentiating responses to adrenaline. The glucocorticoids alter vascular tone by suppressing the production of agents which dilate the blood vessels such as prostacyclin and nitric oxide, whereas the constricting affect which will raise blood pressure is brought about by enhancing the effects of adrenaline. These effects on nitric oxide may impact on erectile function in males adding to the fertility issues we described in Chapter 8, Part 4.

In Figure 8.46 we summarise in more detail the way that glucocorticoids and mineralocorticoids affect blood vessel function. In this example, we show the effects when the corticosteroids are under replaced leading to reduced contraction of the muscle in the blood vessels and increased relaxation of the endothelial cells leading to lower blood pressure.

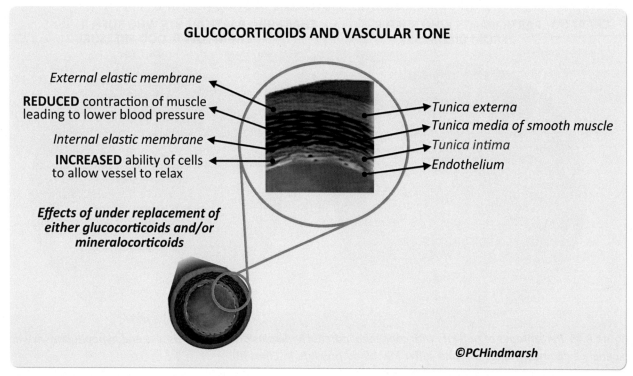

Figure 8.46 *Effects of under replacement of glucocorticoids and/or mineralocorticoids on muscle function in the middle of the wall of blood vessels as well as relaxation of the endothelial cells on the inside of the blood vessels all leading to lower blood pressure.*

Both glucocorticoids and mineralocorticoids affect heart function. The effect of mineralocorticoids is greater because they alter blood pressure which alters the work the heart has to do, so this effect is indirect. If there is mineralocorticoid under replacement, then the heart will have to beat faster and pump harder to maintain blood pressure. However, this can only happen if the glucocorticoid replacement is adequate.

The situation with glucocorticoids and the heart is more complicated. Whilst hydrocortisone also leads to a certain amount of water retention which will tend to increase blood pressure, excess hydrocortisone when present, will lead to some retention of water and if the heart is not in a very good state can lead to under function and heart failure. This is more of a problem for older adults whose cardiac function may be less able to increase output, compared to children and younger adults.

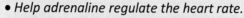

CORTICOSTEROIDS AND CARDIAC FUNCTION

GLUCOCORTICOIDS
- *Help adrenaline regulate the heart rate.*
- *Deficiency of cortisol is associated with a fast heart rate initially to compensate for the altered cardiac function and blood volume.*
- *Facilitate cardiac muscle contraction.*
- *Deficiency associated with weak pulse as heart contracts weakly when in a severe adrenal crisis.*

MINERALOCORTICOIDS
- *Indirect effect by altering blood pressure.*
- *If the blood pressure is raised, this leads to increased work needed to be done by the heart.*
- *If blood pressure low then the heart also needs to work harder to maintain circulation but if cortisol is low, this cannot happen.*
- *Falling sodium and rising potassium in mineralocorticoid deficiency can lead to dangerous cardiac arrythmias.*

©PCHindmarsh

Figure 8.47 *Effects of corticosteroids on the heart. The situation described relates to under replacement of either glucocorticoids and/or mineralocorticoids.*

Under replacement with glucocorticoids is more of an important issue because the heart function, particularly the heart rate and to a certain extent how hard it forces blood into the circulation, is very dependent on the amount of glucocorticoid present (Figure 8.47). In people who do not have any glucocorticoid present, the heart rate can be extremely slow which will lead to problems with fainting and dizziness, but this is a late effect.

Generally, the heart rate is fast as it is trying to maintain the circulation of blood and it is only in an extreme adrenal crisis that it becomes very slow. Like in the blood vessels, glucocorticoids act in conjunction with and enhance the effect of adrenaline, so that both of these agents contribute to the problems associated with glucocorticoid under replacement.

Dizziness is often a sign of low blood volume and this can also occur in hypopituitarism where arginine vasopressin is missing. Careful checking of plasma and urine osmolality will help in this situation. In all cases it is important to have a good water intake each day, in other words good hydration. Daily intake for adults should be 2 to 3 litres per day.

Finally, we must not forget that dizziness can occur during episodes of hypoglycaemia. This is in addition to the signs and symptoms we described in Chapter 8, Part 2 such as sweating, feeling shaky, heart beating fast and irritability.

Checking blood glucose with a meter system is a good idea and careful consideration of cortisol replacement based on 24 hour cortisol and glucose profiles is the way to pinpoint the problem and make the necessary changes to cortisol delivery.

HEADACHES

Glucocorticoids have been associated with headaches in the sense that they have been used to manage migraine headaches, particularly a migraine that lasts for more than 72 hours which is also called status migrainosus. Certainly, in our survey of patients with adrenal insufficiency the side effect, daily headaches, accounted for 17% of the CAH population, 29% of those with hypopituitarism and 54% with Addison's (Figure 8.48). The distribution of the doses was similar to those with low blood pressure and dizziness, leading to the feeling that this particular symptom was a reflection of suboptimal dosing. As with the general population and often experienced in diabetes, low headaches can be the first sign of low blood glucose. In the case of adrenal insufficiency, this can occur when doses are too far apart and cortisol levels drop low or are undetectable between doses. Interestingly, although the percentage of participants with CAH who suffered daily headaches was 17%, their dosing schedules were twice a day dosing or 3 doses spread inappropriately throughout the 24 hours.

This was evident in the blood glucose data, with the CAH patients dosing twice a day with their last dose time being 6 pm (18:00). Of note, there were several comments from the participants with hypopituitarism who did not know and never had their blood glucose levels checked despite the increased risk of hypoglycaemia in those with the condition. Whilst mineralocorticoids may play a part, it is more likely that the headaches represent cortisol deficiency given how important cortisol is in regulating blood vessel tone. So, the first task in dealing with such recurrent headaches is to optimise glucocorticoid replacement.

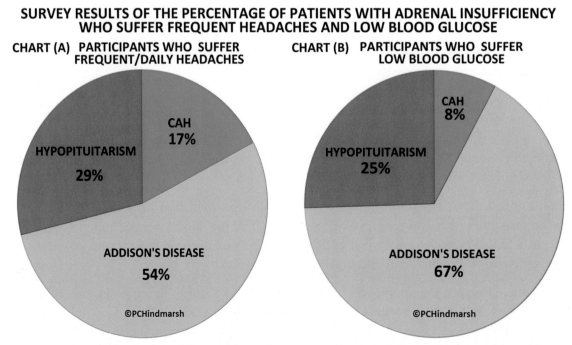

SURVEY RESULTS OF THE PERCENTAGE OF PATIENTS WITH ADRENAL INSUFFICIENCY WHO SUFFER FREQUENT HEADACHES AND LOW BLOOD GLUCOSE

CHART (A) PARTICIPANTS WHO SUFFER FREQUENT/DAILY HEADACHES

CHART (B) PARTICIPANTS WHO SUFFER LOW BLOOD GLUCOSE

CAH 17%
HYPOPITUITARISM 29%
ADDISON'S DISEASE 54%
©PCHindmarsh

CAH 8%
HYPOPITUITARISM 25%
ADDISON'S DISEASE 67%
©PCHindmarsh

Figure 8.48 *Chart (A) Percentage of patients with congenital adrenal hyperplasia, Addison's disease and hypopituitarism who complain of frequent/daily headaches and those with low blood glucose in Chart (B).*

The headaches can be quite severe and almost migrainous in nature. There is a wide literature which considers the role of dilation of blood vessels in the migraine process. The precise relationship is not clear. Glucocorticoids play an important role in enhancing adrenaline action to narrow blood vessels and if glucocorticoids are low, blood vessels widen (vasodilation). Headaches will relate therefore, in part to how adequate mineralocorticoid dosing is, what the sodium or salt intake is and whether there is cortisol deficiency due to under replacement or poor dose distribution of glucocorticoids. Severe headaches in adrenal insufficiency are also common in those who do not require fludrocortisone therapy, pointing to an important role for glucocorticoids in maintaining blood vessel function.

In hypopituitarism with diabetes insipidus, alterations in blood volume from treatment with DDAVP can lead to headaches. In this situation monitoring of blood and urine osmolality can determine adequacy of DDAVP replacement. For patients on glucocorticoid replacement therapy, individualising treatment with 24 hour cortisol profiles has been very helpful in patients with persistent headaches, as getting the glucocorticoid replacement right in all cases led to resolution of the headaches.

Over replacement with glucocorticoids is also likely to produce headaches probably due to increased blood volume and raised blood pressure so headaches cannot be used to guide changes to replacement doses. Only 24 hour cortisol profiles will provide the data to optimise dosing schedules.

It is always useful to note if there is a specific time of the day the headaches occur. What we have often found in our practice, is that many patients who develop headaches have been on three doses of hydrocortisone per day and once changed to four doses per day the headaches abated. Remember that hydrocortisone lasts 6 hours in the circulation, so a three times daily treatment programme leaves the individual with no cortisol for a period of 6 hours.

Finally, as we mentioned with dizziness, dehydration can lead to headaches due to a reduction in blood volume. A good intake per day is needed ranging between 2.5 and 3 litres per day for adults with a minimum set at 1.5 litres. For children, the amount varies with age: 1 to 3 years, 1 litre; 4 to 8 years 1.2 litres and over 9 years 1.5 litres. People with diabetes insipidus should work with their endocrinologist to determine what their daily intake should be. This is even more important in those with diabetes insipidus and loss of thirst, where fixed daily intakes need to be determined with their endocrinologist.

DEHYDRATION

A note now on dehydration as it is referred to in this Chapter and will appear again in Chapters 12 and 14, so we will cover some broad principles here.

There are various grades of dehydration and we are more used to the severe end of the spectrum as we see in adrenal crises, or when there is marked water loss in diabetes insipidus. We consider the hormonal response to changes in blood volume and water intake in Chapter 14.

What happens when water is lost from the circulation is that the blood becomes more concentrated as the blood volume decreases. This change in the blood is picked up in the hypothalamus by the osmoreceptors which when the plasma sodium concentration starts to rise to 145 mmol/l, switch on thirst so the person seeks water to drink. At the same time the posterior pituitary releases arginine vasopressin. Arginine vasopressin acts on the kidneys via its receptor or docking station leading to increased reabsorption of water so that we see this as a reduction in urine output and a deeper coloured urine. These two effects of thirst and arginine vasopressin return blood volume back to normal and this can be measured by the plasma osmolality.

HYDRATION AND URINE COLOUR

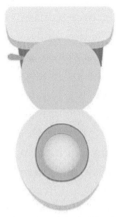

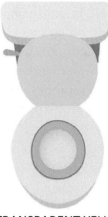

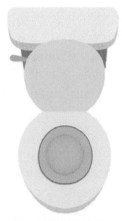

NO COLOUR, TRANSPARENT
Might be drinking too much water and may need to cut back a little on consumption.

TRANSPARENT YELLOW
Normal, healthy and well hydrated.

HONEY OR AMBER
DRINK WATER NOW!
Sign your body is not getting enough water.

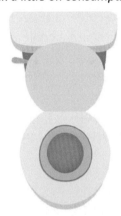

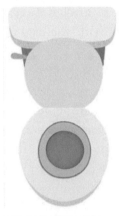

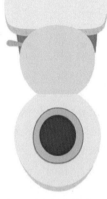

BROWN ALE OR SYRUP COLOUR
DRINK WATER NOW!
This is a sign of severe dehydration or a sign you could have liver disease. See your doctor, it your urine continues to be this colour.

REDDISH/PINKISH
This could be due to something you have eaten, such as beetroot. However, it could be blood in the urine, so contact your doctor.

COLA COLOURED
This occurs from Rhabdomyolysis, muscle breakdown after being bedbound for a long period of time, having done heavy exercise or major trauma.

©PCHindmarsh

Figure 8.49 *Top panel shows changes in the colour of urine depending on how much is passed. Very dilute urine occurs (top panel left) when too much water has been drunk but also in diabetes insipidus. Moving across to the right of the top panel shows more concentrated urine indicating a need for more fluid intake. This can progress to the picture on the left of the lower panel where the urine is very dark like brown ale and this implies severe dehydration and that needs a consultation with your doctor. Other examples of urine colour include in the middle of the lower panel red coloured urine which can reflect beetroot ingestion but could also be blood so again a consult is needed. Cola coloured urine means that there is rhabdomyolysis or muscle break down usually when bedbound for a long period, done heavy exercise, had a crush injury or a major trauma. This needs urgent medical attention.*

Signs and Classification of Dehydration

We can gain quite a lot of insight into the state of body hydration from observing the amount and colour of the urine. There are other things we can learn too as shown in Figure 8.49. Other information can come from the colour of urine ranging from very dilute as occurs in diabetes insipidus, through normal pale yellow colour to very dark (Figure 8.49). Very dark urine, which is passed in small volumes indicates, if persistent, marked dehydration.

SIGNS OF DEHYDRATION

DEHYDRATION PARAMETERS	NO DEHYDRATION	SOME DEHYDRATION	SEVERE DEHYDRATION
GENERAL APPEARANCE	Normal, well alert	Thirsty, restless, or lethargic irritable	Drowsy, limp, cold, sweaty, lethargic, floppy
THIRST	Drinks normally, not thirsty	Thirsty, drinks eagerly	Drinks poorly or unable to drink
EYES	Normal	Sunken	Very sunken
MOIST LINING OF MOUTH & EYES	Moist	Sticky	Dry
TEARS	Present	Decreased	Absent
URINE	Normal volume light yellow	Less frequent with dark yellow colour	Very little and dark brown
SKIN	Normal elastic rebound when pinched	Slow rebound when pinched	Remains standing up when pinched and/or doughy feel and goes back very slowly
ACTION		Increase fluid input & monitor	If showing symptoms above need to go to A&E immediately

©PCHindmarsh

Figure 8.50 *Classification of dehydration based on appearance, eye tone, presence of thirst and skin tone. Note, signs of dehydration may be less obvious in the over 65 year age group.*

We can then take these observations of the amount of urine passed as well as the colour and combine with how the person looks, the skin tone, whether the eyes are sunken or not and how moist the lining of the mouth is. This allows us to decide whether we are well hydrated right through to severe dehydration and what action is needed (Figure 8.50).

CONCLUSION

Dizziness and headaches were common symptoms in our survey. Both can indicate under replacement with glucocorticoids and/or mineralocorticoids and arise due to alterations in blood vessel tone as well as a reduction in blood volume. Adequate daily fluid intake is important as is adjusting mineralocorticoid acting on the basis of plasma renin or renin activity and by checking the dose and distribution of glucocorticoid by 24 hour cortisol profiles. We also need to remember that hypoglycaemia can manifest with dizziness and headaches and is particularly likely when there are large gaps between doses, for example when the last dose of the day is at 6pm (18:00). This is particularly so in illness which we cover in Chapter 12 and in children.

FURTHER READING

Dehydration - National Health Service, 2023. https://www.nhs.uk/conditions/dehydration.
Oray, M., Samra, K.A., Ebrahimiadib, N., Meese, H., Foster, C.S., 2016. Long-term side effects of glucocorticoids. Expert Opin Drug Saf 15, 457—465.
Ullian, M.E., 1999. The role of corticosteroids in the regulation of vascular tone. Cardiovascular Res 41, 55—64.
Yang, S., Zhang, L., 2004. Glucocorticoids and vascular reactivity. Curr Vasc Pharmacol 2, 1—12.

CHAPTER 8.8

Sleep, Mood and Cognitive Affects

GLOSSARY

Central clock A collection of cells predominantly within the suprachiasmatic nucleus of the hypothalamus which respond to the light/dark cycle altering expression of several genes that control metabolic function and generate circadian rhythm generation of cortisol, temperature, and blood pressure. The central clock synchronises the peripheral clocks present in various tissues and organs of the body enabling a coordinated response of these tissues and organs.

Depression A clinical condition characterised by disturbances in mood, appetite and sleep.

Light/dark cycle Cyclicity in the function of a number of brain components which appear to follow light and dark, rather than an exact linkage to a 24 hour clock.

SLEEP

In a detailed questionnaire covering reported side effects associated with glucocorticoid use in 226 patients with adrenal insufficiency, the frequency of difficulties with sleep, particularly trouble falling asleep was 25% in the CAH participants, 27% in those with hypopituitarism and 48% in those with Addison's disease (Figure 8.51).

This disparity between the CAH and hypopituitary participants and those with Addison's is difficult to understand.

There has been a long tradition in endocrinology which has implicated glucocorticoids and particularly late evening dosing with glucocorticoids, in the difficulties that people associated with getting off to sleep. Whether this is in fact glucocorticoid related, we will assess in this section.

SURVEY RESULTS OF THE PERCENTAGE OF PATIENTS WITH ADRENAL INSUFFICIENCY WHO HAVE TROUBLE FALLING ASLEEP

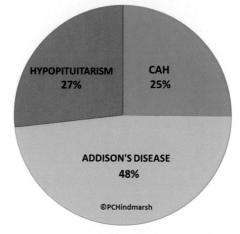

Figure 8.51 *Percentages of patients with different forms of adrenal insufficiency having trouble falling asleep.*

Replacement Therapies in Adrenal Insufficiency. https://doi.org/10.1016/B978-0-12-824548-4.00023-1

Conventionally, sleep is broken down into various stages depending upon brain activity which is usually recorded using an electroencephalogram. Depending on the classification there are 4 stages of sleep, starting in Stage 1 with a relatively light stage of sleep which is a transition period between wakefulness and sleep. This lasts only 5 to 10 minutes. The second stage lasts for approximately 20 minutes and is associated with a decrease in body temperature and heart rate. By the time Stage 3 sleep is reached, the person is less responsive and extraneous events such as noises may fail to generate a response. In Stage 4, sleep dreaming takes place and there is also associated rapid eye movements (REM). Breathing rate is increased and brain activity also.

The amount of time spent asleep and in these different stages of sleep varies. Infants will spend more time sleeping and this sleep is spent in Stage 4 compared with older children and adults. Babies also do not have a circadian cortisol rhythm until 3 months of age and tend to have a constant level of cortisol which does not seem to impact on their ability to sleep.

Sleep also has a close relationship with hormones. Figure 8.52 shows the relationship between time of day and the circulating concentrations of melatonin and cortisol. Melatonin is produced by the pineal gland, situated at the base of the brain attached to the roof of the third ventricle by a stalk and appears to be important in sleep onset. In adults, the melatonin starts to increase when cortisol is low and with aging, the production of melatonin declines and is shifted to the later hours so that it tends to overlap with the onset of the rise of cortisol from midnight. It should be pointed out however, that cortisol concentrations are always detectable in the evening, it is just that they are lower than encountered at different times of the day.

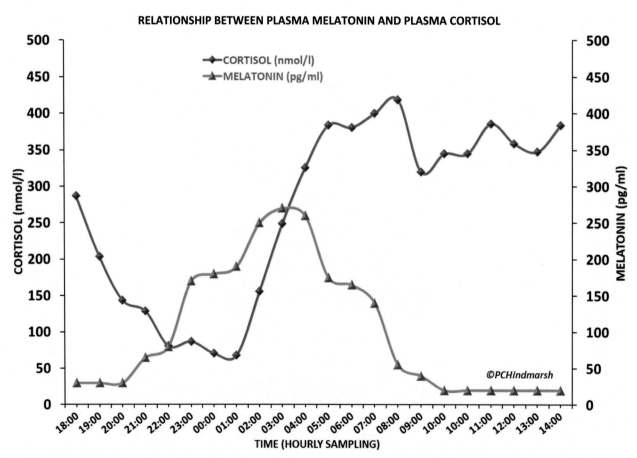

Figure 8.52 *Relationship between plasma melatonin (orange line) and plasma cortisol (blue line) showing that melatonin starts to rise late evening as cortisol reaches its lowest level. There is also the suggestion that as cortisol levels rise melatonin production is switched off. Note cortisol measurements are never 'undetectable' in the blood.*

Melatonin appears to be extremely important in setting the trigger to go to sleep. This has been used to great advantage by the pharmaceutical industry, in manufacturing melatonin as a support for people who find it difficult to get off to sleep and also to assist individuals with sleep problems associated with jetlag. It is important to note that melatonin simply gets the individual off to sleep but it will not maintain sleep thereafter. Of interest in Figure 8.52 is that as soon as cortisol starts to rise from midnight melatonin levels fall which may be important in enabling people to wake up.

Sleep and cortisol affect electrical activity in the brain especially during the transition between sleep stages and variations in cortisol during its circadian rhythm. This is particularly the case for seizure activity which was originally thought to occur randomly, but appears to be driven physiologically by both sleep and cortisol with cortisol through the light/dark cycle acting independently of the sleep/wake cycle.

Sleep is also associated with the release of other hormones. Growth hormone tends to be released during Stage 4 sleep. ACTH and cortisol tend to increase during Stage 3/Stage 4 sleep (Figure 8.53). However, the relationship between sleep stages and ACTH and cortisol release is not clear cut and ACTH and cortisol are more attuned to the light/dark cycle than sleep itself. The clock genes we mentioned in earlier chapters in the hypothalamus which regulate ACTH release, work almost independently of sleep itself, receiving their cues from day/night lengths.

The association of sleep with the release of many hormones, for example ACTH, cortisol and growth hormone is close, but sleep itself does not necessarily trigger the release of these hormones.

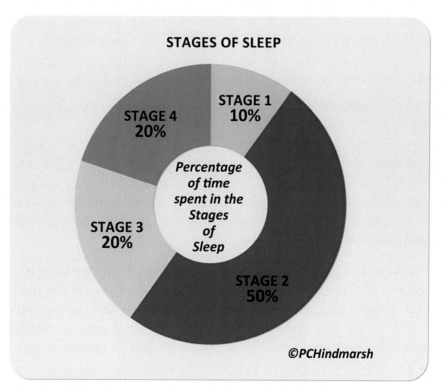

Figure 8.53 *Representation of the percentage of time spent in the four stages of sleep.*

We also do not understand if the converse is true. Do the hormones themselves influence the stages of sleep or rather the time spent in various stages of sleep?

The situation is complex because not only do we have all these interactions taking place between hormones and also the central clock, but our natural day/night rhythm is not actually 24 hours and more like 23 hours which means we need to readjust every now and again to fit the 24 hour cycle. If this does not happen, then the sleep/wake cycle gradually gets out of synchrony and we experience difficulties getting off to sleep or going to sleep at different times of the day. This is quite a problem in the elderly where this disrupted pattern is common and a major problem for night shift workers.

As already mentioned, when considering melatonin there are two major issues with respect to understanding sleep problems:

1. The first, is whether the problem is regarding getting off to sleep?
2. The second, is sleep being maintained or disrupted at a later stage of the night?

As previously discussed, the first group responds well to melatonin therapy. The second group is more complicated to treat as melatonin does not seem to work very well and the best treatments seems to be the benzodiazepine group of drugs, (the class of sleeping tablets such as Valium). These are not without their own problems and side effects, but they are effective in this particular group of individuals.

Returning now to the issue of receiving glucocorticoids and having problems falling asleep. This concept is very ingrained in adult endocrine practice such that patients are advised to take their last dose of medication no later than 6 pm (18:00). This raises the question as to whether the way in which glucocorticoids are replaced, affects how people sleep.

Studies have shown that in people without adrenal problems, cortisol concentrations are naturally going to be at their lowest at the time when people are going off to sleep. However, it may be important that there is some, albeit low, amounts of cortisol present. This raises two possibilities:

1. There should be no cortisol present which would be the adult endocrine practice dosing argument.
2. Or there needs to be some cortisol present in the circulation, albeit a small amount in the region 50 to 100 nmol/l.

This is an important question which needs to be resolved because if you dose at 6 pm (18:00) with hydrocortisone, you will be without cortisol in the bloodstream for a very long period of time and there will be no cortisol present from midnight, which is the time cortisol levels naturally start to rise. The duration of hydrocortisone in the bloodstream is 6 hours although this varies between individuals depending on their metabolism.

In children, many of the treatment regimens use a midnight dose. If we now look at the effect of dosing with hydrocortisone at 6 pm (18:00) which is shown in Figure 8.54, we see the peak is achieved quite quickly and the peak is quite high. However, by the late evening there is very little cortisol present such that the patient does not have cortisol levels above the critical value of 50 - 100 nmol/l in the bloodstream and from 23:00 (11 pm) onwards until the next dose in the morning, there is no cortisol measurable so they are without cortisol for a period of 9 hours.

If you look at the dashed line in Figure 8.54 you can see an example of the normal circadian rhythm which we are trying to mimic and in people with primary adrenal problems such as CAH or Addison's disease, this would mean that the strong ACTH drive at this period of time would make the adrenal glands produce a lot of adrenal androgens in the case of CAH. In fact, in both conditions ACTH concentrations would be high and explains why patients with primary adrenal insufficiency complain of increased pigmentation, because this occurs when ACTH concentrations are high.

It is not just the pigmentation that would be an issue, but the very high ACTH concentrations may lead to the development of adrenal rests in the testes and this occurs in patients with CAH and Addison's disease. It will not occur in individuals with hypopituitarism because ACTH production is absent.

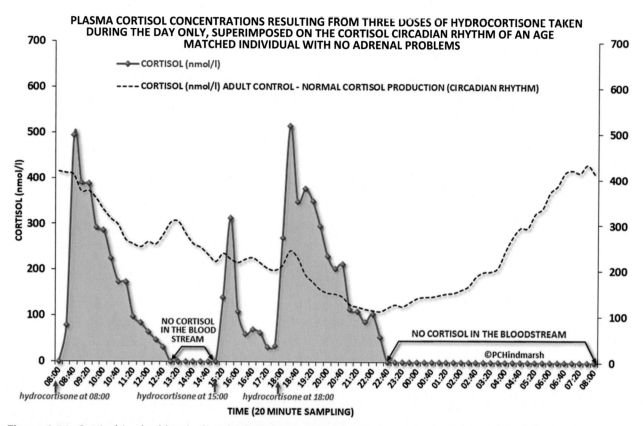

Figure 8.54 *Cortisol in the blood after the last dose of the day (hydrocortisone) is given at 18:00 (6 pm). Note the periods of time 13:00 to 15:00 (1 to 3 pm) and from 23:00 (11 pm) to the morning dose at 08:00 (8 am) where there is no measurable cortisol in the bloodstream compared to the cortisol production (dashed blue line) of an individual who has no adrenal problems. Remember the amount of cortisol differs between individuals, however the pattern of production is constant. Please note this is the natural production in an individual of a similar age to the person receiving hydrocortisone.*

Additionally, the dosing schedule shown in Figure 8.54 shows all the doses are taken between 08:00 (8 am) and 18:00 (6 pm), resulting in cortisol only being in the system from 08:00 (8 am) until approximately 23:00 (11 pm). This is not mimicking the circadian rhythm as it:

- Delivers the total daily replacement dose during the day with quite high peaks

- Leaves periods of time, 2 hours between 13:00 to 15:00 (1 pm to 3 pm) and 9 hours from 23:00 to 08:00 (11 pm to 8 am), therefore 11 hours, where there is under exposure

- Creates the situation where the individual oscillates between periods of over and under treatment.

It is true it can be difficult getting the timing of the late evening dose correct and we look at this aspect in more detail in Chapter 9. There is no doubt that moving the dose as close as possible to midnight or 01:00 (1 am) provides the best outcome. One useful point is that the dose at night is metabolised differently so that the profile is almost one of slower delivery and longer presence in the circulation (Figure 8.55).

PHARMACOLOGY OF MORNING AND EVENING DOSES OF HYDROCORTISONE

PARAMETER	MORNING DOSE	EVENING DOSE
T_{max} (minutes)	**60** (20 - 80)	**100** (60 - 120)
TIME to 50 - 100 nmol/l (minutes)	**220** (140 - 250)	**315** (255 - 540)

©PCHindmarsh

Figure 8.55 *Pharmacology of similar doses given first in the morning usually between 06:00 to 07:00 (6 am to 7 am) and last dose at night at 00:00 (midnight) in patients with congenital adrenal hyperplasia. The time to the peak (T_{max}) was longer at night and this resulted in a longer time that cortisol levels were above 50 to 100 nmol/l (P = 0.01 for significance).*

We do need to consider if there is any evidence that sleep is really disrupted with glucocorticoids. Over the years there have been a number of carefully constructed sleep studies which have investigated this question. The message is very clear. It does not matter if you take hydrocortisone medication late in the evening, the time of sleep onset, sleep quality and duration of sleep, is not affected and that is irrespective of the reason you are taking hydrocortisone tablets.

Several conditions have been associated with high cortisol levels. One such situation is insomnia. Having difficulty getting to sleep or staying asleep for long enough to feel refreshed the next morning is called insomnia. Again, careful evaluation has shown that in insomnia there is a state of hyperarousal of the nervous and metabolic systems and that any increase in cortisol production is secondary to the state of hyperarousal. This really important information means we can replace cortisol as close to the circadian rhythm as we possibly can without worrying about sleep issues.

This point is also supported by the questionnaire data which we introduced this section with. Figure 8.56 (page 221) shows the answers to how people with CAH, Addison's disease, and hypopituitarism cope with sleep. The important point here is it does not matter what time the last dose is taken, there is no difference in ability to get off to sleep. Possibly the group which has the least problems in falling asleep was the CAH group who always take their medication as late as is possible. Many of these are children who have a fair amount of cortisol in the bloodstream before going off to sleep and wake at midnight to take a further dose of hydrocortisone before going straight back to sleep. To put this all in perspective in the United Kingdom and United States of America insomnia is a common problem thought to regularly affect around one in three people, and is particularly common in elderly people. These proportions are similar to those found in our survey (Figure 8.51, page 251) with the exception of the patients with Addison's disease. Finally, studies in patients with Addison's disease show that it is the condition per se, not the treatment which leads to sleep problems and that poor quality of life follows from poor sleep. It is also possible that patients with Addison's disease are older than those with CAH or hypopituitarism. Sleep patterns change with age in the general population so that it is harder to fall asleep and once asleep waking is more frequent (3 to 4 times) during the night. Total sleep time stays the same or is slightly decreased (6 to 7 hours per night) and less time is spent in deep sleep.

There does not appear to be any good reason to take the last dose at 18:00 (6 pm) and the last dose should be given as late as is possible and ideally around midnight, as this would better mimic the circadian rhythm. Melatonin can be quite helpful in assisting with sleep onset and needs to be taken approximately an hour before going to bed. Stimulants such as caffeine before bed should be avoided.

DOSE TIMING AND SLEEP PROBLEMS IN A SURVEY OF PATIENTS WITH ADRENAL INSUFFICIENCY

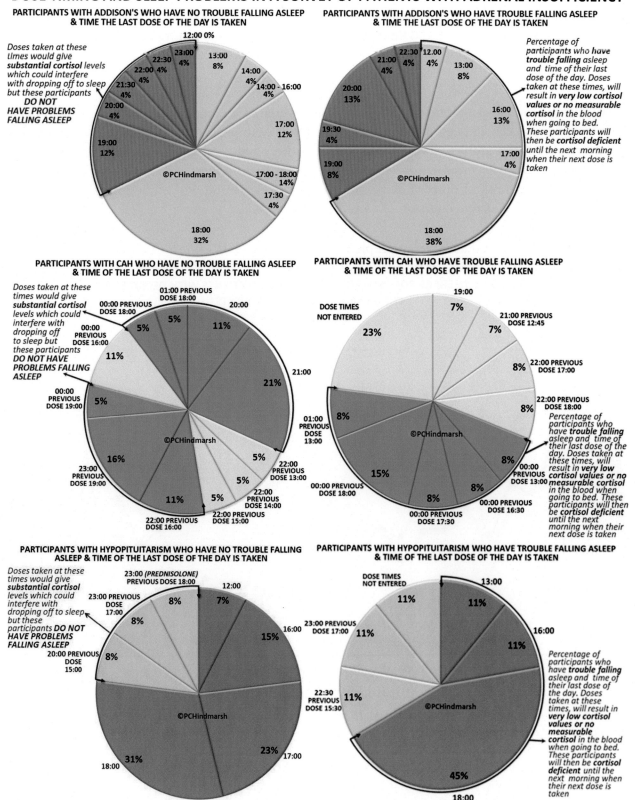

Figure 8.56 *Effect of timing of last dose taken at night and difficulty in falling asleep in 82 patients with Addison's disease (upper), 77 patients with congenital adrenal hyperplasia (middle) and 67 patients with hypopituitarism (lower).*

MOOD ALTERATIONS

The adult psychiatry literature contains a large number of publications showing that in conditions such as depression, cortisol concentrations are altered and an example is shown in Figure 8.57 comparing cortisol levels in patients with depression and those without. The circadian pattern is remarkably similar between the two, but overall the depressed patients produce 20% more cortisol during the 24 hour period than the control group.

Is it the depression that causes the raised cortisol or vice versa? We cannot say definitively, but studies to dissect out this chicken and egg situation are ongoing. For example, a similar question existed for sleep and depression. Sleep problems were long thought to be a result of depression. More recent studies combining genetics with measures of sleep and depression have shown that short sleep duration alone carries with it a high risk of onset of depression over an 8 year period. Hopefully such approaches will help determine the causative direction of cortisol and depression.

For more details on mood and depression please refer to Chapter 16.

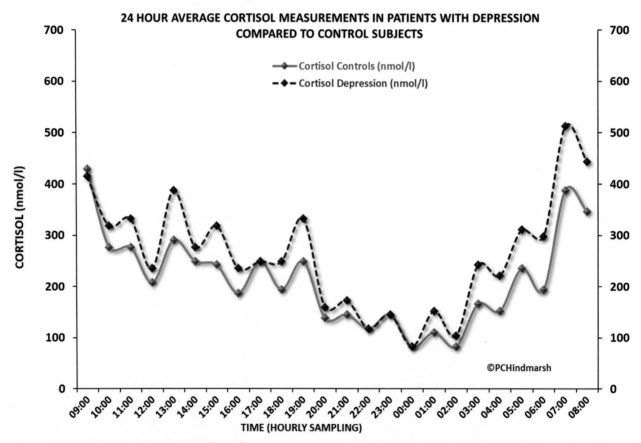

Figure 8.57 *24 hour average cortisol profiles in 15 patients with depression (purple dashed line) compared to 22 subjects without depression (blue line).*

Chronic stress is another situation where clinical studies show that cortisol concentrations are raised as a result of the stress. This would imply it is the event that alters the cortisol rather than the other way around. Having said that, in Cushing's disease there is an increased production of ACTH from the pituitary gland and this ACTH is present at high levels throughout the 24 hour period. Cushing's disease can often be associated with depression which usually reverses once the condition has been treated.

This would suggest persistent high levels of glucocorticoids can lead to mood alterations such as depression. This certainly can be seen with the more potent glucocorticoids as both prednisolone and dexamethasone appear to have high rates of mood changes associated with their use.

The beginning of the appearance of symptoms induced by glucocorticoids varies. It might arise at the start of treatment, usually the first 5 days. This is slightly different of course to the situation we are looking at, which is more long term exposure to glucocorticoids.

The number of individuals affected appears to be quite small in that only 2% to 4% of patients develop depression, anxiety or become apathetic. These overall effects however, are dose dependent and are particularly associated with the use of the more potent glucocorticoids such as dexamethasone and prednisolone.

The reaction people manifest can be quite different. With oral prednisolone, several studies have reported that there is an unusual sense of wellbeing which is often called 'steroid euphoria,' characterised by a reduced sense of anxiety and depression when compared with patients not on prednisolone or taking placebo. The literature on the more severe phases of depression vary from the low numbers suggested above to incidences of 40%. Emotional mood swings and irritability do appear to be the more common symptoms. Altered consciousness and disorientation are rarely observed.

COGNITIVE AFFECTS

Prolonged treatment with high dose glucocorticoids has been associated with cognitive defects, difficulty to maintain concentration and poor memory. This type of problem appears to be associated with dysfunction at the hippocampal level in the brain. The hippocampus is particularly involved in short term memory and is an area which is extremely rich in glucocorticoid receptors, so it would be an area highly susceptible to the effects of glucocorticoids.

This observation is of interest because many individuals consider examinations as stress. Whilst they are certainly stressful and there is a fear of the unknown in what is likely to happen, this fear or anxiety is more an adrenaline effect rather than an effect of heightened cortisol production. It would be tempting to increase the dose of cortisol to cover this 'stressful period.' That would probably not be the best thing to do because the increased amount of glucocorticoid is likely to impair short term memory and in particular short term memory recall which would be counterproductive in an exam situation!

Finally, it is also worth pointing out that under treatment can lead to problems in a number of ways. Lack of cortisol is associated with a general slowing in activity and reduced energy levels. It is also associated with low blood glucose and this in itself can lead to mood changes, irritability, loss of concentration and lethargy as well as anger.

Hypoglycaemia can impair cognitive function, particularly mathematical tasks as well as fine motor activities such as writing. Hypoglycaemia is a particular problem in secondary adrenal insufficiency where many anterior pituitary hormones are missing (Chapter 8, Part 2). Ensuring adequate replacement therapy helps guard against hypoglycaemia and blood glucose monitors can be helpful if this is a recurrent problem even when hormone replacement is optimised.

Cognitive problems are also associated with primary adrenal insufficiency due to X-linked adrenoleukodystrophy where they may represent involvement of parts of the brain in the disease process. Regular MRI brain scans are helpful for early detection of changes and any changes in academic performance should be reported to the metabolic team managing the condition.

In secondary adrenal insufficiency, there can be associated central hypothyroidism (Chapters 1 and 2). Untreated hypothyroidism, particularly from birth is associated with cognitive defects such as information processing, mathematical skills and coordination. This is because thyroxine is involved, particularly in the last 12 weeks of pregnancy, in forming multiple small connections between nerve cells called dendrites.

The effects are less severe than seen in patients with severe congenital hypothyroidism where the thyroid gland does not form. In secondary or central hypothyroidism, the thyroid gland forms normally and can produce a small amount of thyroxine. What is lost in secondary or central hypothyroidism, is the regulation of thyroxine production by the thyroid-stimulating hormone which is produced by the pituitary gland. In either case, the changes are not reversible on introducing thyroxine treatment.

Adults developing hypothyroidism may experience a general slowing in mental function and if left untreated for long episodes of time can develop myxoedema coma. Over replacement with thyroxine can lead to tremors, poor concentration, irritability and anxiety (Chapters 1 and 2).

In Chapter 1 we considered causes for secondary adrenal insufficiency. The congenital forms are often associated with defects in genes that code for developmental proteins which are involved not only with pituitary gland development, but also with the development of particular regions of the brain including hearing and the eyes. This means that neurodevelopmental and cognitive problems may not simply be due to the effects of the missing hormones e.g., hypoglycaemia, but may reflect a broader issue in brain development. This is important because the clinician needs to address not just the hormone replacement that is required, but the social and educational needs of the patient which may be extensive in terms of hearing, speech, language and vision as well as autism and learning difficulties. These are not remediable simply by replacing the hormones that are missing. For the effects of hypoglycaemia in hypopituitarism please see Chapter 8 Part 2.

Treatment of primary and metastatic brain tumours includes high dose radiation to the brain. Understanding the effects of irradiation are complicated by additional factors such as brain surgery and any associated chemotherapy and hormone deficiencies. Intracranial radiotherapy leads to permanent and significant cognitive disability in 50% to 90% of patients and the situation is worse in children. The cause of these problems is poorly understood although immediate inflammation plays a role. Overall brain tumours and/or their treatment are associated with impaired verbal learning and memory, attention and working memory, processing speed and executive functioning. Radiotherapy exacerbates these problems. This means that for many people with secondary adrenal insufficiency secondary to brain tumours and their treatment, the cognitive problems are almost certainly due to the radiotherapy used. However, optimising cortisol and thyroxine replacement is important in order to maximise brain function.

MEMORY

The hippocampus in the brain plays an important role in memory and is particularly sensitive to plasma cortisol levels. Adrenal steroids affect this structure by fast metabolic changes and slower effects on the genes within the hippocampus. Both mineralocorticoid and glucocorticoid receptors are found in the hippocampus.

The relationship between optimal cognitive functioning and circulating glucocorticoids follows an inverted U-shape (Figure 8.58), so that detrimental effects on memory consolidation can result from both deficiency and excess of circulating glucocorticoids, in this case when given acutely just before testing was undertaken.

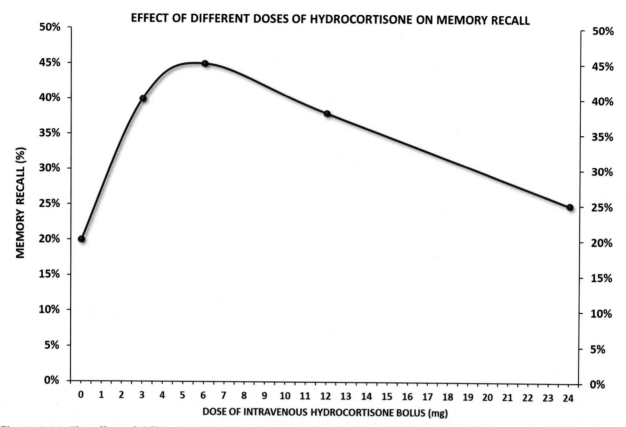

Figure 8.58 *The effect of different intravenous bolus injections of hydrocortisone given before memory recall tests in adult subjects demonstrating an optimum dose (6 mg) of intravenous hydrocortisone. Lower or higher doses are associated with reduced performance. Redrawn from data presented in Schilling, T.M., Kölsch, M., Larra, M.F., Zech, C.M., Blumenthal, T.D., Frings, C., Schächinger, H., 2013. For whom the bell (curve) tolls: Cortisol rapidly affects memory retrieval by an inverted U-shaped dose-response relationship. Psychoneuroendocrinology 38, 1565–1572.*

The effect on memory when agents such as prednisolone are administered can be observed during both short term (3 months) and long term (1 year) treatment. Memory is complex and the type of memory differs such as recollection of facts (what is the capital of the United Kingdom?) as opposed to the recollection of processes e.g., riding a bike. Glucocorticoids seem to particularly affect the former.

There is a complex age related and treatment duration interaction, suggesting that older individuals experience more dramatic memory changes when treated for shorter periods of time. This might explain the results from our questionnaire survey where 7% of people with CAH, 47% with Addison's disease and 46% with hypopituitarism complained of short term memory problems (Figure 8.59).

Both the Addison's disease and hypopituitary group were older but did not necessarily have longer years of treatment than the CAH group who were younger. The use of twice or three times daily dosing was more common in those with Addison's disease and hypopituitarism especially as the last dose was taken at 6 pm (18:00). This would produce the inverted U-shape described above with periods of both over and under treatment.

**SURVEY RESULTS OF THE PERCENTAGE OF PATIENTS WITH ADRENAL INSUFFICIENCY
WHO HAVE TROUBLE WITH SHORT TERM MEMORY**

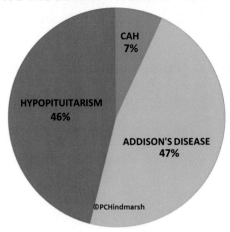

Figure 8.59 *Percentage of people with congenital adrenal hyperplasia, Addison's disease and hypopituitarism who had problems with short term memory.*

These observations of acute and chronic glucocorticoid effects on memory and memory recall are important when considering whether exams are a stress event and need extra dosing with glucocorticoid (see Chapter 12 for full discussion). Yes, they do generate an adrenaline response, but they do not need dosing with extra glucocorticoid as the onset of action is too slow and well after the person has settled into the exam.

Glucocorticoids in high doses do have negative effects on memory retrieval which is not the desired outcome in this situation and is illustrated in Figure 8.58. Handling exams is quite complex and we provide more detail in Chapter 12. Generally, we do need to ensure there is enough cortisol during the exam and if the dose is taken 3 to 4 hours before, then a small extra dose could be taken 30 mins before the exam to ensure there is enough in the system. For example, if the morning dose is taken at 06:00 (6 am) and the exam is at 10:00 (10 am) with the next dose due at 12:00 (noon) then a small dose can be taken before the exam starts as cortisol levels will have dipped lower by the time the lunchtime dose is due. This plan needs to be worked through with the endocrinologist.

BRAIN FOG AND POOR CONCENTRATION

Brain fog is a term that has been used frequently by many with adrenal insufficiency. Brain fog covers a number of symptoms including difficulty learning new things, poor concentration, forgetfulness, difficulty processing instructions and maths problems and poor recall of words. In our questionnaire survey, we did not ask about brain fog but we did ask about poor concentration and the response in all groups was quite high: 43% of those with CAH, 73% of those with Addison's disease and 67% in those with hypopituitarism (Figure 8.60). Babies and young children were not included in the analysis so the effect may also be one of age as well.

It is a little hard to understand all these symptoms, but it is a bit like, in part, the situation where you are in a rush and go to a cash machine to draw out money and you cannot quite remember the PIN and a queue forms and you become agitated which makes it all worse. A lot of the cash machine problem is adrenaline driven but it gives an idea of what people are referring to. What is less clear is how these symptoms relate to cortisol in particular.

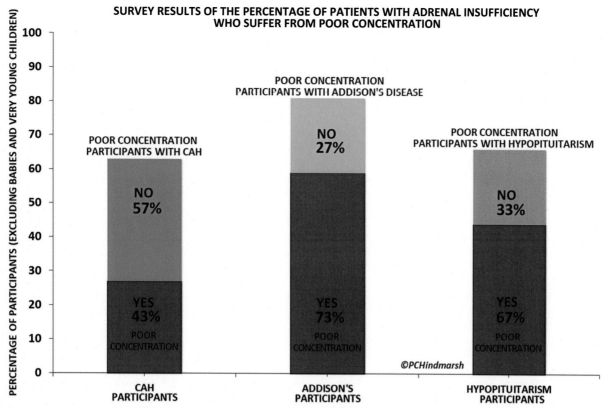

Figure 8.60 *Percentages of survey participants with congenital adrenal hyperplasia, Addison's disease and hypopituitarism who complained of poor concentration. Babies and very young children excluded. Poor concentration (red boxes) was reported in 43% of participants with congenital adrenal hyperplasia, 73% with Addison's disease and 67% with hypopituitarism.*

Changes in cortisol production have not been clearly established. In those with adrenal insufficiency who experience brain fog, adjusting the cortisol dose and distribution throughout the 24 hour period does improve these symptoms which would be expected given what we know about the diverse effects of cortisol on areas of the brain.

This particular issue could become increasingly important in conditions such as long Covid following infection with Covid-19. Many of the features of long Covid are similar to many of the cognitive problems which we have just described and there are reports of brain fog and adrenal insufficiency with Covid-19. The Covid-19 virus can be found in the adrenal cortex and there is a pathological pathway which would explain how the virus affects adrenal function. The role that dexamethasone administration for Covid-19 respiratory problems might play is unclear but needs to be considered as the doses used have been high. There is no doubting the beneficial effects which glucocorticoids have ranging from their life saving role in people with adrenal insufficiency, through to the improvement in symptoms when used as anti-inflammatory agents.

CONCLUSION

Sleep is divided into four stages and cortisol increases in the bloodstream from low values in the evening during Stage 3/Stage 4 of sleep. It is not clear if the sleep cycle affects the production of cortisol, as cortisol is more attuned to the light/dark cycle than sleep itself. It has been suggested taking glucocorticoids late in the evening causes problems in trying to fall asleep. Hence many patients are advised to take the last dose of glucocorticoid at 18:00 (6 pm), but this leads to long periods of time without cortisol overnight. Careful sleep studies have shown the time at which sleep starts, quality and duration of sleep is not affected by the timing of hydrocortisone dosing. Cortisol plays an important role in mood and cognitive function and these can be affected when high doses of glucocorticoids, particularly those with high potency such as prednisolone and dexamethasone are used.

FURTHER READING

Alderson, A.L., Novack, T.A., 2002. Neurophysiological and clinical aspects of glucocorticoids and memory: A review. J Clin Exper Neuropsychol 24, 335–355.

Basta, M., Chrousos, G.P., Vela-Bueno, A., Vgontzas, A.N., 2007. Chronic insomnia and stress system. Sleep Med Clin 2, 279–291.

Belvederi Murri, M., Pariante, C., Mondelli, V., Masotti, M., Atti, A.R., Mellacqua, Z., Antonioli, M., Ghio, L., Menchetti, M., Zanetidou, S., Innamorati, M., Amore, M., 2014. HPA axis and aging in depression: Systematic review and meta-analysis. Psychoneuroendocrinology 41, 46–62.

Collaer, M.L., Hindmarsh, P.C., Pasterski, V., Fane, B.A., Hines, M., 2015. Reduced short term memory in congenital adrenal hyperplasia (CAH) and its relationship to spatial and quantitative performance. Psychoneuroendocrinology 64, 164–173.

De Winter, R.F., Van Mehert, A.M., De Rijk, R.H., Zwinderman, K.H., Frankhuijzen-Sierevogel, A.C., Weigant, V.M., Goekoop, J.G., 2003. Anxious-retarded depression: Relation with plasma vasopressin and cortisol. Neuropsychopharmacology 28, 140–147.

García-Borreguero, D., Wehr, T.A., Larrosa, O., Granizo, J.J., Hardwick, D., Chrousos, G.P., Friedman, T., 2000. Glucocorticoid replacement is permissive for rapid eye movement sleep and sleep consolidation in patients with adrenal insufficiency. J Clin Endocrinol Metab 85, 4201–4206.

German, A., Suraiya, S., Tenenbaum-Rakover, Y., Koren, I., Pillar, G., Hochberg, Z., 2008. Control of childhood congenital adrenal hyperplasia and sleep activity and quality with morning or evening glucocorticoid therapy. J Clin Endocrinol Metab 93 (12), 4707–4710.

Hamilton, O.S., Steptoe, A., Ajnakina, O., 2023. Polygenic predisposition, sleep duration, and depression: evidence from a prospective population-based cohort. Transl Psychiatry 13, 323. https://doi.org/10.1038/s41398-023-02622-z.

Henry, M., Thomas, K.G.F., Ross, I.L., 2021. Sleep, cognition and cortisol in Addison's disease: a mechanistic relationship. Front Endocrinol (Lausanne) 12, https://doi.org/694046.10.3389/fendo.2021.694046.

Henry, M., Wolf, P.S.A., Ross, I.L., Thomas, K.G.F., 2015. Poor quality of life, depressed mood, and memory impairment may be mediated by sleep disruption in patients with Addison's disease. Physiol Behav 151, 379–385.

Machin, P., Young, A.H., 2004. The role of cortisol and depression: exploring new opportunities for treatment. Psychiatric Times. From. http://www.psychiatrictimes.com/articles/ role-cortisol-and-depression-exploring-new-opportunities-treatments.

Makale, M.T., McDonald, C.R., Hattangadi-Gluth, J., Kesari, S., 2017. Brain irradiation and long-term cognitive disability: Current concepts. Nat Rev Neurol 13, 52–64.

Marinelli, I., Walker, J.J., Seneviratne, U., 2023. Circadian distribution of epileptiform discharges in epilepsy: Candidate mechanisms of variability. PLOS Computational Biology | https://doi.org/10.1371/journal.pcbi.1010508.

National Institutes of Health: National Heart, Lung and Blood Institute, 2022. Sleep deprivation and deficiency. https://www.nhlbi.nih.gov/health/sleep-deprivation.

Oray, M., Samra, K.A., Ebrahimiadib, N., Meese, H., Foster, C.S., 2016. Long-term side effects of glucocorticoids. Expert Opin Drug Saf 15, 457–465.

Samuels, M.H., 2014. Psychiatric and cognitive manifestations of hypothyroidism. Curr Opin Endocrinol Diabetes Obes 2, 377–383.

CHAPTER 8.9

Growth and Development Issues Which Occur in Adrenal Insufficiency

GLOSSARY

Adrenal androgen Male like hormones with a structure similar to testosterone. The two main adrenal androgens are dehydroepiandrosterone and androstenedione.

Aromatase inhibitors A class of drug which block the conversion of testosterone to estradiol and androstenedione to estrone by inhibiting the aromatase enzyme which undertakes this conversion. Estrogens are the main factors in maturing the skeleton and advancing bone age.

Cortisol profile Measurement of cortisol in the blood at one hourly intervals to build up a profile of what levels are achieved from treatment with hydrocortisone.

Gonadotropin-releasing hormone analogue Hormone which is produced by the hypothalamus and directs the pituitary gland to produce luteinising and follicle-stimulating hormones. Analogues (an analogue has a similar biochemical structure to the native molecule and is often altered slightly to enhance or decrease biological action), stay attached to the pituitary gland for long periods of time and cause the pituitary gland to stop producing luteinising and follicle-stimulating hormone.

Height velocity The rate of gain in height over a time period, usually 1 year.

Non-classical Congenital Adrenal Hyperplasia (NCCAH) Also known as late-onset CAH (LOCAH). Mildest form of CAH and often not detected until late childhood/adolescence or sometimes as late as adulthood.

Proteoglycan matrix Proteoglycans are proteins to which a large amount of glucose is attached. They form a major part of the 'space' between cells. Proteoglycans can join with other proteoglycans to form large complexes. When proteoglycans join with fibrous proteins like collagen they form cartilage which is a major component of joints.

Simple Virilising Congenital Adrenal Hyperplasia (SVCAH) Presents in childhood with rapid growth, body hair development and body odour. Cortisol production is maintained by high ACTH drive.

From the early use of glucocorticoids, it was apparent they had effects in children on both weight and height. Height is a sensitive marker of child health and can be described using the height growth charts which are available for boys and girls. Growth in height can be split into three. The infancy component from 0 to 3 years of age displays a rapid gain in height followed by the childhood component from 3 to 10 years of age which displays more steady accumulation of height at a rate of 5 cm per year. At variable times after this, the pubertal growth spurt is superimposed on the childhood component and adds a further 25 to 30 cm of height in boys and 20 to 25 cm in girls.

OVERTREATMENT

Overtreatment with glucocorticoids lead to the suppression of growth. The amount of height added on a year by year basis is less than normal and if this went on for a very long period of time, then adult height would be reduced. This is where steroids gained their bad name from in terms of growth. However, it has to be remembered that this effect is seen when very high doses of very powerful steroids such as dexamethasone are used. When glucocorticoid therapy is replaced to mimic what happens naturally, the possibility that growth might be supressed is reduced.

Replacement Therapies in Adrenal Insufficiency. https://doi.org/10.1016/B978-0-12-824548-4.00024-3

Glucocorticoids upset the growth process when given in high doses by disrupting the architecture of the growth plate as discussed in Chapter 8 Part 1. Normally, the cells which are increasing in size in the growth plate are aligned in columns and held in this position by a proteoglycan matrix, glucocorticoids disrupt the proteoglycan matrix impairing the careful arrangement of the expanding cells. There is a critical dose of glucocorticoid which will supress height gain and this is at a total hydrocortisone dose of greater than 30 mg/m^2 body surface area/day. If we suspect the glucocorticoids dose is too high, then this will be reflected in weight gain and poor gain in height as exemplified in Figure 8.61. When this happens, we need to check with a 24 hour cortisol profile what is happening with the distribution of cortisol as a result of hydrocortisone administration. Are the cortisol peaks too high? Is the level of the cortisol in the blood too high generally over the 24 hours? Are the doses taken correctly distributed?

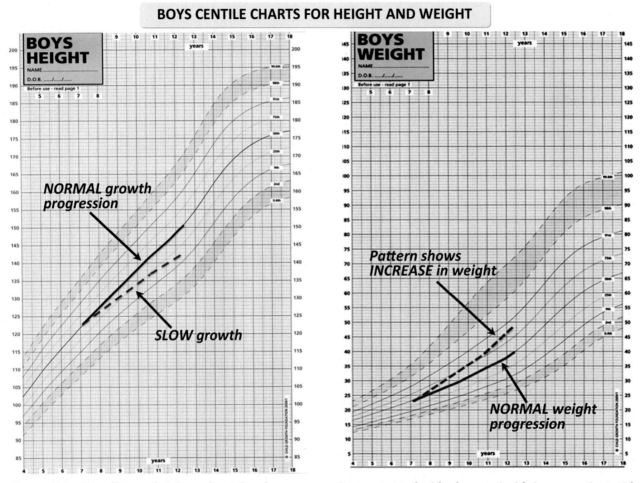

Figure 8.61 *The effect on height and weight when someone is over treated with glucocorticoids in any patient with adrenal insufficiency shown by the dashed lines. Charts copyright Child Growth Foundation reproduced with kind permission.*

The effect of overtreatment will also be reflected in the bone age. Bone age tells us the percentage of growth which has taken place and in situations of overtreatment, the bone age will be delayed and if the doses used are too high, damage to the growth plates can occur, leading to a loss in the adult height achieved. Poor height gain is a consistent feature of overtreatment, no matter what the cause of the adrenal insufficiency is.

We use bone age as a measure of how much skeletal growth has taken place and therefore how much is still to come. To estimate bone age we take an x-ray of the hand and wrist. We use the hand and wrist as it contains a large number of growing areas which we can give a certain score to depending on their size and shape.

Figure 8.62 shows the hand x-ray from the same person at ages 3 and 6.5 years. Some of the growth areas appear over time and also there is a change in shape. These scores can be used to determine the maturity of the skeleton and this is expressed as a bone age. It is not really a measure of age which is based on time rather it is a measure of maturation of the skeleton, but it is easier to understand in terms of years.

In Figure 8.62 the bone age is delayed slightly by a year compared to the chronological age which means the person has extra time in which to grow.

HAND AND WRIST X-RAYS TO ESTIMATE BONE AGE

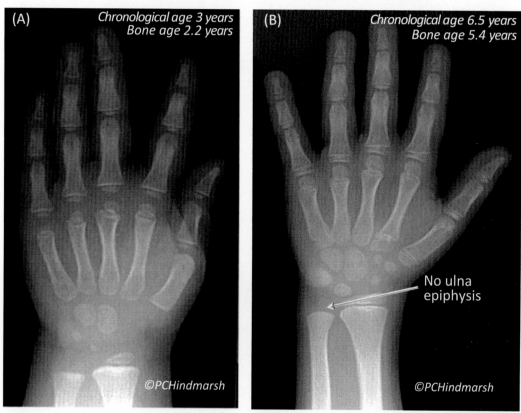

Figure 8.62 *Two hand x-rays from the same girl aged (A) 3 years with a bone age of 2.2 'years' and again at (B) the age of 6.5 years with a bone age of 5.4 'years'. Note the difference in shape and size of the epiphyses with several absent in (A). Even the ulna epiphysis has not appeared in (B).*

In Figure 8.63 there are three x-rays from children 12 years of age, but with different bone ages that are either commensurate with the chronological age, or advanced or delayed. An advanced bone age means that there is less time available to grow which means that adult height might be reduced compared to where we might have expected it to be.

We can use bone age further when we think of it in terms of this idea of skeletal maturation. In Figure 8.64 we see the percentage of final height completed at different chronological ages. We can substitute chronological age with bone age which will tell us how much growth is left to come for any given bone age.

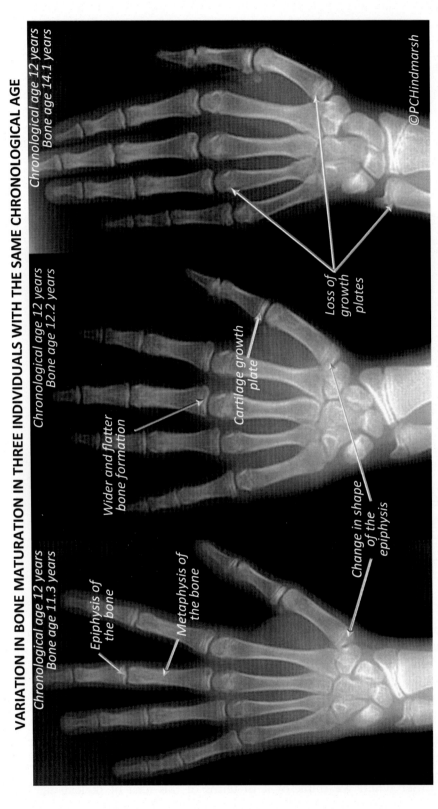

Figure 8.63 *Hand and wrist x-rays from three girls aged 12 years showing the variation in bone maturation. In the middle picture the bone age is 12.2 'years' and on the left 11.3 'years.' The bone is made up of the central part the metaphysis and at the end of the bone the newly grown bone the epiphysis. Separating the two is the cartilage growth plate. The differences between the left and central x-ray are due to changes in the shape of the epiphyses and in the fingers the growth plate becomes wider and flatter. On the right the bone age is 14.1 'years' and is characterised by the loss of the distinct black line of the growth plate as fusion of the growth plate is taking place which will unite the epiphysis and metaphysis as a single bone structure.*

By the time of menarche (a girl's first period) at a chronological age of 12.5 to 13 years, 96% of growth in height has taken place and there is only another 5 to 7 cm left to come. In boys, at the same age, because the puberty growth spurt starts later, there is still 16% of growth to come. If bone age advances quickly as in early puberty, then there is less and less time in which to complete growth and the end result is a reduction in adult height compared to what would have been expected had puberty occurred at the normal time.

The converse, where puberty is delayed, bone age is also delayed but this does not alter adult height unless the pubertal growth spurt is very delayed towards 17 or 18 years of age when height gain is attenuated.

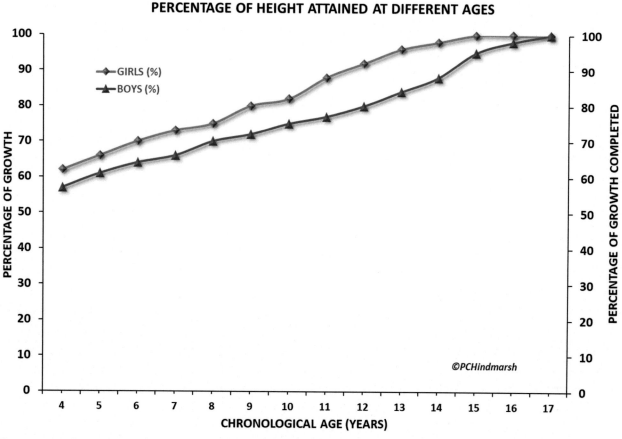

Figure 8.64 *Percentage of total growth in height at different chronological ages. Chronological age can be substituted by bone age to give a generalised projection from how much growth has taken place to how much is left to come.*

In individuals with hypopituitarism, there is the additional problem of growth hormone deficiency. In this situation growth hormone can be replaced by daily injections of biosynthetic human growth hormone, but this will only be effective in promoting growth provided the glucocorticoid dose is carefully balanced and does not exceed the critical hydrocortisone daily dose of 30 mg/m² body surface area/day. Growth hormone and the sex steroids, testosterone or estradiol, contribute fifty percent each to the pubertal growth spurt which amounts to approximately 30 cm in boys and 25 cm in girls. Of interest is the situation we see in individuals who do not have pituitary problems, where growth hormone and cortisol are secreted out of phase with each other. It is unclear how important this effect is in maximising growth, but it would suggest growth hormone doses should be given in the evening and before the usual midnight dose of hydrocortisone.

Growth Hormone and Cortisol

One of the important points about growth hormone treatment is that when it is used in individuals who also have adrenal insufficiency, care needs to be undertaken with the hydrocortisone dosing. The reason for this is growth hormone decreases the conversion of cortisone to cortisol by reducing the activity of the 11beta-hydroxysteroid dehydrogenase type 1 isoenzyme in the liver. In most individuals there is a balance between the activity of this isoenzyme and the type 2 isoenzyme in the kidney which converts cortisol to cortisone. We looked at this system in Chapter 6 (Figure 6.7). If the type 2 isoenzyme functions normally, then cortisol will be converted to cortisone, but if the type 1 isoenzyme is less active then the pool of cortisol in the blood will reduce. In individuals with an intact hypothalamo-pituitary-adrenal axis, this does not matter because the pituitary can increase the production of ACTH, thereby increasing the amount of cortisol in the circulation. However, in adrenal insufficiency where we use fixed amounts of hydrocortisone on a daily basis, reduced activity in the type 1 isoenzyme will mean a reduction in the amount of cortisol in the circulation and a readjustment of the hydrocortisone dose will be required.

DELAYED PUBERTY

Delayed puberty happens commonly in the general population, particularly in boys. The reasons for this are unclear, but it may relate to how the body clock, which is involved in setting the timing of puberty, works. This clock is very susceptible to changes particularly in individuals with longstanding illnesses because the clock gets reset to start late. This is often seen in children with asthma who have a pattern of pubertal delay, so the onset of puberty is late but once it gets underway, they have a normal pubertal growth spurt and normal adult height. The mechanism is unclear, but a similar pattern can be seen in children who are diagnosed with Addison's disease in the prepubertal years and who often have a delayed onset of puberty. Whether the adrenal androgens play an important part in setting the timing of puberty is unclear. In Addison's disease with a prepubertal onset, the adrenal androgens are not present and it could be speculated this is the reason for the pubertal delay seen in these individuals.

The converse can also happen in CAH when adrenal androgen production may be high, particularly in the simple virilising type of CAH which often does not present until 5 or 6 years of age. In this situation, early puberty is often a consequence of the condition or treatment. We will consider this a bit more below in the section on early puberty. We cover fertility in more detail in Chapter 8, Part 4.

Delayed puberty will also be a consequence in hypopituitarism due to the lack of luteinising hormone (LH) and follicle-stimulating hormone (FSH) production. This is also the case in adrenal hypoplasia congenita. In this situation of delay, puberty may need to be induced with estrogens in girls and testosterone in boys. The doses used start low and build up which maximises the pubertal growth spurt, also allowing normal pubertal growth of the uterus in girls. In girls with hypopituitarism and delayed puberty, long term fertility is good although assistance will be needed in order to induce ovulation. In males with hypopituitarism however, fertility outcomes are not as good as in females.

Puberty delayed by around 12 to 18 months does not usually need anything to be done. In some instances, particularly in boys with Addison's disease, the timing of puberty can be quite late by 2 to 3 years and because the puberty growth spurt is later in boys than girls, they can lag a long way behind their peers in terms of height. Sometimes, it is useful to induce puberty in a similar way to that undertaken in hypopituitary children. In either case, considerable care needs to be taken because if the dose of sex steroids used are too high, then rapid acceleration in the bone age might take place which would lead the individual to be shorter than they might have otherwise been, had no intervention taken place.

UNDERTREATMENT

In hypopituitarism and forms of primary adrenal insufficiency other than CAH, undertreatment with glucocorticoids rarely presents a problem from the pubertal standpoint. This is not the situation in CAH because in the two most common forms, (21 hydroxylase (CYP21) deficiency, 11beta-hydroxylase (CYP11B1) deficiency), the point at which there is a block in cortisol formation means the compensatory increase in ACTH production from the pituitary, leads to accumulation of precursors before the enzyme block which include the adrenal androgens DHEA (dehydroepiandrosterone) and androstenedione.

If replacement therapy with hydrocortisone is low or we are actually dealing with non-classical CAH which is also known as late-onset CAH (LOCAH), which presents later in life and not at birth, then growth will accelerate as will bone age maturation due to exposure to excess androgen production from the adrenal glands for a long period of time. This advance in bone age means there is less time available to complete growth.

When this situation occurs in an individual with classical CAH, 24 hour cortisol and 17 OHP profiles will help us calculate the exact distribution of hydrocortisone during the 24 hour period and determine periods where the individual might be undertreated. We can then readjust the hydrocortisone dosing to improve cortisol coverage.

In an individual with LOCAH, we introduce hydrocortisone treatment to reduce the ACTH drive to the adrenal glands and thereby reduce adrenal androgen production. This can be extremely effective in its own right but is often associated with the onset of true puberty. This occurs because the adrenal androgens appear to prime the hypothalamus, so it functions like a more mature system in puberty. In this situation, the pubertal process can be held up using a gonadotropin-releasing hormone analogue to switch off the secretion of LH and FSH until a more appropriate time of onset of puberty around 11 years of age.

Going back to the situation in the more classical forms of CAH where bone age is advanced because of under replacement with hydrocortisone, people sometimes try to improve the situation again by holding up the entry into puberty using the analogue approach. This is not as effective as might seem to be the case because the contribution of the pubertal growth spurt is relatively fixed, so altering this towards the end of growth, is unlikely to make major changes to adult height because the amount needed to be manipulated is greater than what is available.

Various attempts have been made to overcome this. Growth hormone therapy has been advocated by some in order to boost growth during the period of time when puberty is switched off, but overall the long term effects do not seem to suggest a major improvement can be expected.

Another approach which may prove to be more successful, is to stop the conversion of the adrenal androgens to female hormones. This takes place by the enzyme aromatase (CPY19) which is present in many parts of the body but particularly in fat cells.

It may come as a surprise to many that bone maturation is dependent on the formation of estrogen in both males and females. There are many examples where estrogens cannot be synthesised or act through the estrogen receptor in males, who go on to develop osteoporosis, but also continue to grow well into adulthood because the growth plates in their skeleton do not fuse.

We can capitalise on this information by using aromatase inhibitors which block the conversion of testosterone to estradiol (Figure 8.65) and the conversion of androstenedione to estrone (Figure 8.66).

AROMATASE INHIBITOR BLOCKING CONVERSION OF TESTOSTERONE TO ESTRADIOL

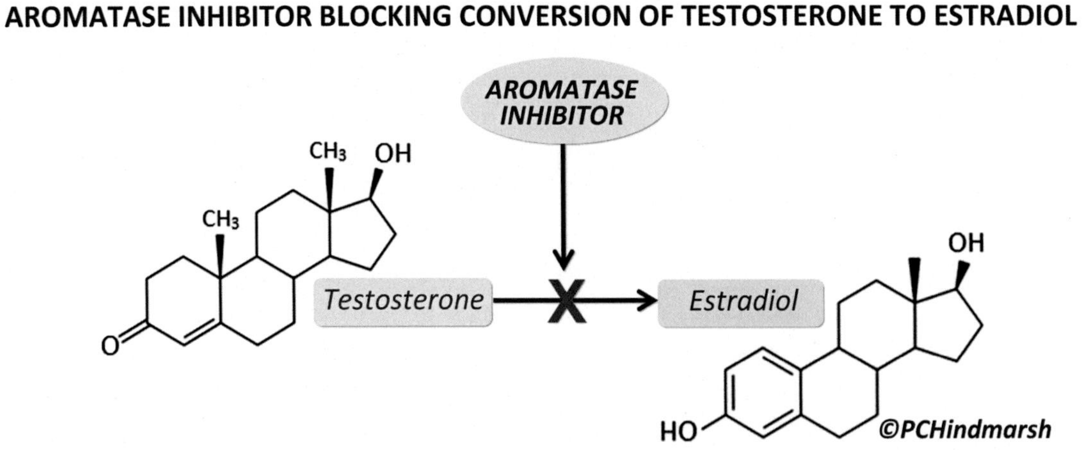

Figure 8.65 *The enzyme aromatase converts testosterone to estradiol and is blocked by aromatase inhibitors.*

AROMATASE INHIBITOR BLOCKING CONVERSION OF ANDROSTENEDIONE TO ESTRONE

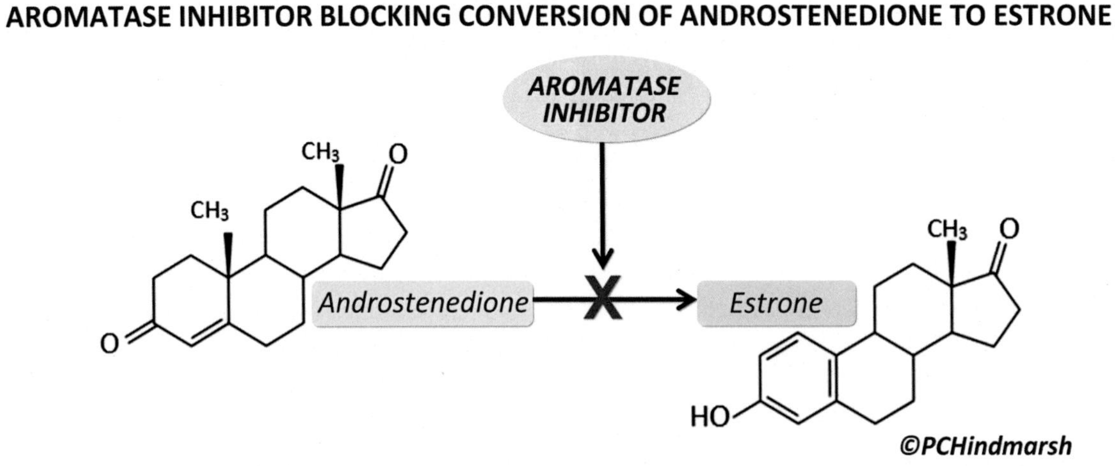

Figure 8.66 *The enzyme aromatase converts androstenedione to estrone and is blocked by aromatase inhibitors.*

There is still a long way to go in understanding the efficacy of this approach and care is needed when using these agents because they can lead to osteoporosis over time. There is a clear problem in using aromatase inhibitors in girls, because it will increase their exposure to androgens.

Several groups have advocated that to overcome this particular problem, androgen receptor inhibitors such as flutamide can be used. This type of approach enters into polypharmacy and the androgen receptor inhibitors are not without problems, particularly with respect to liver function.

CONCLUSION

In paediatrics, growth is a good indication of general health and when we are considering the treatment of adrenal insufficiency, changes in height and weight can reflect over and under treatment, particularly in CAH. Although height and weight do reflect the effects of glucocorticoid dosing, they take some time to manifest in either direction, so should be used in conjunction with 24 hour profile data. Over treatment can lead to weight gain and slow growth and if high doses of glucocorticoids, particularly those that have high potency, are used for long periods of time, damage to the growth plate can take place. Puberty can occur early or late in these conditions and is likely to be late in secondary adrenal insufficiency due to loss of gonadotropin secretion. In this situation, puberty will need to be induced with exogenous estrogen or testosterone. Early puberty occurs in simple virilising CAH (SVCAH) and non-classical CAH which is also known as late-onset CAH (LOCAH) which present later than the classic salt-wasting form as the adrenal glands have been producing androgens for some time.

When hydrocortisone and cortisone acetate were introduced in the late 1940s as replacement therapy for adrenal insufficiency, the main problems centred on issues with weight and growth - excess weight gain and not enough gain in height. Over time it became apparent that both over and under treatment were associated with a number of short and long term problems and we have begun to realise this is also apparent in areas such as fertility, bone health and cardiovascular disease. To prevent these problems an understanding of how to optimise cortisol replacement is necessary, so it might be worth reviewing the ideas outlined in Chapter 6 before reading further. Careful adjustment of the dose and duration of exposure to hydrocortisone can be best achieved using the 24 hour blood profile approach which we will look at further in the next section of the book.

FURTHER READING

Dattani, M.T., Hindmarsh, P.C., 2009. Normal and abnormal puberty. In: Brook, C.G.D., Clayton, P., Brown, R. (Eds.), Brook's Clinical Paediatric Endocrinology, fifth ed. Blackwell Publishing, Oxford.

Hindmarsh, P.C., 2009. Management of the child with congenital adrenal hyperplasia. Best Pract Res Clin Endocrinol Metab 23, 193—208.

Rivkees, S.A., Danon, M., Herrin, J., 1994. Prednisolone dose limitation of growth hormone treatment of steroid induced growth failure. J Pediatr 125, 322—325.

Smith, E.P., Boyd, J., Frank, G.R., et al., 1994. Estrogen resistance caused by a mutation in the estrogen-receptor gene in a man. N Engl J Med 331, 1056—1061.

Tanner, J.M., 1989. Foetus into Man. 2nd edition. Castlemead Publications, Ware.

SECTION 3

In Section 2 we noted some of the short and long term problems which can arise from glucocorticoid use. In this section we look at how we dose with glucocorticoids and especially how we determine the dosing schedule over the 24 hour period is optimal in terms of:

1. Dose - by establishing and considering the cortisol peak values attained by each dose.

2. Metabolism of each dose - how quickly or slowly each dose is absorbed into and cleared from the bloodstream.

3. Distribution of each dose - where we consider if there is any remaining cortisol from a previous dose onto which the next dose is stacked, as well as if there are any periods where there is no cortisol in the bloodstream.

4. How close we approximate the circadian rhythm of cortisol.

5. What to do when unwell or facing stressful situations such as surgery.

It is worth reiterating a central principle of endocrinology which is to replace the hormone that is missing, with a synthetic version, in the same way it would be normally produced. In adrenal insufficiency the missing hormone is cortisol, so this needs to be replaced with the synthetic form of cortisol, hydrocortisone, which should be given in a dosing schedule to mimic as closely as possible, the normal circadian rhythm of cortisol. To assess how well the cortisol is replaced, we measure the cortisol achieved from the dosing regimen and compare it with the circadian rhythm of cortisol. Ensuring the circadian rhythm cortisol replacement is correct is important, as this is likely to avoid over and under treatment.

A lot of our thinking on cortisol replacement has come from our work with hydrocortisone pumps (Chapter 11), detailed analysis of well over three hundred 24 hour cortisol profiles in children, adolescents and young adults with adrenal insufficiency, clinical studies of natural cortisol production in adults and children, as well as formal studies on cortisol replacement in prepubertal, pubertal and post pubertal patients.

The information we present is applicable to all with adrenal insufficiency receiving glucocorticoid replacement therapy. In the following chapters we will occasionally refer to cortisol and 17-hydroxyprogesterone (17OHP) as these are hormones present in congenital adrenal hyperplasia (CAH). This is an advantage due to the correlation between cortisol and 17OHP, as we can use 17OHP as a measure of what the hypothalamus and pituitary are doing in the face of the feedback they receive from the cortisol which is being replaced. This gives us extra information to assist us with our replacement therapy. There is a caveat however, as elevated 17OHP levels can originate from adrenal rests, polycystic ovaries or even from painful blood tests or cannula insertion. Due to the lag in effect of the replacement cortisol on 17OHP, you cannot use this as a sole marker in replacing cortisol in CAH. However, 17OHP levels are a useful marker in assessing how active the adrenal glands are. The function of the adrenal glands is driven by ACTH production, so when there is too little glucocorticoid replacement the adrenal glands enlarge because there is not enough cortisol feedback to reduce ACTH production and 17OHP levels rise. However, if there is over replacement with glucocorticoids, ACTH production is suppressed and the adrenal glands shrink which results in no 17OHP secretion. We cover this in Chapter 9, Figures 9.1-9.3.

In other forms of primary adrenal insufficiency, the marker we could use is ACTH, which would need to be frequently measured which is not feasible because we would need large blood samples at least every 30 minutes and the sample processing has to be rapid. In secondary adrenal insufficiency, there is no ACTH production. In both situations we apply our knowledge of what happens in CAH to these conditions. This means all these chapters are as relevant to anyone with adrenal insufficiency as they are to those with CAH. In addition, because we can also measure blood glucose, we can also use this measurement as a marker of adequacy of cortisol replacement in adrenal insufficiency.

It is often suggested in children that we can use growth and bone age as measures of how well the condition is being treated but these elements are slow to change, so any problem is well established before any changes are seen, let alone rectified. Our aim is to prevent the side effects occurring with carefully calculated and individualised dosing schedules.

Finally, please remember cortisol measurements vary in all individuals not only in those without adrenal problems, but also those on replacement hydrocortisone due to differences in metabolism. Hydrocortisone is the synthetic form of cortisol and easily measured in the blood, whereas the other more potent glucocorticoids are not. However, this is also not without challenges as the result is also dependent on the cortisol assay used. The vast majority of blood measurements used in this book are using the Immulite assay (including clinical trials), so it is important to know which assay is being used when considering results. When cortisol data is superimposed on the circadian rhythm, these are average values, taken from published, peer reviewed studies and it is the pattern of the circadian rhythm which is important. Solu-Cortef (sodium succinate) which has recently been renamed in the UK to Hydrocortisone Powder for Solution for Injection or Infusion (sodium succinate), has been used for the intravenous and intramuscular studies.

CHAPTER 9

Dosing with Glucocorticoids

GLOSSARY

Circadian rhythm Changes in hormone levels, in this case cortisol, throughout the 24 hour period where values peak in the morning and reach low levels late evening.

Cortisol replacement dose This is worked out in relation to the normal cortisol production rate over 24 hours and considers cortisol which is lost through the gut.

Enteric coated Enteric coatings are polymers that coat certain tablets (such as prednisolone) to prevent them from dissolving in the acid of the stomach or damaging the lining of the stomach. The coating allows the tablets to survive intact as they pass through the acid in the stomach. Once in the small intestine which is less acidic, they are broken down and absorbed.

Metabolism of cortisol The way cortisol is absorbed, carried around the blood and cleared from the circulation.

Over stacking The phenomenon which happens if the timing of doses is incorrect. Occurs where the dose is taken too early and builds onto the cortisol remaining from the previous dose, leading to higher cortisol levels than expected.

Stacking The addition of a dose upon another dose within a certain time frame, usually the time the drug is in the circulation.

Under stacking The phenomenon which happens if the timing of doses is incorrect. Occurs where the dose is taken too late and leaves periods of time between doses when there is no cortisol.

Useful stacking Cortisol is added when cortisol drops to a desired level, which not only prevents levels dropping too low but also allows a smaller amount to be added to give the optimal peak.

GENERAL

In this section we are going to consider the use of hydrocortisone, which is the synthetic preparation of cortisol and is the preferred glucocorticoid replacement therapy for cortisol in adrenal insufficiency. The information we presented in Chapter 6 is what we use to determine replacement therapy. The aim is to replace cortisol as closely as possible, to the normal circadian rhythm to avoid the well documented side effects encountered in adrenal insufficiency, which relate to either over or under treatment with glucocorticoids. This is not only just a dose effect but also relates to the distribution of cortisol throughout the 24 hour period.

From a historical perspective the total daily hydrocortisone dose was originally split into two doses, morning and evening. Results from many studies suggested splitting the total daily dose into three per day was better than twice daily and this stemmed from assessing 17-hydroxyprogesterone (17OHP) in individuals with congenital adrenal hyperplasia (CAH). Improved dosing was associated with less of an increase in body weight and other recognised side effects. In these studies, 17OHP was used as a marker of adequacy of cortisol replacement rather than determining how much cortisol was delivered by the treatment regimens. The focus was and is still today in many centres, solely on 17OHP levels, without examining the amount or distribution of cortisol. However, the pharmacology of hydrocortisone tells us the duration of time hydrocortisone is present in the circulation as cortisol, is on average 6 hours and this would suggest dosing four times a day would give a better distribution of cortisol over the 24 hour period.

Replacement Therapies in Adrenal Insufficiency. https://doi.org/10.1016/B978-0-12-824548-4.00020-6

A further benefit of dosing four times per day, is it allows for smaller doses at appropriate times which approximate better to the normal cortisol circadian rhythm. Whatever we do, we must appreciate the clearance and absorption of the glucocorticoid needs to be tailored to the individual and using a blanket formula for all, will not give optimal cortisol coverage.

In this chapter we will consider average cortisol levels but throughout the chapter and this book, we need to be mindful of individual variation (See Chapter 6 Figure 6.5). Above all, remember when we use CAH, it is as a useful model for assessing cortisol replacement as the principles are applicable to anyone with adrenal insufficiency from whatever cause. Once normal 17OHP production is attained in CAH through optimal cortisol replacement (Figure 9.1), the replacement requirements will be the same for all with adrenal insufficiency.

Before we discuss dosing further, we can recap using Figures 9.1, 9.2 and 9.3 as to what we want to achieve with our dosing in the various forms of adrenal insufficiency. Getting replacement optimal is important not just from a side effects viewpoint, but also quality of life as well as excluding treatment as a possible cause for symptoms.

In considering Figures 9.1, 9.2 and 9.3 it is important to remember there are many causes of primary and secondary adrenal insufficiency and the most common cause is the administration of exogenous glucocorticoids which we review in Chapter 15. There can also be considerable variation in the manifestation of each of the causes between individuals.

A good example of this is the effect of excess androgen production in CAH due to 21-hydroxylase deficiency. Adrenal androgens in the untreated state may be similar between two individuals but the degree of virilisation may differ between the two. This is because we have to introduce an additional variable, the androgen receptor. The androgen receptor gene contains a series of CAG (cytosine, adenine, guanine) repeats. Cytosine, adenine, guanine and thymine are the four main components of DNA. In the androgen receptor, the number of repeats affect receptor function. Few repeats lead to increased receptor sensitivity to the circulating androgens and more repeats lead to decreased receptor sensitivity. Receptor variants play an important role in determining tissue responsivity as we have observed in Chapter 6.

This variation between individuals which includes the variations between individuals in drug bioavailability and clearance outlined in Chapter 6, adds to the complexity of drug dosing and understanding the manifestations of side effects between individuals. These observations heighten the need to tailor replacement therapies to the metabolism of the individual and not to assume a one size fits all approach.

Variation is not just confined to how an individual metabolises a drug or in its action but there is variation even in the actual dose of the drug within a tablet. Although the drug packaging may say that there are 10 mg of drug in each tablet, it is known that this can vary by $\pm$ 10% between manufacturers which amounts to quite a difference at either end of the range. Another point to consider is not only can different brands vary in the actual dose of the drug within each tablet, but there are potential differences in the bioavailability between brands. And this is before we introduce potential drug interactions!!

From this, there is a need to consider many facets in the determination of the right drug to deliver. To this, we need to add the principles of pharmacology covered in Chapter 6 which help us not only to decide the dose to use but also the timing of administration.

EXAMPLE 1

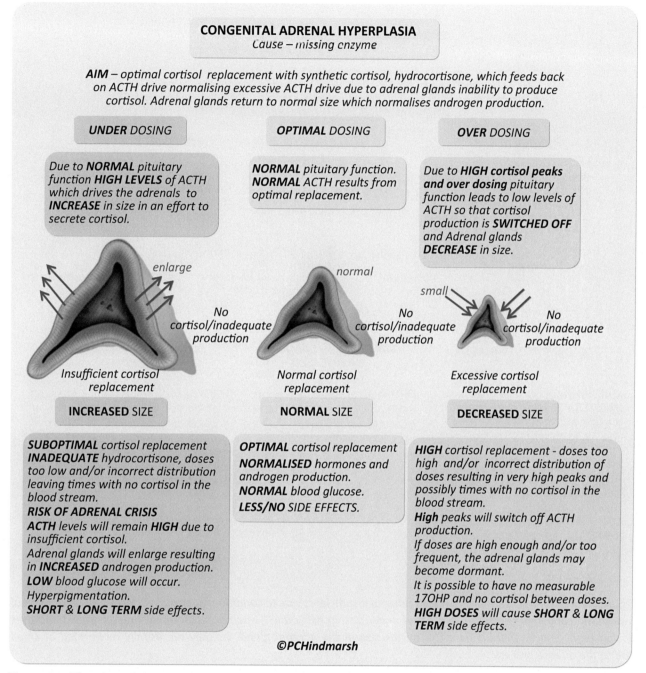

Figure 9.1 *The aims of therapy in primary adrenal insufficiency due to congenital adrenal hyperplasia showing the effect of under dosing (left panel), optimal replacement (middle panel) and over dosing (right panel) on the size of the adrenal glands and side effects associated with the different dosing scenarios.*

In CAH, the loss of cortisol production leads to a compensatory rise in ACTH which results in the enlargement of the adrenal glands along with an increase in adrenal androgen and 17OHP levels. This arises because of the trophic effects of ACTH on cells in the adrenal cortex. Replacement with cortisol in the form of hydrocortisone leads to a normalisation of ACTH levels, a reduction in the size of the adrenal glands and normalisation of adrenal androgen and 17OHP levels. If cortisol is over replaced, the ACTH production from the pituitary gland is switched off and the adrenal glands shrink in size with suppression of adrenal androgens and 17OHP.

EXAMPLE 2

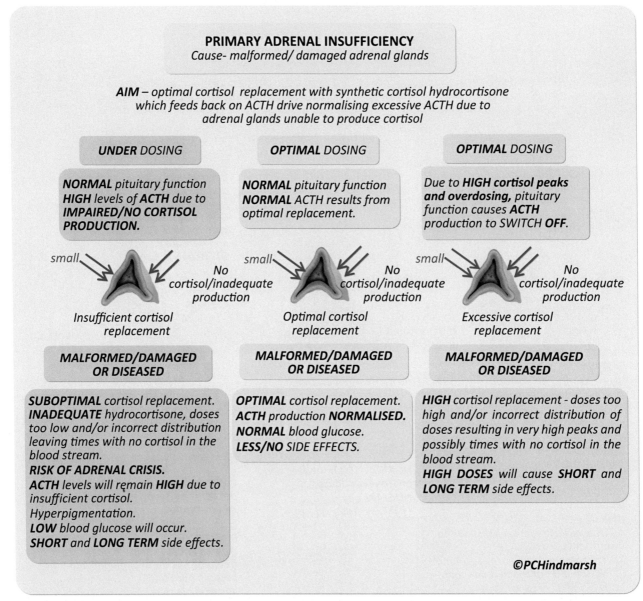

Figure 9.2 *The aims of therapy in primary adrenal insufficiency due to conditions such as Addison's disease or adrenal hypoplasia congenita showing the effect of under dosing (left panel), optimal replacement (middle panel) and over dosing (right panel). There is no effect on the size of the adrenal glands as they are usually malformed or small due to the disease process.*

In primary adrenal insufficiency, the loss of cortisol production leads to a compensatory rise in ACTH, but in contrast to the CAH situation because the adrenal glands are damaged or not formed properly, there is no increase in adrenal gland size. In addition, because the pathways to the formation of cortisol and the adrenal androgens are also damaged there is no associated increase in the adrenal androgens and 17OHP.

Replacement with cortisol in the form of hydrocortisone leads to a normalisation of ACTH levels but there is no effect on adrenal androgen and 17OHP levels. Equally, when there is over replacement with hydrocortisone, adrenal androgens and 17OHP will be low anyway as they cannot be formed due to the damaged adrenal glands, although ACTH will be low/suppressed.

EXAMPLE 3

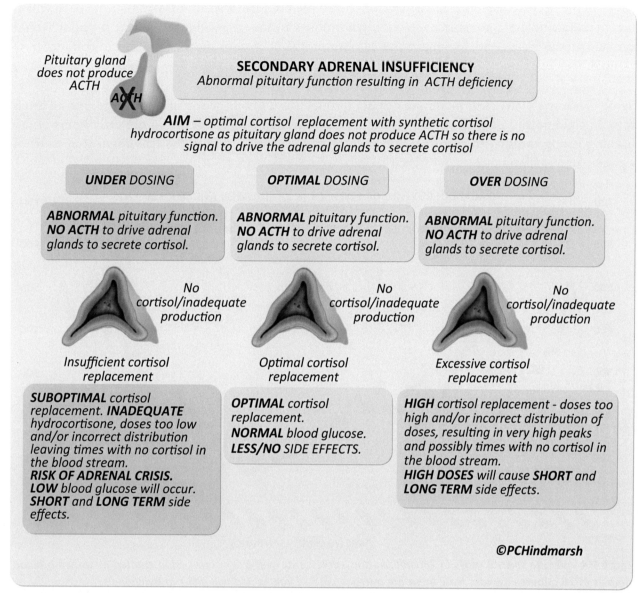

Figure 9.3 *The aims of therapy in secondary adrenal insufficiency showing the effect of under dosing (left panel), optimal replacement (middle panel) and over dosing (right panel) on the size of the adrenal glands and side effects associated with the different dosing scenarios. Although the glands are structurally normal without the trophic effect of ACTH, they shrink. This is similar to the effect of exogenous glucocorticoids which will switch off ACTH production and after 6 weeks of exposure the adrenal glands will also shrink.*

In secondary adrenal insufficiency due either to hypopituitarism or treatment with exogenous glucocorticoids, there is no ACTH production and the adrenal glands are small or atrophied. None of the parameters we have mentioned in primary adrenal insufficiency are measurable in any situation of over or under treatment nor when cortisol replacement is normalised. This makes assessing the adequacy of replacement therapy difficult as there are no markers of what is happening at the pituitary or adrenal levels.

The best that can be attained is to approximate as closely as possible the cortisol delivery from hydrocortisone with the natural circadian rhythm of cortisol.

THE CIRCADIAN RHYTHM OF CORTISOL

Earlier in the book (Chapters 1 and 2) we considered the circadian rhythm of cortisol. One of the main rules of endocrinology is to replace the missing hormones as close as possible to the way the body would naturally produce them. So, looking at the 24 hour profile of cortisol allows us to start to consider how we might achieve this.

Figure 9.4 shows a very clear rhythm in cortisol through the 24 hour period in the average cortisol levels from 28 children and adolescents. The profile starts with high concentrations in the early hours of the morning lasting through to 8 am (08:00), with a gradual decline during the day down to a nadir of between 50 and 75 nmol/l.

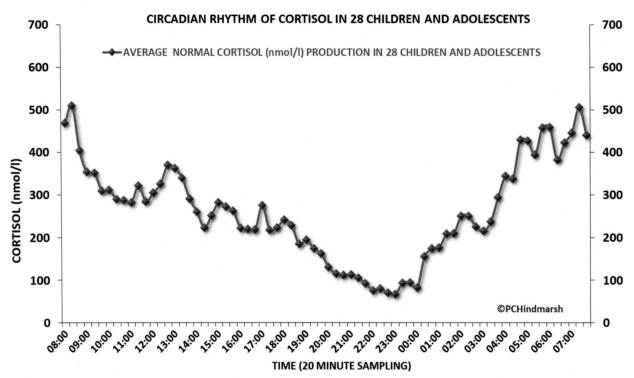

Figure 9.4 *Average cortisol levels in 28 children and adolescents over a 24 hour period created by drawing blood samples at 20 minute intervals. Note these are average cortisol values and will differ in individuals.*

There are also several points to consider:

1. The body is not without cortisol at any time although values are low at around 10 pm (22:00). Note the data in Figure 9.4 are averaged from 28 children and adolescents and the timing of the nadir differs in adults whereas the peak timing does not.

2. From this very low value in the evening the amounts of cortisol in the blood start to rise progressively until they reach a peak in the early hours of the morning between 6 am to 8 am (06:00 – 08:00). This is due to the increased drive of ACTH from the pituitary.

3. The decrease during the day is punctuated by small bursts of cortisol, which are driven by ACTH, particularly around 4 pm (16:00).

To mimic this physiological situation, we need to take different doses of hydrocortisone throughout the 24 hour period. How often the hydrocortisone should be taken is determined by how long the cortisol derived from the hydrocortisone is present in the bloodstream.

Impact of gender and age on the Cortisol Circadian Rhythm

For many medications, gender and age influence dosing. The first question to consider is do cortisol levels differ with gender and age? The cortisol production rate when expressed in terms of body surface area, does not change with age or gender once the circadian rhythm becomes established after the first three months of life. It remains fixed on average between 8 and 10 mg/m^2 body surface area/day. Figure 9.5 shows the change in average cortisol from birth.

CORTISOL AND AGE

AGE	MEAN CORTISOL (nmol/l)
Cord blood	360
Preterm baby	140
Term baby	180
Infant at 4 weeks	250
Child from 3 months onwards	330
	©PCHindmarsh

Figure 9.5 *Change in mean cortisol from birth to childhood.*

Figure 9.6 illustrates there is no difference in cortisol levels at different ages between older adults and children. We looked at this in Chapter 2 Figure 2.8 but it is worth another look, as this is an important point which influences our thinking on dosing. Re-emphasising what we said previously, the only noticeable point is the difference in timing of the rise from the nadir which is slightly later in adults. This probably relates to the fact that children go to bed earlier than the adults. If we look in more detail at the adults, in younger adults, the lowest concentrations are usually encountered between 00:00 (midnight) and 02:00 (2 am) and then rise progressively to reach a peak at the same time as the children and older adults.

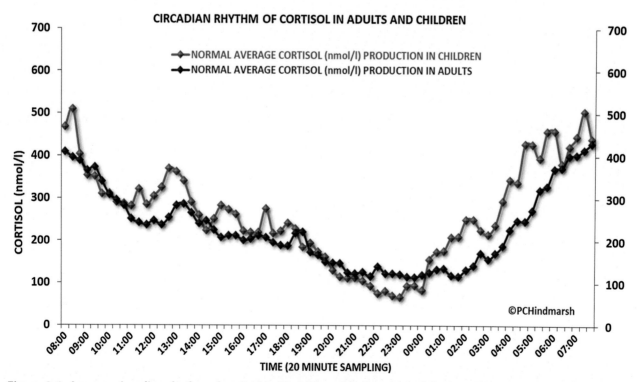

Figure 9.6 *Average circadian rhythm of cortisol in 28 children (blue) and 80 adults (purple) without adrenal problems. The profile shows overlap of cortisol levels in the different age groups with the only difference being the later rise in cortisol from the nadir between 22:00 (10 pm) and 23:00 (11 pm) in children and 00:00 (midnight) in adults. Note these are average cortisol values and will differ in individuals.*

The impact of gender on the circadian rhythm in boys and girls and adult men and women is shown in Figure 9.7.

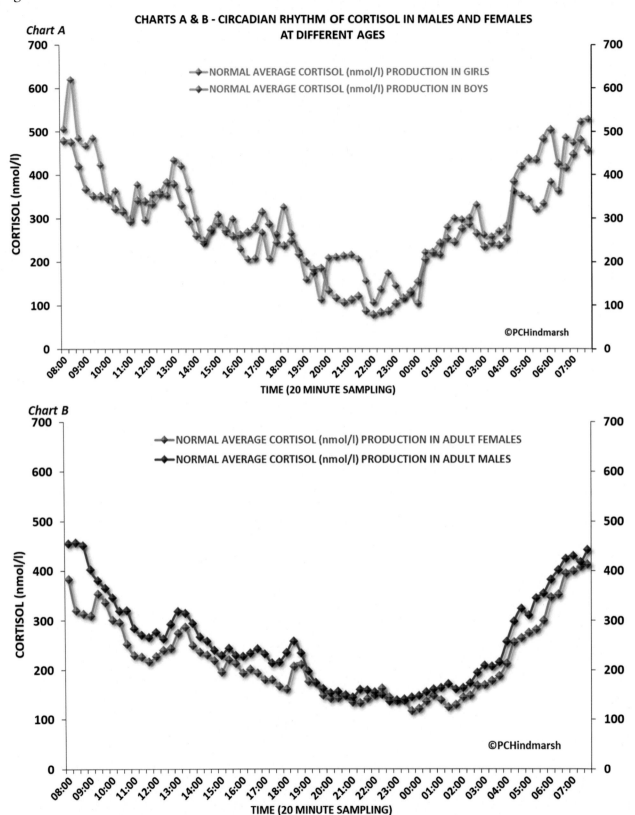

Figure 9.7 *Chart A shows the average 24 hour cortisol levels in boys (light blue) and girls (pink) showing similar peak and trough levels and with similar timing of peaks and the morning rise. In Chart B data from adult males (blue) and females (purple) is shown with similar cortisol levels and timings throughout the 24 hour period of peak and nadir. Note these are average cortisol values and will differ in individuals.*

In both children and adults there is no discernable difference in the average cortisol patterns between males and females. The circadian pattern is superimposable between the males and females irrespective of age. There is no real difference between the genders, as to when the peak and trough cortisol concentrations occur or the value of these peaks and troughs.

It needs to be reiterated that individual cortisol levels values will be different and what is presented here, are average values. However, the pattern does not differ.

This very important information does make replacement therapy a little easier. It means we can use a standard representation of the circadian rhythm to aim for in males and females and for any age. It also shows cortisol is always present in the bloodstream. In fact, our studies have determined cortisol values rarely fall below 50 nmol/l and this information gives us good measures to aim for when we start cortisol replacement using hydrocortisone.

This is not quite the end of the story because we still need to remember the absorption and clearance of hydrocortisone, as we explained in Chapter 6. These are very important factors which we also need to consider when calculating doses to attain cortisol values which best mimic the circadian rhythm.

REPLACEMENT DOSING WITH HYDROCORTISONE

Individualising hydrocortisone dosing is our aim as this will reduce over and under dosing that can arise with a one dose fits all approach. To help with this aim the following points should be considered:

1. Cortisol measurements achieved from each dose of hydrocortisone vary in individuals.

2. Individual half-life and clearance will influence dose and timing (Chapter 6).

3. Several factors may influence cortisol levels achieved such as other medications for example, the oral contraceptive pill (see Chapters 6 and 13). It is important to take measurements of cortisol whilst on the medication you need to take daily. If you stop these medications, then you will need to have a re-evaluation of your dosing schedule, as dose amounts and dose timings may need to be altered.

4. If you always take your medication with food, then do so during the test because any influence on cortisol levels will be detected and will give a better indication of the cortisol values achieved every day.

5. When evaluating the changes to a dose, it is important to realise that simply increasing the dose will only increase the peak and not how long the dose will last for. This is due to the patient's individual cortisol half-life (see Chapter 6 Figure 6.5 for the variance in cortisol half-life of 75 patients). Figure 9.8 illustrates an example of this, where an increase in the morning and afternoon doses achieve higher peaks but does not achieve a longer duration). Increasing the dose does not give better cortisol cover during the 24 hours. The only way to do that is to dose more frequently. Double dosing is important however for different reasons when unwell (Chapter 12).

6. In many patients, the late night dose takes much longer to peak and lasts longer in the body. This is most likely due to body functions naturally slowing down.

7. Please note the amount of cortisol gained from each dose will be different in each person. There can be many influencing factors such as height, weight, absorption, clearance, half-life, the time of day the medication is administered (early morning versus late evening), other medications being taken, along with certain foodstuffs for example, grapefruit juice, liquorice and a low carbohydrate containing diet (see Chapters 10 and 13).

We have already discussed that simply increasing a dose of hydrocortisone does not make it last longer, it will simply give a higher peak of cortisol. Figure 9.8 illustrates an occasion where the lunchtime and morning doses were increased due to the side effects the patient was experiencing. The increase in dose simply increased the cortisol peak values in both instances and the individual still had periods of time without any cortisol in the blood and the side effects did not abate. The evening dose was lowered and again we see an example of the dose taking longer to peak than at previous times of the day, the reduction in the dose gives a more appropriate cortisol peak.

Note we have not quoted the actual doses as the peak values and duration will differ between individuals.

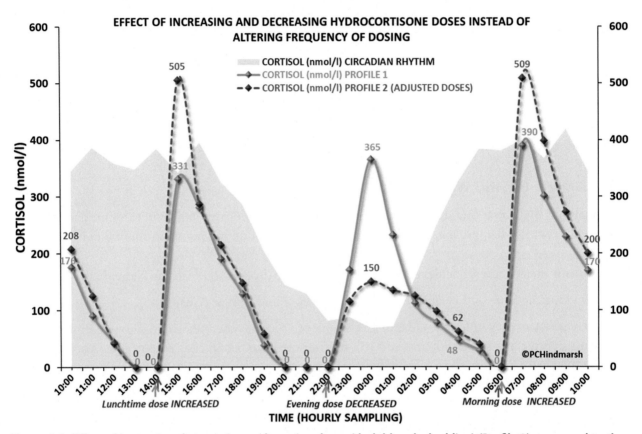

Figure 9.8 *Effect of increasing the morning and evening doses (dark blue dashed line) (Profile 2) compared to those obtained previously in Profile 1 (light blue solid line). All that has happened is that the increase in dose only increased the peak values attained without altering the duration cortisol is in the circulation. Cortisol is zero for the same 4 hour blocks in each profile. Note that decreasing the dose at 22:00 (10 pm) does not alter duration either but gives a more appropriate peak at that time. Data are superimposed on the average circadian rhythm (light blue shaded area) constructed with 20 minute sampling in adults and children without adrenal problems. Note the average circadian cortisol values will vary in individuals, however the circadian pattern remains constant. Profile starts at 10:00 (10 am) and runs through to 10:00 (10 am) the following day.*

What the data in Figure 9.8 tells us, is that this patient's dosing schedule needs to be carefully revised in terms of amount and timing of doses. The data indicate that 4 doses of hydrocortisone a day would give better cortisol distribution and a new dosing schedule needs to be calculated with an additional sample taken 30 minutes after each dose, to ensure the cortisol peak is not missed.

Again, remember the time the cortisol peak varies in individuals and sometimes an extra sample needs to be taken 45 minutes post dose.

When we get the situation as illustrated in Figure 9.9 with similar cortisol values in concurrent samples, this often indicates the peak may have occurred between the two points and we have not detected it, or it sometimes reflects slower absorption, although it is even more difficult to be certain without more frequent sampling.

The more likely explanation is that the peak has been missed which is also supported by the fact that this scenario occurred twice in the same person/profile between two different doses and that the likely peak was around 45 minutes after the dose was taken. This helps guide us to the most appropriate time to take samples around the doses for the patient.

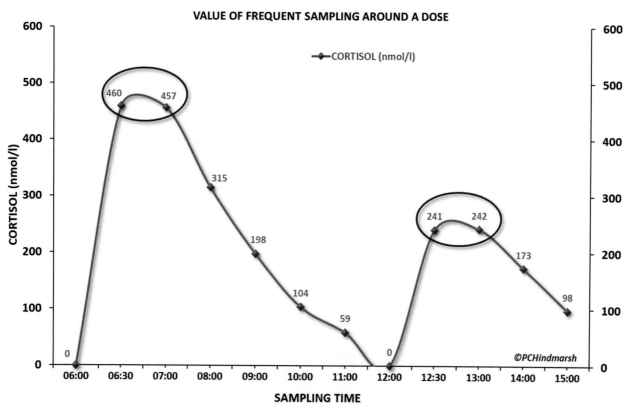

Figure 9.9 *Cortisol concentrations obtained from two doses of hydrocortisone given at 06:00 (6 am) and 12:00 (noon). Similar values are highlighted in the red circles suggesting either slower absorption or more likely that the peak occurred between the two sampling points and was higher than the values in the circles. A sample taken 45 minutes after the dose would help identify this.*

One final point to re-emphasise is there is a great deal of individual variation in how doses are metabolised as shown in Figure 9.10:

- The person receiving 25 mg of hydrocortisone has an earlier and lower peak compared to the one who took 15 mg and whose measured cortisol could be detected for a slightly longer period (60 minutes).

- Even the same dose of 22.5 mg of hydrocortisone in two people produced different peaks albeit occurring at the same time.

This means that although we can generalise on treatment, we do need to know what happens in the individual, especially as these doses are taken every day and both under and over dosing can cause long term side effects which may only become obvious many years down the line, such as osteoporosis.

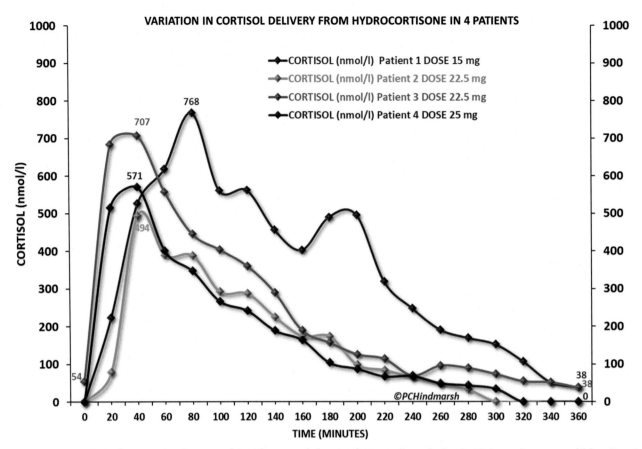

Figure 9.10 *Cortisol concentrations resulting from oral doses of 15 mg (purple line), 22.5 mg (green and blue lines) and 25 mg (red line) of hydrocortisone given to four individuals. Notice the difference in peaks obtained as well as the timing of those peaks and how different people have different durations when cortisol is measurable after a dose. (From Congenital Adrenal Hyperplasia: A Comprehensive Guide).*

TIMING OF EACH HYDROCORTISONE DOSE

We can build on the information that we have just considered about dose and timings. The first task is to look at what the different dose timings achieve.

The original dosing schedule used a twice a day regimen and the cortisol profile resulting from such an approach is shown in Figure 9.11, where the cortisol concentrations achieved are superimposed on the circadian rhythm of cortisol averaged from our studies in normal individuals. In this example, we use the data from a study performed on patients with CAH because we can see the effect cortisol has on the adrenal glands. The data in the figure reveals too much cortisol will switch off the hormone 17OHP and the adrenal glands decrease in size and become dormant as can be seen in the over dosing column in Figure 9.1 as well as in Figure 9.11.

In CAH the focus has always been to 'control' androgen and 17OHP production and in an attempt to do this, two high doses of hydrocortisone per day have been used. Cortisol levels are not usually measured and treatment was to increase the doses of hydrocortisone if the 17OHP levels increased. Androgen production was switched off, but the high doses of glucocorticoids caused long term side effects as did the periods where there was no cortisol present in the blood. As hydrocortisone lasts on average 6 hours, this dosing schedule leaves the patient without cortisol for up to 12 hours. This leads to the situation of over and under treatment taking place during the 24 hour period.

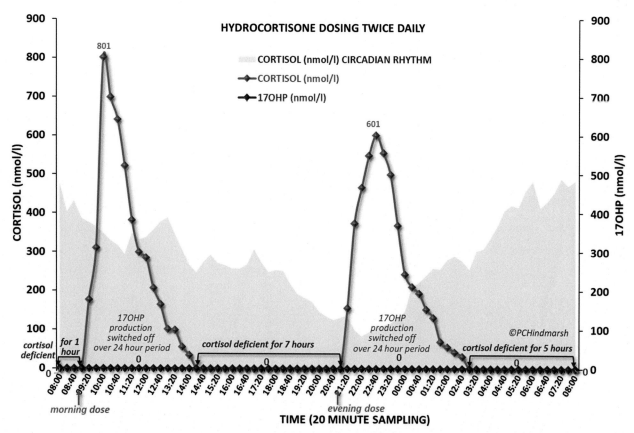

Figure 9.11 *24 hour cortisol (blue line) profile from an individual with congenital adrenal hyperplasia receiving twice daily hydrocortisone doses and the 17-hydroxyprogesterone levels (purple line) are undetectable. Data are superimposed on the average circadian rhythm (light blue shaded area) constructed with 20 minute sampling in adults and children without adrenal problems. Note the average circadian cortisol values will vary in individuals, however the circadian pattern remains constant. Profile starts at 08:00 (8 am) and runs through to 08:00 (8 am) the following day. Note the higher scale on the y-axis compared to Figure 9.8.*

If this patient was on replacement therapy for any other type of adrenal insufficiency, the cortisol gained from the doses would be the same. The high peaks would cause the same side effects. Figure 9.11 shows doses that deliver quite high peaks of cortisol which do not last very long and for more than 12 hours of the 24 hour period, the cortisol concentrations fall below our target of 50 - 100 nmol/l with periods where the cortisol is often unmeasurable. This means at night, the ACTH production will rise and reach high levels as there is no cortisol feedback to switch off the ACTH from 03:00 (3 am) until the next tablet is taken at 09:00 (9 am). However, in this case as can be seen in Figure 9.11, there is no measurable 17OHP throughout the 24 hour profile, indicating the adrenal glands have become inactive as a result of the high doses taken which not only switched off 17OHP but also subsequently switched off ACTH production.

This scenario occurs again during the period 14:00 (2 pm) until 21:00 (9 pm) where no cortisol is present. These periods where there is no cortisol present will result in symptoms of under treatment and will place the individual at risk of an adrenal crisis, particularly in illness.

We have in fact a classic situation during the 24 hour period of both under and over treatment occurring. In CAH and in Addison's disease, hyperpigmentation may result due to the high ACTH (Chapter 8, Part 4.) This could be a particular problem if the adrenal glands have been removed, which sometimes transpires to manage Cushing's disease, due to the high ACTH secretion. Approximately 7% of patients with Cushing's disease are treated with bilateral adrenalectomies usually because of other comorbidities which prevent a pituitary operation to be undertaken.

In this situation, if the cortisol replacement is not delivering good coverage, this would allow the pituitary to continue to produce ACTH, leading to an increase in the ACTH tumour size in the pituitary and very marked hyperpigmentation. This is often referred to as Nelson's syndrome.

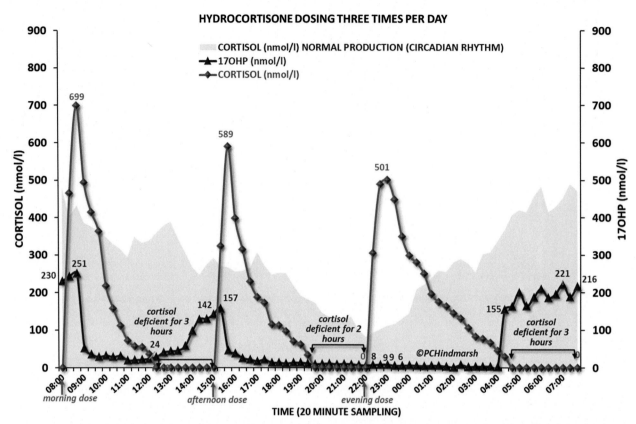

Figure 9.12 *24 hour profile of cortisol (blue line) measurements in a person receiving hydrocortisone 3 times per day and 17-hydroxyprogesterone (17OHP) levels (purple line). Data are superimposed on the average circadian rhythm (light blue shaded area) constructed with 20 minute sampling in adults and children without adrenal problems. Note the average circadian cortisol values will vary in individuals, however the circadian pattern remains constant. Profile starts at 08:00 (8 am) and runs through to 08:00 (8 am) the following day.*

The next development was to try three times per day dosing therapy as shown in Figure 9.12.

This had the following effects:

- It improved the distribution of cortisol through the 24 hour period however all three doses do produce high peaks

- Reduced the time without cortisol in the bloodstream.

- However, notice, no cortisol stacking is taking place as the period between dosing times is 7 to 8 hours and is longer than the duration of hydrocortisone in the circulation, which is on average 6 hours. This leads to periods between doses where there is no cortisol.

- Did not lead to over suppression as the figure clearly demonstrates that ACTH can still be produced as reflected in the rise in 17OHP, proving that cortisol is needed at those time points.

- Define cortisol levels below 50 nmol/l in this person as critical level, as below this value 17OHP starts to rise as ACTH production from the pituitary commences.

The 17OHP begins to fall after the very high morning dose but then rises when there is no cortisol, although this is not always the case as it depends on the activity of the pituitary gland which differs at various times of the day. The high evening dose dampens the 17OHP down, but then the ACTH surges back at 04:00 (4 am) raising the 17OHP. You can also see the delay of the effect of cortisol on the 17OHP as the levels take time to fall. These observations tell us what the ACTH production is doing at different times of the day and night. Cortisol is, therefore, needed over the full 24 hours as without it:

- ACTH levels naturally rise. This occurs in people without adrenal problems and in anyone with primary adrenal insufficiency from whatever cause.

- In CAH, without considering the cortisol replacement and focusing only on the 17OHP concentrations, leads to both over and under treatment as not only are peaks important but keeping the cortisol troughs above 50 nmol/l keeps the system under control by the negative feedback mechanism.

With this in mind we now look at a profile where dosing four times per day has been used (Figure 9.13).

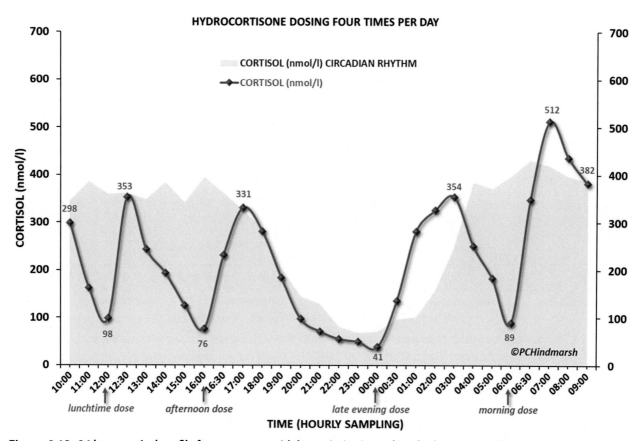

Figure 9.13 *24 hour cortisol profile from a person with hypopituitarism taking hydrocortisone four times per day with the fourth dose taken at midnight. Data are superimposed on the average circadian rhythm (light blue shaded area) constructed with 20 minute sampling in adults and children without adrenal problems. These are average values for the circadian rhythm which will differ in individuals. Profile starts at 10:00 (10 am) and runs through to 09:00 (9 am) the following day.*

When dosing four times per day the amount of time within our target (more appropriate peak values and cortisol concentrations that do not fall below 50 nmol/l) is further improved. In this example cortisol concentrations fall below 50 nmol/l for only approximately an hour at most and there are no periods where there is no cortisol present. The peaks are appropriate and now we see episodes of useful stacking taking place. In this example, we have more successfully captured the pattern of normal cortisol production. It is important to realise everyone will achieve different cortisol values as they are determined on the dose used, body size, absorption and clearance which is why we have not shown the dose amounts. However, the circadian rhythm is more constant, which is the main aim of replacement. Only carefully calculated individualised dosing schedules, checked by means of 24 hour cortisol profiles, make this achievable.

In some individuals, five doses per day are necessary and is usually required for those who have a faster than normal clearance. The way to address proven fast clearance (see Chapter 6) is to give doses more frequently and not to simply increase the dose, as this will not lead to a longer duration of cortisol in the circulation (see Figure 9.8).

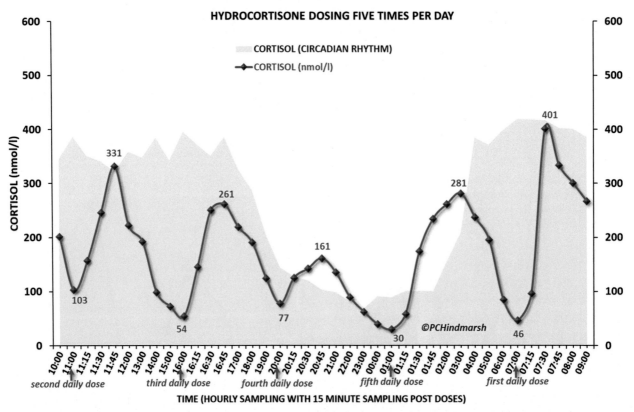

Figure 9.14 *24 hour cortisol profile from person taking hydrocortisone five times per day with dosing during the night. Data are superimposed on the average circadian rhythm (light blue shaded area) constructed with 20 minute sampling in adults and children without adrenal problems. Note the average circadian cortisol values will vary in individuals, however the circadian pattern remains constant. Profile starts at 10:00 (10 am) and runs through to 09:00 (9 am) the following day.*

Figure 9.14 shows the results of an individual on a five times per day dosing schedule in a 24 hour profile, which illustrates how close we can achieve the circadian rhythm by such an intervention without either over or under treatment. Previously, this patient was on 3 high doses a day and was suffering both weight gain and headaches. With the distribution of cortisol implemented in Figure 9.14, the side effects the patient was experiencing which were very frequent headaches, disappeared and weight gain which had been a problem, stabilised. Note, blood samples were taken every 15 minutes for an hour post dose to best identify the actual cortisol peak attained in this situation. The cortisol peak occurred approximately 45 minutes after taking the dose, except for the fifth (late evening dose). The late evening dose taken at 01:00 (1 am) peaked approximately 2 hours after the dose was taken. This example again highlights the need for individual dosing schedules and cortisol replacement is not one size fits all!

So far, we have looked at dosing which covers the 24 hour period but what happens if we start to compress the dosing into a smaller time frame. This is done in adult practice where the last dose is often given at 18:00 (6 pm) because of 'unsubstantiated' problems with going to sleep. However, as we discussed in Chapter 8, Part 8 there is no evidence that hydrocortisone given in the late evening affects the ability to get off to sleep, as the number of people saying they had problems were the same as those without problems and this was irrespective of the timing of the last dose. Several patients stated they slept better and felt better when they took a dose at midnight. When the last dose is taken at 18:00 (6 pm), cortisol cover particularly in the early hours of the morning when cortisol is naturally rising, is zero, as is shown in Figure 9.15.

This places the person at risk of nocturnal hypoglycaemia as well as side effects during the day due to the concentration of all the doses over a short period, particularly if the person has a slow clearance of cortisol. What is more important is that in primary adrenal insufficiency, from any cause, no cortisol overnight means there is no negative feedback on ACTH production, resulting in a surge of ACTH production which probably explains why the problems we have discussed such as hyperpigmentation and the development of adrenal rest tissue, occur. In patients with CAH the high ACTH drive would, in addition, increase production of the adrenal androgens with an increased risk of all the effects of excess androgen exposure.

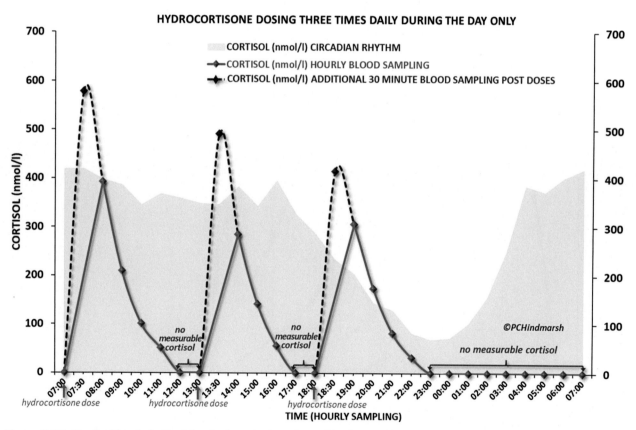

Figure 9.15 *Cortisol levels in the blood when the last dose of hydrocortisone is given at 18:00 (6 pm) compared to the cortisol production of an individual with the same body mass index but without any adrenal problems shown as the light blue shaded area. Note over the 24 hour period, in this example, the patient who is on replacement hydrocortisone is without any cortisol in the circulation for 10 hours. Please also note that every individual without adrenal problems will achieve different cortisol concentrations and it is the pattern, the circadian rhythm which we are highlighting. The blue line shows the cortisol measured at hourly intervals and the red dashed line shows the additional measurements made in this person 30 minutes after each dose.*

What Figure 9.15 also demonstrates is the importance of sampling frequently around a dose. If we did not have the additional 30 minute cortisol measurements and based adjustments on the hourly sampling only, the cortisol peaks attained from the morning and afternoon dose are good, however the evening dose would need a slight reduction. If the patient still complained of symptoms, it would be incorrectly concluded their symptoms were not related to their doses. However, when we consider the 30 minutes sampling, the data clearly show all the doses peak too high and in fact all three doses need to be reduced, not just the evening dose.

Going back to periods of under treatment, the period without cortisol becomes even more problematic in illness as it leaves the patient particularly at risk of an adrenal crisis, because even doubling the dose at 18:00 (6 pm) as shown in Figure 3.10, will not double the length of time, only increase the cortisol peak value. So, in fact there will be no cortisol during the early hours of the morning, blood glucose will fall, and the patient will be at risk of an adrenal crisis. Note, this is the time when most fatal adrenal crises occur. This is why Professor Hindmarsh started a More@4 AM campaign in illness (see Chapter 12).

We can take this a step further and look to see how our evening dose will last if we give this at different times of the evening starting at 18:00 (Figure 9.16).

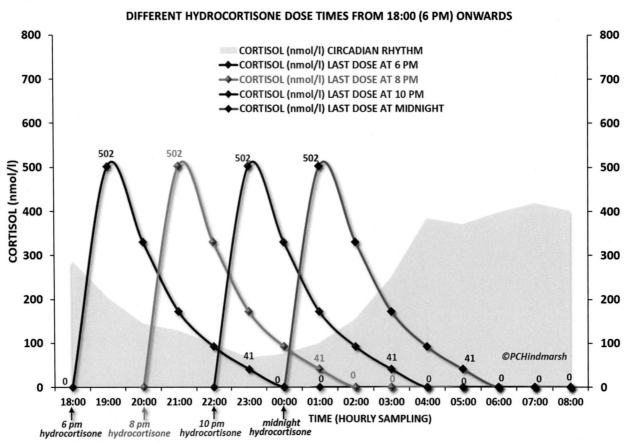

Figure 9.16 *Hypothetical illustration of how the same dose given at different times of the evening lasts in the circulation. The original dose was given at 18:00 (6 pm) and this dose has then been constrained to be given at 20:00 (8 pm) or 22:00 (10 pm) or 00:00 (midnight). This is to show the range of time the individual will be without cortisol and when cortisol levels fall below 50 nmol/l, whilst taking the same dose at different dose times, based on the next dose being taken at 06:00 (6 am). Data are superimposed on the average circadian rhythm (light blue shaded area) constructed with 20 minute sampling in adults and children without adrenal problems. These are average values for the circadian rhythm which will look different in an individual. The illustration is centred on a start at 18:00 (6 pm) and runs through to 08:00 (8 am) the following day.*

Figure 9.16 is a hypothetical illustration using the same post dose profile originally given at 18:00 (6 pm), but with the result of dosing at different times constructed from 18:00 (6 pm) with 2 hourly intervals until midnight. We have taken the cortisol profile following the 18:00 (6 pm) dose and then started it at 20:00 (8 pm) or 22:00 (10 pm) or 00:00 (midnight) instead of 18:00 (6 pm). This is to illustrate the period the person is without any cortisol or the concentration falls below 50 nmol/l until the next dose is taken at 06:00 (6 am). This varies from 7 hours when dosing at 18:00 (6 am), to 2 hours when the dose is taken at midnight.

The shaded blue area depicting the normal circadian rhythm, tells us that ACTH production will be rising from midnight onwards and it is important to prevent this rise in primary adrenal insufficiency as already mentioned, as this will lead to hyperpigmentation and adrenal rest development, as well as creating a period when the person is at increased risk of an adrenal crisis and/or hypoglycaemia.

This illustration was taken from a profile, and we must remember that the midnight dose in most people is slower to absorb and clear, although this does vary between individuals. This is just an illustration of the same dose taken at different times, to demonstrate the period without cortisol when a dose is taken at 18:00 (6 pm), 20:00 (8 pm) or 22:00 (10 pm).

ESTIMATING THE DISTRIBUTION OF CORTISOL
What is the difference between a Diurnal and a Circadian rhythm?
The two terms diurnal and circadian are often used interchangeably but have different meanings.

Diurnal means activity or something happening during daylight hours. This is in distinction to nocturnal, which means of the night. Circadian is made up of two words circa meaning around and Dian which means of the whole day or 24 hour period. Diurnal and nocturnal are words derived from Greek and Latin whereas circadian was constructed in the 1950s to describe patterns which vary on a 24 hour basis. Hence, we talk about the 'circadian' cortisol rhythm which means a rhythm which repeats itself once every 24 hours.

Finally, you may come across the word ultradian which means having a period of recurrence shorter than a day but longer than an hour. An example of this, are heartbeats. There are even longer rhythms such as monthly, for example the menstrual cycle and circannual, yearly, such as the shedding and regrowth of deer antlers!!

Circadian Dosing
Following on from the consideration of the circadian rhythm and dose timing, we can start to think how to use all this information and knowledge discussed in Chapter 6, to calculate dosing schedules.

Circadian dosing is simply a way of administering hydrocortisone which distributes the amount of cortisol gained from each dose, at specific times to mimic the normal circadian rhythm. Central to this idea, is understanding how cortisol is produced and distributed through the 24 hour period and along with the knowledge of the individual's absorption and clearance rate, we can start to work out both the dose amount and timing.

The 24 hour profiles in this chapter so far, show what is happening to the concentration of cortisol in the blood at points in time. At any point in time in people with normal adrenal function, the cortisol concentration measured is dependent on the amount of cortisol secreted by the adrenal glands and how fast the cortisol is cleared from the circulation. We know from pharmacology, the half-life of cortisol from hydrocortisone is on average 80 minutes and from this we can work backwards to determine what the secretion of cortisol would be at any time point, to produce a certain cortisol concentration given that we know how it is removed from the circulation. The process is called deconvolution analysis. It is a very powerful tool in that if we know the individual cortisol half-life of the person, we can calculate with a degree of precision the actual cortisol production that they would naturally produce in a normal day.

Using this technique, we have been able to determine two important points in people with normal adrenal glands. First, the average total production rate of cortisol by the adrenal gland is about 8 to 10 mg per meter square body surface area per day (mg/m^2/day). This immediately gives us a target dosing schedule to aim for. We could say that we need to equal this total production rate of cortisol with our replacement therapy. The situation is not as quite as easy as that, because we are also using an oral preparation which is influenced by how well it is absorbed through the gastrointestinal system and how much is metabolised by the liver and excreted back into the gut — the enterohepatic circulation. (See Chapter 6, Figures 6.10 and 6.12).

When we think about replacement therapy for CAH, we often talk about doses between 10 to 12 mg/m^2/day, as this leads to switch off of ACTH secretion from the pituitary gland but also accounts for the enterohepatic circulation of cortisol. In replacing cortisol for other forms of adrenal insufficiency, we would aim for a similar total daily dose, although it could be argued that we do not quite need as much because there are no adrenal androgens which need to be suppressed. The marker in primary adrenal insufficiency would ideally be ACTH but this is not practical to measure frequently, so for primary and secondary adrenal insufficiency, matching to the normal 24 hour cortisol circadian profile becomes the goal. Just as we observed the variation in absorption and clearance of hydrocortisone, it would be expected there will also be a variation in the total daily production of cortisol by the adrenal glands and this can range from 8 to 16 mg/m^2/day. This is largely due to individual clearance which is also very variable.

The total daily dose gives us a rough estimate of the amount of hydrocortisone we might expect an individual to need. The exact amount, however, can only be worked out by a careful study of how cortisol is delivered into the bloodstream from oral hydrocortisone and the half-life of hydrocortisone in the individual. To achieve this, we need to obtain 24 hour profile measurements.

The second important observation which we can make from deconvolution analysis, is to work out what the cortisol distribution derived from the total daily dose should be between certain times. To achieve optimal dosing times, we would need to consider the way the individual metabolises hydrocortisone. We can see the percentage of the total cortisol daily production in given time frames in Figure 9.17A. To create this figure we analysed all the profiles undertaken in adults and children. We then averaged the production for each time block to illustrate an overall effect for both adults and children. This tells us, for example, that on average for adults and children between 06:00 (6 am) and 12:00 (noon) approximately 35% of the total daily amount of cortisol is produced. The time blocks illustrated in Figure 9.17A give us an indication of the amount of hydrocortisone needed to deliver the cortisol required for each 6 hour period. This might be what is needed, if we were using a four doses per day dosing schedule. If we wanted to dose at different frequencies, for example, three or five times per day then we would need to recalculate the percentage of cortisol within the new time blocks.

Please note this is only appropriate as a base for an oral dosing schedule and cannot be applied to other ways of administering hydrocortisone, such as pump therapy.

We now have two components to emulate the circadian rhythm:

1. The total amount of hydrocortisone we would need to give in mg/m^2/day and now we have to add to this, the second point.

2. How the total daily hydrocortisone dose should be divided in terms of percentages, during the 24 hour period. Using the deconvolution analysis data in Figure 19.17A which is an averaged percentage of cortisol produced by the adrenal glands by all ages during four time frames that would allow us to divide up our daily dose to give similar proportions.

In fact, we can go one step further in terms of the distribution if we consider the variation in the known timing difference between adults and children.

We noted this earlier in the chapter when we looked at the timings of peak and nadir cortisol levels when we observed that:

• In children and adults the timing of the peak in the morning was similar

• The nadir in the evening differed being earlier in children than adults.

These differences are important because if we continue with the same time blocks used in Figure 9.17A, then because of the differences in the timing of the nadir between children and adults, the average percentages will change for the children and adults (Figure 9.17B).

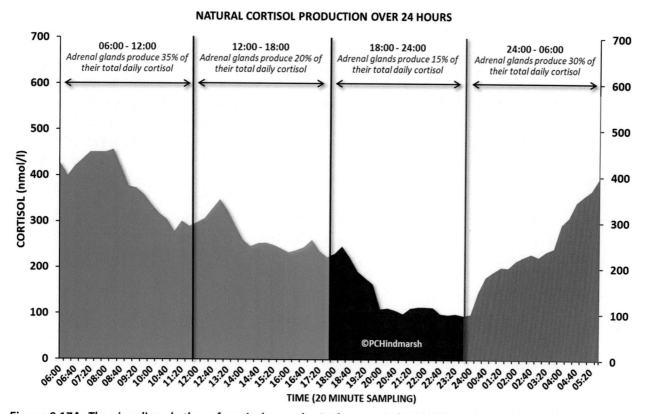

Figure 9.17A *The circadian rhythm of cortisol over the 24 hour period with blue representing daytime, dark blue evening period and grey midnight through the early hours of the morning. The day is split into six hour segments and the amount of cortisol delivered over each time block is expressed as a percentage of the total daily amount of cortisol produced by the adrenal glands in adults and children. The data from adults and children have been pooled to create this chart which is why the percentages differ in Figure 9.17B.*

CORTISOL PRODUCTION OVER 24 HOURS

TIME SEGMENT	PERCENTAGE OF TOTAL CORTISOL SECRETION DURING TIME SEGMENT	
	CHILDREN	ADULTS
06:00 – 12:00	38.4	26.4
12:00 – 18:00	21.2	21.2
18:00 – 24:00	10.7	7.2
24:00 – 06:00	29.7	45.2

Figure 9.17B *The average percentage of the total daily amount of cortisol produced in four time segments for children and adults.*

However, we need to be aware this is the average percentage of the cortisol distribution needed in these time frames and to achieve these, we also need to consider the way the individual metabolises hydrocortisone in terms of clearance and absorption which may also vary in these time blocks. If we want a peak at 06:00 (6 am) then we have to give the medication orally at 05:00 (5 am) because it takes about an hour to get to the peak, (again this varies in individuals). Figures 9.17A and 9.17B show cortisol production that goes from the adrenal gland straight into the blood as these data come from people without adrenal problems. In clinical practice we do modify these percentages. Although, as we can see the lowest total average cortisol produced in adults and children is from 6 pm (18:00) to midnight (15% of the total daily dose is needed), (Figure 9.17A), the late afternoon dose is usually given at 4 pm (16:00) because there is a natural surge of ACTH and cortisol around this time. This raises cortisol which then peaks approximately an hour later and then slowly declines in the early hours of the evening until 10 pm (22:00) in children and midnight (00:00) in older adults and 2 am (02:00) in younger adults. We do check this with a 24 hour profile to ensure we know how much cortisol we are stacking the dose on, as well as checking the most appropriate time to stack the next dose. Individuals with a very fast clearance may need more doses of hydrocortisone per day and those with a very slow clearance may need less, but the aim is to mimic the percentage of cortisol produced in these time frames by tailoring the dose and timing of the dose, to achieve the percentage. The values in Figures 9.17A and 9.17B are a guide therefore and as they are averages, will vary between individuals because everyone is different and this is what individualising doses is all about.

These observations answer the question as to why hydrocortisone is used in preference to the longer acting glucocorticoids available. The pharmacology of hydrocortisone can best approximate the natural cortisol circadian rhythm. Prednisolone has a longer glucocorticoid presence of approximately 8 hours, and it would still need to be given 3 times a day. Dexamethasone has an even longer glucocorticoid presence in the circulation of approximately 12 hours and would need to be given twice a day, but because it lacks the 'peakiness' of hydrocortisone and prednisolone, it becomes extremely difficult to match the times of the day when the peaks and troughs are required. In addition, its duration of action as an anti-inflammatory agent is more than 24 hours so overlapping of effects will occur. Due to these points, it becomes very difficult to avoid over or under treatment when using dexamethasone.

In fact, with both prednisolone and dexamethasone, it is very difficult to manage their longer action as a glucocorticoid because they were developed as anti-inflammatory agents. This is particularly an issue in paediatrics where both these preparations are known to suppress growth (Chapter 6, Figure 6.20). In adult endocrinology, the relevant potencies of dexamethasone and prednisolone need to be considered, particularly in terms of bone mineral density (Chapter 8 Part 1). Finally, a further advantage is we can simply measure hydrocortisone as cortisol in the blood, but for prednisolone or dexamethasone it is more difficult in routine laboratory practice.

Cortisol Stacking and the Importance of Timing of the Dose

We are now in the position to consider the most appropriate time to administer each dose. We have already considered the duration of cortisol which is in the circulation following ingestion of hydrocortisone and we have seen how much we will need on a daily basis, coupled with an idea of how the total daily dose should be distributed throughout the 24 hour period. In addition, factors such as absorption and clearance of hydrocortisone will play an important role, especially when it comes to checking what we have achieved with our treatment using 24 hour cortisol profile assessments.

Rather than just considering the timing of the dose, what we want to actually do is make sure we have optimal coverage during the 24 hour period and this is where the idea of stacking plays an important role. We have considered stacking in the section on pharmacology (Chapter 6). We previously mentioned if the dose of hydrocortisone is given too early, for example after 4 hours in a person who has a slow clearance, or if the person has a very slow clearance and takes a dose at a normal 6 hourly interval, the cortisol level achieved when the dose is taken will be increased, which in turn will generate a higher peak than expected, as the cortisol resulting from the dose will add or stack onto the amount of cortisol remaining in the blood. This is an important concept in dosing, and it is worth a revisit here.

Recognising that cortisol is present in the circulation for approximately 6 hours after ingestion of hydrocortisone, tells us immediately that problems could be encountered for whatever reason if we shorten or lengthen the time between doses, unless we know the amount of cortisol in the bloodstream at that time. This is seen when doses are all delivered during the daytime with no doses to be taken after 18:00 (6 pm). This dosing regimen is common in adult endocrine practice, where the total daily dose of cortisol is administered between 07:00 (7 am) and no later than 18:00 (6 pm).

Leaving aside the fact this leaves the whole of the late night and early morning without cortisol cover at a time when cortisol is naturally present, this concentrates 100% of the total daily doses given between these time points of 07:00 (7 am) and whenever the cortisol last dose is given based on no later than 18:00 (6 pm), leaving the patient without any measurable cortisol after the last dose given is out of the system. The example in Figure 9.18 illustrates this point as the last dose is given at 18:00 (6 pm) and by 00:00 (midnight) there is no cortisol present, whereas Figure 9.17B shows during this time interval we would expect a normal adult without adrenal problems, to produce approximately 45% of their total daily cortisol. This point is also discussed with respect to Figure 8.54 in Chapter 8, Part 8.

This is likely to lead to over exposure to glucocorticoids during the daytime and under exposure during the late night and early morning. Side effects are likely, particularly with respect to glucose and insulin, where the insulin antagonistic effects of the glucocorticoids are likely to provide long term stress and strain on the beta cells in the pancreas.

Notice in Figure 9.18 that the two 10 mg hydrocortisone doses give a similar peak in the 700's but the 5 mg hydrocortisone dose does not deliver a peak half that value. This is due to differences during the day in handling hydrocortisone particularly once cortisol binding globulin is saturated, as it would be with the first two 10 mg doses, when free cortisol would be cleared very rapidly so that the true peak, if we could saturate cortisol binding globulin even more, would have been higher than the 700's. Again, it is important to appreciate the peaks attained from these doses would vary in individuals, due to body size and clearance.

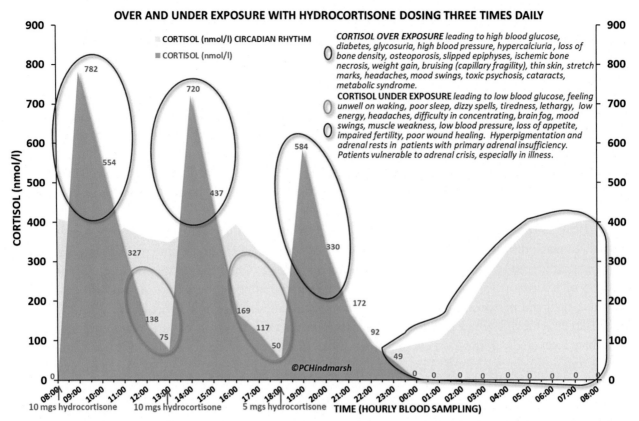

Figure 9.18 *24 hour cortisol profile illustrating cortisol values achieved in this patient who has taken all their daily replacement doses cortisol between 08:00 (8 am) and 18:00 (6 pm). This dosing schedule leaves this individual without any cortisol for a long period of time (purple circled area) compared to the normal circadian rhythm (light blue area) as well as areas where over exposure (circled in red) occurs. In this individual whose clearance is within the normal range, under stacking also occurs where cortisol levels drop low between doses (numbers circled in green). Note, the cortisol values attained from the stated doses are relevant to this patient only as cortisol values achieved will be determined by patient body size and individual absorption and clearance of hydrocortisone.*

Under stacking occurs when the time gap between doses is too long and/or the person clears cortisol quickly, as can be seen in the two and three daily dosing examples, Figures 9.11 and 9.12.

As a reminder, over stacking occurs when:

- The time gap between the doses is too short
- Or the person clears the dose slowly and another dose is added in too soon.

In essence, the next dose is added onto cortisol values remaining in the blood, which are higher than expected/known and consequently this will:

- Increase the cortisol peak values which will be much higher than anticipated.
- Lead to side effects which may not be immediately or obviously attributed to the dosing schedule, for example, weight gain and long term side effects such as osteoporosis.

Both over and under stacking demonstrates the importance of knowing the best time to add in a dose.

In Figure 9.19 we explore different scenarios where we superimpose a second smaller dose onto the first dose of the day. Firstly, we use the classic dosing schedule of taking hydrocortisone every 6 hours and this is shown by the solid blue lines.

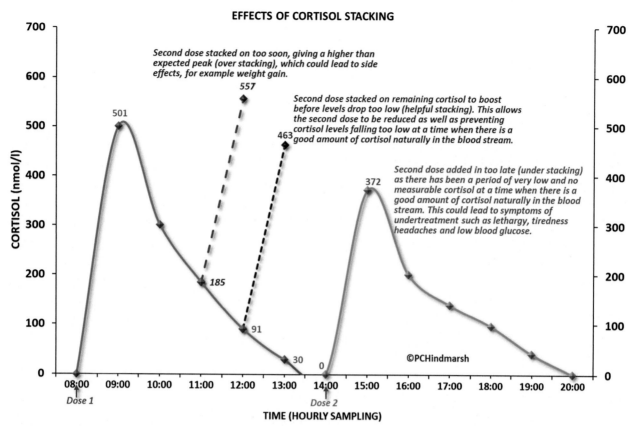

EFFECTS OF CORTISOL STACKING

Second dose stacked on too soon, giving a higher than expected peak (over stacking), which could lead to side effects, for example weight gain.

Second dose stacked on remaining cortisol to boost before levels drop too low (helpful stacking). This allows the second dose to be reduced as well as preventing cortisol levels falling too low at a time when there is a good amount of cortisol naturally in the blood stream.

Second dose added in too late (under stacking) as there has been a period of very low and no measurable cortisol at a time when there is a good amount of cortisol naturally in the blood stream. This could lead to symptoms of undertreatment such as lethargy, tiredness headaches and low blood glucose.

©PCHindmarsh

Figure 9.19 *The phenomenon of cortisol stacking. The solid blue lines show classic dosing (Dose 1 in dark blue line followed by a lower dose, dose 2 in light blue line) with a time interval of 6 hours. This often includes time when cortisol is undetectable which is under stacking. Over stacking (red dashed line to the peak of 557 nmol/l) occurs when doses are given too close together leading to a higher peak than expected. If this happens regularly then over exposure to cortisol will occur with side effects. Useful stacking (purple dashed line to peak of 463 nmol/l) is when one dose is built on a lower cortisol value leading to an appropriate peak without over exposure but a more prolonged overall cortisol exposure. The dashed lines connect to the peaks and the down swing from the peak has been removed for clarity.*

Under stacking:

When the smaller second dose is given 6 hours after the first dose, (solid darker blue line) there is a period when the cortisol concentrations drop below 100 nmol/l. This occurs just before the 12:00 (noon) cortisol measurement of 91 nmol/l onwards. In fact, the cortisol value drops to 30 nmol/l at 13:00 (1 pm) and there is then no measurable cortisol prior to the second dose taken at 14:00 (2 pm).

This occurs at a time of the day when there is normally good amounts of cortisol present in the bloodstream, however, for approximately an hour and a half before the second dose is taken, the cortisol levels fall below the lowest replacement target of 50 nmol/l, thus indicating the second dose should be taken earlier.

Over stacking:

If the second dose is taken too soon after the first dose, the dose will stack onto the remaining cortisol from the first dose, resulting in a higher than expected cortisol peak concentration. In this example the second dose illustrated by the red dashed line, which is a lower dose of hydrocortisone than the first dose, stacks on the remaining cortisol value of 185 nmol/l, resulting in a cortisol peak value of 557 nmol/l which is too high for that time of day and even higher than the morning peak of 501 nmol/l. This over stacking will lead to over exposure at this point and if the timing of the dose is not corrected, then this over exposure day after day will lead to short and long term side effects.

As the time interval between dose administration shortens, the resulting cortisol concentration from the second dose gradually increases, therefore increasing the cortisol peak value. This is an important point as we move to more frequent hydrocortisone dosing regimens of four times per day or more.

Useful stacking:

A careful look at Figure 9.19 tells us this phenomenon can be used to the advantage of the individual. If the timing of the second dose is carefully worked to be added at a time to avoid periods without cortisol, we call this useful stacking (purple dashed line). Often, another beneficial effect is that a lower dose can be used to reach the appropriate cortisol concentrations at a time more in line with the circadian rhythm.

In this example, if the second dose is moved to an earlier time where the cortisol level from the first dose falls to 91 nmol/l which is at 12:00 (noon), the period of very low/no cortisol is avoided, which occurs between 13:00 (1 pm) and 14:00 (2 pm). Also, if the second dose is taken at 12:00 (noon), a peak cortisol value of 463 nmol/l occurs at 13:00 (1 pm) which is between the peak value of the first dose of 501 nmol/l and 372 nmol/l where the second dose is taken at 14:00 (2 pm). Even though a small surge of ACTH occurs naturally around 12:00 (noon) the peak concentration of 463 nmol/l is still slightly high for this time of the day. As a result, the second dose could be reduced to achieve a lower cortisol peak whilst also maintaining a reduced time without cortisol in the bloodstream.

One additional point to reiterate with useful stacking, is often a lower dose of hydrocortisone is required to attain good cortisol coverage because the dose is added onto the cortisol remaining from the previous dose. One final point is that these data serve to illustrate the points about stacking and timing of the dose. They do not say that doses in everyone have to be taken at the times that we have used in Figure 9.19, the timing and the dose can only be determined from knowledge of how the individual handles hydrocortisone and that will depend on many things, such as body size and whether they are fast, normal or slow absorbers and clearers.

Everyone is different, so dosing schedules need to reflect that.

The aim is to get the cortisol replacement, this being hydrocortisone, distributed in the way to avoid the short and long term side effects from both under and over treatment.

These observations illustrate doses must be taken at fixed times and these times need to be worked out based on time of day and how quickly the person clears the drug from the circulation. Having said this, we should clarify exactly what we mean.

Although pharmacology tells us that hydrocortisone lasts as cortisol in the blood for 6 hours, this does not mean that the dosing frequency is always four times per day. If we assumed this, then we could have periods of time when cortisol was too low, and symptoms might result. Studies have proven there is always cortisol present in the circulation in people without adrenal problems and cortisol levels should be no less than 50 – 100 nmol/l. This means we really need to dose five times per day, but again this is dependent on how quickly/slowly the patient clears hydrocortisone. Yes, we will need fixed times, but the times may not be equally spread for example, if we work towards useful stacking then dosing times might be more like 06:00 (6 am), 11:00 (11 am), 16:00 (4 pm) and 00:00 (midnight).

We will only know the exact most suitable timing once we start to check what we are achieving with 24 hour cortisol profile studies.

Could we use preparations that last longer? The answer is no as the currently available ones, prednisolone and dexamethasone, were designed for their anti-inflammatory properties and not as adrenal replacement therapy. They are more prone to causing the short and long term problems we describe in Chapter 8.

There are two types of 'longer acting' hydrocortisone currently available. A dual-release preparation (Plenadren ®) and a slow/delayed release one (Efmody ®). Plenadren has a high peak followed by a long tail not much different from prednisolone. It comes in two doses 5 mg and 20 mg which does not allow for much flexibility. Dosing is a single dose in the morning but this does not provide for any cortisol after 17:00 (5pm) if the dose is taken at 09:00 (9 am) and there is no cortisol rise overnight.

Efmody is a capsule with an enteric coat. How it is taken in consideration to meal times needs careful planning as the morning dose needs to be taken on an empty stomach at least an hour before any food is consumed and the evening dose needs to be taken at bedtime, at least 2 hours after the last meal of the day, which may make fitting into daily routines difficult. There is a slow rise to a cortisol peak and the medication needs to be given twice daily. However, the profile lacks the natural cortisol peaks of the circadian rhythm, for example the rise in cortisol precipitated by the natural ACTH increase that occurs at 4 pm which is important in cortisol signalling.

As with all replacement cortisol, no matter what method or medication used, Efmody and Plenadren needs more detailed work to tailor them to the individual, as absorption will differ between individuals due to variable gut transit times as well as the known variation in clearance. 24 hour cortisol profiles will be valuable as with standard hydrocortisone, to calculate the optimal dose (peak values), the best time to dose, (stack the next dose) thus ensuring good cortisol distribution to prevent side effects which will occur if these parameters are incorrect.

Long term data will be required to answer these questions, as well as to evaluate the effects on and of the bowel and gut microbiome (Chapter 6), along with cost effectiveness compared to standard therapy.

Careful thought is needed for sick days as Plenadren will not cover the 24 hour period and the onset of action of Efmody may be too slow in delivering the hydrocortisone, so reversion to four times per day using standard hydrocortisone may be required when ill as the body needs hydrocortisone quickly. Neither medication will be particularly suitable for those with altered absorption or clearance.

The data from a 24 hour profile helps guide us to when the best time to stack cortisol and also show the level achieved. This guides us to what dose we should use to gain optimal cortisol levels. The aim is to prevent the common problem of over and under stacking, which tend to occur when doses are not individualised and lead to the short and long term side effects of over or under treatment.

Remember you can have both over and under treatment in the same day!!

CONCLUSION

One of the central principles of endocrine practice is to replace the hormone which is missing as closely as possible to its natural production. In the case of cortisol, this means mimicking as closely as possible the circadian rhythm of cortisol. Considering the total daily dose of hydrocortisone to be administered is important, as is how each dose will be distributed throughout the 24 hour period. These are the first two steps in determining the dose of hydrocortisone to be used and this has to be followed with a careful appraisal of how the individual absorbs and clears cortisol from the circulation. Two situations need to be avoided. First, is over stacking where doses are given too close to each other and second, the need to avoid periods of time without cortisol (under stacking). Detailed 24 hour profiles are the way in which we can elicit this information and subsequent chapters will consider how to obtain such information and how we interpret it in order to optimise cortisol replacement with hydrocortisone.

FURTHER READING

Charmandari, E., Matthews, D.R., Johnston, A., Brook, C.G.D., Hindmarsh, P.C., 2001. Serum cortisol and 17 hydroxyprogesterone interrelation in classic 21-hydroxylase deficiency: is current replacement therapy satisfactory? J Clin Endocrinol Metab 86, 4679–4685.

Hartmann, A., Veldhuis, J.D., Deuschle, M., Standhardt, H., Heuser, I., 1997. Twenty-four hour cortisol release profiles in patients with Alzheimer's and Parkinson's disease compared to normal controls: ultradian secretory pulsatility and diurnal variation. Neurobiol Aging 18, 285–289.

Hindmarsh, P.C., Charmandari, E., 2015. Variation in absorption and half-life of hydrocortisone influence plasma cortisol concentrations. Clin Endocrinol 82, 557–561.

Hindmarsh, P.C., Honour, J.W., 2020. Would cortisol measurements be a better gauge of hydrocortisone replacement therapy? Congenital adrenal hyperplasia as an exemplar. Int J Endocrinol. Article ID 2470956. https://doi.org/10.1155/2020/2470956.

Kenney, F.M., Malvaux, P., Migeon, C.J., 1963. Cortisol production rate in newborn babies, older infants and children. Pediatrics 31, 360–373.

Oosterman, J.E., Wopereis, S., Kalsbeek, A., 2020. The circadian clock, shift work, and tissue-specific insulin resistance. Endocrinology 161, 1–11.

Peters, C.J., Hill, N., Dattani, M.T., Charmandari, E., Matthews, D.R., Hindmarsh, P.C., 2013. Deconvolution analysis of 24h serum cortisol profiles informs the amount and distribution of hydrocortisone replacement therapy. Clin Endocrinol (Oxf) 78, 347–351.

Sarafoglou, K., Addo, O.Y., Hodges, J.S., Brundage, R.C., Lightman, S.L., Hindmarsh, P.C, Miller, B.S., 2022. The evidence for twice-daily hydrocortisone dosing in children with congenital adrenal hyperplasia is lacking. Horm Res Paediatr 95, 499–504.

Van Cauter, E., Leproult, R., Kupfer, D.J., 1996. Effects of gender and age on the levels and circadian rhythmicity of plasma cortisol. J Clin Endocrinol Metab 81, 2468–2473.

CHAPTER 10

Monitoring Replacement Therapy

GLOSSARY

Bioavailability The fraction of the dose administered (usually oral or intramuscular) that reaches the systemic circulation as an intact drug.

Stacking The addition of a dose upon another dose within a certain time frame, usually the time that the drug is in the circulation.

GENERAL

Following on from the previous chapters, it is clear we need to be able to monitor the replacement therapy of glucocorticoids and mineralocorticoids. We consider the latter in detail in Chapter 14. Both over and under dosing with hydrocortisone or any glucocorticoid, leads to many of the problems which have been summarised in the previous chapters. The most important point in adrenal insufficiency, is to appreciate we are replacing the hormone which is missing, namely cortisol and we are doing this with cortisol, usually in the synthetic form of hydrocortisone and therefore a measure of our replacement should be cortisol in the blood.

This means we need to understand how best to get the information we require to optimise changes in dosing in terms of how much and how often. We do not have a single simple measure that will tell us what we are achieving, so we need to test the effect of each dose we give in terms of how high the peak is, how long it remains in the bloodstream and as a result, how well is cortisol replaced over the 24 hour period. We also have to try to distribute the missing cortisol in a way which mimics the circadian rhythm. In order to achieve all these goals, we need to undertake 24 hour cortisol profiles, as this is the only way we can obtain a complete picture of replacement. This principle applies to all causes of adrenal insufficiency where we are replacing the missing hormone, cortisol, with its synthetic form, hydrocortisone.

WHAT IS MISSING, WHAT WE ARE REPLACING WITH AND WHAT WE SHOULD CHECK

In endocrinology, the basic principle is to replace the missing hormone with as close a synthetic preparation as possible and administered in a way in which it would naturally have been produced. In adrenal insufficiency, the missing glucocorticoid is cortisol and what we are replacing it with, is synthetic cortisol namely hydrocortisone. If we follow the argument from other areas of endocrinology, for example hypothyroidism, we would replace the missing thyroxine with the synthetic form of thyroxine and our measurements would entail either the measurement of free thyroxine (T4) and/or thyroid-stimulating hormone (TSH). If we are thinking about testosterone replacement, we would adopt a similar strategy. Why this does not happen with glucocorticoid replacement is rather more complicated because of the need to mimic the circadian variation of cortisol which necessitates the replacement therapy to be given several times during the 24 hour period and with varying doses.

Replacement Therapies in Adrenal Insufficiency. https://doi.org/10.1016/B978-0-12-824548-4.00026-7

METHODS OF MONITORING CORTISOL REPLACEMENT

There are different methods of measuring cortisol, for example, using various immunoassays for different body fluids such as blood, saliva or measuring the breakdown products in the urine, which we covered in Chapter 4. For further comprehensive information we recommend the recently published book by Dr John W Honour (details can be found at the end of this chapter). In Figure 10.1 we have summarised the body fluids commonly used in clinical practice when measuring cortisol concentrations, listing the advantages, disadvantages and practical points.

MONITORING CORTISOL REPLACEMENT

	BLOOD	SALIVA	URINE
Advantages	• Direct measure • Easy to relate to dose and timing • Easy to obtain samples • Sample volume is small • Cortisol and all relevant hormones can be measured at strategic times • Sampling can be timed so peaks and troughs can be measured • Values measured are showing amount of cortisol being taken to the organs • A detailed set of relevant measures obtained allowing full evaluation of cortisol replacement and fine tuning as well as individualised dosing schedule	• Easy to get sample in cooperative person • Can be done at home • Good for diagnosing situations of cortisol excess	• Easy to get sample in cooperative person • Easy to obtain samples • Can be done at home • Good for diagnosing situations of cortisol excess
Disadvantages	• Needs hospital admission at present	• Indirect measure via cortisone so dependent on salivary 11 beta hydroxysteroid dehydrogenase type 2 activity • Assumes constant saliva flow • Low levels not so easy to detect due to cortisol binding globulin effect • Works well when cortisol levels are high • Not easy to relate to dose as time lag in the system • Easily contaminated by any acid in the mouth • Sample does not show how much cortisol going to the organs but rather that which has been through salivary glands • Salivary flow varies during the day and with ambient temperature	• If using urine steroid profile then needs to relate break down products to cortisol • Not easily related to cortisol in blood • Needs good urine flow • Timing difficult to correlate with dosing • If use urine free cortisol influenced by cortisol binding globulin so only good when cortisol high • 24+ urine samples at specific times throughout 24 hour period impossible to achieve • Sample does not show how much cortisol going to the organs but rather that which has been through metabolic processes
Practical points	• Needs cannula for samples • Frequent samples every hour	• Needs good hydration and mouth clean of hydrocortisone or acidity • Frequent samples needed • Sample needs to be collected carefully and duration of collection influences result	• Needs good hydration • Cannot do frequent samples as best is 4-6 hourly ©PCHindmarsh

Figure 10.1 *Summary of the advantages, disadvantages and practical points on the various methods of measuring cortisol.*

Saliva

Saliva is produced by three glands around the mouth as shown in Figure 10.2.

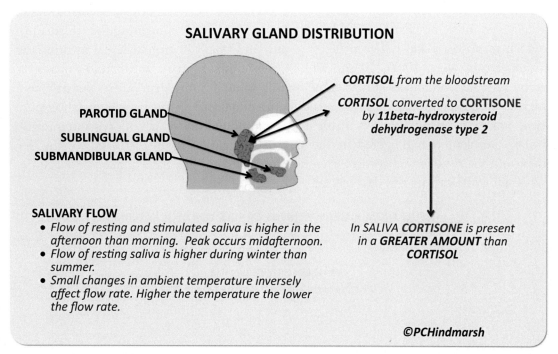

Figure 10.2 *The salivary glands and the handling of cortisol by them with a note on factors influencing flow of saliva.*

To recap, using the saliva method is easy to carry out, but the relationship between the measures in the saliva and what is actually happening closer to the dosing schedule in the blood, is far from clear. The reason for this is twofold.

Firstly, in saliva, cortisol or cortisone in the free state is measured and to measure the free cortisol, the amount of cortisol in the blood has to exceed the binding of cortisol to the binding protein, cortisol binding globulin. This means overall, only high peaks of cortisol will be measured which is not what we are only interested in. The information needed are the measurements of the high and low cortisol values, how long they remain in that state, how the replacement cortisol is distributed over the 24 hours and the levels on which doses are 'stacked' in its various forms (helpful and unhelpful). Although saliva measurements can sometimes be a guide, it is not precise enough to allow for subtle dosing changes. It is much better when used to test for high cortisol levels as seen in Cushing's disease. The variations in salivary flow also affects the results obtained and careful mouth preparation is essential to avoid contamination of samples. There are further problems and we have reviewed these in Chapter 4.

Secondly, cortisone is easier to measure because there is more present in saliva, however this is dependent on the enzymatic activity of 11beta-hydroxysteroid dehydrogenase type 2 in the salivary glands. This will vary between individuals making interpretation very complex. Finally, there is no comparison between frequent blood and saliva sampling to understand the lag between dosing and the measurement in saliva. This is highlighted in a recent study where salivary cortisol pharmacokinetics were not related to hydrocortisone dose, probably reflecting in part, first-pass metabolism in the salivary gland. At this stage salivary measurements for drug monitoring should be viewed as experimental.

Urine

Urine measures are also appealing but they are more difficult to interpret because urine is often collected over very long periods of time and so the precise relationship to the time and amount of hydrocortisone taken is difficult to define.

Generally, urine measurements can only average the effect over a period of several hours and that is not what we want when we are thinking about the close interaction between dose and what levels of cortisol are being delivered in the circulation. This becomes very clear when comparing the circadian rhythm of cortisol, which in plasma peaks between 06:00 (6 am) and 08:00 (8 am), whereas in urine the highest excretion rates are between 10:00 (10 am) and 14:00 (2 pm). Urinary free cortisol measurements are influenced by stress, alcohol intake, a high urine output volume (more than 5 litres per day) and in some reports, high sodium excretion. Urine also introduces an additional factor, namely metabolism of cortisol in the liver, which is an additional variable between individuals which makes interpretation more complex. This problem is highlighted in the next two figures. Figure 10.3 shows the result of a measurement of the 24 hour free cortisol excretion in the urine. We have a value and a normal range. Exactly what information does this data tell us?

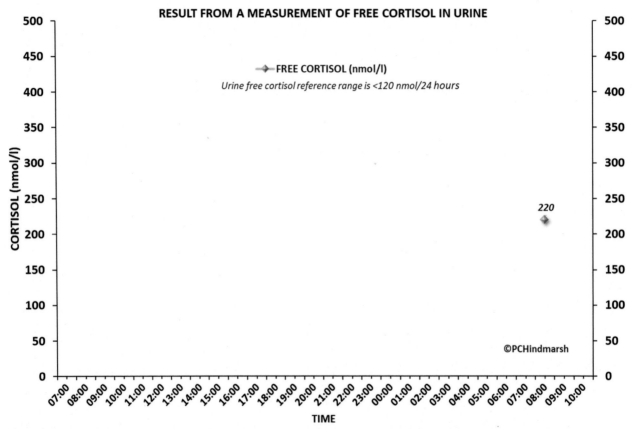

Figure 10.3 *Results of a 24 hour urine free cortisol measurement compared to the normal range at the top of the chart.*

To make it easier we have added when the hydrocortisone doses were given in Figure 10.4. When we study the data in Figure 10.3 and Figure 10.4 where we have more detail about the start and finish time of the collection and the dosing times, can we answer the following questions?

1. Which dose do we need to alter?

2. How can we see or even judge how high or when the doses peak?

3. Can we tell if cortisol levels fall too low, or in fact how long the dose is lasting?

4. Can this information show us which dose to adjust as we can see the result is above the normal range?

5. Do we need to adjust the timings of the doses, due to 'over stacking'?

6. Are there periods of over or under treatment, or are all the doses too high?

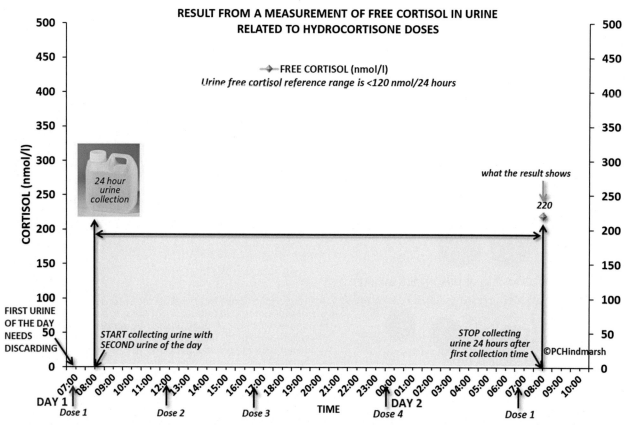

RESULT FROM A MEASUREMENT OF FREE CORTISOL IN URINE RELATED TO HYDROCORTISONE DOSES

Figure 10.4 *Results of a 24 hour urine free cortisol measurement showing the technique for timing the sample along with the associated hydrocortisone dosing schedule which shows 4 doses of 5 mg each.*

The quick answer is that we cannot do anything with the information other than say the amount of cortisol is probably high at some point. We might be able to refine this if we collect urine samples between the doses but that is going to be a major exercise in bladder control and going to the toilet on demand.

Too much or too little fluid intake can affect the results as can getting the start and finish time out of synchrony with the first dose.

Blood

This leaves us with blood tests which can be broken down into classic venepuncture or blood draw through a cannula and blood spots. Blood spots have been predominantly used for the measurement of 17-hydroxyprogesterone (17OHP) in congenital adrenal hyperplasia (CAH), but suffer from the limitation in the number of tests that can be easily obtained over a 24 hour period. 17-hydroxyprogesterone measurements, however, do not tell us how much cortisol is in the bloodstream and remember it is cortisol which is being replaced in CAH. 17-hydroxyprogesterone is a hormone which rises when the adrenal glands increase in size, however 17OHP can be elevated for other reasons, such as adrenal rests or polycystic ovaries, or from the stress of the blood spot test itself. In addition, 17OHP can also be switched off completely which leaves you with no measurable 17OHP and sometimes, as we have seen in profiles, with no measurable cortisol.

Figure 10.5 illustrates some of the problems which can arise with blood spot collection which has to be from a free flowing site and collected carefully to cover the spot and soak through. A free flowing blood sample is essential. If you test blood glucose twice on the same glucose meter a minute apart you get a different reading, as the first drop of blood you squeeze out of your finger is different to the next drop of blood as it may contain more interstitial fluid because of the squeezing, which can give a lower reading by diluting the sample. This is an issue with glucose which is measured in mmol/l, so it is likely to be an even bigger issue with 17OHP measured in nmol/l which is a million times less to measure and will be more susceptible to dilutional effect. Finally, you can get a similar effect if hands are not properly dried before the test.

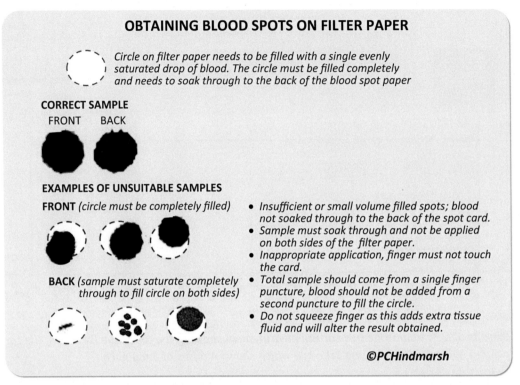

Figure 10.5 *Blood spot filter paper collection showing the correct method at the top where the spot is covered and the blood is absorbed right through to the back. Below this are examples of unsuitable samples and a comment on the need for good sample collection and factors which can lead to erroneous results.*

In addition, there are also concerns over how much steroid is actually measured in the spot particularly when assays other than mass spectroscopy are used. Even then, there may be an under reading of some 20% to 50% for cortisol and 25% for 17OHP.

As previously mentioned, if we restrict measurement to 17OHP in CAH this gives no indication of the level of cortisol at that moment in time. We also know there are large lag effects between dosing with cortisol, the cortisol peak and the effect on the subsequent 17OHP concentrations as described in Chapter 6.

Several other problems which can arise from using this method, for example, is when the result from a blood spot shows a high 17OHP level, the preceding dose is usually increased to bring the 17OHP to a level that 'feels' clinically appropriate. In fact, there is not a lot of agreement on what the 17OHP value should be, with some centres feeling it should be in the normal range, others between 10 and 20 nmol/l, others anything up to 40 nmol/l and a few centres accept the morning 17OHP value to be as high as 80 nmol/l. The simple answer is that it is likely to be high and certainly not in the normal range unless large doses of glucocorticoid are used, or the cortisol distribution has been carefully titrated using 24 hour profiles to optimise and individualise the cortisol replacement. Our knowledge of the pharmacology of hydrocortisone helps us explain why solely using measurements of 17OHP is difficult to interpret and what could be done about it. Cortisol affects 17OHP, but a normal 17OHP does not necessarily mean that cortisol is adequately replaced as the amount of cortisol needed to normalise/suppress 17OHP, is less than the normal daily production rate. Therefore, measuring 17OHP only may give an incorrect impression of how well a patient's cortisol is being replaced as we all differ in how we handle hydrocortisone.

Figure 10.6 illustrates the 17OHP values derived from blood spots carried out before each dose is taken. This patient is on 3 doses of hydrocortisone per day. Exactly what information does this data tell us? Not much at all — only the 17OHP levels at that moment in time.

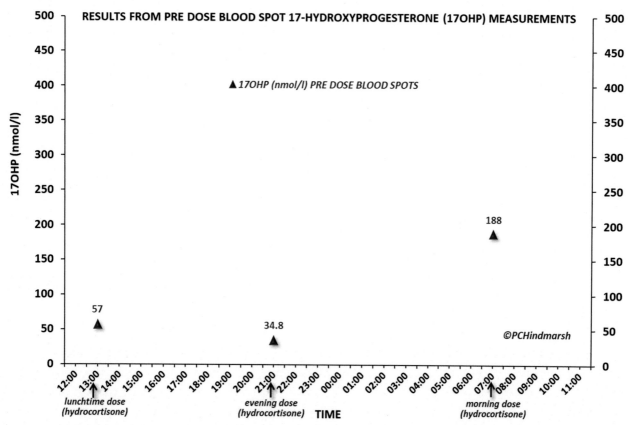

Figure 10.6 *17-hydroxyprogesterone (17OHP) results in a person with congenital adrenal hyperplasia from blood spots obtained before each oral dose of hydrocortisone is taken over a 24 hour period.*

As mentioned, the morning 17OHP 'within range' value very much depends on what each centre decides is acceptable, however for the rest of the day, the aim is to have 17OHP values below 10 nmol/l. The normal range in people without CAH is below 5 nmol/l.

Most centres accept the morning 17OHP value will be high due to the previous evening dose running low with the surge of ACTH which occurs in the early morning. As the adrenal glands are unable to produce cortisol, the replacement cortisol levels fall and ACTH rises. This ACTH surge occurs in anyone with primary adrenal insufficiency and if ACTH levels remain high and are not adequately suppressed, hyperpigmentation and adrenal rests will occur (See Chapter 8 Part 4) and 17OHP levels increase, resulting in a very variable acceptable range. This early morning surge of ACTH also occurs in other forms of primary adrenal insufficiency. However as the adrenal glands are either damaged or unable to function properly, they do not enlarge. The side effects of lack of cortisol at this time, with high ACTH, lead to the same side effects, except for no androgen production.

For reference, Figure 10.7 illustrates the average hourly 17OHP values over 24 hours of 4 post pubertal individuals who do not have any adrenal problems.

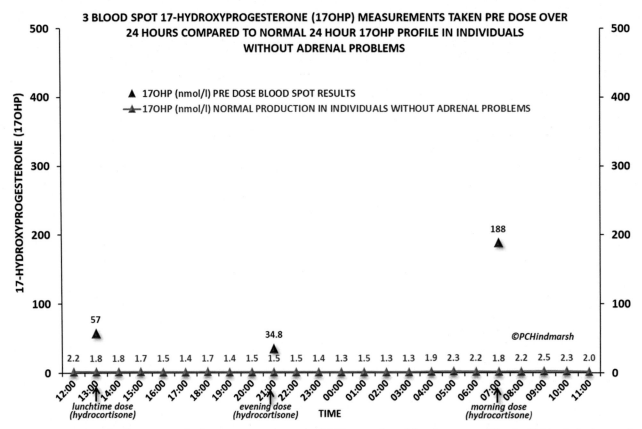

Figure 10.7 *Results from a 17-hydroxyprogesterone (17OHP) pre dose blood spot profile (individual dark purple triangles) superimposed against the average 17OHP concentrations of 4 individuals without adrenal problems (light purple triangles and line).*

The blood spot results indicate all the 17OHP values are high which suggest all the hydrocortisone doses need to be increased. However, as we discussed in Chapter 9 and illustrated in Figure 9.5, increasing a dose simply increases the peak value and in this case if the doses were increased, the 17OHP levels would decrease as can be seen in the example in Figure 9.6, although in the example the two high doses of hydrocortisone switch off the 17OHP production altogether. Remember, we have no idea of how much cortisol is in the blood at any given time, never mind how high the peak values are, because only 17OHP is being measured. Simply increasing the doses, without knowing the cortisol values could lead to all the well known and well documented short and long term side effects of over treatment, particulary weight gain.

We have established in CAH and other forms of primary adrenal insufficiency, the adrenal glands are unable to produce cortisol and the treatment is to replace this with a synthetic form of cortisol, which is hydrocortisone. We have also discussed that in CAH when there is not enough cortisol present, the adrenal glands increase in size which in turn increases both the production of 17OHP and adrenal androgens. We also know there is a lag in the effect of cortisol on the 17OHP which we cover extensivley in our book on this condition. It is very well documented that cortisol production has a circadian rythmn and we show several examples of this in Chapter 9 when we discuss dosing. So when we look again at the blood spot values, this information leads us to believe cortisol levels are too low due to the high 17OHP levels and this patient needs more cortisol! We have absolutley no idea how much cortisol is in the blood, is this correct? Figure 10.8 shows the value and the reasons we believe in measuring cortisol in CAH, or for that matter any form of adrenal insufficiency, over the 24 hours. The data reveals the cortisol peaks are too high and there are several periods where the indivdual is without cortisol, consequently both under and over treatment is occuring.

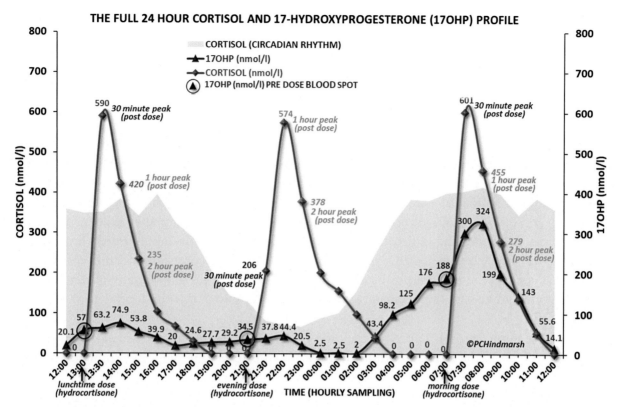

Figure 10.8 *The detailed information a 24 hour profile (sampling every hour with additional samples at 30 minutes around the actual doses of hydrocortisone) for cortisol (blue line) and 17-hydroxyprogesterone (purple line) compared to the 17-hydroxyprogesterone blood spots (red circles) and the average circadian cortsiol rhythm (light blue shaded area).*

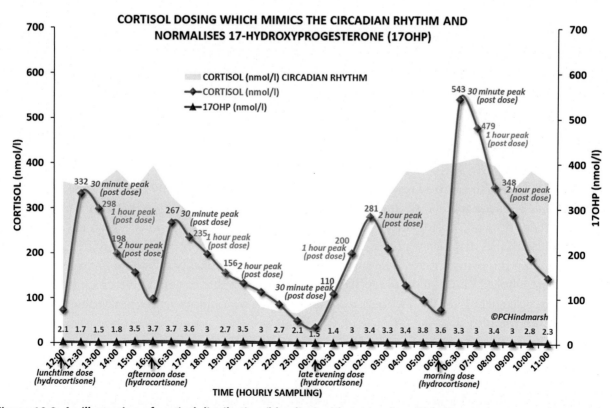

Figure 10.9 *An illustration of cortisol distribution (blue line) with appropriate 17-hydroxyprogesterone levels (purple line) calculated using the criteria described in Chapter 9. Average circadian cortisol rhythm shown as light blue shaded area. Note the additional information provided by the extra 30 minute samples after each dose.*

Using the pharmacology data from Chapter 6 and the criteria for dosing in Chapter 9, we achieve the result in Figure 10.9 which is close to what we would want to see as we mimic the circadian rhythm. Good distribution with no periods of over or under treatment and all cortisol values above 50 nmol/l. Notice how we stack the 06:00 (6 am) and 16:00 (4 pm) doses.

SINGLE CORTISOL BLOOD TESTS

There is no doubt it would be preferrable if a single measure could be used to determine replacement cortisol, in fact, several attempts have been made to achieve this by using molecular genetic markers. As exciting as this may sound, it is unfortunately unlikely this will ever achieve our goal which is a marker to alter the individual doses to match the circadian rhythm, the difficulty being due to the individuality in metabolism of hydrocortisone as well as uniqueness of natural cortisol values in those without adrenal problems. The molecular marker may give an idea of overall long term exposure, but the time lags in the system between exposure to a dose of hydrocortisone and the change in the molecular marker may be too long to be of value. This highlights the importance of mimicking the circadian rhythm and keeping replacement cortisol values in line with this rhythm.

Many centres monitor cortisol replacement in adrenal insufficiency by using a single blood test. The blood sample is often taken at random times and not timed to catch the highest cortisol concentration, which would be difficult to achieve even if the individual had the blood test an hour after a dose was ingested, as the peak might be missed. In this individual (Figure 10.9) the peak occurs 30 minutes after ingestion, however the time a dose takes to peak not only differs in individuals but varies throughout the 24 hours. As an example see Chapter 9 Figure 9.14 where the dose taken at 07:00 (7 am) peaks at 30 minutes, the 11:00 (11 am) dose at 45 minutes, the 16:00 (4 pm) dose at 45 minutes, 20:00 (8 pm) dose at an hour and the 01:00 (1 am) dose peaks 2 hours after it was taken. Figure 9.15 illustrates how the peak occurs regularly at 30 minutes in this individual. Further examples can be seen in Figure 6.14 where the timing of the peak depends on the frequency of blood sampling. If more frequent blood sampling takes place, the more accurately we can identify the timing of the peaks and this is also evident in Figure 10.9. Dose amounts differ throughout the day with the largest in the morning and smallest late evening. In most people, the late evening dose is absorbed and metabolised more slowly resulting in the dose taking longer to reach its highest cortisol concentration and lasting longer (see Chapter 9), this is also evident in Figure 10.9. Even the current quoted 09:00 (9 am) normal cortisol range from 133 – 537 nmol/l in the UK, is very broad.

Figure 10.10 illustrates the cortisol result from a single blood test taken at 10:00 (10 am). The individual's dosing schedule is 10 mg at 07:00 (7 am), 5 mg at 12:00 (noon) and 2.5 mg at 18:00 (6 pm), resulting in a total replacement dose of 17.5 mg for the 24 hours. The patient reports side effects such as weight gain, dizziness and headaches despite a reasonable cortisol level at 10:00 (10 am). What decisions can we make when we consider this cortisol value? The answer as you will have probably guessed is not many!!! In fact, if we judge the whole 24 hours cortisol replacement on this one value, it could give us a misleading idea that cortisol replacement over the 24 hours is ideal, however we cannot see the peak value or the ideal time to stack on the next dose.

The reason is the system we are looking at is dynamic, changing during the day and night and because of the pharmacology of hydrocortisone, frequent dosing will always be required. Even with slow release preparations, we still need a number of blood tests to determine the peak and trough concentrations resulting from administration of the slow release preparation. This would most likely require the same number of samples over a 24 hour period as needed for oral hydrocortisone.

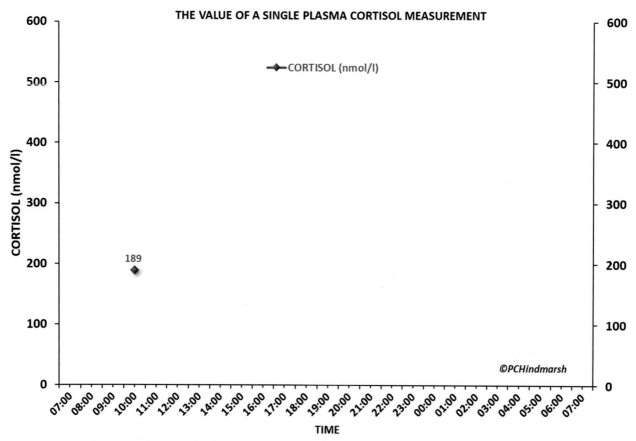

Figure 10.10 *Data obtained from a single blood test taken and from which daily cortisol replacement is assessed.*

We have already seen the marked variation in terms of absorption, half-life and clearance of hydrocortisone (Chapter 6) and this is likely to remain an issue no matter what preparation hydrocortisone comes in, as it has to be metabolised by the liver, circulated through the gut and these times are influenced by many factors, such as gastric emptying and gut motility. Even if we had one single measure, it might tell us doses need changing, but which dose/doses need altering by amount or timing is not clear.

DAY CURVES AND 24 HOUR PROFILES

A day curve is often performed on patients with adrenal insufficiency. Patients are asked to arrive at the hospital without taking their morning dose, they then take their morning dose at 08:00 (8 am) as soon as they have had their first blood sample taken. The time frame between each blood sample differs in each centre, but generally most centres take samples every 2 or 4 hours with the last sample taken usually at 16:00 (4 pm).

Figure 10.11 shows the results of a day curve which started at 08:00 (8 am) with samples drawn every 2 hours.

In Figure 10.12 we have added all this information to aid interpretation.

We can see the 2 hour value is good at 365 nmol/l, however we do not know what the morning peak value is, as the morning dose is normally taken at 07:00 (7 am) not 08:00 (8 am) and it is likely that the true peak occurred before the 10:00 (10 am) sample! So, it could be concluded based on this information, no dose adjustments are necessary and the side effects the patient complains of are nothing to do with the dosing schedule.

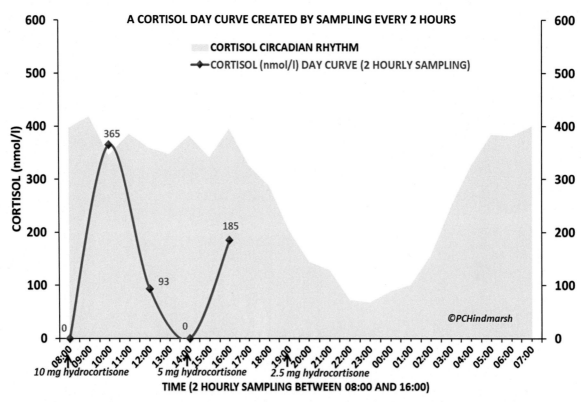

Figure 10.11 *Day curve in patient on three doses of hydrocortisone per day. The morning dose has been delayed to the start of the profile at 08:00 (8 am) when normally given at 07:00 (7 am) and the 14:00 (2 pm) dose would normally be given at 13:00 (1 pm). The average circadian rhythm of cortisol is shown in the blue shaded area for reference.*

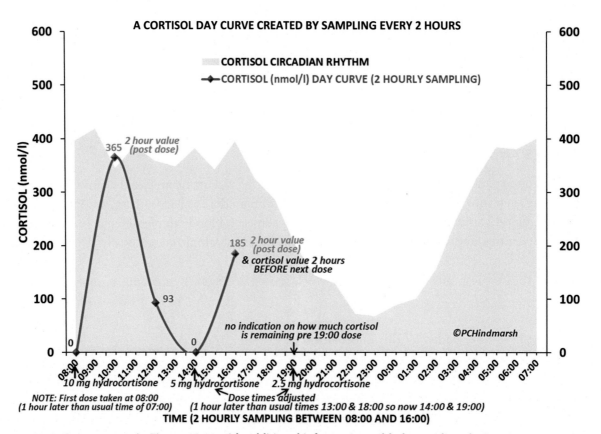

Figure 10.12 *Day curve as in Figure 10.11 with additional information added regarding dosing times superimposed on the average circadian rhythm of cortisol in the blue shaded area.*

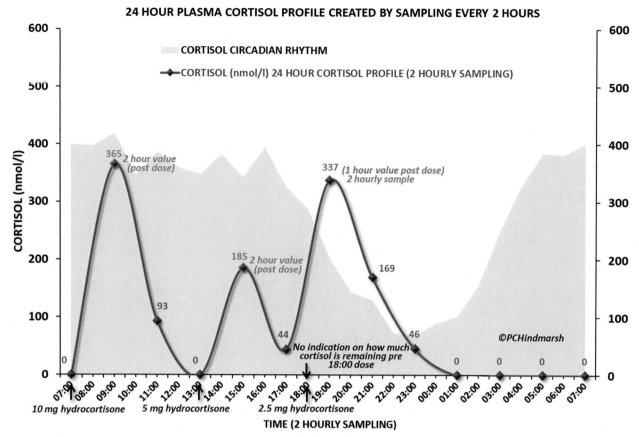

24 HOUR PLASMA CORTISOL PROFILE CREATED BY SAMPLING EVERY 2 HOURS

Figure 10.13 *The full 24 hour cortisol profile of which Figures 10.11 and 10.12 form a part. This has been constructed with 2 hourly sampling to match the day curve but the dosing is now at the timings normally used by the patient.*

Next, we look at the information a 24 hour profile gives when the sampling is taken 2 hourly over 24 hours (Figure 10.13).

Almost the same data is obtained as the day curve, except we can now see the following:

- The dose taken at 13:00 (1 pm) is running low at 17:00 (5 pm) and an hour after the dose is taken at 18:00 (6 pm), there is a value of 337 nmol/l.

- The 18:00 (6 pm) dose drops very low by 23:00 (11 pm) and there is no cortisol present from 01:00 (1 am) until 07:00 (7 am) when the next dose is taken.

Would hourly sampling really make that much difference in helping with optimising the dosing schedule? Figure 10.14 illustrates the extra information gained from hourly sampling.

The hourly sampling shows us there is now a peak of 509 nmol/l at 08:00 (8 am) and although we see the circadian rhythm superimposed behind the data, it is important to remember the data is based on the average cortisol production from 90 individuals without any adrenal problems and used as a guide.

Some of those individuals will produce higher and lower cortisol values than the graph indicates and what we aim to achieve is the pattern of the circadian rhythm over the 24 hours. It is easier in CAH to determine what is an appropriate peak or not, because we can measure feedback effects on ACTH or 17OHP and androstenedione. The latter two are not without problems in situations where there are adrenal rests or polycystic ovaries. For other adrenal conditions where we do not have these measures we have to extrapolate from what we achieve in CAH with hydrocortisone doses. We could measure ACTH in primary adrenal insufficiency, although practically this is difficult due to the sample volume needed and the need to transport quickly on ice to the laboratory.

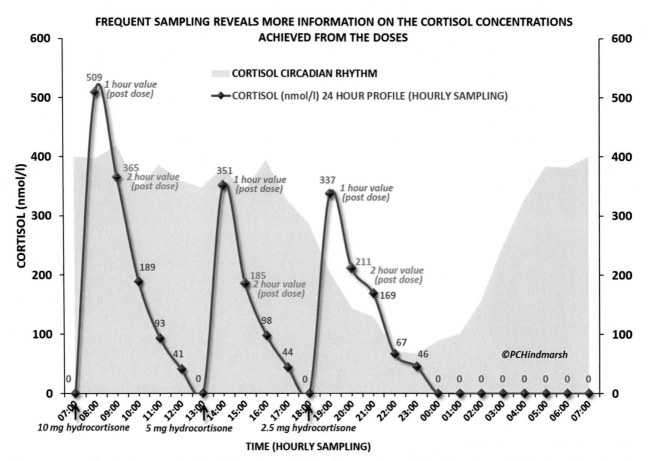

Figure 10.14 *The 24 hour cortisol profile as it was originally constructed showing the cortisol values for 2 hourly sampling with the peak value in green and now with one hourly sampling with the peak value in orange. The average circadian cortisol rhythm is shown in the background as the light blue area.*

Does this 24 hour profile give us all the information we need?

As discussed, there is a vast variation in the way individuals metabolise hydrocortisone, this includes absorption rate and individual half–life (see Chapter 9 Figure 9.10). If we are to take this into account, then we need some additional sampling around each dose and Figure 10.15 shows our profile data with the results from sampling 30 minutes after each dose has been taken.

The data clearly show:

- A much higher peak concentration of 763 nmol/l occurs 30 minutes after the dose taken at 07:00 (7 am).

- This individual absorbs hydrocortisone very quickly. This is apparent because the peak concentration also occurs at 30 minutes after the doses taken at 13:00 (1 pm) 626 nmol/l and 18:00 (6 pm) 498 nmol/l.

- Without these 30 minutes samples, the peak concentrations would be completely missed and lead to both short and long term side effects, which would not be attributed to the replacement doses.

- There are periods of over and under treatment.

Please note, these high cortisol peak values are not apparent in any of the previous data we have just looked at (Figures 10.11 to 10.14).

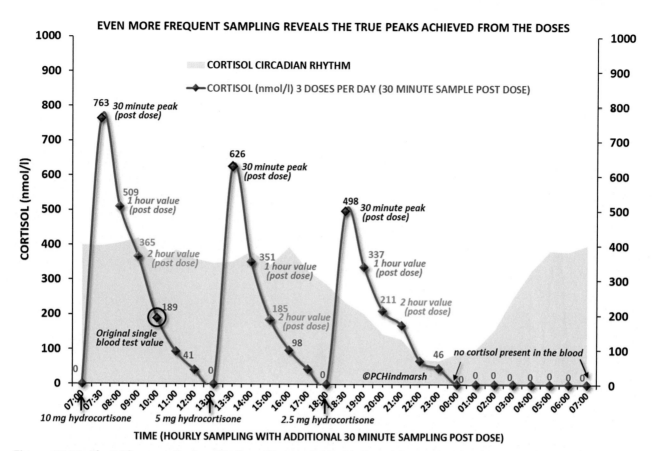

EVEN MORE FREQUENT SAMPLING REVEALS THE TRUE PEAKS ACHIEVED FROM THE DOSES

CORTISOL CIRCADIAN RHYTHM

CORTISOL (nmol/l) 3 DOSES PER DAY (30 MINUTE SAMPLE POST DOSE)

763 *30 minute peak (post dose)*

626 *30 minute peak (post dose)*

498 *30 minute peak (post dose)*

509 *1 hour value (post dose)*

365 *2 hour value (post dose)*

351 *1 hour value (post dose)*

337 *1 hour value (post dose)*

189 *Original single blood test value*

185 *2 hour value (post dose)*

211 *2 hour value (post dose)*

41

98

46 *no cortisol present in the blood*

0   0   0   0   0   0   0   0   0   0

©PCHindmarsh

CORTISOL (nmol/l)

TIME (HOURLY SAMPLING WITH ADDITIONAL 30 MINUTE SAMPLING POST DOSE)

10 mg hydrocortisone   5 mg hydrocortisone   2.5 mg hydrocortisone

Figure 10.15 *The 24 hour cortisol profile from Figure 10.14 with the addition of samples drawn 30 minutes after each dose was given shown in blue, the cortisol peak values from 2 hourly sampling in green and one hourly sampling peak value in orange. The average circadian cortisol rhythm is shown in the background as the light blue area.*

We can establish the following from this analysis:

- 30 minute samples show high peak values – all doses are too high.

- No cortisol is present before each dose is taken, demonstrating all the doses do not last until the next dose is taken.

- From midnight there is no cortisol in the bloodstream until the morning dose is taken.

- Side effects experienced are related to dosing.

- Dosing schedule is not following the known circadian rhythm of cortisol as there is no cortisol from midnight which is when cortisol levels naturally slowly begin to rise.

- There are periods during the day between doses where cortisol levels drop very low and periods where there is no cortisol.

- The dosing schedule has periods of excess glucocorticoid (over treatment) and periods where there is no cortisol present (under treatment). In illness, sick day rules need to be followed, however periods where there is no cortisol will remain zero or at very low concentrations unless the frequency of dosing is changed, particularly in the early hours of the morning leaving individuals at risk of adrenal crisis and particularly in children, hypoglycaemia.

This scenario often occurs and the peak cortisol concentrations from each dose are missed. As we have seen in previous examples, the same dose taken at different times of the day often results in a different peak cortisol concentration, this is due to variations in absorption and clearance, particularly at night.

Although it is appreciated that not all the common symptoms are related to dosing, once the dosing schedule is individualised to the patient and checked with a carefully planned 24 hour profile, the cortisol replacement can be excluded as a cause.

It is evident that not only the dose amounts need changing but also the timing of the doses need to be altered. Figure 10.16 puts all these graphs together so that you can check the points that have come out of our analysis.

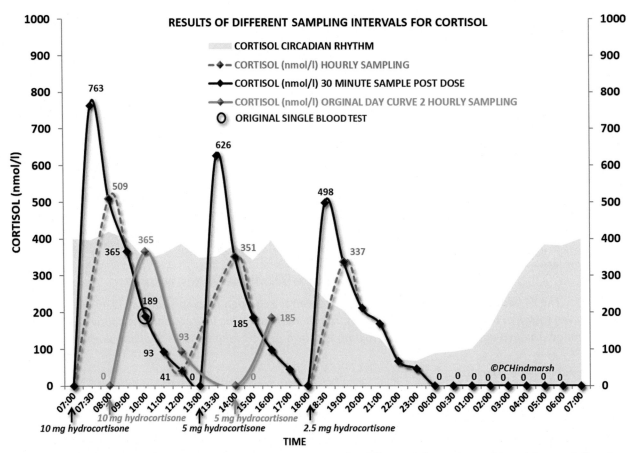

Figure 10.16 *Composite of Figures 10.11 to 10.15 comparing the different information achieved from a full 24 hour profile with the normal dosing schedule starting at 07:00 (7 am) with hourly (orange dashed line) and half hour post dose (solid blue line) sampling when superimposed on the original day curve with 2 hourly sampling (solid green line) which was started later than the usual dosing time at 08:00 (8 am).*

Figure 10.17 shows the results of a 24 hour profile undertaken once adjustments have been made to the dose amounts and times. We see helpful stacking occurring where each dose is taken and the individual is never totally without cortisol, although levels do drop low.

Again, we see the difference in the way the body handles the late night dose taken at midnight, which is due to slower drug metabolism at this time. The peak is only reached 2 hours after ingestion compared to the other three doses which peak 30 minutes after drug administration.

We have not missed the peak as we sampled 30 and 60 minutes after the dose so this is a true representation of what is happening. The total daily dose (17.5 mg) has not changed but is optimally distributed. This case study emphasises the importance of a systematic analysis of 24 hour plasma cortisol profiles.

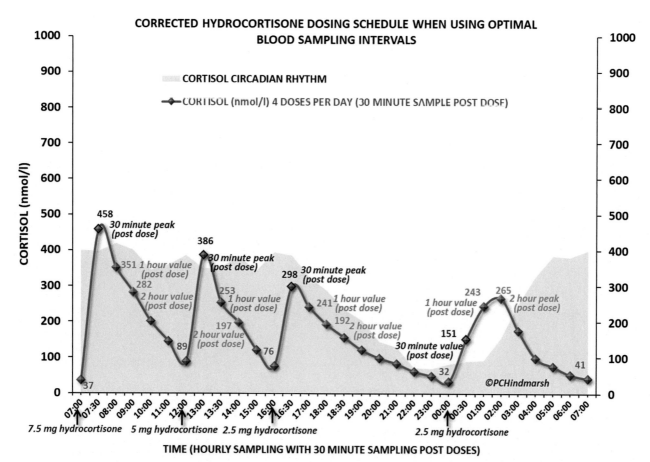

Figure 10.17 *24 hour cortisol profile showing cortisol peak measurements using 30 minute sampling post dose (in blue) and hourly sampling obtained after adjustments were made, based on the analysis from the profiles summarised in Figure 10.16. Peak values are shown if sampling was undertaken hourly in orange and 2 hourly in green. Note that although the total daily dose is the same, it has been redistributed across the 24 hour period to give a profile which is a good approximation of the average cortisol circadian rhythm shown as the light blue area. Note cortisol values achieved from doses are particular to this individual and will differ in people.*

Figure 10.18 illustrates the difference between the three and four times per day dosing schedules, illustrating the importance of dose distribution which impacts also on the dose chosen to be delivered at each time point. Considering information provided from a single blood test (Figure 10.10) (circled in red in Figure 10.18), day curve (Figure 10.12), or even a 1 or 2 hourly 24 hour profile, none of these could highlight completely the periods of over and under treatment this individual experienced whilst taking 3 doses of hydrocortisone per day.

BLOOD SAMPLING INTERVALS

In all cases of adrenal insufficiency, more detailed blood profiles which can be done in a hospital by taking blood samples every one to two hours with an extra sample around the dose time, give a much clearer picture of what is happening and helps us establish the close relationship between cortisol and hydrocortisone dosing. This enables us to identify the precise point at which changes to the dose or frequency of hydrocortisone administration can be made.

The profiles also allow us to gain an idea of how high the cortisol peaks, as well as how low it drops and for how long it remains in the circulation, how long there are periods of cortisol deficiency and when best to administer the next dose.

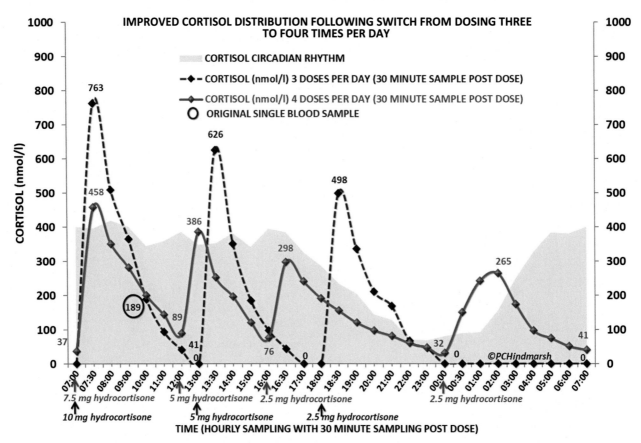

Figure 10.18 *A composite of the three doses daily (dashed blue line) and the four times per day regimen (solid blue line) to illustrate the more physiological cortisol delivery from the four times per day regimen compared with the average cortisol circadian rhythm shown in light blue.*

As can be seen in the examples we have discussed, the number of samples required to give the necessary information to base dose changes needs to be carefully considered. There is no place for taking random samples because that does not help us understand what changes are needed to the hydrocortisone dose, even when other measures are taken — such as ACTH and 17OHP. Instead, careful matching of the blood test to the time the hydrocortisone dose is given is required. A sample must be taken just before the tablet is given which will allow us to see how much cortisol is in the circulation and how much if any, the dose to be taken will stack on. Therefore tablets should always be taken at the set time they are usually taken, even before arriving at hospital and especially when having a profile. There is no need to fast and it is important to take any other medication which is routinely taken, also at the usual time it is taken. This allows us to detect if any of these factors influence the cortisol levels, (see Chapter 6 Figure 6.8) and if any are discovered, these can be factored into the calculations of normal daily dosing schedules. The classic example is the effect of the oral contraceptive pill which increases cortisol binding globulin and leads to an increase in total plasma cortisol that is measured (see Chapter 13, Figure 13.2).

We can follow on now with a little more detail about what is happening after the ingestion of a dose. In our original studies taken at 20 minute intervals, we gained a large amount of information regarding the appearance of cortisol in the blood following oral ingestion of hydrocortisone. Using hourly or two hourly sampling we lose some of this detail and what we have now moved towards, is to introduce 30 minute sampling for a 1 to 2 hour period after the ingestion of a dose. This has helped us better define the peak concentrations which are attained following oral dosing and has also presented us with an interesting observation about the absorption and peaks obtained during the 24 hour period. The data we have shown as examples (Figures 10.16 and 10.18), demonstrate that the true peak following the

07:00 (7 am) dose was 763 nmol/l when we sampled 30 minutes after the dose, 509 nmol/l (33% less) when we used one hourly sampling and 365 nmol/l (52% less) with 2 hourly sampling. We might conclude, depending on the value we recorded, that the dose was too high, satisfactory, or too low. When we have looked at this in more detail in our profiles, we find on average that 1 hourly sampling underestimates the cortisol peak by 15% to 25% and 2 hourly by even more (25% to 45%) (Figure 10.19).

EFFECT OF SAMPLING INTERVAL

SAMPLING INTERVAL (MINUTES)	PERCENTAGE REDUCTION IN PEAK COMPARED TO SAMPLING 30 MINUTES AFTER THE DOSE IS GIVEN
Every 60 minutes	15% – 25%
Every 120 minutes	25% – 45% ©PCHindmarsh

Figure 10.19 *Effect of sampling interval after a dose on the peak cortisol concentration detected using the 30 minute sample as the reference point for comparison.*

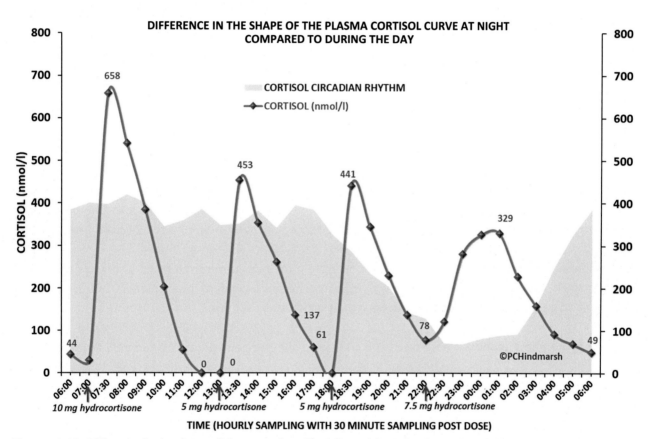

Figure 10.20 *Difference in the shape of the cortisol profile delivered from the dose taken at 22:00 (10 pm) compared to the three daytime doses. Note that the 22:00 (10 pm) dose of hydrocortisone is 7.5 mg which is midway between the 10 and 5 mg doses during the day so we might expect a peak midway between the two. The bioavailability of hydrocortisone during the day is lower at 94% compared to at night (128%).*

What this sampling approach also reveals, is the hydrocortisone dose gives very different patterns when taken late evening/midnight compared to other times of the day (Figure 10.20). This varies between individuals. The late evening/midnight dose has less of a peak with a greater spread of the dose over the ensuing hours. This leads to differences in several pharmacology parameters. Relative bioavailability (evening compared to morning hydrocortisone doses (Chapter 6)) is greater (128% versus 94%), the time to the peak is longer (100 versus 60 minutes) and the time to reach a cortisol concentration between 50 and 100 nmol/l, is longer (315 versus 220 minutes) at night compared to during the day. In Figure 10.20 it is not until 05:00 (5 am), 7 hours after the dose. Those of you who appreciate our cortisol stacking principle, will also notice that the evening dose has been stacked on a cortisol concentration of 78 nmol/l, emphasising how different the resulting cortisol levels achieved are compared to the rest of the day. It is important to say that every patient derives different amounts of cortisol from each dose, this is due to the way they metabolise hydrocortisone. So, in essence, people will achieve different peak levels/times from the same dose, which is why 24 hour profiles are the only way to fine tune doses.

The precise reason for the difference in the handling of cortisol is not clear. The rapid rise in the morning might reflect taking the hydrocortisone on an empty stomach. More likely, it is the high peak that saturates cortisol binding globulin which means that a lot of the cortisol will be in the free state and therefore cleared quickly, which will cause the high value to drop very fast.

The prolonged manner in which cortisol can be measured in the evenings may reflect different clearance and handling of free cortisol by the kidneys in the recumbent position or perhaps even circadian variation in the metabolism of cortisol in the liver and the kidneys. However, it is unclear what alters the relative bioavailability at night compared to the day. This is an area worth exploring further as there may be factors that are modifiable which will enhance this phenomenon. It is also important to understand, because of the introduction of delayed release hydrocortisone formulations which will also be subject to these overnight effects.

This again stresses the importance of understanding what we are achieving by our dosing regimen.

Finally, a pre and 2 hour post dose blood sample sounds attractive but it is better overall to extend this so that we can determine not just the peak attained from the dose, but also how long that dose actually lasts and whether there are periods of time not covered with cortisol in the blood. It is tempting to do pre and 2 hour post dose blood samples and it is certainly better than nothing, but is a poor substitute for a full 24 hour profile.

Understanding how the body handles hydrocortisone after oral administration is also important as it helps us stack doses in a helpful way. We refer to this in several of our chapters but it is worth looking at again as it is such a useful concept when it comes to working out the timing of doses.

Stacking is the phenomenon where one dose adds onto the previous dose to generate a cortisol level.

This stacking may be unhelpful either as under stacking (it does not occur because the time interval is too great between doses), or over stacking (the time interval is too short between doses and the second dose gives a much higher cortisol level than would have been otherwise expected).

Figure 10.20 illustrates helpful stacking where the 22:00 (10 pm) dose, stacks on the cortisol from the previous dose which has not fallen to zero and we get a profile close to the natural circadian rhythm with lower doses for each dose and the same daily total dose compared to previously with the three times per day regimen.

It is all about getting the dose and distribution right.

Dose Timing makes a Difference

People often ask if taking a dose earlier or later than they usually do would make a difference. In Figure 10.21 we can see what happens when dose times are altered. Although in this example the dose times have been altered to gain better cortisol coverage, there are many facets to consider.

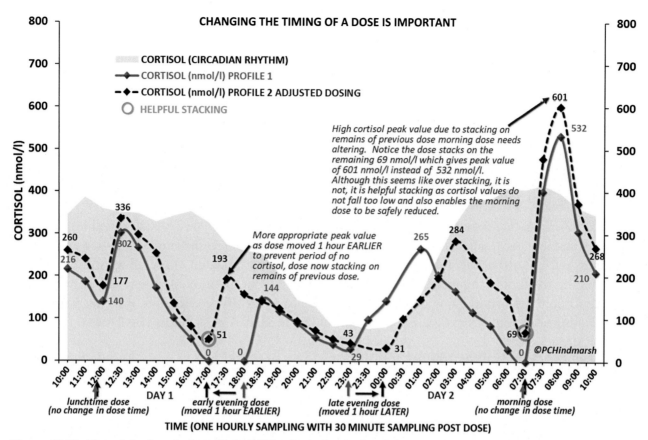

CHANGING THE TIMING OF A DOSE IS IMPORTANT

Legend:
- CORTISOL (CIRCADIAN RHYTHM)
- CORTISOL (nmol/l) PROFILE 1
- CORTISOL (nmol/l) PROFILE 2 ADJUSTED DOSING
- ○ HELPFUL STACKING

High cortisol peak value due to stacking on remains of previous dose morning dose needs altering. Notice the dose stacks on the remaining 69 nmol/l which gives peak value of 601 nmol/l instead of 532 nmol/l. Although this seems like over stacking, it is not, it is helpful stacking as cortisol values do not fall too low and also enables the morning dose to be safely reduced.

More appropriate peak value as dose moved 1 hour EARLIER to prevent period of no cortisol, dose now stacking on remains of previous dose.

©PCHindmarsh

TIME (ONE HOURLY SAMPLING WITH 30 MINUTE SAMPLING POST DOSE)

lunchtime dose (no change in dose time) — early evening dose (moved 1 hour EARLIER) — late evening dose (moved 1 hour LATER) — morning dose (no change in dose time)

Figure 10.21 *The original cortisol profile (solid blue line) obtained with four times per day dosing showing times when there is no cortisol present in the circulation and cortisol peaks following the 07:00 (7 am) and 23:00 (11 pm) doses are higher than our average reference cortisol circadian rhythm shown in light blue shading. Moving (dashed dark blue line) the 18:00 (6 pm) dose to 17:00 (5 pm) and the 23:00 (11 pm) dose to dose to 00:00 (midnight) helps by preventing periods of time with no cortisol and allows helpful stacking to take place at 17:00 (5 pm) on the cortisol value of 51 nmol/l. The midnight dose has a more appropriate distribution and allows us to stack the morning dose on the 69 nmol/l at 07:00 (7 am). The peak value is now 601 nmol/l which will allow us in turn to reduce the morning hydrocortisone dose.*

If we look firstly at both days, then we can see the benefit of taking a crossover timed sample at the start and end of a profile as:

- Profile 1 on Day 1 has a value of 216 nmol/l and a similar value on Day 2 of 210 nmol/l at 10:00 (10 am).

- Profile 2 on Day 1 has a value of 260 nmol/l and a similar value on Day 2 of 268 nmol/l at 10:00 (10 am).

The start and end cortisol values of each profile are very similar on Day 1 and Day 2 and this would be expected because we are replacing the cortisol with the same dose at the same time on consecutive days, which is why careful attention needs to be taken when sampling and of course, when the tablet is ingested. Because this is reproducible, this gives us a guide to how much cortisol this individual will have on a daily basis at this time. If we now follow the solid blue line Profile 1 of Day 1, the first dose we come across at 12:00 (noon) is stacking helpfully on the tail of the morning dose. It does, however, decline to zero by 17:00 (5 pm) and remains at zero for an hour, until the next dose at 18:00 (6 pm) is taken. The late evening dose is taken at 23:00 (11 pm) which gives a peak of 265 nmol/l at 01:00 (1 am), which is higher than we would see in the natural circadian rhythm and because we gave the dose at 23:00 (11 pm), cortisol falls below 100 nmol/l just after 05:00 (5pm) and is undetectable by 07:00 (7 am) when the morning dose is taken. Of note, this dose peaks a little high.

On Day 2 (dashed blue line Profile 2) adjustments were made to fine tune the dosing. The timing of the afternoon dose was moved to be taken an hour earlier from 18:00 (6 pm) to 17:00 (5 pm) and the late evening dose was moved to be taken an hour later, from 23:00 (11 pm) to 00:00 (midnight). This did not affect the cortisol concentrations resulting from the lunchtime dose, however we achieved the following:

- avoided both periods where cortisol values went down to zero.
- allowed helpful stacking to occur on both the 07:00 (7 am) and 17:00 (5 pm) doses.
- brought the cortisol from the late evening dose into the circadian rhythm range.
- the helpful stacking which occurred at 07:00 (7 am) will allow in turn a small reduction in the morning dose to be made.

Periods of over and under treatment which occur on a daily basis, each and every day, will lead to both short term and long term side effects. In all forms of adrenal insufficiency, the aim is to replace the missing hormones and to avoid the side effects which are well documented. Careful measuring of the replacement is paramount to prevent these known side effects which commonly occur and allow patients with adrenal insufficiency to enjoy good health and quality of life. If we wanted to dose say 5 times per day, then further adjustments to dose and timing would be needed. Again, checked by 24 hour profiling.

Additional valuable testing and monitoring

24 hour profiles give us detailed information on the distribution as well as the cortisol values attained from each dose, allowing us to fine tune the doses. We can also assess further the effect of the doses by measuring the following hormones:

- 17-hydroxyprogesterone (17OHP) for individuals with CAH. Not only does this measurement allow us to see the effect the hydrocortisone has on 17OHP production, but it also determines how active the adrenal glands are. These measurements along with measurements of androstenedione which vary throughout the 24 hour period, allow us to determine whether production of 17OHP is from the adrenal glands or from adrenal rests in the testes or ovaries. Without these serial measurements it is impossible to tell based on single 17OHP or for that matter androstenedione measurements. We are also able to establish whether raised 17OHP levels are from a painful canula insertion or blood draw.

- ACTH measurements are valuable in both CAH and Addison's disease. Samples for ACTH can be taken at strategic times where we know the body naturally produces a surge. This helps guide us particularly in Addison's disease, because it also indicates that the feedback on the pituitary is correct from our hydrocortisone dosing. Too much hydrocortisone will suppress ACTH and too little at times of the day will lead to high ACTH.

- Blood glucose measurements over the 24 hour period also indicate the effect of cortisol replacement, high levels can be investigated which may be due to diet, as well as low measurements indicating in patients, particularly those where there are no markers, such as those with hypopituitarism, that their replacement dose may need to be increased.

We can also add in other measurements, and these include:

- Fasting insulin which in conjunction with fasting glucose, allows us to compute insulin sensitivity and whether the pancreas is having to work excessively hard to maintain normal blood glucose (Beta cell function).

$$\text{Insulin sensitivity } = \text{ fasting insulin (mU/l) * fasting glucose (mmol/l) / 22.5}$$

$$\text{Beta cell function} = \text{fasting insulin (mU/l) * 20/fasting glucose (mmol/l)} - 3.5$$

- Plasma renin or renin activity measurements taken after a period of lying down (usually at 06:00 (6 am)) and then taken standing after a period of activity (1 hour). These can be combined with blood pressure measurements both lying and standing at these times and overnight. Blood pressure naturally declines by 10% during the night and loss of this dip is one of the first signs of hypertension. Taken together, these measurements inform whether alterations in the fludrocortisone dose is required.

- Urea and Electrolytes to monitor sodium and potassium in the blood.

- Pituitary hormones such as the gonadotropins (luteinising and follicle-stimulating hormones) as well as sex steroids such as testosterone, estradiol in both genders and growth hormone. Gonadotropin measurement can be helpful if puberty is in question.

- Paired plasma and urine osmolalities pre and 2 hours post doses of DDAVP in those with cranial diabetes insipidus.

- Thyroid function tests in those with hypopituitarism on thyroxine replacement.

All this gives us a broad overview of what we are achieving with our therapies, providing information which helps us decide dosing and distribution and also allows us to check the impact of other therapies on our hormone of interest, cortisol.

CONCLUSION

Monitoring of hydrocortisone replacement is extremely important in order to avoid over and under treatment in the long term. There is no easy way to obtain a measure of how well we are doing in terms of cortisol replacement, as unlike many of the hormones we measure for replacement therapy, using a single blood test is not applicable in this very dynamic situation. In order to get replacement therapy correct, we need to understand the pharmacology of hydrocortisone and we also need to understand the mathematics of defining replacement therapy in a system where concentrations vary throughout the 24 hour period. We also need to sample frequently to identify peaks and troughs and get the drug distribution through the 24 hours correct. All these observations bring an additional level of complexity to our understanding of what we are achieving with current dosing schedules, but they are essential in order that we can appreciate better what we are achieving with glucocorticoid replacement therapy and ultimately help us to avoid over and under treatment, with all the problems which arise with both.

FURTHER READING

Charmandari, E., Johnston, A., Brook, C.G.D., Hindmarsh, P.C., 2001. Bioavailability of oral hydrocortisone in patients with congenital adrenal hyperplasia due to 21-hydroxylase deficiency. J Endocrinol 169, 65—70.

Han, L., Tavakoli, N.P., Morrissey, M., Spinks, D.C., Cao, Z.T., 2019. Liquid chromatography-tandem mass spectrometry analysis of 17-hydroxyprogesterone in dried blood spots revealed matrix effect on immunoassay. Anal Bioanal Chem 411, 395—402.

Hindmarsh, P.C., Honour, J.W., 2020. Would cortisol measurements be a better gauge of hydrocortisone replacement therapy? Congenital adrenal hyperplasia as an exemplar. Int J Endocrinol. https://doi.org/10.1155/2020/2470956. Article ID 2470956.

Honour, J.W., 2023. Steroids in the Laboratory and Clinical Practice. Elsevier, Cambridge, USA.

Matthews, D.R., 1988. Time series analysis in endocrinology. Acta Paediatr Scand Suppl. 347, 55—62. PMID: 3254034.

Ross, I.L., Lacerda, M., Pillay, T.S., et al., 2016. Salivary cortisol and cortisone do not appear to be useful biomarkers for monitoring hydrocortisone replacement in Addison's disease. Horm Metab Res 48, 814—821. https://doi.org/10.1055/s-0042-118182.

Saevik, A.B., Wolff, A.B., Bjornsdottir, S., et al., 2021. Potential transcriptional biomarkers to guide glucocorticoid replacement in autoimmune Addison's disease. J Endocr Soc 5, bvaa202. https://doi.org/10.1210/jendso/bvaa202.

CHAPTER 11

Hydrocortisone Pump Therapy to Mimic the Circadian Rhythm

GLOSSARY

Basal rates The rates on a pump that deliver cortisol. These can be changed every half hour if necessary but by varying the rates a circadian pattern can be built up. Increases as low as 0.025 mg per hour can be given.

Bolus function A feature on a pump that allows a bolus of subcutaneous hydrocortisone to be delivered rather like an emergency injection of hydrocortisone.

Circadian rhythm Changes in a hormone in this case cortisol through the 24 hour period where values peak in the morning and reach low levels late evening/early hours of the morning.

Clearance The efficiency of the irreversible elimination of a drug from the body.

'Double' or 'triple' rates pattern A pump function available to deliver increased basal rates compared to the standard day to day rates in illness. Although called 'double' and 'triple' basal rates they are actually 2.5 and 3.5 times respectively the standard rate because of the effect of cortisol binding globulin on the cortisol levels achieved. A bolus should be given when switching to either the 'double' or 'triple' rate.

Professor Peter Hindmarsh formula Formula based on scientific and complex mathematical calculations incorporating the pharmacokinetics of hydrocortisone and the individual's metabolism. Using this method Professor Peter Hindmarsh was the first in the world to successfully mimic the circadian rhythm of cortisol in adrenal insufficiency and in congenital adrenal hyperplasia, successively normalising ACTH and 17OHP levels.

Solu-Cortef Recently renamed in the UK to Hydrocortisone Powder for Solution for Injection or Infusion (sodium succinate). There is no change to the excipients.

Standard basal rate These are the basal rates that over 24 hours create the cortisol circadian rhythm which is used on a day to day basis and which is used as the basis for the increased patterns during illness.

17OHP 17-hydroxyprogesterone is an intermediary steroid in the formation of cortisol from cholesterol. It is the substrate for the enzyme CYP21 which converts 17OHP to 11-deoxycortisol and also progesterone to deoxycorticosterone. Loss of enzyme function leads to a build up of 17OHP.

24 hour cortisol and 17OHP profiles Measures of cortisol and 17OHP in the blood over a 24 hour period created by blood sampling every hour to establish how basal rates are working.

GENERAL

Throughout this book we have regularly referred to the circadian rhythm of cortisol. We have looked at how this is generated in individuals who do not have adrenal insufficiency and also considered how we give hydrocortisone in tablet form to try and mimic as closely as possible, the natural circadian rhythm of cortisol. At all points we have stressed that mimicking the circadian rhythm is extremely important, as it is the one way we can ensure that we have achieved good replacement, as well as the proper distribution of cortisol throughout the 24 hour period. In addition, we know optimal cortisol replacement will help avoid over and under treatment with the associated side effects which can occur from either extreme, therefore the distribution of cortisol is important in this regard. It is as important to achieve the correct cortisol peaks during the day as it is to have correct concentrations during the period when cortisol levels are naturally low.

Replacement Therapies in Adrenal Insufficiency. https://doi.org/10.1016/B978-0-12-824548-4.00022-X

In Chapters 9 and 10 which cover hydrocortisone replacement, we have demonstrated with the data from the 24 hour profiles for oral replacement, that we do not achieve exactly the true circadian rhythm of cortisol. If the dosing and distribution of cortisol derived from the tablets is correct, we come very close to mimicking the circadian rhythm but we still run the risk of over and under treatment throughout the 24 hour period. It also means patients need to take their medication at an exact time with precise doses, 4 to 5 times a day to allow for helpful stacking. This is particularly the situation in the early hours of the morning, when no matter how hard we try with oral hydrocortisone dosing, it is very difficult to ensure good cover between 04:00 (4 am) and 06:00 (6 am). This is a critical period and one way we can be confident in achieving the correct cortisol distribution, is either to give the last dose of hydrocortisone at 01:00 (1 am) or else to have a way of administering the hydrocortisone at 04:00 (4 am). Various approaches have been considered to try to improve the situation. These range from slow as well as delayed release cortisol preparations, through to using devices to deliver cortisol so the amount delivered into the circulation accurately and precisely replicates the circadian rhythm of cortisol.

The accurate and precise replication of the cortisol circadian rhythm can be achieved using a continuous subcutaneous hydrocortisone infusion. This approach uses what is known from insulin pump therapy in diabetes, but instead of using insulin, hydrocortisone is substituted and the rate of delivery of hydrocortisone is varied to give the characteristic circadian rhythm. We have previously discussed the individual nature of the half-life of hydrocortisone and all glucocorticoids (Chapter 6, Figure 6.13) and we can use this to our advantage in tailoring hydrocortisone delivery exactly for the individual. Not only can we start to really fine tune cortisol delivery, but the hydrocortisone pump systems have taught us a lot about getting oral dosing right not just for congenital adrenal hyperplasia (CAH) which is where we started, but for anyone with adrenal insufficiency.

PRINCIPLE OF THE HYDROCORTISONE PUMP

The basic principle of pump therapy is to vary the amount of cortisol delivered during a 24 period. This needs to be carefully individualised considering many factors, such as the variation in the clearance of hydrocortisone which we have mentioned in previous chapters (Chapter 6, Figure 6.5). The absorption of hydrocortisone when using the pump is 100% as it gets straight into the subcutaneous tissues and then into the veins, so in this situation, how the individual clears cortisol becomes the most crucial factor.

There are a variety of pumps available but they all preform two functions. Firstly, they deliver a background amount of drug, in this case hydrocortisone, throughout the 24 period. This is known as the basal hydrocortisone infusion rate.

The background or basal rate which we refer to in this chapter as the standard rate can be varied at any time and it can be changed every 30 minutes if required although this is actually rarely needed, even in diabetes and even less so in cortisol replacement. The basal rates can be adjusted to deliver very small increases and decreases (0.025 mg/hr increments!!) when needed which is impossible with other therapies, not only because of the oral preparations used but also because we are delivering essentially directly into the bloodstream.

We do not need to worry about the immediate (first pass) metabolism in the liver which occurs when we use the oral route, as we bypass this giving the hydrocortisone instead into the subcutaneous tissue which takes it straight into the veins and then around the body without going through the liver initially. The pump allows for accurate dosing without having to round up or down doses as can happen with tablet therapy.

The second feature of the pump is not only can this background rate be varied, but it also can be temporarily increased which is immensely valuable in hydrocortisone replacement because it means we can more accurately tailor the dosing of hydrocortisone during episodes when people are unwell. This component of pump therapy is called the temporary background rate. In fact, there is an even more advantageous aspect of pump therapy where you are able to set different patterns to deliver different amounts of hydrocortisone. Therefore, you can have a standard pattern for day to day activities and also a double and a triple pattern which allows for increased dosing during illness. However, as we know a double dose does not achieve double the cortisol concentration, consequently we need to programme the pump to deliver two and a half times the normal daily basal amount in order to achieve a 'double' pattern for illness.

If we want to 'triple' the cortisol concentration value, then three and a half times the normal daily basal amount would be needed. This is because of the effect of cortisol binding globulin (see Chapters 6 and 12). In this chapter we refer to 'double' and 'triple' to mean these increases of either 2.5 times standard or 3.5 times standard. A lot about what we know on double and triple dosing, has come from what we have learned from profiling on the pump. Figure 11.1 shows an example of 'triple' dosing where the cortisol concentration achieved is just about doubled and this is similar to oral double dosing where you do not get double cortisol in the circulation.

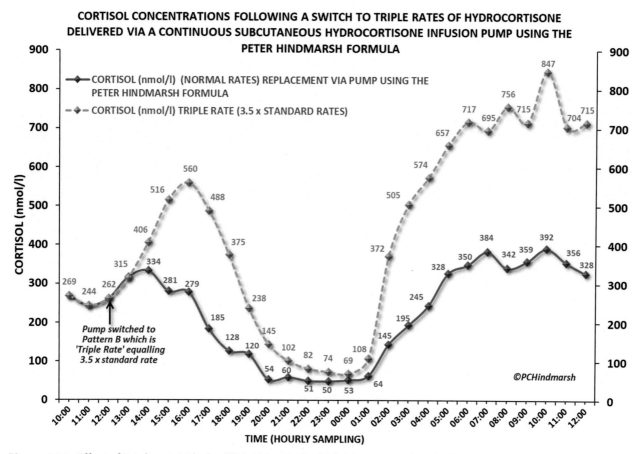

Figure 11.1 *Effect of 'triple rate' (dashed light blue line) which is 3.5 times the standard hydrocortisone infusion rates switched in at 12:00 (noon) on plasma cortisol concentrations thereafter. Note the triple rates only doubles the cortisol concentration compared to the standard day rate (blue solid line) achieved because of saturation of cortisol binding globulin once plasma cortisol concentrations start to exceed 500 nmol/l. Hydrocortisone delivered via continuous subcutaneous hydrocortisone infusion pump with the rates calculated using the Peter Hindmarsh formula.*

This figure also illustrates a further critical point about pump therapy. When we switch the infusion rate to 'triple' at 12:00 (12 noon) it takes about 2 hours for the cortisol to build up (compare the values at 12:00 (noon), 13:00 (1 pm) and 14:00 (2 pm)). This is why in illness or trauma it is important to give a bolus dose via the pump or take an oral dose when switching to 'double' or 'triple' rates. From this the levels will rise quickly and you do not get periods where the cortisol falls between doses as you do with oral dosing.

There is inevitably a lag between the change we make and what we see in the blood because we are using the subcutaneous route, which introduces a short lag because absorption has to take place from the site into the bloodstream and the extra cortisol given then has to mix in the blood volume before we can measure the change.

You may recall in Chapter 6 we introduced the idea of volume of distribution. This was a rather odd term but has a very important role to play because it tells us the amount you would have to bolus before commencing an intravenous infusion in order to fill up the 'volume' and get to a steady state more quickly. We make this point again in Chapter 12 when we talk about hydrocortisone infusions for covering types of surgery. The same is true as Figure 11.1 demonstrates when switching up to 'double' (Pattern A) or 'triple' (Pattern B) dose patterns and before each switch is made, a bolus dose is required, this generally being 10 to 15mg, which can be given via the pump bolus function or orally. Although higher bolus amounts can be given using the bolus function, we recommend giving 5 mg at a time, to prevent problems occurring with the cannula site, so it is best to give two or three 5 mg boluses prior to switching to Pattern A or Pattern B, in illness. A bolus dose can be given by using the bolus function on the pump. This priming of the system is extremely important and helps the individual get good, raised cortisol concentrations immediately during illness.

The pump delivers hydrocortisone into the subcutaneous tissue through a small cannula inserted through the skin into the layer of subcutaneous fat (Figure 11.2). This subcutaneous fat is well supplied with blood vessels which quickly absorb hydrocortisone from the infusion site. Both the subcutaneous and intramuscular sites of administration of hydrocortisone are very efficient in terms of hydrocortisone delivery into the bloodstream. It does not appear to matter what site is chosen as long as the cannula can be easily inserted into the underlying fat.

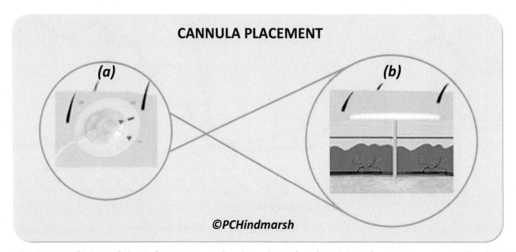

Figure 11.2 *Illustrative figure of the infusion cannula placed on the skin (a) with a cross section (b) showing the slim cannula through the layers of the skin with the tip in the subcutaneous fat layer (shown in yellow) through which the hydrocortisone is infused.*

If we look a little closer at the bolus function (Figure 11.3), using this gives a very similar profile to giving an emergency injection in the way it delivers a rapid increase in cortisol concentrations. In the illustration we used a full 25 mg hydrocortisone bolus all in one go. In practice, as such a large bolus can damage the infusion site, it is safer to give several smaller bolus doses such as 5 to 10 mg. We always advise the pump user to carry an emergency injection kit and tablets because of any potential pump failure and also there may not be adequate hydrocortisone left in the pump reservoir to cover what you would need in an emergency situation.

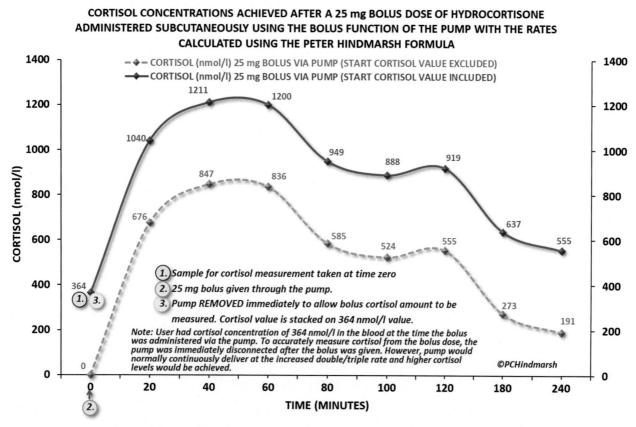

Figure 11.3 *Effect of a bolus of 25 mg of hydrocortisone delivered by the pump subcutaneously. The bolus was given and the pump switched off to show what cortisol concentrations were achieved from the bolus alone (solid blue line). Normally the pump would not be disconnected and continue to stack the bolus on top of the ongoing increased double/triple basal rate of hydrocortisone. The dashed turquoise line shows the cortisol values subtracting the start value of 364 nmol/l. Continuous hydrocortisone subcutaneous infusion pump delivery rates calculated using the Peter Hindmarsh formula.*

Figure 11.3 shows the cortisol concentrations achieved after the bolus dose of 25 mg was given via the pump. Immediately after the bolus, the pump was disconnected, to allow us to estimate the amount of cortisol which was delivered by the bolus. We started from a cortisol concentration of 364 nmol/l (already in the blood) on which the bolus stacked (blue line). If, however, had we started from a zero cortisol level, the cortisol concentration would have been much lower and of course we would not have disconnected the pump, so the pump would have continued to deliver cortisol and the cortisol concentrations achieved would have been much higher. This clearly shows the advantage of using the bolus function to rapidly get cortisol into the circulation, which in illness must be followed by a change to the 'double' or 'triple' basal pattern rate, allowing this to be superimposed (stacked) on the cortisol from the bolus which will result in an additional rise in the cortisol concentrations in the blood.

As always, it is important to appreciate that in this patient, an adult male, these cortisol values achieved by the bolus via the pump are specific to him. The exact levels achieved with any dose will vary in every patient as it will depend on the body mass index of the patient and how they metabolise cortisol. However, a bolus of this amount will keep a patient safe allowing the patient to call for help. If the patient is unable to self-administer, they should be given an emergency hydrocortisone injection.

Delivery Rates

The delivery rates are calculated by understanding the way in which the hydrocortisone is cleared in the individual. The pump delivery formula devised by Professor Peter Hindmarsh, is very different to that for oral hydrocortisone and is based on how the individual metabolises hydrocortisone. As discussed in Chapter 6 there is a vast variation in the half-life of hydrocortisone in individuals and therefore, also in the clearance of it from the circulation. This knowledge is essential because from this information, we then work backwards to determine the amount of hydrocortisone we would need to give at any point in time, to achieve a particular concentration of cortisol in the blood. We do this throughout the 24 hour period, in time blocks usually of 4 to 6 hours. In doing this, we build up varying rates throughout the 24 hour period which generate cortisol in the circulation at cortisol concentrations which we want at any particular point in time. So, for example if we want to create low cortisol concentrations at 22:00 (10 pm), there would be a rate change coming in at 21:00 (9 pm) which would probably be the lowest rate of the day to mimic the nadir at this time of the evening.

We always start the change in dose about an hour before we want it to occur because there is a slight delay in the pump delivering the change in cortisol subcutaneously and then absorption from that site into the circulation. In essence in this scenario, it will take time for the cortisol levels to decrease. Also remember, this is totally different to the delivery of cortisol from oral dosing. Oral dosing schedules cannot be used to programme rates into the pump. The successful peer reviewed formulae published by Professor Peter Hindmarsh, calculate an individual's metabolism of hydrocortisone to precisely mimic the circadian rhythm.

USE AND BENEFITS OF HYDROCORTISONE PUMP THERAPY

Currently we use hydrocortisone delivered through the pump system in two important situations. Firstly, in those individuals who have a very fast clearance of hydrocortisone from the blood, which is often present in individuals as part of their genetic makeup where hydrocortisone is metabolised much more quickly than normally. This is reflected in the wide variations of half-lives we have already alluded to in this book (Chapter 6, Figure 6.5) ranging from 40 minutes to 225 minutes.

For people with very fast half-lives, hydrocortisone is removed very quickly from the bloodstream which leaves the individual under treated for considerable periods of time. There is often the temptation to get round this by increasing the dose of hydrocortisone but no matter how high the peak reaches, it still does not prolong the duration of exposure very much as we discuss in Chapter 6. For a person with a half-life of 50 minutes, doubling the dose will only increase the duration cortisol is in the blood by 50 minutes which is not much when we want the dose to cover something like 300 minutes. Treating the situation with higher and higher doses leads to very little other than concomitant over and under treatment.

Secondly, the pump is also very useful for those individuals who have developed gastric problems following exposure to hydrocortisone, or in particular when prednisolone has been used. Individuals can have quite severe stomach problems ranging from gastritis through to relative immobility of the stomach to contract properly. The overall effect of this is to reduce how easy it is to absorb hydrocortisone when taken in tablet form. The pump, because it delivers the hydrocortisone into the subcutaneous tissues, bypasses the stomach and eliminates this particular problem.

One final use of the pump that may come to the fore in future years, is for those individuals who have been on long term glucocorticoids for non endocrine conditions where the adrenal glands have become suppressed. Weaning such people off the glucocorticoids can be slow and difficult because of the low doses that we need to achieve and the need to miss doses out the lower we go. Pump therapy could help here because we could provide lower round the clock hydrocortisone and more gradually reduce the amount allowing a safer recovery of adrenal function.

Problems of clearance and absorption can affect anyone with adrenal insufficiency, so pump usage is not just confined to patients with CAH although this was the first patient to receive such therapy. It can be used in anyone that needs it as we shall now see. Congenital adrenal hyperplasia has the advantage that we can easily measure how the hypothalamo-pituitary-adrenal axis is responding to the delivery of hydrocortisone. This is less easy to do in primary adrenal insufficiency as we cannot measure ACTH frequently enough and in secondary adrenal insufficiency there is of course no ACTH to measure. The best we can do is to apply what we have learned from the CAH model to best approximate the circadian rhythm in primary and secondary adrenal insufficiency. We do however, measure blood glucose over the 24 hours along with cortisol to ensure blood glucose levels do not fall too low or rise too high.

Pump use in congenital adrenal hyperplasia

We will use CAH as the exemplar from which we apply the knowledge gained, to patients with Addison's disease or hypopituitarism. Figure 11.4 shows a 24 hour profile from a young male with salt-wasting CAH, showing optimal cortisol replacement with excellent normal and non suppressed 17-hydroxprogesterone (17OHP) concentrations, superimposed within the cortisol profiles of two males with no adrenal problems.

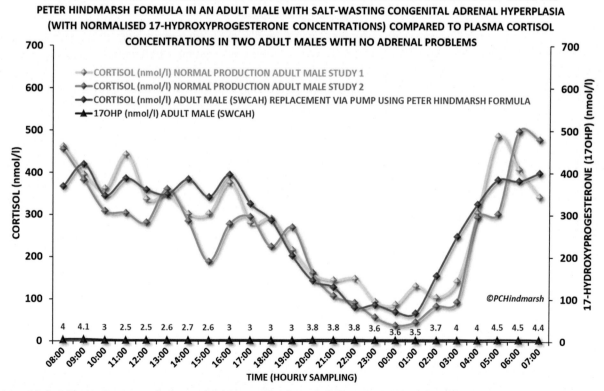

Figure 11.4 *24 hour plasma cortisol concentration profiles in two adults without adrenal problems (green and yellow lines) and in an adult male with salt-wasting congenital adrenal hyperplasia (SWCAH) (blue line) receiving hydrocortisone via a continuous subcutaneous hydrocortisone infusion pump with rates calculated using the Peter Hindmarsh formula. The profile derived from pump administration of hydrocortisone is identical to the two males without adrenal problems. The 17-hydroxyprogesterone (purple line) is normalised by this method and is not suppressed because the cortisol concentrations are normal.*

Many say the 17OHP is suppressed in this situation. It is not. It is actually within the normal range as we compare in Figure 11.5 the 17OHP from the patient on the pump and the average from people who have normal adrenal function. Normal 17OHP concentrations are low and sometimes undetectable at times, in individuals without adrenal problems. This is achieved with the normal cortisol profile seen in Figure 11.4.

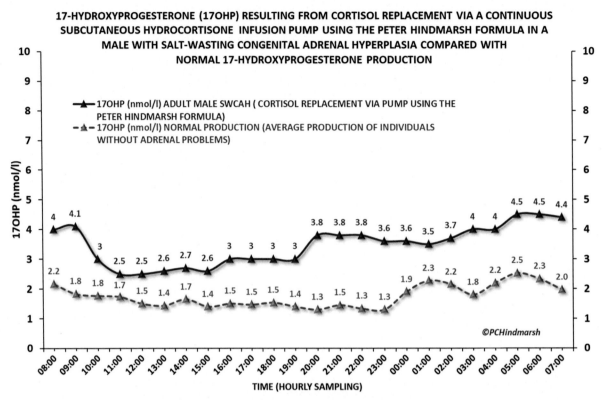

Figure 11.5 *24 hour plasma 17-hydroxyprogesterone (17OHP) profiles in an adult male with salt-wasting congenital adrenal hyperplasia (SWCAH) (purple line) receiving hydrocortisone via continuous subcutaneous hydrocortisone infusion pump with rates calculated using the Peter Hindmarsh formula compared to the average 17OHP of individuals without adrenal problems (dashed light purple line). The 17OHP is normalised and not suppressed by this method.*

In Figure 11.6 we show a similar situation in a young female with salt-wasting CAH. It is almost impossible to tell the difference between the cortisol production of the normal controls and the cortisol infused via the pump using the Professor Peter Hindmarsh method. As the increments in infusion rates are so small, we can very easily fine tune the pump rates to deliver the desired amount and we can readjust by very small amounts to get the cortisol levels absolutely correct. For example, there is a natural increase in ACTH at around 16:00 (4 pm) and even this increase can be factored into the delivery rates. Using the very small increments in basal rates we can even mimic the evening nadir plasma cortisol of 50 nmol/l. In this example we have included blood glucose measurements which are all within the normal range as these can be a helpful indication of when cortisol replacement values are too low or too high.

The pump therapy was developed some 18 years ago initially for a patient who presented with a very rapid clearance of hydrocortisone. Formal testing showed a half-life of 40 minutes for hydrocortisone and in this individual, there was a rapid large conversion of cortisol to cortisone by the shuttle. Not only were there problems in terms of the clearance of hydrocortisone but the bioavailability was also reduced to 45%, so there were two problems, firstly absorption and secondly increased clearance. To bypass these issues, hydrocortisone was then delivered using an insulin pump with infusion rates calculated to this individual's metabolism. Initially, quite high doses were used because at that stage in this individual with CAH, the adrenal glands were enlarged which needed to be decreased in size.

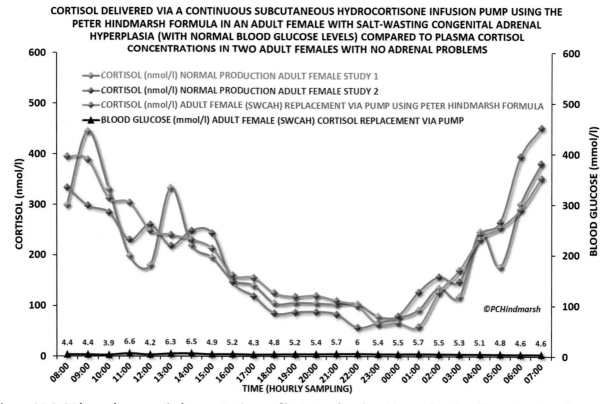

Figure 11.6 *24 hour plasma cortisol concentration profiles in two females without adrenal problems (purple and turquoise lines) and in an adult female with salt-wasting congenital adrenal hyperplasia (SWCAH) (light blue line) receiving hydrocortisone via continuous subcutaneous hydrocortisone infusion pump with the rates calculated using the Peter Hindmarsh formula. The profile derived from pump administration of hydrocortisone is identical to the two females without adrenal problems. In this instance a normal blood glucose profile from the patient on pump therapy is shown as the red line.*

Enlarged adrenal glands are a common problem when cortisol replacement has been suboptimal in individuals with CAH but is not the case in other forms of primary or secondary adrenal insufficiency because the glands are not present or not stimulated by absent ACTH respectively. However, in this individual this was an important consideration as the person had struggled for many years with replacement therapy and the increased ACTH drive led to adrenal enlargement. When this occurs, it needs to be addressed by using higher pump rates to deliver higher amounts of hydrocortisone initially, to shrink down the adrenal glands and switch off androstenedione generation. Simply starting with the calculated rates from the clearance studies will not bring about a quick return to normal size of the adrenal glands, as the ACTH drive will remain too high.

In CAH, the size of the adrenal glands influence the amount of 17OHP and androstenedione produced which is why both hormones are used as markers, although relying on these hormone values only, does not give an accurate picture of the amount of cortisol present in the blood. With under treatment, the glands enlarge and more 17OHP and androstenedione are produced, leading to high blood values. With over treatment, the adrenal glands decrease in size and the production of 17OHP and androstenedione falls so the amounts that can be measured, are low. In some cases when over replacement occurs, the adrenal glands switch off production completely, even when there is no cortisol present. This is why we stress the importance when we normalise the cortisol with pump therapy that we are not over treating, as we can continue to measure normal amounts of 17OHP and androstenedione. This is illustrated in Figure 11.7 (Chart A) where initially on the first day of introducing pump therapy, a high daily dose of infused hydrocortisone was implemented to shrink the adrenal glands which were enlarged due to CAH. After the initial post pump start a further 24 hour profile was carried out, based on these results and subsequent profiles, the rates were slowly decreased resulting in the adrenal glands returning to a normal size, normalising 17OHP, androstenedione (Figure 11.10) as well as all other hormones.

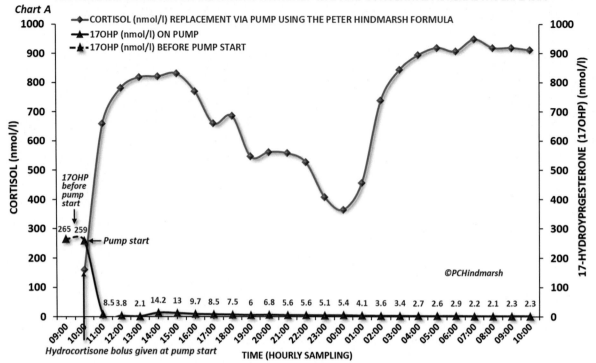

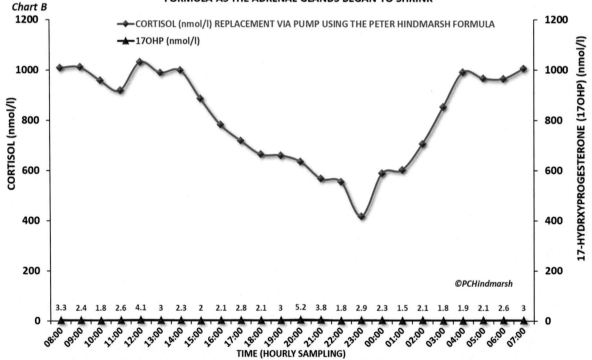

Figure 11.7 *24 hour cortisol and 17-hydroxyprogesterone profiles in a male teenager with salt-wasting congenital adrenal hyperplasia. In Chart A high infusion rates (80 mg per day) delivered via a continuous subcutaneous hydrocortisone pump infusion with rates calculated using the Peter Hindmarsh formula generated high cortisol levels (blue line) which were needed to shrink the adrenal glands. Note that even these higher values did not switch off 17-hydroxyprogesterone production. Chart B shows a profile one month after the pump start initiating a reduction in basal rates. Note despite the high cortisol concentrations (Chart B), 17-hydroxyprogesterone levels were still not over suppressed.*

Note that even when we started on high infusion rates the 17OHP was not suppressed indicating how active the system is when the adrenal glands are large.

What is of further interest is as we were able to reduce the infusion rates, the 17OHP remained unchanged indicating that normal feedback was attained at these lower total daily doses once the adrenal glands size was normalised. Understanding this principle allowed us to take a similar approach in patients receiving oral therapy and we explore this further in Chapter 15. Over the next few months, the dose was reduced further and the profile resulting is shown in Figure 11.8 which shows a normal cortisol circadian rhythm and 17OHP concentrations within the normal range.

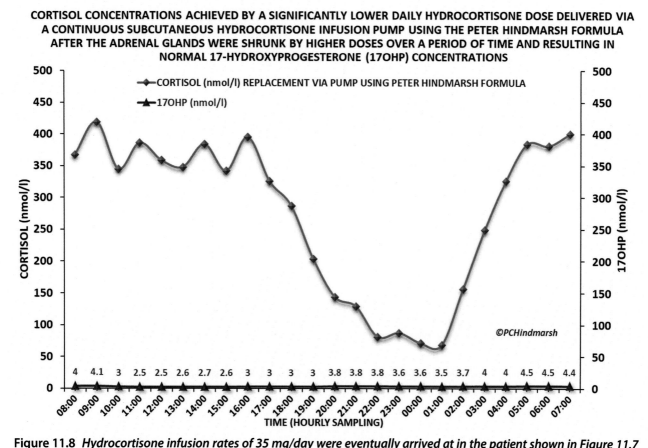

CORTISOL CONCENTRATIONS ACHIEVED BY A SIGNIFICANTLY LOWER DAILY HYDROCORTISONE DOSE DELIVERED VIA A CONTINUOUS SUBCUTANEOUS HYDROCORTISONE INFUSION PUMP USING THE PETER HINDMARSH FORMULA AFTER THE ADRENAL GLANDS WERE SHRUNK BY HIGHER DOSES OVER A PERIOD OF TIME AND RESULTING IN NORMAL 17-HYDROXYPROGESTERONE (17OHP) CONCENTRATIONS

Figure 11.8 *Hydrocortisone infusion rates of 35 mg/day were eventually arrived at in the patient shown in Figure 11.7 once the adrenal glands had been reduced in size. This patient had a very fast clearance of hydrocortisone, so the dose was individualised to overcome this. This dosing was appropriate as indicated by the normal cortisol rhythm, normal 17-hydroxyprogesterone level and the maintenance of a normal body weight. The continuous hydrocortisone pump infusion rates were calculated using the Peter Hindmarsh formula.*

What was amazing with this intervention, was the side effects of over and under treatment with cortisol disappeared as soon as the hydrocortisone infusion normalised the cortisol concentrations in the blood. These included severe headaches which this young person had suffered from for the best of 14 years, all hyperpigmentation disappeared, the gut problems caused by the high doses of dexamethasone and prednisolone which had been tried prior to starting the pump therapy settled, growth resumed as this had previously stopped and over the years bone density normalised. Prior to commencing pump therapy he was very underweight. With the introduction of the initial high doses and then dose titration based on careful profiling and testing, his weight returned to normal which has remained stable over the years with no extra weight gain. This is similar to the experience in the patient shown in Figure 11.6.

The patient was able to return to school, go on to university and holds down a very demanding and responsible managerial role. He partakes in sport, such as surfing and sea swimming, goes to the gym regularly and lives a very full active life.

The basal rate of hydrocortisone delivery via the pump is central to the creation of the plasma cortisol concentrations that constitute the circadian rhythm. Once established care must be taken if altering the rates. A small change (particularly an increase during the day when cortisol levels are higher than the evening) will lead to a cumulative effect increasing the cortisol level.

As an example, an increase in the basal rate of 0.2 mg/hour on a rate of 3.6 mg/hour does not sound very much (5.5 % increase) but if the rate is set for 4 to 5 hours, this equates to an additional 0.8 mg to 1.0 mg respectively. If the clearance is 25 l/hour and the pump is running a rate of 3.6 mg/hour, this will achieve a plasma cortisol concentration of 400 nmol/l. Therefore, if we increase the rate by 0.2 mg/hour the plasma cortisol concentration will increase to 412 nmol/l. Remember, this effect applies to each hour of the new rate. Additionally, when this rate changes to the next programmed rate, the cortisol level delivered will be stacked onto a higher plasma cortisol concentration resulting from the earlier rate increase. This amplification will then continue for the rest of the day.

The pump delivers very small doses which can be altered with very small increments and even very small incorrect adjustment to the rates can have a profound effect. Figure 11.9 shows three examples of profiles in an individual where very small adjustments have been made to the rates. Chart A shows a profile undertaken on an individual with a fast clearance using rates to deliver 32.6 mg per day. A small adjustment was made to address the slight increase in the early morning rise of 17OHP.

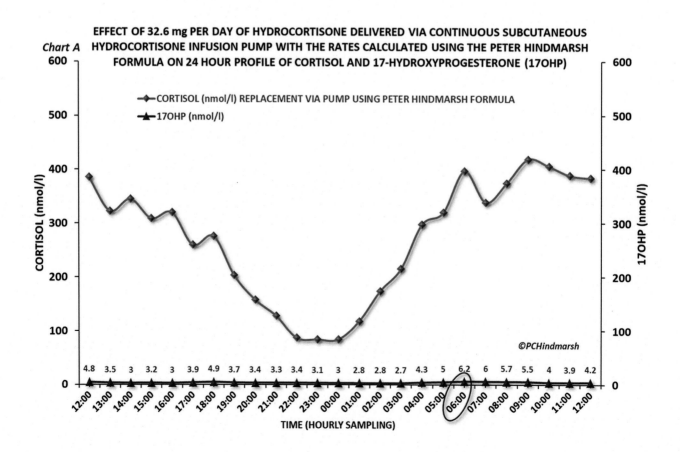

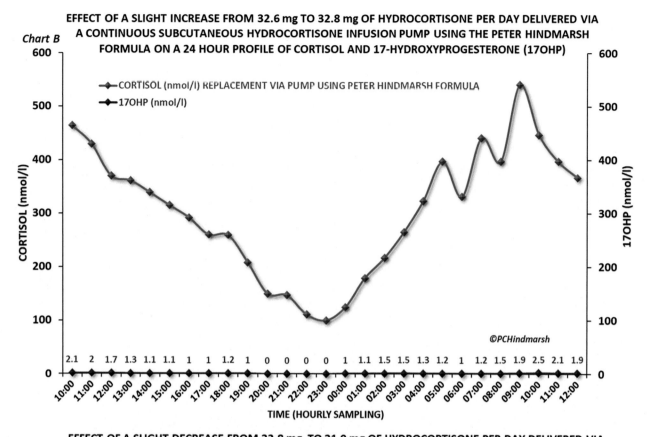

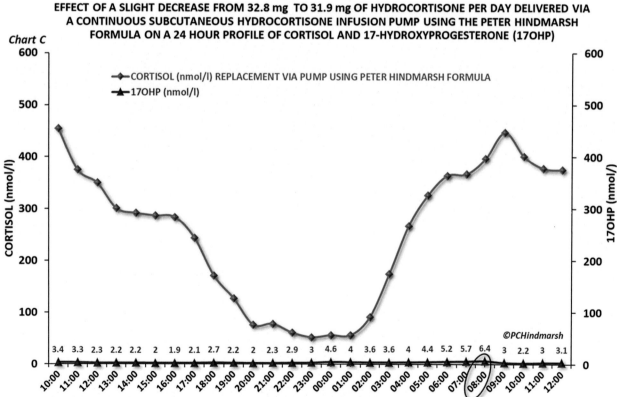

Figure 11.9 *24 hour plasma cortisol profiles on three total daily doses of hydrocortisone delivered via continuous subcutaneous hydrocortisone infusion pump with the rates calculated using the Peter Hindmarsh formula where minor adjustments have been made to the dose with the small increments implemented at different times. Profile doses per day were 32.6 mg (Chart A), 32.8 mg (Chart B) and 31.9 mg (Chart C) in a patient who has a fast clearance. See text for full discussion. Note how the changes also reflect in the timing of the peak 17-hydroxyprogesterone shown in the red circles.*

Chart B shows the result of a slight increase of 0.2 mg to the daily dose which is now 32.8 mg per day. Overall, there is an increase in the cortisol achieved, the peak attained is higher and as we can see the 17OHP is now much lower, with periods of time where there is no production.

This is due to the cumulative change over the whole 24 hours.

Chart C shows a follow up profile where the rates were reduced to deliver 31.9 mg and once again, we can see this small adjustment had an effect on the overall delivery of cortisol over the 24 hours. Note the adjustment was applied only to one rate time and not to each time change, however, as can be seen in Chart C where the increase was applied to a different time than the decrease was made, there is also a slight change in pattern which still follows the circadian rhythm. Any adjustment to a rate will have a short term effect at that point but it will take time for this to happen and this change will be carried through the 24 hour period.

It is important to appreciate the adjustment of any rate not only has a cumulative effect over the 24 hour period but the time the adjustment is made also affects the cortisol pattern. You can see this in the way that the peak 17OHP (circled in red in Charts A and C) has moved from 06:00 (6 am) initially to 08:00 (8 am). This means that the time frame the change is implemented, is effective and changes the whole day as can be seen in the change in the pattern of the 17OHP and the cortisol pattern and values. The effect is not really immediate due to the slight delay in absorption from the subcutaneous site and is illustrated by the values in the red circles of the 17OHP.

Unless the rates are calculated for the individual, cortisol concentrations will not follow the circadian rhythm.

It is important to get the rates correct and there is no substitute for checking with detailed 24 hour cortisol profiles which ensures this therapy delivers exactly the appropriate amount of hydrocortisone at the correct time for the individual.

What this approach demonstrates very clearly is as cortisol concentrations are normalised, in other words mimic the circadian rhythm, then in the case of CAH, pituitary ACTH production is regulated properly and the increased production of 17OHP (Figure 11.4) and androstenedione is normalised (Figure 11.10).

In a sense, CAH is a useful model in which to study this intervention because we are able to measure androstenedione and 17OHP at multiple time points which give us insight into how the pituitary gland is functioning and this gives added confirmation that we are not over suppressing the system.

We could not do that if we only measured ACTH because it is technically difficult to do. This is for three reasons:

- The half-life of ACTH in the circulation is very short (10 minutes) so frequent sampling would be required every 10 minutes.
- ACTH is degraded quickly so samples need to be transported on ice immediately to the laboratory and processed quickly.
- Currently the blood sample volume is still quite high compared to the low sample volumes needed on assay platforms that measure the steroid family. Even in an adult, a frequent sampling approach would need a considerable amount of blood to be drawn over the 24 hour period.

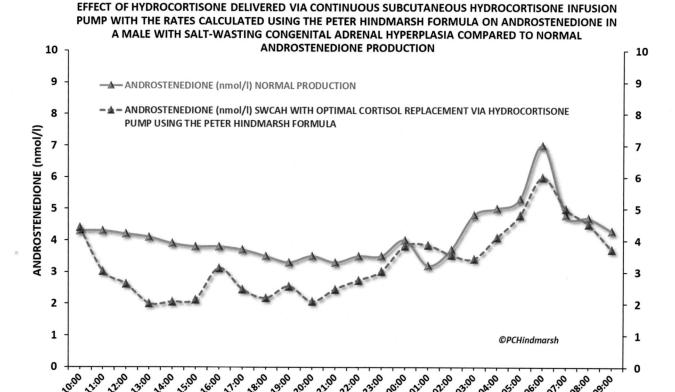

Figure 11.10 *Hydrocortisone delivered via continuous subcutaneous hydrocortisone infusion pump with the rates calculated using the Peter Hindmarsh formula in a patient with salt-wasting congenital adrenal hyperplasia (SWCAH) leads to androstenedione levels (dark green dashed line) like those observed in individuals without adrenal problems (solid green line). 17-hydroxyprogesterone levels measured at the same time were all normal between 1 and 8 nmol/l.*

As already mentioned, it is often said that CAH patients need higher doses of glucocorticoids, however when using the pump method with all levels optimised, the replacement doses are on a par with other forms of adrenal insufficiency, because the adrenal glands remain a normal size with the constant tailored dose infused mimicking normal production. The optimal dose and distribution needed is dependent on 24 hour profile testing to allow for doses and rate times to be individualised.

Addison's disease

Now that we have the model where we know that our infusion rate formula delivers cortisol to mimic the circadian rhythm and in doing so does not lead to suppression of the hypothalamo-pituitary-adrenal axis, we can use the principles in other conditions leading to primary or secondary adrenal insufficiency. In Addison's disease, we can achieve a cortisol profile that is again exactly like that seen in people without an adrenal problem as shown in Figure 11.11 and when plotted against individuals without adrenal problems (Figure 11.12). The pump rates are calculated in exactly the same way they are for CAH. An interesting parallel with CAH is that ACTH levels may be very high as well at the start of pump therapy and higher starting pump rates may be required.

Monitoring should be done with 24 hour profiles and ACTH measures at 08:00 (8 am) until the rates deliver the exact normal cortisol circadian rhythm levels. Again, all that we have done is to take what we know are optimum rates from our CAH work and transpose to this situation in a patient with Addison's disease.

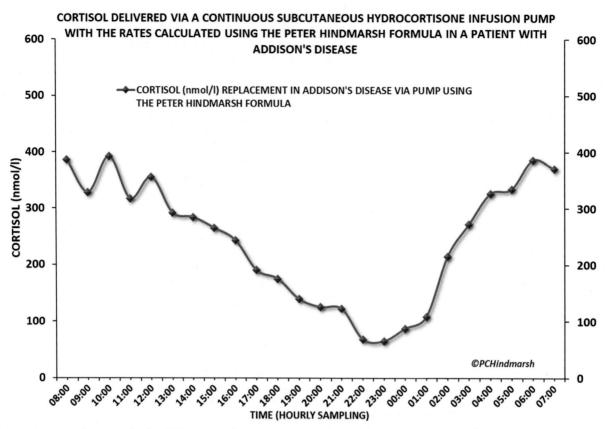

Figure 11.11 *24 hour cortisol profile in an adolescent patient with Addison's disease receiving hydrocortisone from a continuous subcutaneous hydrocortisone infusion pump with rates calculated using the Peter Hindmarsh formula.*

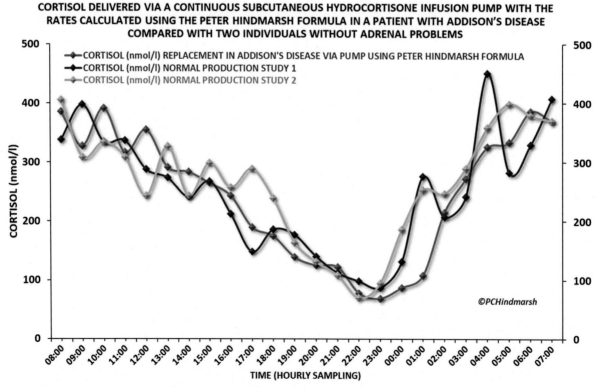

Figure 11.12 *24 hour plasma cortisol concentration profiles in 2 individuals without adrenal problems (purple and turquoise lines) superimposed on the profile of the adolescent patient (blue line) depicted in Figure 11.11 receiving hydrocortisone via a continuous subcutaneous hydrocortisone infusion pump with the rates calculated using the Peter Hindmarsh formula.*

In Figure 11.13 we have superimposed the results of an adult male who underwent a bilateral adrenalectomy resulting in adrenal insufficiency, against the profiles of the normal cortisol production of two adult males. As with the patient with SWCAH, clearance testing showed this patient had a very fast clearance of cortisol. Using the Peter Hindmarsh formula to calculate the appropriate pump rates, a normal circadian rhythm of cortisol was achieved as can be seen in Figure 11.13 dark blue line. After the adrenalectomy the patient was left with a poor quality of life, however, once on the pump he was able to return to his physically demanding work and now lives a normal and very active life.

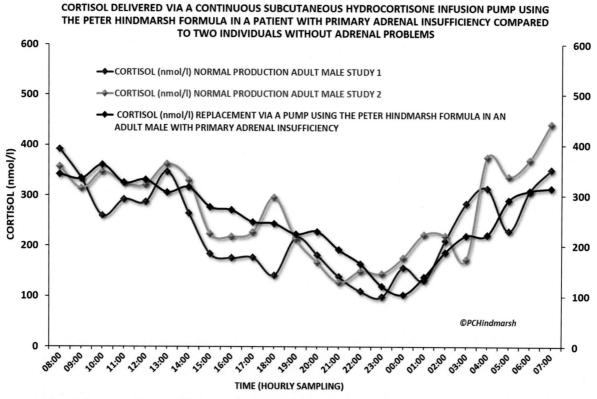

Figure 11.13 *24 hour cortisol profile in an adult male with primary adrenal insufficiency using a continuous subcutaneous hydrocortisone infusion pump with the rates calculated using the Peter Hindmarsh formula (dark blue line) compared to two subjects (green and purple lines) without adrenal problems. Clearance study showed this patient who had undergone a bilateral adrenalectomy had a fast clearance of hydrocortisone.*

Hypopituitarism

In secondary adrenal insufficiency there are fewer parameters to measure. We cannot measure ACTH as there is no production and there are no adrenal androgens. However, armed with what we have learned on pump hydrocortisone delivery from our work in CAH, we can arrive at rates that will deliver a normal cortisol circadian rhythm which we can check with 24 hour profiles. We can also add in measurements of blood glucose along with cortisol to exclude episodes of hypoglycaemia which is a potential problem because of the loss of growth hormone, cortisol and adrenaline (see Chapter 8, Part 2). This is an important measure in hypopituitarism due to the loss of these glucose counterregulatory hormones. Weight gain is also an issue in these patients so achieving a normal cortisol profile lessens the risk of weight gain due to glucocorticoid administration. In this situation with no other markers to measure against, the rates were constructed using the Peter Hindmarsh Formula to mimic the average cortisol circadian rhythm which has been achieved with the profile in Figure 11.14 Chart A, along with blood glucose measurements over the 24 hour profile. The blood glucose levels show there are no very high values which gives evidence that cortisol levels are not too high. In Figure 11.14 Chart B, the profile is nestling within two profiles from adult men without adrenal problems. We measure blood glucose levels similar to our model of CAH (Figure 11.6).

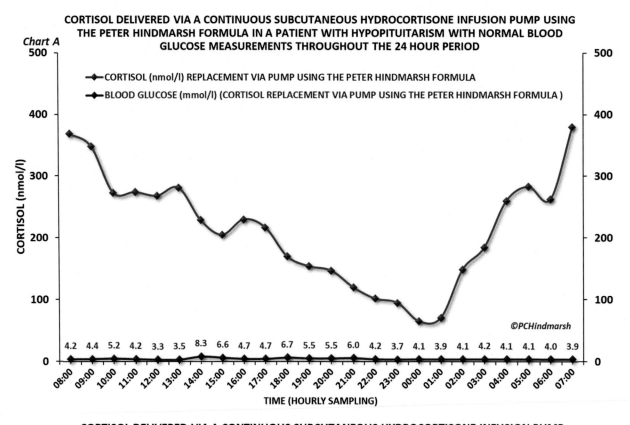

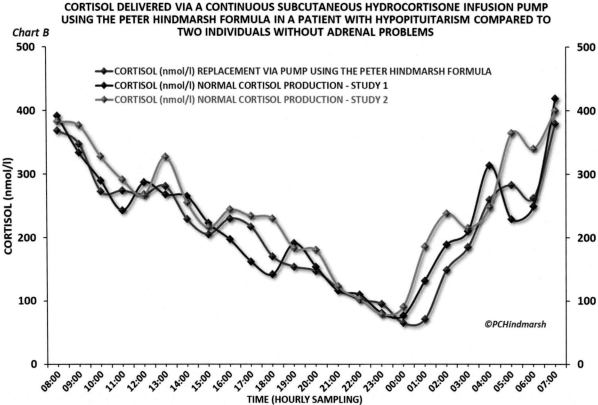

Figure 11.14 *24 hour profile of the individual with hypopituitarism (Chart A) showing optimal cortisol replacement (blue line) with blood glucose measurements (red line). Chart B shows this profile superimposed within the normal cortisol production of two males (orange and purple lines) with no adrenal problems. Continuous subcutaneous hydrocortisone infusion pump with rates calculated using the Peter Hindmarsh formula.*

Pump use in Adrenal Insufficiency

Finally, in Figure 11.15 we have put together the profiles obtained from hydrocortisone pump therapy in three patients with adrenal insufficiency. Please note:

- The patients all have different forms of adrenal insufficiency, this being either congenital adrenal hyperplasia, Addison's disease, or hypopituitarism.

- Each individual has a very different clearance of hydrocortisone, but by carefully calculating the infusion rates for each person, the daily cortisol replacement mimics the circadian rhythm and is very similar in each person.

- Each patient had clearance and half-life studies. Their rates were calculated using the Professor Peter Hindmarsh formula and full 24 hour profile were done pre pump on oral medication, as well as a profile once on the pump. This is very important as without these tests the cortisol replacement cannot be accurately assessed and over and under treatment can occur. Based on the profile results, the rates can then be adjusted if necessary.

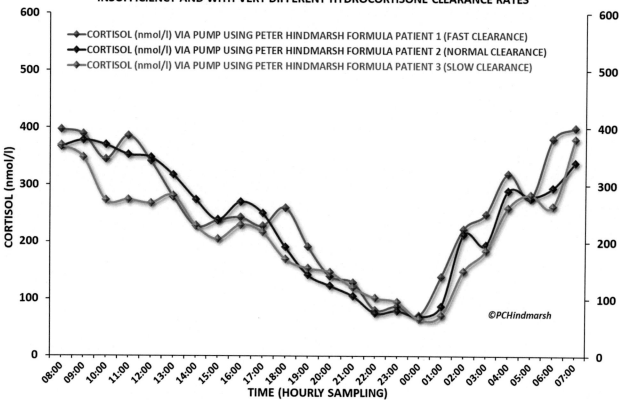

CORTISOL DELIVERED VIA A CONTINUOUS SUBCUTANEOUS HYDROCORTISONE INFUSION PUMP USING THE PETER HINDMARSH FORMULA IN PATIENTS WITH THREE DIFFERENT FORMS OF ADRENAL INSUFFICIENCY AND WITH VERY DIFFERENT HYDROCORTISONE CLEARANCE RATES

Figure 11.15 *24 hour cortisol profiles from three patients with different diagnoses and clearance rates (Patient 1 with salt-wasting congenital adrenal hyperplasia and fast clearance (blue line), Patient 2 with Addison's disease and normal clearance (purple line), Patient 3 with hypopituitarism and slow clearance (orange line)) showing how similar cortisol profiles can be generated by cortisol delivery via a continuous subcutaneous hydrocortisone infusion pump using the Peter Hindmarsh formula.*

Note, each of these patients oral dosing schedules prior to pump therapy were totally different to the calculated dosing rates on the pump. In fact oral dosing schedules would not have given the results which can be seen in Figure 11.15 or any of the examples shown in this chapter. Each person documented an improvement in their quality of life and general health.

PRACTICAL POINTS WHEN USING THE PUMP

Siting the cannula

The pump system delivers hydrocortisone into the subcutaneous tissues. The small plastic cannula through which the hydrocortisone is infused, needs to be changed every three days in order to prevent possible infection occurring at the site of entry. Inserting the cannula is relatively painless and very quick to do and there are a number of user friendly auto inserter disposable devices available which insert the fine cannula extremely quickly. The type available depends on the pump model used.

There are a number of places where the cannula can be placed (Figure 11.16). The cannula should be sited in either the bottom or stomach areas. Arms and legs are not suitable when using the pump for hydrocortisone delivery as there is simply not enough subcutaneous tissue available.

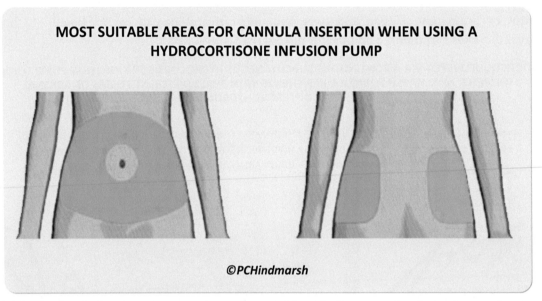

MOST SUITABLE AREAS FOR CANNULA INSERTION WHEN USING A HYDROCORTISONE INFUSION PUMP

©PCHindmarsh

Figure 11.16 *Sites for placing the pump cannula are shown in blue. The best areas for absorption are the stomach and bottom. We do not recommend using the arms or legs.*

To keep infusion sites healthy here are some useful tips:

- Rotate sites every 2 to 3 days. Previous insertion sites should be given a minimum of 1 week to heal before the area is used again.

- Clean the skin with an oil free soap and dry thoroughly. Do not use a moisturiser containing oil on the area.

- Do not insert the cannula immediately after a shower/bath or in a steamy bathroom. The adhesive is less likely to stick.

- Solid or spray antiperspirant may help with skin prone to sweating. Apply a thin layer, wait 10 to 15 min and wipe off excess.

- When the cannula is removed check the skin. If the skin is intact moisturizing lotion may be applied to sooth and protect the skin. If the skin is intact but irritated, additional anti-inflammatory or anti itch compounds may be applied to the skin. If the surface is broken then avoid the area until healed. The latter is a very rare occurrence and usually arises when the cannula has been removed too forcefully.

This is important, as similar to pump use in diabetes, very occasionally in some people an abscess can occur at the pump site. These should be treated immediately with antibiotics. To prevent these from occurring, it is important to rotate the sites, change the site regularly and ensure hands and site are clean before inserting the cannula.

Obtaining the data to set the rates

As mentioned throughout this chapter, before starting pump therapy, the really important step is to know the clearance of hydrocortisone from the blood and as we have illustrated in Chapter 6, Figure 6.5, clearance is extremely variable in each and everyone. To calculate clearance requires a specific study to be undertaken which consists of giving an intravenous bolus of hydrocortisone, followed by taking very frequent blood samples at specific intervals over a period of 2 to 3 hours, through a different cannula than the cannula used for the IV hydrocortisone administration to avoid cross contamination, although once flushed well this can be used if the second cannula becomes problematic.

From these precisely timed results, a series of calculations are used to work out the clearance of cortisol from the blood and these are detailed in Chapter 6. Once this value is determined, the clearance information is placed in a set of equations which allows us to establish the appropriate amount of hydrocortisone required, to produce a specific concentration of cortisol in the blood. Once the clearance has been established and the calculations undertaken to determine the rates needed, then it is a simple matter of programming these values into the pump in the appropriate time blocks over the 24 hour period. We use multiple rates, calculated using the individual's clearance and half-life to cover the 24 hour period with each rate designed to deliver the plasma cortisol concentration expected at that time of day.

Hydrocortisone preparation

The hydrocortisone preparation we recommend and use is Solu-Cortef which in the UK, has recently been renamed to Hydrocortisone 100 mg Powder for Solution for Injection or Infusion. It comes in powder form which is made into a liquid by adding sterile water for injection. The Solu-Cortef comes as a 100 mg vial so you simply dissolve the 100 mg in 1 ml of water which corresponds to the increments which are in the pump system. This is important, as not only does it make running the pump system easier, but there are also issues regarding the dilution of the solution as not only is there less solution to deliver when the dilution is 100 mg to 1 ml, the cortisol levels achieved are higher.

Figure 11.17 shows an example of the differences in the cortisol concentrations achieved in the circulation using the different solution strengths of the Solu-Cortef, 100 mg in 1 ml and 100 mg in 2 ml. We always use Solu-Cortef in the UK because it does not tend to cause skin reactions which is a problem we encountered when using hydrocortisone sodium phosphate, (previously known as Efcortesol). The hydrocortisone sodium phosphate seems to cause local skin reactions, small lumps develop under the surface of the skin and ultrasound studies showed these to be pooling of the hydrocortisone sodium phosphate, which is probably due to the viscosity of this ready mixed liquid preparation.

Care needs to be taken in other countries, for example some batches of the ACT-O-VIAL® product can cause skin irritation if the pH of the solution is not correct and the dilution is often not 100 mg in 1 ml. It is best to always use the 100 mg of Solu-Cortef vials, as when diluting vials containing more than this introduces errors and makes working out the rates to be programmed more difficult.

Any change in dilution or rates or both, needs to be checked with a 24 hour profile as we have already demonstrated in Figure 11.9, a small change in the rates affects the delivery of hydrocortisone i.e. the cortisol concentrations over the 24 hour period.

A number of studies have demonstrated that hydrocortisone is stable in the reservoir for at least 7 days and at temperatures up to 35° C but we recommend changing every 3 days using the 100 mg Solu-Cortef in 1 ml of water dilution.

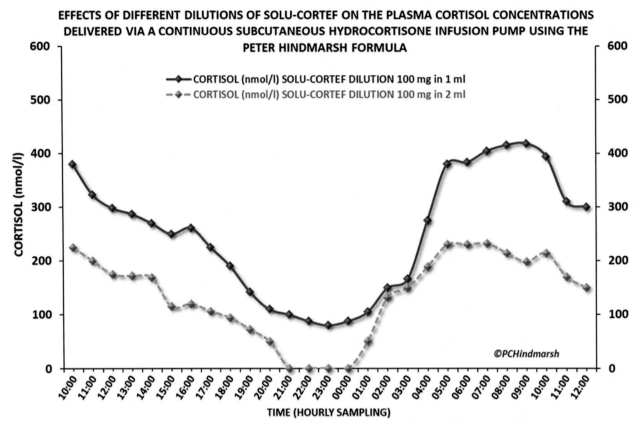

Figure 11.17 *Effects of different dilutions of Solu-Cortef 100 mg in 1 ml water for injection (dark blue line) and 100 mg in 2 ml water for injection (blue dashed line) on the cortisol levels delivered via a continuous subcutaneous hydrocortisone infusion pump using the Peter Hindmarsh formula, the same rates in the same individual were used.*

Finally, prednisolone and dexamethasone should not be used in the pump system.

The pharmacology of these drugs is completely different from hydrocortisone and their duration of action markedly different. In addition, it is not possible to measure either glucocorticoid in plasma which means that it is not possible to determine what is being delivered into the circulation so we cannot be certain whether treatment is optimal or represents over or under treatment.

Reservoirs and cannulas

The cannula and tubing need to be attached to the reservoir containing the hydrocortisone and filled with hydrocortisone. Reservoirs come in different sizes depending on which pump system is used and it is always best to fully fill the reservoir at each change. The cannula is then inserted under the skin. Once the cannula insertion needle is removed the cannula has to be primed otherwise when immediately switching on, there will be a period of time whilst the empty space created by removing the needle fills and no hydrocortisone is delivered into the individual.

This is an important step in setting up the pump. Depending on the cannula system used the 'dead-space' can be 0.6 ml which in a child or adolescent on low infusion rates can represent a considerable period of time without hydrocortisone whilst the space fills.

We recommend to always set the pump up or change the reservoir and the cannula first thing in the morning, so if there are any problems with the cortisol delivery, you can identify them and deal with them during the day.

If the pump is not delivering it should alarm, however the symptoms to watch out for if the pump is not working properly are those of adrenal insufficiency such as headache, lethargy and nausea. If in doubt, an oral dose of hydrocortisone should be taken (use the usual morning tablet dose). The oral dose may need checking and recalculating from time to time by your endocrinologist. Then check the plaster at the site to see if it is damp or wet, which may mean the cannula bent on insertion, which is less of a problem with the new quick inserters. Change the site immediately, remember to always rotate the site. Along with the fresh cannula and particularly if the removed cannula is not bent, also change the reservoir. Check the pump history which will also show how much has been delivered daily. The pump will alarm if the pump is not delivering or if the battery is low. Once the above checks have been carried out and the pump is still not delivering, contact the pump supplier for assistance. You can also check your blood glucose levels and if they are below 4 mmol/l, have a sugary drink, or a high calorie snack.

Basal Settings/Patterns

This is the main part of the pump function. In the basal settings menu, you can create three basal patterns:

1. There is standard day which runs all the time which we call standard rate in this chapter.

2. Pattern A which is 'double' dose for sick days which needs to be 2.5 times the standard rate.

3. Pattern B which is 'triple' dose for sick days when body temperature is over 39 °C, which is 3.5 times standard rate.

Note that the rates are more than double or triple because simply doubling or tripling does not achieve double or triple cortisol concentrations in the blood due to the cortisol binding globulin effect (see Chapter 3).

Note all calculations have been evaluated and based on the potency of 100:1 (100 mg Solu-Cortef diluted in 1 ml of water for injections).

In illness, a bolus should be given when changing patterns to boost levels of cortisol. This can be calculated from the volume of distribution which comes from the hydrocortisone clearance study. We discuss this in Chapter 6. Essentially, to reach a plasma cortisol of 800 nmol/l which is a reasonable value for illness, the bolus that you would give on average when switching patterns, would be 10 mg in a prepubertal child and 15 mg in an adolescent or adult. This will vary between individuals and can be worked out from the clearance study for each person. An oral dose may be taken if there is no vomiting.

It is preferable to use the Pattern A or B in illness rather than increase by a percentage, for example 200%, using the temporary basal option as the maximum time you can deliver a temporary basal rate is 24 hours and you then have to reset again. 200% will however, not give double the cortisol concentrations, you would need to use 250%. This is difficult to do however as the maximum pump setting is usually 200% therefore a new pattern would need to be created, so it is better to use Patterns A and B. Using the Pattern A or B settings is safer as you will get longer term delivery, but you do need to remember to switch back to the standard rate when appropriate. This is usually 48 hours after the temperature has settled to cope with residual inflammation.

Bolus

General points on the bolus function. It is not necessary to give a bolus dose when the pump site/pattern is changed, unless ill, or pump is disconnected for more than one hour.

Important points:

- When giving a bolus dose it is best to do this in amounts of 5 mg, so as not to damage the site.

- If an emergency bolus is ever needed, then give several 5 mg boluses and call for an ambulance, it is still safer to give an intramuscular hydrocortisone injection.

- Always carry an emergency injection in case there is not enough hydrocortisone in the reservoir to bolus. The intramuscular injection of hydrocortisone is a more direct way of getting hydrocortisone into the body quickly.

Figure 11.18 provides a useful comparison of bolus administration via different routes which we looked at in Chapter 6 (Figure 6.15). To those data we have added the cortisol concentrations resulting from a 25 mg hydrocortisone bolus given subcutaneously with the pump. Note that the time to peak differs depending on the route of administration as well as the duration in the circulation. After 100 minutes, the levels of cortisol are reasonably spread out but if we continue to 240 minutes then because of the effect of half-life (Chapter 6), the resulting concentrations are similar, particularly when comparing the intramuscular injection with the subcutaneous bolus via the pump.

The point here is that intravenous, intramuscular and the pump all get cortisol into the bloodstream and to a peak, quickly.

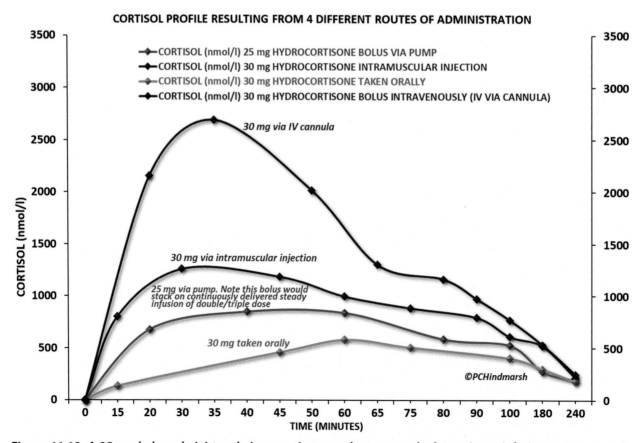

CORTISOL PROFILE RESULTING FROM 4 DIFFERENT ROUTES OF ADMINISTRATION

- CORTISOL (nmol/l) 25 mg HYDROCORTISONE BOLUS VIA PUMP
- CORTISOL (nmol/l) 30 mg HYDROCORTISONE INTRAMUSCULAR INJECTION
- CORTISOL (nmol/l) 30 mg HYDROCORTISONE TAKEN ORALLY
- CORTISOL (nmol/l) 30 mg HYDROCORTISONE BOLUS INTRAVENOUSLY (IV VIA CANNULA)

30 mg via IV cannula

30 mg via intramuscular injection

25 mg via pump. Note this bolus would stack on continuously delivered steady infusion of double/triple dose

30 mg taken orally

©PCHindmarsh

Figure 11.18 *A 25 mg bolus administered via a continuous subcutaneous hydrocortisone infusion pump using the bolus function (blue line) compared with the data shown in Figure 6.15 where 30 mg of hydrocortisone was given by an intravenous bolus (red line), 30 mg intramuscular injection (purple line), or 30 mg orally (green line).*

Surgery

A bolus via the pump can be very useful for managing the stress of surgery. If the patient is having surgery, an intravenous bolus before and after surgery should still be given.

The data in Figure 11.19 is derived from samples taken at induction of general anaesthesia and whilst the patient was undergoing major surgery, due to the complexity of the surgery, limited sampling of cortisol and 17OHP were undertaken.

This patient was known to have a very fast clearance of cortisol, due to a problem with the cortisol shuttle where there was rapid conversion of cortisol to inactive cortisone.

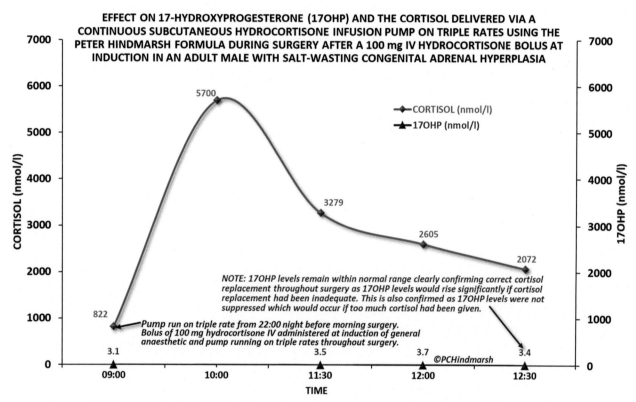

Figure 11.19 *Cortisol (blue line) and 17OHP (purple line) levels after a 100 mg bolus of IV hydrocortisone at induction of general anaesthesia prior to the start of surgery superimposed upon an already established 'triple rate' (3.5 x normal basal rate infusion) derived via a continuous subcutaneous hydrocortisone infusion pump using the Peter Hindmarsh formula. Good cortisol coverage was provided with good management of the stress response as indicated by the normal and not suppressed 17OHP levels.*

At midnight the night prior to surgery the pump was switched to deliver 'triple rate' (Pattern B), a sample before induction measured a cortisol concentration of 822 nmol/l and 17OHP of 3.1 nmol/l. The pump continued to deliver cortisol throughout the surgery on the 'triple rate.'

A cortisol measurement of 5700 nmol/l was obtained one hour into surgery (post one hour after the 100 mg bolus) and this was followed with a value of 3279 nmol/l one and half hours later. Cortisol levels remained elevated an hour later when sampling stopped.

Note the 17OHP levels remain unchanged and normal throughout despite the constantly high levels of cortisol, indicating that the stress response was well managed. If it were not, the ACTH drive from the pituitary resulting from the surgical stress would increase the 17OHP, but as 17OHP levels remained in the normal range, enough cortisol was given. Furthermore, over the three and a half hour sampling period, the l7OHP remained at a constant level with no fall in concentration values indicating there were no periods of over suppression. The cortisol replacement pattern is similar to that achieved from an intravenous hydrocortisone infusion and the cortisol values match those encountered on intensive care. The 'triple rate' continued for 24 hours after surgery and then reduced to 'double rates' for 48 hours and then back to normal standard rates thereafter. During this time the patient also received an intravenous glucose drip with sufficient sodium added to deliver 2 mmol/kg body weight/day. The latter is important as fludrocortisone was stopped until oral intake was recommenced. Plasma sodium and potassium were within the normal range before and after surgery and the patient made a good recovery. This approach kept the patient safe before, during and after surgery, due to the constant infusion keeping cortisol concentrations increased but still mimicking the circadian rhythm whereas with oral medication this is not possible due to the half-life of hydrocortisone.

Safety

On all pumps there are safety alarms. The pump alarms when it is not delivering, as well as to warn when the hydrocortisone in the reservoir is running low. It will not stop alarming until these problems are rectified. The pump also records the delivery of the hydrocortisone, so you can keep check on the daily amounts it has delivered. In addition, the pump delivery data and settings can be downloaded using special software which is useful backup information should the pump fail in any way. It also alarms when the battery is getting low. All these features are to keep the patient safe.

We view it as essential and good practice to undertake several profiles when first starting on pump therapy. Experience has shown that as the body adjusts to the pump delivery of cortisol, particularly in CAH, the adrenals reduce to a normal size, androgen levels drop to normal values and often less hydrocortisone is needed. This is probably less of an issue in other forms of primary and secondary adrenal insufficiency. Once the rates are set, the pump will require a check profile every 6 months for the first couple of years, but once stable rates are established then an annual profile is sufficient.

At the start of pump therapy, weight and height measurements are taken and these are carefully monitored along with body mass index calculated from height and weight. During the 24 hour profile, blood pressure measurements are taken both lying and then standing 4 hourly, blood glucose and other relevant hormone measurements are included in the blood sampling.

Finally, some general advice to keep the patient safe on pump therapy. The patient should always carry hydrocortisone tablets and an emergency kit. As time goes on, the consultant must remember to recalculate oral doses as they grow and/or based on any changes in pump rates in case tablets are needed. The patient should always have an oral dosing schedule in case it is needed for any reason. Patients, particularly adolescents and adults, know when they do not feel their best and recognise symptoms of low cortisol and it is important they receive good training on what to do.

We also provide a protocol outlining the steps to take in illness. The pump itself needs a label to indicate it is using 'hydrocortisone for adrenal insufficiency, not insulin. It is best to issue a dedicated emergency treatment letter Figure 11.20 along with a pump card and Standard Operating Procedures for emergency management (Figure 11.21) and for gastrointestinal problems (Figure 11.22). A key point to remember with diarrhoea is the particular problem of fluid loss and oral rehydration solutions such as Dioralyte should be used. Check urine output and colour (see colour guide Chapter 12 Figure 12.11). Always seek medical advice early especially if there are any of the following: a fever, blood in the stool, the person becomes confused, the diarrhoea does not stop after 24 hours or there is associated vomiting.

EMERGENCY CARE LETTER FOR A PERSON ON A HYDROCORTISONE PUMP

Hospital letterhead with
relevant telephone contact numbers

EMERGENCY CARE FOR PATIENTS WITH ADRENAL INSUFFICIENCY
USING THE PUMP METHOD

PATIENT NAME:

HOME ADDRESS:

POST CODE:

DATE OF BIRTH:

HOSPITAL NUMBER:

NEXT OF KIN CONTACT NUMBER:

To Whom It May Concern:

The above patient has adrenal insufficiency and wears a diabetic pump which delivers **HYDROCORTISONE.**

... must be seen by a medical physician **IMMEDIATELY**. *Time in a waiting room or triage situation is* **INAPPROPRIATE**.

... is on replacement steroids and is at risk of a life-threatening adrenal crisis if not treated quickly. A crisis will occur when there is an electrolyte imbalance with febrile illness, fluid depletion from vomiting and diarrhoea, burns, serious illness and injury. Signs of an impending crisis can include, weakness, dizziness, failure to respond, nausea and vomiting, hypotension, hypoglycaemia, pallor, and clammy sweating.

1. ***INSERT IV CANNULA***
2. ***URGENT BLOOD TESTS REQUIRED***
   - *Basic metabolic panel including: - sodium, potassium, chloride, and bicarbonate, urea, glucose, creatinine and calcium.*
   - *Cortisol to get idea of current status.*
   - *Check capillary blood glucose level and perform any other appropriate tests.*
3. ***TREATMENT***
   STAT: Hydrocortisone injection IV or IM, if NOT already administered
   Dose: *Standard emergency hydrocortisone dosing schedule should be used:*
   0 – 1 year 25 mg, 1 to 5 years 50 mg and over 5 years including adults 100 mg
   DO NOT DISCONNECT THE PUMP UNTIL ESTABLISHED ON IV HYDROCORTISONE INFUSION
4. ***IV FLUIDS***
   1. *Commence IV fluids Infusion of 0.45% sodium chloride, 5% glucose at maintenance rate (extra if patient is dehydrated). Add potassium depending on electrolyte balance.*
   2. *Commence hydrocortisone infusion (50mg in 50 ml 0.9% sodium chloride) via syringe pump.*
   3. *Monitor for at least twelve hours before discharge.*
   4. ***IMPORTANT*** *If blood glucose is <2.5 mmol/l give bolus of 2ml/kg of 10% glucose.*
   5. *If patient is drowsy, hypotensive and peripherally shut down with poor capillary return give 20ml/kg of 0.9% sodium chloride stat. Otherwise once sodium is at 120 mmol/l raise it slowly at a rate of no more than 0.3 mmol/l/hour.*
   Contact Dr .... on .... for further information.

Issued for the use of the above named patient only.

©PCHindmarsh

Figure 11.20 *Example of an emergency care letter generated by Professor Hindmarsh for use in Accident and Emergency Department. Such letters should be on hospital headed paper and signed and dated by the responsible physician.*

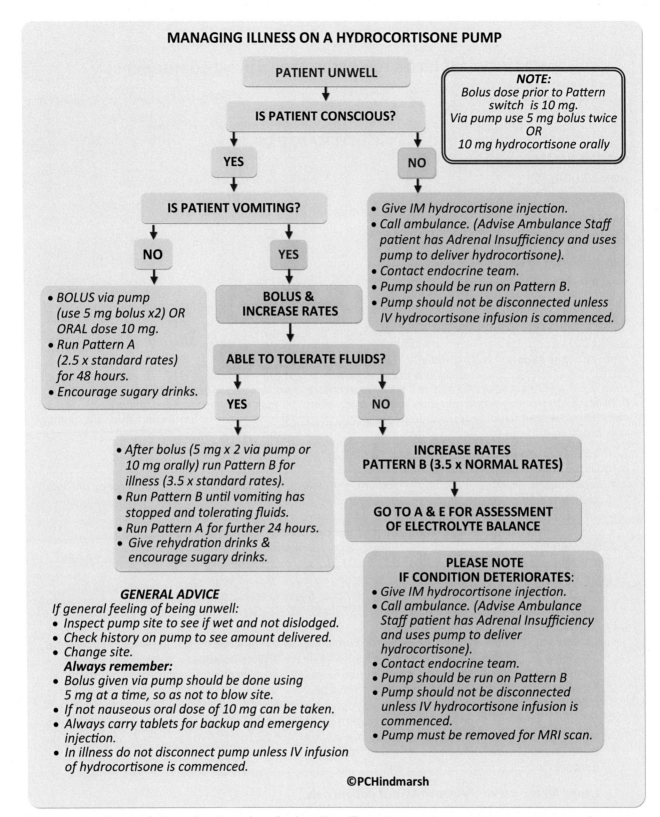

Figure 11.21 *Standard Operating Procedure for handling illness in a patient receiving continuous subcutaneous hydrocortisone infusion pump therapy.*

MANAGING DIARRHOEA AND DEHYDRATION ON A HYDROCORTISONE PUMP

CHECK: DEHYDRATION SCORE	0	1	2
GENERAL APPEARANCE	*Normal*	*Thirsty, restless, or lethargic but irritable when touched*	*Drowsy, limp, cold, sweaty*
EYES	*Normal*	*Slightly sunken*	*Very sunken*
MOIST LINING OF MOUTH & EYES	*Moist*	*Sticky*	*Dry*
TEARS	*Present*	*Decreased*	*Absent*
URINE	*Normal volume light yellow*	*Less frequent with dark yellow colour*	*Very little and dark brown*
SKIN	*Normal elastic rebound when pinched*	*Slow rebound when pinched*	*Remains standing up when pinched. If doughy feel, then go to A&E immediately*

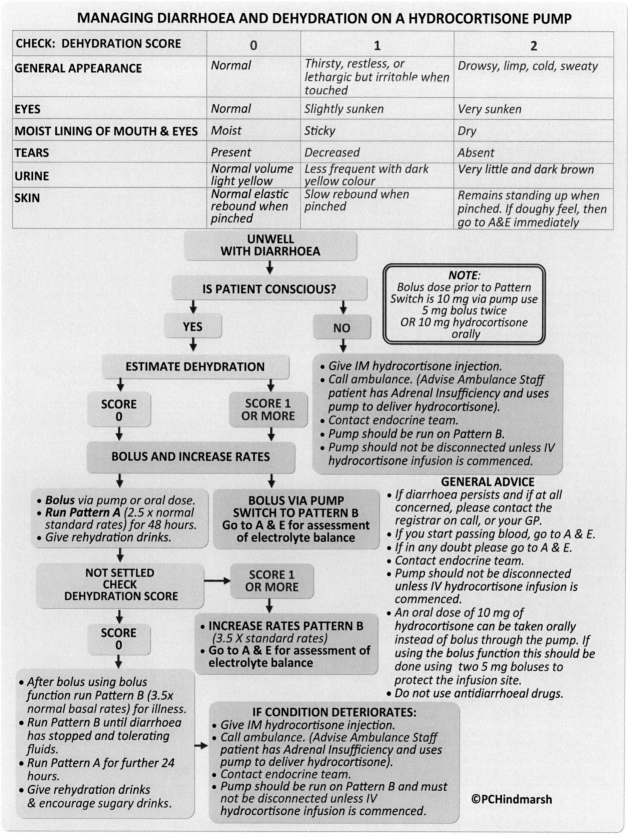

UNWELL WITH DIARRHOEA

IS PATIENT CONSCIOUS?

NOTE:
Bolus dose prior to Pattern Switch is 10 mg via pump use 5 mg bolus twice OR 10 mg hydrocortisone orally

YES → **ESTIMATE DEHYDRATION**

NO →
- *Give IM hydrocortisone injection.*
- *Call ambulance. (Advise Ambulance Staff patient has Adrenal Insufficiency and uses pump to deliver hydrocortisone).*
- *Contact endocrine team.*
- *Pump should be run on Pattern B.*
- *Pump should not be disconnected unless IV hydrocortisone infusion is commenced.*

SCORE 0 / **SCORE 1 OR MORE**

BOLUS AND INCREASE RATES

- ***Bolus** via pump or oral dose.*
- ***Run Pattern A** (2.5 x normal standard rates) for 48 hours.*
- *Give rehydration drinks.*

BOLUS VIA PUMP SWITCH TO PATTERN B Go to A & E for assessment of electrolyte balance

NOT SETTLED CHECK DEHYDRATION SCORE → **SCORE 1 OR MORE**

SCORE 0

- **INCREASE RATES PATTERN B** (3.5 X standard rates)
- **Go to A & E for assessment of electrolyte balance**

- *After bolus using bolus function run Pattern B (3.5x normal basal rates) for illness.*
- *Run Pattern B until diarrhoea has stopped and tolerating fluids.*
- *Run Pattern A for further 24 hours.*
- *Give rehydration drinks & encourage sugary drinks.*

GENERAL ADVICE
- *If diarrhoea persists and if at all concerned, please contact the registrar on call, or your GP.*
- *If you start passing blood, go to A & E.*
- *If in any doubt please go to A & E.*
- *Contact endocrine team.*
- *Pump should not be disconnected unless IV hydrocortisone infusion is commenced.*
- *An oral dose of 10 mg of hydrocortisone can be taken orally instead of bolus through the pump. If using the bolus function this should be done using two 5 mg boluses to protect the infusion site.*
- *Do not use antidiarrhoeal drugs.*

IF CONDITION DETERIORATES:
- *Give IM hydrocortisone injection.*
- *Call ambulance. (Advise Ambulance Staff patient has Adrenal Insufficiency and uses pump to deliver hydrocortisone).*
- *Contact endocrine team.*
- *Pump should be run on Pattern B and must not be disconnected unless IV hydrocortisone infusion is commenced.*

©PCHindmarsh

Figure 11.22 *Standard Operating Procedure for handling diarrhoea and dehydration in a patient receiving continuous subcutaneous hydrocortisone infusion pump therapy.*

EMERGENCY CARD FOR HYDROCORTISONE PUMP USERS

EMERGENCY MANAGEMENT PROTOCOL

Emergency management protocol for arrival at A & E

1. Insert an IV cannula. DO NOT DISCONNECT PUMP.
2. Take blood for urea and electrolytes.
3. Check capillary blood glucose level.
4. Give appropriate bolus dose of hydrocortisone intravenously:
   0-1 year:25mg, 1-5 years:50mg, over 5 years:100mg (The bolus dose is not needed if the intramuscular hydrocortisone injection has already been given).
5. Monitor blood pressure.
6. Commence IV infusion of 0.45% sodium chloride and 5% glucose at maintenance rate (extra if patient is dehydrated). Add potassium depending on electrolyte results.
7. Run pump on PATTERN A (2.5 X normal rates) or PATTERN B (3.5 X normal rates) or commence hydrocortisone infusion. Contact endocrine team to discuss rates and setting up infusion. If IV infusion is run, then disconnect pump.
8. Perform any other appropriate tests such as urine culture etc. *Monitor for at least six hours before discharge.*
9. All pump rates are calculated on 100mg hydrocortisone to 1ml.

IMPORTANT!

* If blood glucose is < 2.5 mmol, give bolus of 2 ml/kg of 10% glucose.
* If patient is drowsy, hypotensive and peripherally shut down with poor capillary return give 20ml/kg of 0.9% sodium chloride stat. Otherwise once sodium is at 120 mmol/l raise it slowly at a rate of no more than 0.3 mmol/l/hour.
* **The fludrocortisone dose should remain the same.**

PUMP MUST NOT BE DISCONNECTED UNLESS REPLACED WITH IV INFUSION PUMP USING HYDROCORTISONE

Name of Endocrine Consultant:

....

Hospital: ....

Telephone: ....

Hospital No: ....

Name of General Practitioner:

....

Telephone:

Allergies or other medical conditions Emergency Services should be aware of:

....

....

....

....

This card is suitable for adults and children using hydrocortisone subcutaneous infusion via a pump.
It is essential to carry a supply of hydrocortisone tablets for backup use. Please keep a check on the expiry date of the tablets. Label the pump with Adrenal Insufficiency Hydrocortisone not insulin.
Always carry an emergency kit.

CARD PRODUCED BY PROFESSOR PETER HINDMARSH

ADRENAL INSUFFICIENCY ON HYDROCORTISONE PUMP

The owner of this card has a medical condition which results in adrenal insufficiency & is on hydrocortisone subcutaneous infusion replacement therapy using the Peter Hindmarsh pump method

Name:...

....

Date of Birth :____/____/____

Address: ....

....   Affix photo here

....

Medical condition: ....

....

Mobile no: ....

Next of Kin: ....

Contact Tel: ....

IN AN EMERGENCY CONTACT:

Name: ....

Contact Tel: ....

EMERGENCY HYDROCORTISONE INJECTION DOSE
.... mg (IF REQUIRED)

GUIDELINES FOR ILLNESS AND INJURIES

Bolus should be given when changing patterns to boost level of cortisol. This should be 10 mg via pump.
* *Mild to moderate illness, e.g. heavy cold with temperature, chesty cough, sore throat, flu, tummy upset, switch to illness rate Pattern B (Pattern A is 2.5 X normal rates).*
* *Temperature of 38ºC give bolus and switch to Pattern A.*
* *Temperature above 39ºC give bolus and switch to illness rate Pattern B (Pattern B is 3.5 X normal rates).*

For the following, give an emergency injection of hydrocortisone and then call for an ambulance. The pump should not be disconnected.
* *If patient is unconscious, has suffered serious burns or severe scalding, broken bones or serious injury.*
For minor injuries bumps and bruises, it is not necessary to give extra hydrocortisone. For burns that blister, give double dose and see GP for assessment.
* *For vomiting illness see flowchart.*

Points to Remember

* *Always carry an emergency injection kit.*
* *Always carry hydrocortisone tablets in case of pump failure.*
* *An IV bolus dose of hydrocortisone must be given pre and post a general anaesthetic.*
* *Double/triple dose of hydrocortisone via the pump must be preceded by the 10 mg bolus as the increased pattern rates build upon the bolus.*
* *Always change reservoir, cannula and sites in the mornings so you can check delivery throughout the day.*
* *It is better to give small frequent bolus doses using the pump rather than large amount which could blow the site.*

QUICK GENERAL GUIDELINES FOR ILLNESS

If concerned always contact your endocrine team

UNWELL

CONSCIOUS?
YES — NO

YES → CHANGE SITE CHECK DELIVERY → VOMITING?

NO → *Give IM hydrocortisone. *Call ambulance. *Advise Ambulance staff patient has Adrenal Insufficiency.*

VOMITING? NO / YES

NO → *Bolus via pump 2x5 mg doses or 10mg ORALLY. *Run PATTERN A (2.5 X standard basal rates) for 48 hours. *Contact endocrine team. *Encourage sugary drinks.

YES → BOLUS and increase rates → Able to tolerate fluids → YES / NO

NO → Go to A & E for assessment of Electrolyte Balance

*After bolus using bolus function giving 2x 5mg doses. *Run PATTERN B (3.5 X normal basal rates) until vomiting has stopped and tolerating fluids. *Run PATTERN A (2.5 X standard basal rates) for FURTHER 24 hours. *Contact endocrine team. *Give rehydration drinks.

*If condition deteriorates: *Give IM hydrocortisone. *Call ambulance. *Advise Ambulance staff patient has Adrenal Insufficiency. *Contact endocrine team. *Pump should not be disconnected until IV infusion of hydrocortisone is started.

STEROID TREATMENT MUST NOT BE STOPPED

MEDICATION	OTHER PRESCRIBED MEDICATION	TIME				
		DOSE				
		NAME				
	CURRENT RATES	RATE				
		TIME				

©PCHindmarsh

Figure 11.23 *Example of emergency card for person with adrenal insufficiency receiving continuous subcutaneous hydrocortisone infusion pump therapy.*

We do not recommend taking an antidiarrhoeal medication as these will not treat the underlying cause (such as an infection or inflammation), but may help with the discomfort that comes from having repeated watery bowel movements. However, you should definitely not take antidiarrhoeal drugs when diarrhoea is accompanied by fever, severe illness, abdominal pain, or if there is blood or pus (mucus) in the stool. This can make the condition worse. These findings mean a medical opinion is needed urgently. Taking the drugs can lead to problems with the gut and the development of dilated sections of bowel which can be dangerous.

As always, the patient must wear medic alert stating, '**Adrenal Insufficiency**, hydrocortisone delivery via pump' and this information can be carried on a card (Figure 11.23).

And most importantly — the pump must be removed for any MRI scan and also not sent through the x-ray scanner at airport security. Wear it through the normal metal detection system, tell the staff what the pump does and they can do their swab testing. A letter is needed from the endocrinologist for customs and Solu-Cortef along with reservoirs, cannulas, emergency hydrocortisone injections and oral hydrocortisone medication should be carried in the hand luggage to prevent loss in luggage that might go astray.

Clock changes and travelling with the pump

The basal standard rates are dependent on clock time for different cortisol delivery rates. This means that when the clocks go forward and back during the year, the time on the pump clock needs to change so that the circadian rhythm is maintained exactly as it should be. You should do this on going to bed or midnight at the latest.

A similar situation also pertains to travel across time zones. This is quite easy on a pump. All that you do is alter the pump clock time to the clock time of the place you arrive in immediately you arrive there. That's it!!

To pulse or not to pulse hydrocortisone using a pump

There has been quite a debate in the literature as to whether the hydrocortisone should be pulsed rather than infused. Whilst many pulses of cortisol can be detected in detailed 24 hour profiles involving very frequent sampling (every 20 minutes) compared to hourly sampling (see Chapter 15, Figure 15.17) in people without adrenal insufficiency, how important it is to mimic on a pump these rises and falls in cortisol levels using the subcutaneous route is unclear, because of the delay in absorption and the variable half-life of hydrocortisone.

We also know that the natural response to pain can trigger a sharp rise in cortisol which falls within minutes, which you cannot emulate with hydrocortisone due to the half-life and clearance of the drug. What we do have evidence of from both oral and particularly pump profiles, is the cortisol derived from treatment does not dramatically fall if pain, or emotional upset occurs. This is because the cortisol binding globulin (CBG) is not affected. However, in CAH, a very painful cannulation can cause 17OHP to rise in response to an increase in ACTH. The 17OHP then returns to the normal range as the system settles down from the painful stimulus and cortisol levels are not affected as they are derived from the drug. However, in illness, the cortisol binding globulin changes shape causing cortisol to drop off which is why we double dose (see Chapter 12). These acute changes as well as these mini bursts are very difficult to mimic by the subcutaneous route. That said, all insulin pumps do actually pulse. Although it is said the pump is delivering 1 mg of hydrocortisone for example, over an hour, the design of the electronics and mechanics is often they give a series of mini bursts of 0.25 mg every 15 minutes, so although it has been thought it was sensible to source a pulsing pump, in fact in actual practice, all insulin pumps pulse anyway and the effect cannot be seen very clearly in 24 hour profiles obtained via the subcutaneous route. Presently, the most up to date insulin pumps, Medtronic 780G and the Tandem T-slim actually do mini bursts every 5 minutes or so to generate the basal pattern. Our data show a very close relationship between the pump cortisol profile data created using Professor Peter Hindmarsh's method and those obtained in individuals without adrenal problems of all ages and all genders (profiles that were sampled every 20 minutes), some examples of which can be seen earlier in this chapter.

RESULTS OF PUMP THERAPY

Pump therapy has been extremely effective in delivering a normal cortisol rhythm. In all the individuals who we have set up and are using pump therapy, the response has been extremely dramatic with a marked reduction in side effects, normalisation of body weight, increased marked unexpected growth in one individual, restoration and normalisation of energy levels, and quality of life leading to a normal life in all individuals. All patients note a marked improvement in general health and a vast increase in their overall stamina. All now partake in sports, such as attending the gym, running, swimming, long distance cycling, skiing, and surfing whereas before using pump therapy their quality of life was poor. For an individual with gastroparesis bypassing the gut using the pump has allowed the stomach and gut to heal which has enabled normal food consumption. Similar results have come from several other published studies including from the National Institutes for Health in the USA. However, patients who have a slow metabolism, do very well on oral medication and enjoy a good quality of life and those who have other underlying health problems may not feel as much benefit from pump therapy as those who have a fast clearance or suffer gut problems. With long term pump use, patients on the pump using the Peter Hindmarsh formula have shown an improvement not only in their quality of life but an improvement in bone density, energy levels, stamina and general health. A more recent study has indicated that the use of cortisol pumps was associated with a 78.5% risk reduction of adrenal crisis compared with oral glucocorticoids. All these patients had problems with absorption of conventional glucocorticoids.

Pump therapy use in CAH has allowed us to refine the basal standard rate delivery calculations by comparing cortisol delivered with feedback at the pituitary gland in terms of ACTH production using the surrogate marker 17OHP. The calculated rates along with confirmation of feedback without ACTH/17OHP suppression allowed us to use this knowledge in conditions where markers such as 17OHP were not available, Addison's disease and hypopituitarism. If we emulate the blood cortisol levels exactly like the normal circadian rhythm and without suppression of the hypothalamo–pituitary–adrenal axis, then the basal rate calculating algorithm derived from half-life and clearance must be correct. As a further step we also check blood glucose levels which drop when cortisol runs too low for periods of time and rise when too much cortisol is in the blood. This is particularly important for those with hypopituitarism where other glucose counterregulatory hormones may be deficient.

Finally, achieving normal cortisol delivery and normal pituitary adrenal axis feedback means that we also normalise the hormones in other systems. In CAH if adrenal androgens run high, then pituitary production of luteinising (LH) and follicle-stimulating (FSH) hormones will be attenuated. Testosterone will be high as it will form from adrenal androgens (i.e. adrenal testosterone). This is what is shown in Chart A of Figure 11.24. Once we get the cortisol right the hypothalamo–pituitary–adrenal axis becomes balanced. Pulsatile secretion of LH returns, FSH also rises and testosterone also rises as it is now generated as it should be from the testes by the action of pulsatile LH secretion (Figure 11.24 Chart B).

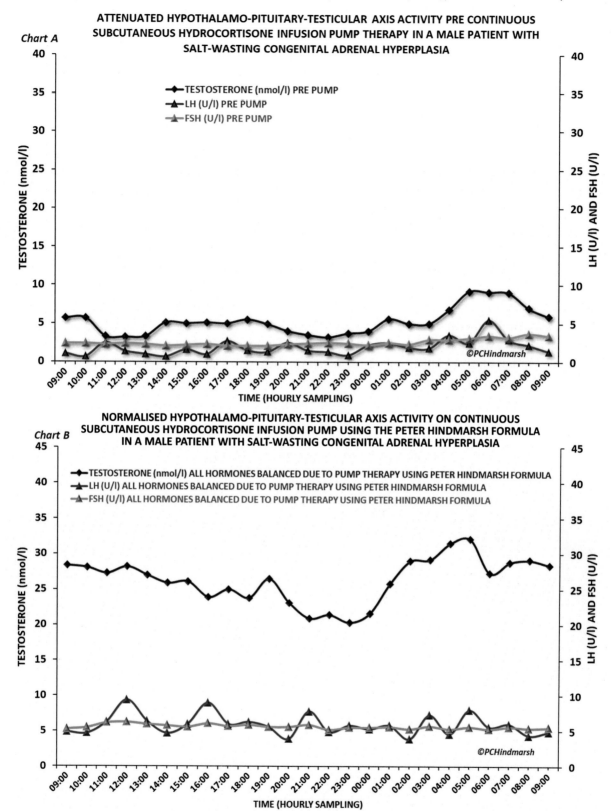

Figure 11.24 *24 hour profiles of luteinising hormone (LH) (blue line), follicle-stimulating hormone (FSH) (green line) and testosterone (red line) in a male with salt-wasting congenital adrenal hyperplasia (CAH) before (Chart A) and after (Chart B) cortisol is normalised and the hypothalamo-pituitary-adrenal axis balanced following the introduction of continuous subcutaneous hydrocortisone infusion pump therapy using the Peter Hindmarsh formula. In CAH if adrenal androgens run high then pituitary production of LH and FSH is attenuated by the testosterone formed from adrenal androgens (i.e., adrenal testosterone). Once cortisol replacement and distribution is optimal over the 24 hour period the pituitary adrenal axis becomes balanced. Pulsatile secretion of LH returns, FSH rises along with testosterone which is now generated as it should be from the testes by the action of pulsatile LH secretion.*

PUMPS AND CANNULA SETS

A number of infusion pumps are available and the most commonly used are the Medtronic 640G, Tandem T-slim and the Omnipod. All pumps display the infusion rates as U/HR (Units/hour) and when using the pump to deliver hydrocortisone, as discussed earlier in this chapter, 1 Unit is equal to 1 mg of hydrocortisone. This is one of the reasons why the dilution of the Solu-Cortef needs to be 100 mg to 1 ml of water which then runs in line as 1 Unit on the pump display equates to 1 mg of hydrocortisone.

Patients should not set themselves up on pump therapy without training on all aspects of the pump and of course without the relevant testing using blood sampling, to calculate individual rates. To reiterate, it is not simply a case of adapting oral dosing schedules, this will NOT work! It is extremely important to have a 24 hour profile when first starting on the pump, which will allow for any adjustments, if necessary. It is not a case of simply increasing a rate because symptoms may appear at a certain time, as the rate which needs adjusting may be in an earlier time frame. As we have demonstrated in Figure 11.9, a small increase or decrease affects the daily pattern. The type of pump should be discussed with the endocrinologist and during training, using the bolus function as well as understanding the alarms on the pump, is important. The pumps either have easy to follow instructions on screen, or a separate handset if the pump is tubeless. Some pumps will display how much hydrocortisone is remaining in the reservoir and all alarm when it is running low and needs changing. The battery status can be clearly seen and again the handset will alarm when the battery needs changing.

In Figure 11.25 we look at several examples of the pumps currently available.

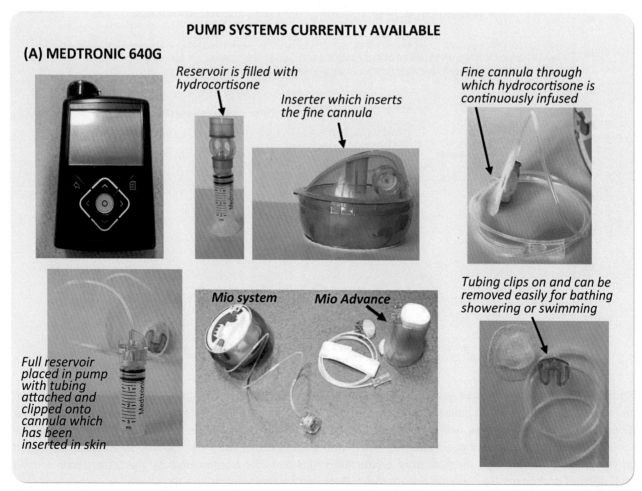

Figure 11.25 (A) *Medtronic 640G pump system showing the pump with reservoir, inserter and cannulas either the Mio or Mio Advance systems.*

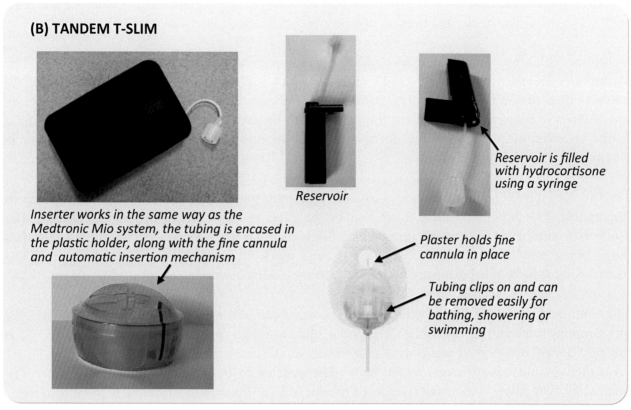

Figure 11.25 (B) *Tandem T-slim showing the pump and reservoir which is filled using a syringe. The inserter system and cannula is similar to the Medtronic Mio. The principles of application are the same but the end attached to the reservoir differs.*

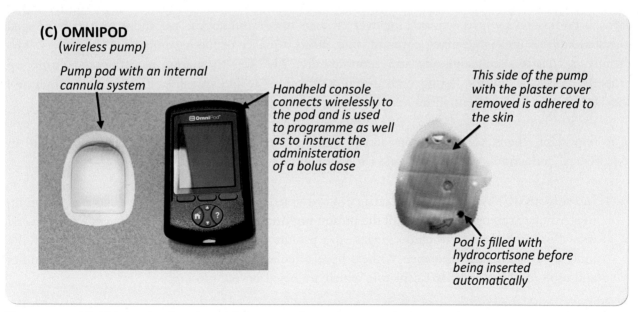

Figure 11.25 (C) *The Omnipod system with pump mechanism contained within the grey pod. There is no tubing and the cannula is inserted automatically after the pod is applied to the body. Basal rates are programmed into the handheld console which also administers any boluses if required.*

One additional factor worth considering when deciding on pump choice, is the total daily dose of hydrocortisone likely to be needed and the size of the pump reservoir. Normally this is not a problem as the reservoir capacity is usually over 1.5 ml which means that it will contain 150 mg of hydrocortisone. This should be enough to last 3 days for most people, which in any event coincides with the point at which the reservoir would need to be changed. During illness when using a 'triple' rate, reservoir changes may be needed every 2 days.

Medtronic 640G have pump menus to set basal rates and patterns as well as to administer boluses. The Medtronic 640G uses an AA battery and a reservoir which is filled manually with hydrocortisone, the reservoir then fits into the pump. The tubing is then connected to the inserted cannula. There are several types of inserters to use to insert the cannula into the areas illustrated in Figure 11.16. Training should be given on how to use the inserters. The tubing can be easily unclipped from the cannula system for bathing and swimming.

Tandem T-slim is a very slim pump and as with the Medtronic pump, the tubing connects the reservoir to the cannula. The pump has menus to set basal rates and patterns as well as to administer boluses. The Tandem T-slim has an induction battery which needs charging like a mobile phone every 2 to 3 days but is best topped up daily. Induction time is quite quick with full charge after 60 minutes. The reservoir needs to be filled manually with hydrocortisone using a syringe.

The Omnipod pump has a pod which inserts into the skin and a handheld phone-like console for programming rates and giving a bolus. The pod of the Omnipod system shown in Figure 11.25 (C) as the grey device, is the actual pump with an internal cannula system which inserts automatically. There is no tubing connecting the pod to the body. The pod has to be loaded with hydrocortisone. The pod has its own power system and is disposed of after 3 days. The handheld device requires batteries.

CONCLUSION

Hydrocortisone pump therapy mimics the normal circadian rhythm of cortisol and avoids periods of over or under treatment. It is, currently, the only method available to mimic the normal circadian rhythm of cortisol. Pump therapy has been used for over 18 years of continuous safe use and is proven to be well tolerated and has prevented many common side effects. Quality of life has improved in all users. The therapy is effective both clinically and economically. The key to success is setting the pump up properly, using the specific testing with careful calculations to individualise the dose rates/times and checking the cortisol concentrations delivered using 24 hour blood cortisol profiles.

It is important, therefore, when considering using the pump method, the expert opinion of an experienced endocrinologist is sought and the following testing must be undertaken:

1. Intravenous (IV) hydrocortisone clearance study which needs to be specifically calculated for pump use. Accurate timing of samples is of the utmost importance. We have had incidences where several individuals calculating clearance suggest the patient is a 'super fast' clearer, when in fact the individual had a slow clearance. Others have calculated rates without any IV clearance studies and using on line formulas/calculators which are based on oral dosing.

2. Two cannulas should be used for the clearance test to avoid blood sample contamination with the IV bolus of hydrocortisone:

   a) Cannula 1 to take blood samples, with the first sample taken prior to the IV administration.

   b) Cannula 2 to be used to administer the IV hydrocortisone and then flushed well to avoid any crossover. This can then also be used as a backup, after careful thorough flushing, if cannula 1 gives problems.

3. Delivery rates must be carefully calculated using an accredited formula which is different to that for oral dose calculations.

4. 24 hour cortisol profile pre pump and then 24 hours after pump start for any fine tuning of the pump rates to achieve the desired cortisol concentrations. If the adrenals are enlarged, as in CAH, then a slow reduction of cortisol basal rates is advised (by using 24 hour profiles to check these changes).

5. Social Media group treatment and advice is strongly not advised as small adjustment in pump rates produce significant changes in delivery.

6. Rates should not be altered without the input of your endocrinologist; the pump rates do not need to be altered at any time unless illness occurs.

7. Finally, it goes to say we do not condone the practice of self pump, or pump treatment by anyone who is not an endocrinologist, or without the proper testing and monitoring.

The system allows for changes to be easily made in terms of sick days and also allows for bolus doses to be delivered as efficiently as a subcutaneous injection, should they be required. In the unlikely event of pump failure which has not occurred in our experience, the individual can always revert to either an emergency injection of hydrocortisone or revert to oral medication (hydrocortisone tablets). It is important that the endocrinologist reviews the total daily dose delivered by the pump on a 6 to 12 monthly basis and readjusts the oral dose recommendation.

Pump therapy when used for individuals who have a very rapid clearance of hydrocortisone or have gastric problems is extremely effective. In the longer term, it may prove to be a valuable intervention for more individuals with adrenal insufficiency, particularly those weaning off high dose glucocorticoids as discussed in Chapter 15.

FURTHER READING

Bryan, S.M., Honour, J.W., Hindmarsh, P.C., 2009. Management of altered hydrocortisone pharmacokinetics in a boy with congenital adrenal hyperplasia using a continuous subcutaneous hydrocortisone infusion. J Clin Endocrinol Metab 94, 3477−3480.

Hindmarsh, P.C., Honour, J.W., 2018. Continuous subcutaneous hydrocortisone pump therapy informs oral hydrocortisone replacement dosing regimens. British Society for Paediatric Endocrinology and Diabetes Meeting, Birmingham.

Hindmarsh, P.C., 2019. Using Hydrocortisone Pumps to Treat Adrenal Insufficiency. Session S56 - S56. Horizon Scanning for Treatments in Adrenal Disease. Endocrine Society Meeting, New Orleans, USA.

Hindmarsh, P.C., 2014. The child with difficult to control Congenital Adrenal Hyperplasia: is there a place for continuous subcutaneous hydrocortisone therapy. Clin Endocrinol (Oxf) 81, 15−18.

Kalafatakis, K., Russell, G.M., Harmer, C.J., et al., 2018. Ultradian rhythmicity of plasma cortisol is necessary for normal emotional and cognitive responses in man. Proc Natl Acad Sci USA 115, E4091−E4100.

Khanna, A., Khurana, R., Kyriacou, A., Davies, R., Ray, D.W., 2015. Management of adrenocortical insufficiency with continuous subcutaneous hydrocortisone infusion: long-term experience in three patients. Endoc Diab Metab, 15-0005.

Khalil A, Ahmed F, Alzohaili O. Insulin pump for adrenal insufficiency, a novel approach to the use of insulin pumps to deliver corticosteroids in patients with poor cortisol absorption. Presented at: American Association of Clinical Endocrinologists 28th Annual Scientific & Clinical Congress; April 24-28, 2019; Los Angeles, CA.

Lovas, K., Husebye, E.S., 2007. Continuous subcutaneous hydrocortisone infusion in Addison's disease. Eur J Endocrinol 157, 109−112.

Mallappa, A., Nella, A.N., Sinaii, N., et al., 2018. Long term use of continuous subcutaneous hydrocortisone infusion therapy in patients with congenital adrenal hyperplasia. Clin Endocrinol (Oxf) 89 (4), 399−407.

Nlla, A.A., Mallappa, A., Perritt, A.F.,, et al., 2016. A phase 2 study of continuous subcutaneous hydrocortisone infusion in adults with congenital adrenal hyperplasia. J Clin Endocrinol Metab 10, 4690−4698.

Oksnes, M., Björnsdottir, S., Isaksson, M., et al., 2014. Continuous subcutaneous hydrocortisone infusion versus oral hydrocortisone replacement for treatment of Addison's disease: a randomized clinical trial. J Clin Endocrinol Metab 99, 1665−1674.

Patel, K., 1993. Stability of adrenocorticotropic hormone (ACTH) and pathways of deamidation of asparaginyl residue in hexapeptide segments. In: Wang, Y.J., Pearlman, R. (eds) Stability and Characterization of Protein and Peptide Drugs. Pharmaceutical Biotechnology, vol 5. Springer, Boston, MA. https://doi.org/10.1007/978-1-4899-1236-7_6.

Rigge, D.C., Jones, M.F., 2005. Shelf lives of aseptically prepared medicines — stability of hydrocortisone sodium succinate in PVC and non-PVC bags and in polypropylene syringes. J Pharm Biomed Anal 38, 332−336.

Sonnet, E., Roudaut, N., Kerlan, K., 2011. Results of the prolonged use of subcutaneous continuous infusion of hydrocortisone in a man with congenital adrenal hyperplasia. ISRN Endocrinol, 219494.

Stewart S, Narendan P, Hudson B, Hindmarsh P, Krone N, Arlt W. Steroid therapy: an unusual alternative to oral replacement via a 24 hour subcutaneous infusion device. British Endocrine Societies 2010 Meeting, Annetee Lousie Seal Memorial Award Winner.

Tuli, G., Rabbone, I., Einaudi, S., et al., 2011. Continuous subcutaneous hydrocortisone infusion (CSHI) in a young adolescent with congenital adrenal hyperplasia (CAH). J Pediatr Endocrinol Metab 24, 561−563.

CHAPTER 12

Dosing for Stress, Sick Days and Surgery

GLOSSARY

Adrenaline effects A rise in heart rate and blood pressure, increased movement of the bowels along with feeling of tension and anxiety.

Adrenal Insufficiency A general term to describe a number of conditions that lead to deficient production or action of cortisol.

Level 1 Level of action needed when there is sickness without vomiting. Double the normal daily hydrocortisone dose with an extra double morning dose given at 4 am (04:00), (More@4 AM).

Level 2 Level of action needed when there is sickness and vomiting. If vomiting occurs 60 minutes after a hydrocortisone dose the medication is likely to have been absorbed and no repeat dose is needed. If vomiting occurs within 60 minutes, then the dose should be repeated. If vomiting occurs again, then an intramuscular injection of hydrocortisone (doses are 0 - 1 year, 25 mg; 1 - 5 years, 50 mg; over 5 years 100 mg) is needed and the person should go straight to hospital.

More@4 AM During periods of illness a double dose equal to the usual morning dose, to be taken at 4 am (04:00), followed by normal double morning dose to be taken at the usual time. This additional dose is taken to prevent hypoglycaemia occurring in the early hours of the morning.

Solu-Cortef Recently renamed in the UK to Hydrocortisone Powder for Solution for Injection or Infusion (sodium succinate). There is no change to the excipients.

GENERAL

Questions about the need to alter the dose of glucocorticoids in various situations constitute most of the consultations we have in endocrine practice. The difficulty is defining what a stressful situation is. We always refer to cortisol as a stress hormone and it is true that in addition to its many roles, higher amounts of cortisol are produced during periods of stress, particularly in association with illness and trauma. We will start in this chapter by looking into the stress response in more detail.

STRESS AND THE STRESS RESPONSE

The human stress response has evolved to allow parts of the body to continue functioning in harmony under conditions of real or perceived stress. Stress is defined as a state of disharmony and is counteracted by an intricate set of physiological and behavioural responses which aim to maintain/reestablish the normal equilibrium.

The stress system receives and integrates a great diversity of sensory (visual, hearing, touch and pain) and blood-borne signals. Acute stress system activation triggers a cluster of time-limited changes, both behavioural and physical. Under normal conditions these changes are adaptive and improve the chances of survival.

Behavioural adaptation includes enhanced arousal, alertness, vigilance, cognition, focused attention, and analgesia.

Replacement Therapies in Adrenal Insufficiency. https://doi.org/10.1016/B978-0-12-824548-4.00025-5

In parallel, physical adaptation mediates an adaptive redirection of energy towards increased availability and reduced storage. Figure 12.1 shows the brain generating an emotional response through a special part of the brain called the amygdala and also how the hypothalamus responds through cortisol and the pathway that operates through adrenaline production.

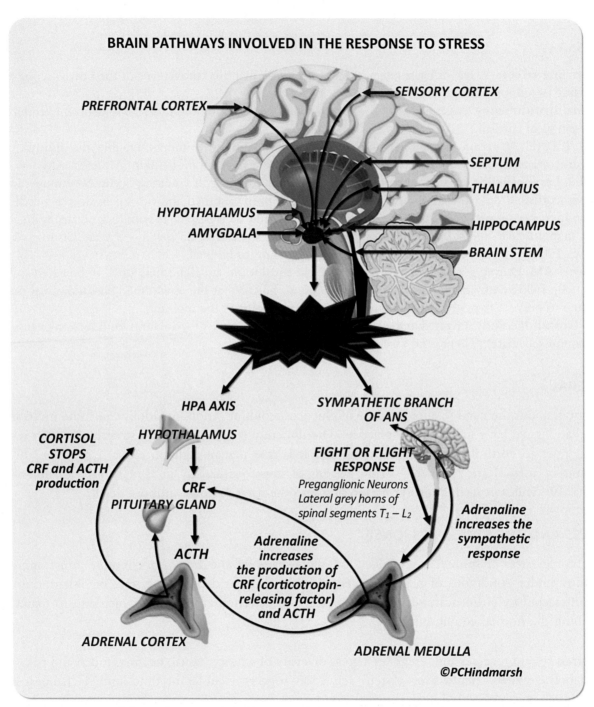

Figure 12.1 *Upper Panel shows the parts of the brain contributing to the emotional response pathway to stress and the lower panel the cortisol and adrenaline pathways for stress responses. Notice that the hypothalamus is in both pathways and is a key player in the overall response. ANS - autonomic nervous system.*

The hypothalamo–pituitary–adrenal (HPA) axis is a vital component of the stress system. The stress response is quite complex and cortisol production via Adrenocorticotropin (ACTH) release from the pituitary is but one component of how we respond to such situations.

The stress pathway also operates through the production of adrenaline, both from the adrenal gland and also within the sympathetic nervous system and we outlined this in Chapter 2, Figure 2.5B.

Adrenaline is a quick response to stress whereas cortisol is a much slower process. When it comes to whether we should be increasing cortisol in certain situations, we need to consider the implications the increase in cortisol will have in the short term and if repeatedly increased when unnecessary, the long term side effects. What we do know, is the important time to double or triple dose is when illness occurs, there is a serious injury, broken limbs, burns and circulatory shock, because these are specific events which are associated with a natural rise in cortisol and there are changes made in the way the body handles cortisol when such episodes occur. Having a fright or watching scary movies are not stresses for which extra cortisol is needed.

It is really important for people with adrenal insufficiency to understand which situation requires extra cortisol and which does not, what an adrenaline rush is, as well as recognise any situation where the body would demand more cortisol. This is because the response of the HPA to stress has different effects depending on how long the person is exposed to stress. During acute stress, cortisol levels rise due to a large surge in ACTH but then settle once the stressor has been dealt with. In chronic stress (durations of weeks, months or even years), hypothalamic activation of the pituitary changes from corticotropin-releasing hormone dominant to arginine vasopressin dominant and cortisol levels remain raised due in part to decreased cortisol metabolism. Acute elevations in cortisol levels are beneficial to promoting survival.

However, chronic exposure to stress results in reversal of the beneficial effects, with long term cortisol exposure becoming maladaptive, which can lead to a broad range of problems including the metabolic syndrome, obesity, cancer, mental health disorders, cardiovascular disease and increased susceptibility to infections. This becomes a very important factor if people with adrenal insufficiency find they constantly need to double dose over long periods of time.

It is more difficult when considering situations such as school, college or university examinations or emotional stresses. Although emotional stress in individuals without adrenal insufficiency, e.g., an interview for a new job, will cause a slight natural immediate increase in cortisol, the cortisol level also naturally comes down very quickly and this whole event, where cortisol rises and falls, occurs in less than an hour.

In adrenal insufficiency, where we are replacing cortisol artificially with hydrocortisone, we know from our discussions in Chapter 6 and other chapters in this book, the drug has to be absorbed and has its own half-life, so it cannot react in the same way as natural cortisol production which can be switched on and off quickly. Our data shows oral hydrocortisone takes on average a good 20 minutes to enter the bloodstream and will peak usually between 60 to 90 minutes later which is well after the event we wish to cover. Essentially, any extra hydrocortisone taken in this situation will not deal with the sudden stress situation. Adrenaline will be released but not as much as in someone with normal adrenal function, because cortisol is involved in adrenaline formation in the adrenal glands as we discussed in Chapter 2. This does not appear to be a problem in the stress response although it can be in the response to a low blood glucose, particularly if low blood glucose happens regularly. This is shown in Figure 12.2 where repeated hypoglycaemia leads to a reduced adrenaline response and therefore a slower recovery from hypoglycaemia. These studies were done in people with intact adrenal function so the situation is likely to be exacerbated in those with adrenal insufficiency where adrenaline production is already attenuated.

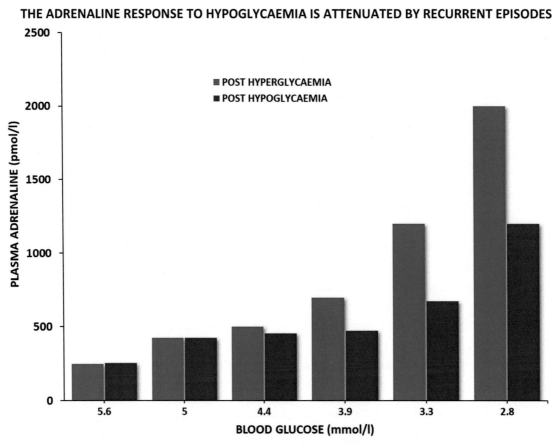

THE ADRENALINE RESPONSE TO HYPOGLYCAEMIA IS ATTENUATED BY RECURRENT EPISODES

Figure 12.2 *The adrenaline response to different blood glucose levels depending upon whether the person had been exposed recently to an episode of high blood glucose (hyperglycaemia) (blue bars) or low blood glucose (hypoglycaemia) (red bars). As blood glucose levels decline prior exposure to a low blood glucose reduces the adrenaline response to blood glucose values below 4.4 mmol/l. (Redrawn from data from Dagogo-Jack, S., Rattarasarn, C., Cryer, P.E., 1994. Reversal of hypoglycemia unawareness, but not defective glucose counterregulation, in IDDM. Diabetes 43, 1426–1434).*

In this chapter, we are going to consider a number of situations where we know cortisol has to be increased. We will separate these from other sudden events where the feelings which are produced are due to adrenaline and the nervous system such as an increase in heart rate, sweating and that uneasy feeling in the stomach. These are due to adrenaline whereas the cortisol response is much slower overall.

EXAMINATIONS

Exams are a problem because of the anxiety associated with them. Figure 12.1 shows the brain involvement and points out that this anxiety is usually adrenaline based. When we are dealing with this particular type of stressful situation in a person's life, we can overcome this by either blocking the effect of adrenaline, or through coaching methods. We would not recommend doubling the hydrocortisone dose because once you are in the examination room and calmed, the feeling of anxiety will subside. This will occur well before any cortisol could get into the circulation. There is also a downside of dosing with high amounts of glucocorticoids in this situation because they do upset short term memory recall which is exactly the situation you do not want to be in during an examination. However, it is important to ensure you consider your dosing time and the examination time, because if you are starting your examination three hours after your last dose, your cortisol levels will be on the decline. In this situation, an extra dose worked out by your endocrinologist can be taken at least an hour to 30 minutes before the start of the exam, to ensure you have good, but not too much cortisol in circulation during the exam.

CORTISOL RESPONSE TO ILLNESS, TRAUMA AND SURGERY

During illness especially where there is an associated fever, trauma and surgery, the body responds by increasing the amount of cortisol produced. Figure 12.3 illustrates the cortisol measured during major and minor surgery in 20 normal individuals. The amount generated does depend on the event, but in intensive care and during severe chest infections, cortisol concentrations can rise up to 800 – 1000 nmol/l.

Interestingly, when cortisol is increased, the body does not keep to the circadian rhythm, instead it tends to move all levels up (increased cortisol concentrations) to these values for the duration of the stress.

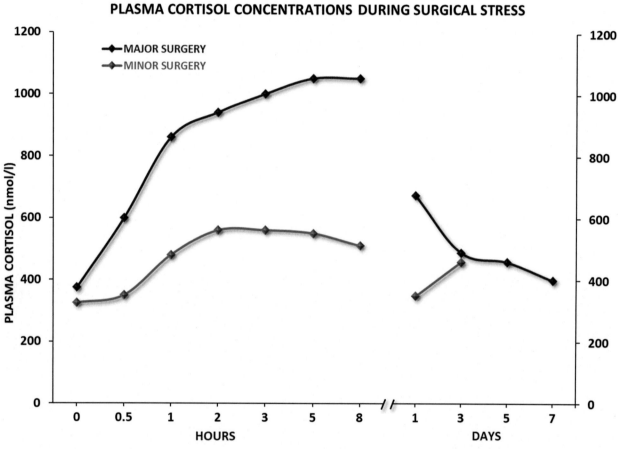

Figure 12.3 *Plasma cortisol responses to major (red line) and minor (blue line) surgery in normal subjects. (Redrawn from Plumpton, F.S., Besser, G.M., 1969. The adrenocortical response to surgery and insulin induced hypoglycaemia in corticosteroid treated and normal subjects. Br J Surg 56, 216–219).*

The situation with a rise in body temperature is quite interesting, because not only is the cortisol concentration in the blood increased naturally (this cannot happen in people with adrenal insufficiency), but the rise in temperature particularly in local tissues, such as the tonsils in the situation of a sore throat, leads to a change in the way cortisol is bound to cortisol binding globulin, so more cortisol falls off the binding globulin into the local tissue or organ where the temperature is elevated. This is quite a useful way for the body targeting certain areas of the body with additional cortisol, to improve the immune response without necessarily subjecting the whole of the body to the potential adverse effects of a rise in cortisol overall. Nonetheless, if we are losing cortisol to a greater degree from cortisol binding globulin, then the amount of cortisol which needs to be produced, or in adrenal insufficiency because we are replacing cortisol with synthetic glucocorticoids, will need to be increased, to cope with the increased tissue demand.

Surgery is slightly different, in that it is only major surgery such as stomach, or chest and heart surgery which really causes a marked increase in cortisol. More minor procedures (procedures lasting less than 90 minutes) don't tend to increase cortisol immediately (Figure 12.3). Cortisol usually tends to rise just after the operation/anaesthetic in these situations. Nonetheless, it is better to err on the side of caution and give extra hydrocortisone before the procedure, as well as immediately after the procedure.

HOW MUCH TO INCREASE THE DOSE?

The advice during illness or after surgery is to double the dose(s) of hydrocortisone taken daily. This is good sound advice, but it is important when we are considering how much cortisol we want to achieve in the blood, to realise there is a limit as to how high you can raise the cortisol concentrations in the blood by increasing the (glucocorticoid) dose.

In Chapter 3 Figure 3.10, we show the effect of increasing a dose from 10 mg to 30 mg to 50 mg. Tripling the dose to 30 mg does not lead to a tripling of the plasma cortisol concentration, in fact, it barely doubles. Going further and quintupling the dose to 50 mg, makes very little difference to the total cortisol which can be measured in the blood. The reason for this is because of the various carrier proteins in blood which the cortisol binds to. As shown in Chapter 6, the cortisol binding globulin rapidly becomes saturated and the additional cortisol is cleared through the kidneys and is lost in the urine. What we are aiming for in illness, are concentrations of approximately 700 – 800 nmol/l and even in intensive care, levels rarely go over 1000 nmol/l so doubling the dose is usually enough. In actual practice, in intensive care because of the other events happening to the individual, it is likely the cortisol would be given as an infusion and the infusion rates can be altered to deliver cortisol at the most appropriate concentration for the individual whilst in that setting.

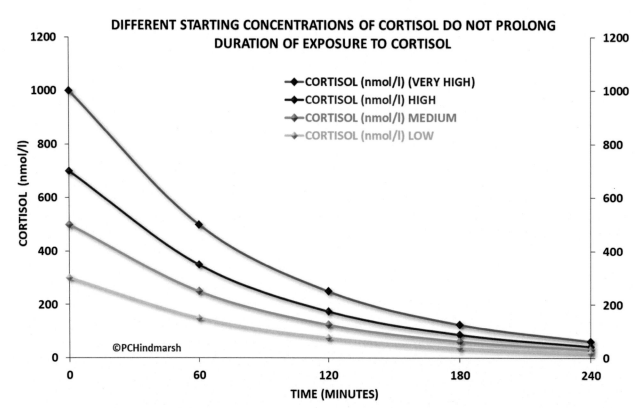

Figure 12.4 *The effect of a half-life of 60 minutes on the amount of cortisol at different time points starting from different peak values ranging from low to very high. At the end of each study despite the different starting cortisol level the cortisol levels are very similar.*

We can explore the fact a double dose of hydrocortisone does not last much longer in the bloodstream by also considering the half-life of hydrocortisone. Higher peak concentrations lead to excess cortisol being passed out in the urine, due to the saturation of cortisol binding globulin as mentioned in the preceding paragraph. Figure 12.4 shows the effect of different starting cortisol concentrations on duration of cortisol in the circulation. If we assume in this instance the half-life of cortisol is 60 minutes, then for a blood peak value of 500 nmol/l (green line) 120 minutes later there would be 125 nmol/l in the blood. If we had doubled the peak to 1000 nmol/l (blue line), then 120 minutes later there would be 250 nmol/l. However, as we can see as we move further to the right of the graph, the actual result after 240 minutes (4 hours) is that the cortisol concentrations in the circulation are all similarly of low value.

Even if the cortisol concentrations remained at the values measured at 120 minutes, these values would be lower than measured in a person without adrenal sufficiency if experiencing the same 'stress' situation where the body would naturally increase cortisol production.

The way we can deal with this is either to give the doses more frequently or ideally if we are in a surgery setting or intensive care area, this would be best achieved by a hydrocortisone intravenous infusion. Overall, a hydrocortisone intravenous infusion is associated with fewer episodes of hyperglycaemia compared to repeated intravenous bolus injections.

MANAGING SICKNESS AT HOME – SICK DAY RULES

With glucocorticoid replacement therapy in adrenal insufficiency, we are heavily dependent on the ease of absorption of hydrocortisone from the gastrointestinal system. Anything which might compromise this absorption, such as gastroenteritis or a vomiting illness, is going to alter the amount of glucocorticoid which is absorbed at a critical point when we would naturally expect an increase in cortisol production. The problem we are trying to avoid is the development of an adrenal crisis, the components of this we have discussed in Chapter 1 where we highlighted the features that you might observe in a patient with primary adrenal insufficiency.

In individuals with secondary adrenal insufficiency, it is slightly different because they retain mineralocorticoid action, so the predominant symptomatology will be those of cortisol deficiency.

ILLNESS

We can classify illness at two levels:

Level 1

There is sickness without vomiting in which case double or triple dosing is needed which mainly depends on the associated temperature. In addition, it is important to give an extra dose overnight/early morning at 4 am (04:00) during illness (More@4 AM).

Level 2

There is sickness and also vomiting.

If vomiting occurs 60 minutes or more after a dose of hydrocortisone, then the medication is likely to have been absorbed and no repeat dose is needed. However, if vomiting occurs within 60 minutes (and no more than 90 minutes ago), then the dose should be repeated. If vomiting occurs again, then an intramuscular injection of hydrocortisone is needed and the person should go straight to Accident and Emergency.

When to double or triple dose with oral hydrocortisone is based mainly on body temperature. A high temperature, a value of 38°C or higher, is usually associated with an infection. The temperature rise results from the immune system attacking the infection and the by-products of these reactions are a series of chemicals known as cytokines (cytokines are a group of small proteins produced by immune cells and aid coordination of the immune cell and antibody response to infection) which are released into the blood and raise the body temperature.

Body temperature does naturally rise and fall throughout the 24 hour period and can rise to 37.5°C at certain times of the day. Normal body temperature varies by person, age, activity and time of day.

What we can be sure of is a temperature of 38°C and above, usually means you have a fever caused by an infection or illness. Between 38°C and 39°C the advice is to double the hydrocortisone doses. If the temperature is 39°C and above, the usual recommendation is to triple the doses. As Chapter 3 Figure 3.10 shows there is little point to increase the dose further than triple.

If on prednisolone then you can double the doses but it is probably better to switch to hydrocortisone when unwell, double or triple dose with the hydrocortisone and add in More@4 AM.

The reason for this is the peak concentration occurs later with prednisolone, particularly if the enteric coated preparation is used. For people using dexamethasone, the situation is more difficult because the profile of dexamethasone is flatter and the attainment of an increased circulating level is slow. So, for both these glucocorticoids it is better to switch to four times per day hydrocortisone with an additional dose at 4 am (More@4 AM see below). The exact dosing schedule should be discussed with your endocrinologist.

Finally, in hypopituitarism there is an additional issue which needs to be considered. Sick days are approached in exactly the same way as any other form of adrenal insufficiency. The difference is:

- If the person is also on DDAVP for diabetes insipidus, because increasing the hydrocortisone can alter water balance and plasma sodium levels.

- Extra hydrocortisone can lead to increased water loss in the urine and this might mean the dose of DDAVP needs to be increased whilst the extra hydrocortisone is taken.

- This can be quite difficult to balance, so if you have hypopituitarism and are on DDAVP as well, it is best to contact your endocrine team to discuss how to manage this situation.

In this discussion and in Figure 12.5 you will notice an extra dose of hydrocortisone is given at 4 am (04:00) (More@4 AM). Figure 12.5 illustrates the steps of how illness can be managed as well as general advice for Accident and Emergency staff.

The advice is during illness an extra double/triple dose of hydrocortisone should be given around 4 am (04:00) (More@4 AM).

- The dose should be the same dose as the usual double/triple morning dose.

- The double/triple morning dose should be given as usual, as the 4 am (04:00) dose is an additional dose.

- The additional 4 am (04:00) dose should be given even if there has been a double dose at 1 am (01:00) or 2 am (02:00).

ADRENAL INSUFFICIENCY - STEPS AND GENERAL ADVICE IN DEALING WITH ILLNESS

PATIENT UNWELL

IS PATIENT CONSCIOUS?

YES → **IS PATIENT VOMITING?**

NO →
- GIVE INTRAMUSCULAR HYDROCORTISONE INJECTION
- CALL AMBULANCE
- ADVISE AMBULANCE STAFF PATIENT HAS ADRENAL INSUFFICIENCY

IS PATIENT VOMITING?

NO:
- Double/triple hydrocortisone dose for the next 48 hours.
- Give an **extra** dose at 4 am (04:00) (MORE@4 AM) equal to double/triple the usual morning dose (this is an **additional** dose so morning double/triple dose must be given as well).
- Encourage sugary drinks.

YES → **WHEN WAS LAST DOSE TAKEN?**

2 – 4 HOURS AGO TOLERATE FLUIDS?

LESS THAN 60 MINUTES AND NO MORE THAN 90 MINUTES AGO

KEEPS DOSE DOWN

REPEAT DOUBLE HYDROCORTISONE DOSE

DOES NOT KEEP DOSE DOWN

- GIVE INTRAMUSCULAR HYDROCORTISONE INJECTION
- CALL AMBULANCE
- ADVISE AMBULANCE STAFF PATIENT HAS ADRENAL INSUFFICIENCY

RECOMMENDED INTRAMUSCULAR HYDROCORTISONE EMERGENCY DOSES

Age range (years)	Dose (mg)
0 – 1	25
1 – 5	50
over 5	100

*If taking **DDVAP** ask your endocrinologist for written advice on what to do when an emergency injection is given.*

GENERAL ADVICE

Advice for going to A & E
- *Tell A & E staff that emergency hydrocortisone has already been administered.*
- *Explain individual has adrenal insufficiency*
- *Get the following measured:*
  1) *Urea and electrolytes*
  2) *Blood glucose concentration*
  3) *Blood pressure*
- *Should any of these levels be abnormal admit for glucose, electrolyte and blood pressure monitoring.*
- *Close monitoring for 6 hours.*
- *Give double dose 4 hours after injection.*
- *Recommend an extra dose at 4 am (04:00) (MORE@4 AM) which is double/triple the morning dose. This dose must be given even if hydrocortisone is being given IV.*
- *Advise that double/triple dose of hydrocortisone does not last longer in the system as cortisol whether given oral or IV, therefore use regular dosing times including the extra dose at 4 am (04:00) (MORE@4 AM).*

*If taking **PREDNISOLONE**, it is better to use hydrocortisone when ill. However, if not prescribed any, then double each dose and add double the morning dose at 4 am (04:00) (MORE@4 AM). This is in addition to the doubled morning dose.*

DIARRHOEA – *double oral doses and give MORE@4 AM. The most important aspect of care is to give fluids using solutions such as dioralyte. Most episodes settle within 24 hours. Make sure there is good urine output. Seek medical advice early especially if there is blood in the diarrhoea, the person becomes confused, the diarrhoea does not stop after 24 hours or there is associated vomiting. Do not use anti-diarrhoeal drugs.*
*IF SUFFERING **BOTH VOMITING AND DIARRHOEA** - get medical help quickly as you cannot be sure that any of the medication has either stayed down or been absorbed. Give IM hydrocortisone injection and go to Accident and Emergency to get checked.*

©PCHindmarsh

Figure 12.5 *Flow chart describing what to do with person with adrenal insufficiency who is unwell and the points at which an emergency injection should be given, guidance on doses to be administered and when to go to the Accident and Emergency Department. Guidance for Accident and Emergency are shown in the bottom left corner in the General Advice section based on British Society for Paediatric Endocrinology and Diabetes 2023 Guidelines.*

The reason why we have introduced this extra dose to be given at 4 am (04:00) (More@4 AM) is because at this time in someone who does not have adrenal insufficiency, the circadian rhythm shows us there is a good amount of cortisol in the system (Figure 12.6).

This cortisol helps keep the blood glucose levels up whilst we are asleep. This is particularly important in young children who are more susceptible to hypoglycaemia as they have reduced stores of glycogen in the liver.

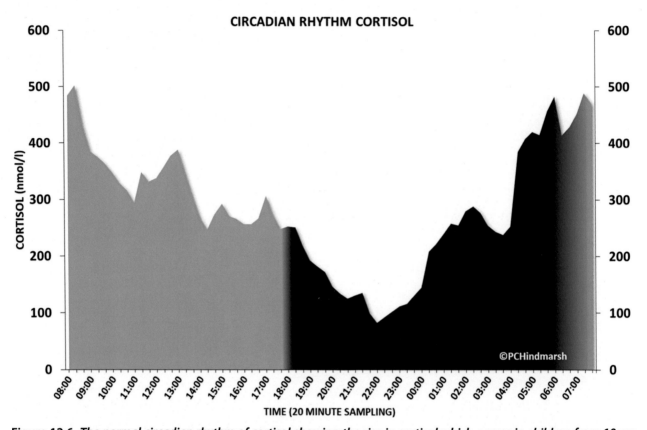

Figure 12.6 *The normal circadian rhythm of cortisol showing the rise in cortisol which occurs in children from 10 pm (22:00) and in adults from midnight (00:00) resulting in a good amount of cortisol in the circulation at 4 am (04:00). The amount of cortisol produced per day per metre squared body surface area is similar between adults and children and between the sexes. Note that the body is never without some cortisol present even at the late evening nadir.*

When using hydrocortisone to replace cortisol, the evening dose or the last dose taken in that period will have dropped to a low level by 4 am (04:00) and in illness this can cause hypoglycaemia (low blood glucose levels).

Hypoglycaemia can be dangerous and lead to unconsciousness. During the early hours of the morning at around 4 am (04:00) is the time when blood glucose in adrenal insufficiency can drop low and it is also the peak time at which an adrenal crisis can occur. Before waking, glucose production and glucose concentrations start to increase, while at the same time glucose utilization is high. This is also the time when blood pressure is at its lowest as is body temperature. For a person with adrenal insufficiency, particularly primary adrenal insufficiency, this is a period of potential compromised body functions.

Cortisol, blood pressure, glucose metabolism and body temperature are all tightly regulated by central and peripheral clocks. We are only beginning to understand the complex interaction between them and this will influence our long term aim of improving the mimicking of the cortisol circadian rhythm as many side effects of replacement therapies may reflect circadian clock disruption.

It is also very important to remember when taking a hydrocortisone tablet, the cortisol takes up to one to two hours to peak, so on taking a double dose when ill, particularly around 4 am (04:00) (More@4 AM) there will then be enough cortisol delivered to cover until the morning dose is due and this will keep the patient safe.

It is important in illness to take this extra double dose, equal to double the morning dose, at 4 am (04:00), even if the last dose was taken at midnight and the next dose is due at 6 am (06:00). This is because the body has starved all night and at this time cortisol levels are naturally high, whereas on oral replacement medication cortisol levels will be waning. Taking the extra hydrocortisone in this situation will not lead to side effects of over treatment as it is only undertaken in situations of illness.

Figures 12.7 and 12.8 show two different examples which illustrate what happens to cortisol concentrations when hydrocortisone is taken at specific times (8 pm (20:00) and midnight (00:00) respectively). Each graph demonstrates the cortisol gap (4 and 2 hours respectively) which commonly occurs during the early hours of the morning. These periods where there is no cortisol will depend on how quickly the individual clears hydrocortisone. For example, if the individual in Figure 12.7 had a very fast clearance of cortisol, they would have low cortisol levels from midnight and would be

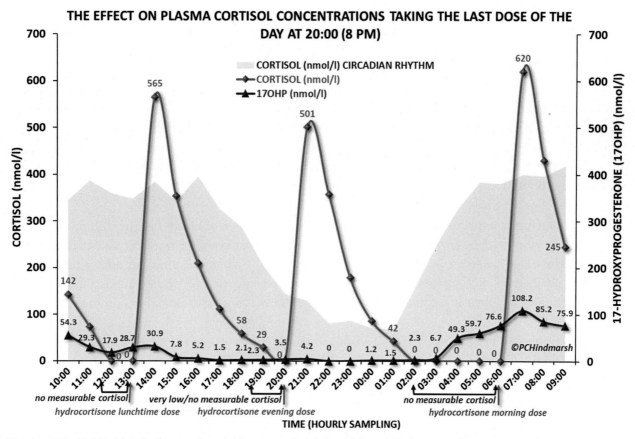

Figure 12.7 *Cortisol levels in a patient with congenital adrenal hyperplasia on a three times daily hydrocortisone regimen with the last dose given at 8 pm (20:00). There is no cortisol in the blood from 2 am (02:00) through to 6 am (06:00) at a time when the circadian rhythm indicates that cortisol should be present and this is evidenced by the rise in 17-hydroxyprogesterone due to the ACTH drive at that time of the night.*

cortisol deficient from 1 am (01:00). In Figure 12.7 the morning dose is taken at 6 am (06:00), however if the dose was taken later it would increase the period when there is no cortisol in the bloodstream.

Interestingly, between 10 pm (22:00) and 11 pm (23:00) there is no measurable 17OHP, yet cortisol levels are higher than those which naturally occur at that time. At 2 am (02:00) there is no cortisol and no 17OHP which again indicates the evening dose is too high for this individual. However, we see a sharp increase in 17OHP at 4 am (04:00) (this may vary between individuals) due to the natural surge of ACTH which continues to drive up 17OHP levels which only start to fall in this instance two hours after a high dose of hydrocortisone is taken at 6am (06:00). Note that 17OHP starts to rise when there is no cortisol (periods of low cortisol between doses) or values drop below a plasma cortisol concentration of 50 nmol/l.

This surge occurs in primary adrenal insufficiency and despite the high cortisol level achieved after the morning dose is taken at 6 am (06:00), the 17OHP production increases after the cortisol peak value, until the effect of the hydrocortisone dampens the ACTH drive. Many centres would increase the hydrocortisone dose at this time. However, in this instance the 24 hour profile has highlighted the over activity of the adrenal glands (increased 17OHP levels) due to the lack of adequate cortisol in the early hours of the morning, which allows the surge of ACTH to drive the adrenal glands to produce 17OHP. In effect what is happening is high cortisol concentrations are being used to treat 17OHP, rather than appropriately replacing cortisol which has a physiological effect on 17OHP by negative feedback.

All these factors show the body naturally needs cortisol during the early hours of the morning and how important it is to get the replacement cortisol distribution optimal. In primary adrenal insufficiency, this results in the normalisation of the ACTH drive and in CAH not only does the 17OHP but also androgen production fall within the normal ranges, unless there are adrenal rests present which would result in normal androgen levels with elevated 17OHP concentrations. In secondary adrenal insufficiency such as hypopituitarism, where there is no ACTH, the cortisol will sustain blood glucose levels and prevent adrenal crises occurring in the early hours of the morning. In essence, optimal cortisol replacement allows the body to function normally as in individuals without any adrenal problems and this highlights the importance of having cortisol present at all times.

In illness as previously explained, even when doubling doses, they would not last much longer, cortisol concentrations would still be low from 1 am (01:00) and there would still be no detectable cortisol left to measure in the blood between 2 am (02:00) until 6 am (06:00), when the morning dose which will be doubled in illness is taken. Data has indicated that in both primary and secondary adrenal insufficiency, the most common time for a fatal adrenal crisis to occur in illness, is during these early hours of the morning.

A similar example can be seen in Figure 12.8 where the patient has taken their evening dose at the later time of midnight (00:00). Again, because the duration of hydrocortisone is 4 to 6 hours, cortisol concentrations drop low and there is little present in the early morning and in this patient, there is no measurable cortisol from around 5 am (05:00).

Before considering the situation of needing an extra dose at 4 am (04:00), an interesting point arises from Figure 12.8. This relates to the duration of action of hydrocortisone. As discussed in Chapter 6, there is a gap between how long hydrocortisone as cortisol lasts in the circulation (approximately 6 hours depending on the individual half-life and clearance of hydrocortisone which we discuss in Chapter 6) and its duration of action. This occurs because glucocorticoids act on cells via their receptor (Chapter 3).

When the glucocorticoids act on the cells there is a time lag between the glucocorticoid attaching itself to the cell and having its effect on the DNA machinery in the cell. This effect on the DNA produces various target proteins, which then all have their own individual effects on the cells close by or sometimes in other parts of the body. This takes time and constitutes what is known as the duration of action.

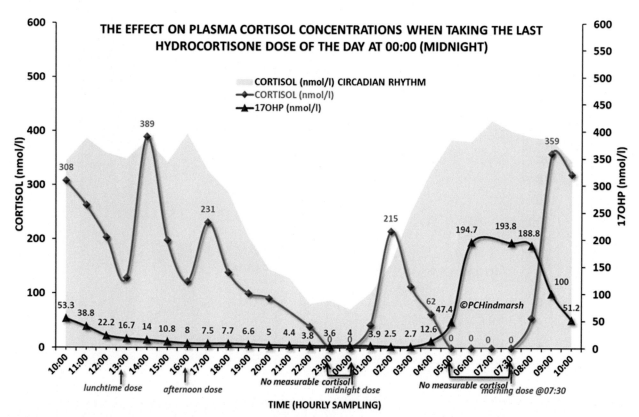

Figure 12.8 *24 hour cortisol profile in a person with congenital adrenal hyperplasia receiving hydrocortisone four times per day. The last evening dose taken at 00:00 (midnight) gives some cortisol at 04:00 (4 am) but it is not sufficient as 17-hydroxyprogesterone is starting to rise.*

Duration of action includes the time we can actually measure the glucocorticoid in the body (often blood) plus the effect on the target cells. The classic measurement of duration of action for the glucocorticoids has been their anti-inflammatory action and for hydrocortisone it is 8 hours. Figure 12.9 summarises the duration of action of hydrocortisone, prednisolone and dexamethasone with respect to their glucose raising properties and their anti-inflammatory action. These differ between the glucocorticoids but also depends on what action we look at. The glucose effect is shorter than the anti-inflammatory action.

The data in Figure 12.9 illustrates the duration of action of each of the glucocorticoids in terms of their effect on raising blood glucose (glucocorticoid action) or dampening down inflammation (anti-inflammatory action). If we now also add in the data in Figure 12.8, we see a different duration of action for the effect of cortisol on ACTH production by the pituitary. High cortisol levels switch off the process regulating ACTH synthesis and its release from the pituitary gland. This is the classic negative feedback loop. What Figure 12.8 shows is there is a different duration of action of hydrocortisone as cortisol on ACTH, as reflected by the rise in 17OHP concentrations at 4 am (04:00). The midnight dose of hydrocortisone keeps the ACTH or rather the 17OHP low until 4 am (04:00) when it starts to rise. This would mean that the duration of action of hydrocortisone on ACTH in this situation, is less than 8 hours and more like 4 to 5 hours. What we can also see, is there appears to be a threshold effect of 50 to 100 nmol/l of cortisol feeding back on ACTH and therefore 17OHP which we discuss in Chapter 6.

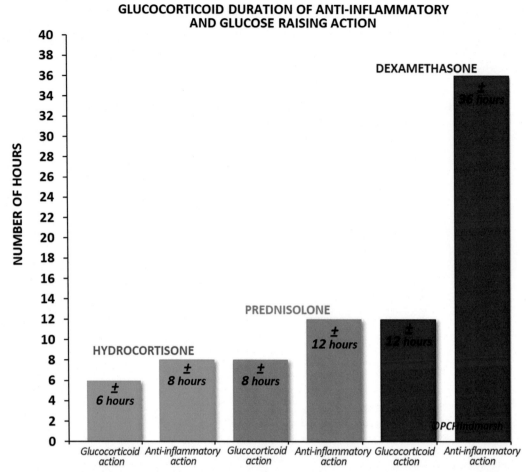

Figure 12.9 *Comparison of hydrocortisone (blue), prednisolone (orange) and dexamethasone (red) in terms of glucose raising action (glucocorticoid) and anti-inflammatory action.*

In Figure 12.8 as mentioned, the dose given at midnight in this individual still delivers a little cortisol at 4 am (04:00), however by 5 am (05:00) there is no measurable cortisol in the bloodstream. We have again used an example from an individual with CAH, in order to illustrate the natural surge of ACTH which drives the adrenal glands to increase cortisol production and in an attempt to do so, the adrenal glands increase their activity resulting in a rise in 17OHP production.

To reiterate, this natural surge of ACTH occurs in anyone with primary adrenal insufficiency, irrespective of the cause. In secondary adrenal insufficiency there is no ACTH production and no 17OHP or cortisol can be produced, but the principles of replacement therapy with More@4 AM are the same. In individuals without adrenal insufficiency, the 17OHP levels would remain within the normal range as the natural cortisol production would feedback on the ACTH, which would prevent the over stimulation of the adrenal glands and in turn there would be no rise in 17OHP.

This early morning natural surge of ACTH which promotes increased cortisol production, is nature's way of preparing the body for the day ahead, as well as keeping blood glucose levels stable as there is no food intake during sleep. In this example as mentioned, we can see the adrenal glands becoming active as the 17OHP concentrations start to increase due to the low cortisol levels and lack of feedback on the ACTH. Interestingly, despite there being no cortisol for the period between 11 pm (23:00) and midnight (00:00), the 17OHP levels remain within the normal range and this is due to good cortisol replacement values earlier in the day.

Having discussed the reason for an extra double dose in illness, taking that extra dose at 4 am (04:00) (More@4 AM) equal to double the usual morning dose would be valuable in preventing an adrenal crisis.

Figure 12.10 illustrates a 24 hour profile of a person with Addison's disease, who has taken their last dose of hydrocortisone at 6 pm (18:00) with the next dose due at 7 am (07:00) the following morning. Cortisol concentrations were measured before all doses were taken and then hourly. The dose taken at 6 pm (18:00) is totally out of the bloodstream with no measurable cortisol in all the samples taken from midnight (00:00) until 7 am (07:00), (note the sample was taken before the morning dose was taken). This dosing resulted in the patient having no measurable cortisol for 7 hours. As the light blue area in the chart shows, this period from midnight (00:00) is when cortisol levels naturally start to increase and reach their highest concentrations. The time of the peak varies in individuals.

Interestingly, this patient presented with hyperpigmentation which disappeared once dosing times were adjusted. General health and quality of life improved.

The vast majority of presentations with adrenal crisis when unwell, occur in the early hours of the morning around 4 am (04:00) probably reflecting the need for cortisol at this time of day, as captured in Figure 12.6, for efficient metabolism and immune function.

Taking the last dose of the day much earlier, as happens in adult practice with dosing schedules suggesting no doses to be taken after 6 pm (18:00), leaves an individual without hydrocortisone for a considerable length of time as we have demonstrated in Chapter 10 and illustrate again in Figure 12.10.

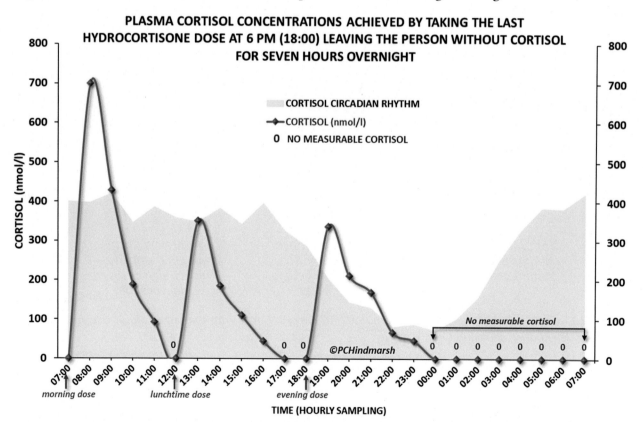

Figure 12.10 *Cortisol profile from patient with Addison's disease on hydrocortisone three doses per day with the last dose given at 6 pm (18:00). Note that by late evening cortisol is undetectable in the circulation for 7 hours until the morning dose is given. This time block covers a period when cortisol concentrations are rising as part of the normal circadian rhythm shown by the light blue shaded area.*

One additional aspect of illness is gastrointestinal infection leading to vomiting and diarrhoea. The combination of vomiting and diarrhoea is a problem in adrenal insufficiency for two reasons:

- The first problem is it is difficult to know how much medication is retained and/or absorbed. If in doubt it is always best to give an intramuscular injection of hydrocortisone and go to Accident and Emergency for review.

- The second problem is dehydration. Dehydration can be scored using the scale illustrated in Figure 12.11 which rates a number of observations such as general appearance and urine colour.

SIGNS INDICATING DEGREE OF DEHYDRATION

Chart A

DEHYDRATION SCORE	0	1	2
GENERAL APPEARANCE	Normal	Thirsty, restless, or lethargic but irritable when touched	Drowsy, limp, cold, sweaty
EYES	Normal	Slightly sunken	Very sunken
MOIST LINING OF MOUTH & EYES	Moist	Sticky	Dry
TEARS	Present	Decreased	Absent
URINE	Normal volume light yellow	Less frequent with dark yellow colour	Very little and dark brown
SKIN	Normal elastic rebound when pinched	Slow rebound when pinched	Remains standing up when pinched. If doughy feel then go to A&E immediately

Chart B   ©PCHindmarsh

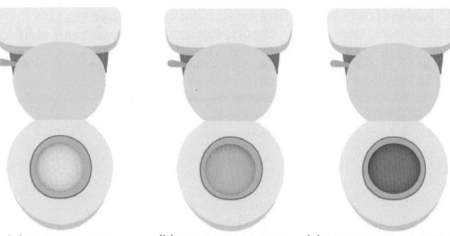

(a) DARK YELLOW
Normal but drink some water soon

(b) HONEY OR AMBER
Drink water now. Your body is not getting enough water

(c) BROWN ALE OR SYRUP COLOUR
Drink some water now!! This is a sign of severe dehydration   ©PCHindmarsh

Figure 12.11 *Chart A Dehydration score from normal (0) through 1 to 2 with the urine colours accompanying the degrees of dehydration shown in Chart B.*

A score of 2 with very brown urine (Figure 12.11 Chart B, picture (c)) would mean the person needs to go to Accident and Emergency for review as this implies marked dehydration and likely to need intravenous fluids.

We can use a similar score for diarrhoea as shown in Figure 12.12. This chart you can use in both directions so that you can decide on severity as you go down the chart but also you can see whether recovery is taking place by going up the chart.

SEVERITY RATING OF DIARRHOEA	
MILD DIARRHOEA	*having a few loose, watery stools in a **single** day*
MODERATE DIARRHOEA	*having more than a few but not more than 10 loose, watery stools in a **single** day*
SEVERE DIARRHOEA	*having **more than 10** loose, watery stools in a **single** day **(24 hours)***

©PCHindmarsh

Figure 12.12 *Severity rating of diarrhoea from mild through moderate to severe.*

Severe diarrhoea would indicate that review by Accident and Emergency is needed. The ratings can be combined so that a dehydration score in the 2 column plus a severe diarrhoea rating would definitely indicate the need for urgent assessment in Accident and Emergency.

Key points with respect to diarrhoea are:

* Diarrhoea is a particular problem due to fluid loss.

* Oral rehydration solutions such as Dioralyte should be used.

* Make sure urine is passed regularly (see colour guide).

* Seek medical advice early especially:

  • If there is a fever

  • Blood in the diarrhoea

  • The person becomes confused

  • The diarrhoea does not stop after 24 hours.

  • There is associated vomiting

* Do not use antidiarrhoeal drugs.

In most cases of diarrhoea, taking an antidiarrhoeal medication will not treat the underlying cause (such as an infection or inflammation), but may help with the discomfort that comes from having repeated watery bowel movements. However, you should not take antidiarrhoeal drugs when diarrhoea is accompanied by fever, severe illness, abdominal pain, or if there is blood or pus (mucus) in the stool. This can make the condition worse. These findings mean a medical opinion is needed urgently. Taking the drugs can lead to problems with the gut and the development of dilated segments of bowel which can be dangerous. We recap all of this in Chapter 16 where we consider what to do if a person develops a vomiting and diarrhoeal illness whilst on holiday. If in any doubt the endocrine team should be contacted for advice and/or assessment sought in an Accident and Emergency Department.

DOSING FOLLOWING ACCIDENTS

Many problems with adrenal insufficiency can be managed at home by increasing the dose of hydrocortisone. Following the sick day rules with the Level 1 and 2 guides can be extremely effective in preventing further deterioration and avoidance of an adrenal crisis. The question now arises how we manage dosing for trauma or other accidents.

This is a particularly important question regarding children who all have falls, scratches, bumps and bruises. Generally, for children, we can say they will not need any extra hydrocortisone if they recover immediately and continue what they were doing before their accident.

We know however, an intramuscular (IM) injection of hydrocortisone is needed immediately for the following events in both adults and children:

- Broken limb

- Bump on the head leading to unconsciousness

- Burn injury (severe or large burn)

- Or if for any reason the person is found in a condition where they are pale, clammy, drowsy and unresponsive

It is always safer in these situations to give the IM injection of hydrocortisone. It will do no harm and it is always better they have the injection as more serious problems may occur if it is not given when needed.

After administering the hydrocortisone injection, the emergency services should be contacted using 999 in the United Kingdom and 911 in the United States of America. In the United Kingdom there is a very clear triage system and the key phrase which triggers the pathway is **'Adrenal Insufficiency'.**

This can be followed with a description, such as 'patient unconscious or unresponsive'. It is now possible to register important clinical details with the ambulance service and this can be flagged by either the patient's address, of which there can be more than one. Most services have now moved to using the registered name of the patient and the location can be easily tracked if using a mobile phone or a landline. This can be organised by the endocrine team.

This reinforces the importance of wearing a medic alert with the wording **ADRENAL INSUFFICIENCY** (Figure 12.18) and also carrying an Adrenal Insufficiency Card which should have the home address details on, the name of your condition and other medications taken such as DDAVP.

Just to recap you should call an ambulance when:

1. You have given an emergency injection of hydrocortisone and there has been no response.
2. If the person is involved in an accident.
3. There is loss of consciousness.
4. The person is vomiting and cannot keep medicines down.
5. If the person is very unwell and you do not have an injection kit or are unable to give the injection.
6. If the patient is unable to travel to hospital to be assessed in order to ascertain the cause of the adrenal crisis and to initiate any treatment that might be required.

We can put all the parts of this section together now into Figure 12.13 which summarises a general guidance for illness and injuries.

GENERAL INFORMATION AND GUIDANCE FOR ILLNESS AND INJURIES

ALWAYS CARRY AN EMERGENCY INJECTION KIT – *If possible, administer injection before calling an ambulance. Advise ambulance staff that the person has 'Adrenal Insufficiency' as this phrase will guide ambulance staff (UK) to the relevant pathway and alerts them to treatment for adrenal crisis. If taking **DDVAP** ask your endocrinologist for written advice on what to do when an emergency injection is given. If taking **PREDNISOLONE**, it is better to use hydrocortisone when ill. However, if not prescribed any, then double each dose and add double the morning dose at 4 am (More@4 AM). This is in **addition** to the doubled morning dose.*

RECOMMENDED INTRAMUSCULAR EMERGENCY INJECTION HYDROCORTISONE DOSES:
25 mg for 0 – 1 year, 50 mg for 1 – 5 years and for over 5 years of age 100 mg.

EMERGENCY INJECTION – *It is always safer, if unsure and depending on the seriousness, to give either an extra double dose or an emergency injection than not to give it. As a one off, it will do no harm even if it wasn't really necessary. Give IM hydrocortisone early if confident to do so. It takes 20 minutes to act, as it has to circulate the body and reach all the cells in the body, to work. Seek help early (Accident and Emergency prefer to see you and send you home than leave it too late). You need to go to Accident and Emergency even if you feel alright after the injection. The reason is that whatever caused the problem may still be present and feeling well may only last until the injection wears off in 4 hours. Give information early i.e., state 'Adrenal Insufficiency' to ambulance staff, reception staff, nurses and doctors. Don't be afraid to keep repeating this. Always carry emergency medicines and any relevant letters/emails or leaflets with your emergency kit and remember **More@4 AM**. If you need to call an ambulance, remember to state, 'Adrenal Insufficiency.' Always wear a medic alert with the words 'Adrenal Insufficiency' on it.*

More@4 AM – *This is an additional dose which should be given at 4 am (04:00). The dose should be equal to double the usual morning dose. The double morning dose should still be given at the usual time. Due to the half-life of hydrocortisone, during the early hours of the morning the evening dose will have run out and the person will be cortisol deficient or have very low cortisol levels.*

MINOR ILLNESSES *such as coughs and colds when there is no increase in temperature – no need to increase dose.*

ILLNESSES – *For temperature, fevers, viral infections and childhood illnesses – double the dose for 24 – 48 hours or until the fever has passed. Give an **extra dose at 4 am (More@4 AM)** which should equal to double usual morning dose, this is an EXTRA dose and double the morning dose should still be given at the usual time. If you wake up at any time with a temperature you can always double dose.*

ILLNESS WITH VOMITING – *Administer double dose immediately even if a dose is not due.*
*If **VOMITING OCCURS 60 MINUTES (1 HOUR)** after a hydrocortisone dose, then the medication is likely to have been absorbed and no repeat dose is needed.*
*If **VOMITING OCCURS WITHIN 60 MINUTES (1 HOUR)** after dose is taken, then the dose should be repeated. If vomiting STOPS continue to double dose for 24 – 48 hours including **More@4 AM**.*
DOES NOT TOLERATE ORAL HYDROCORTISONE – *If vomiting occurs again within 1 hour, then an intramuscular **injection of hydrocortisone** is needed and the person should go straight to Accident and Emergency.*
*If showing signs of hypoglycaemia (low blood sugar) such as very pale, clammy, seem glazed, lethargic, confused or cannot be roused, then administer glucogel by rubbing it inside of the cheek. The emergency **injection should be administered first.***

DIARRHOEA – *Double oral doses and give **More@4 AM**. The most important aspect of care is to give fluids using solutions such as dioralyte. Most episodes settle within 24 hours. Make sure there is good urine output. Seek medical advice early if there is blood in the diarrhoea, the person becomes confused, the diarrhoea does not stop after 24 hours or there is associated vomiting. Do not use anti-diarrhoeal drugs.*
BOTH VOMITING AND DIARRHOEA – *Get medical help quickly as you cannot be sure that any of the medication has either stayed down or been absorbed. Give **IM hydrocortisone injection** and go to Accident and Emergency to get checked out.*

MINOR INJURIES *such as minor bumps and scrapes - an increase in dose should not be necessary.*

SERIOUS INJURIES – *For serious injuries such as a head injury with loss of consciousness, broken bones, serious burns, or **any injury which shows signs of shock**, then administer hydrocortisone injection and phone for an ambulance. **More@4 AM** should also be given for 24 – 48 hours.*

FOR MINOR BURNS – *For minor burns which are small surface burns, give double dose equal to double the usual morning dose and hold the affected area under cold running water for at least 10 minutes. If in doubt, give a double hydrocortisone dose as stated above and seek medical advice or take the patient to A & E for assessment.*

SERIOUS & DEEP BURNS – *All deep burns of any size will require urgent hospital treatment. The hydrocortisone doses will need to be doubled for 48 hours with **More@4 AM**. It is likely if the person has a deep burn, they will need quite intense treatment so hydrocortisone will be given intravenously.*

If you have any concerns contact your endocrine team.   **©PCHindmarsh**

Figure 12.13 *General information for illness and injuries management.*

MANAGEMENT IN ACCIDENT AND EMERGENCY

If an ambulance has been called and the patient is taken to hospital, the ambulance crew will alert accident and emergency it is on its way and relay details of the patient's condition. As a proactive step, if possible, the patient/parent/carer should contact the endocrine team to alert them of what has happened as they will then be able to liaise with the accident and emergency team and assist with what needs to happen next. If the patient goes to accident and emergency by other means, the triage system (UK) in the department will deal with the patient and for children this has to be a turnaround within 15 minutes after arrival. Currently in the UK there is no national protocol for managing adrenal insufficiency in accident and emergency departments, but steps are being taken to improve this issue.

It is extremely important the patient is seen by a doctor immediately after triage and the medical staff should be alerted that the person has **ADRENAL INSUFFICIENCY** and given an outline of the underlying cause.

The important steps which need to be followed are:

1. An intravenous cannula should be inserted so glucose and salt replacement can be given.

2. Urgent blood tests are required including:

   - Sodium, potassium, chloride, bicarbonate, urea, glucose, creatinine and calcium.

   - A cortisol measurement is always helpful for a retrospective review of how the incident was managed.

   - A capillary blood glucose level should be performed immediately.

3. Treatment should be started with an intravenous or intramuscular injection of hydrocortisone if not previously administered by the patient or paramedic.

The emergency hydrocortisone injection doses are shown in Figure 12.14.

4. Intravenous fluids should be started and these need to be administered carefully. This is because of the problems which can follow correcting a low plasma sodium concentration too quickly. The way in which this needs to be managed is outlined in Chapter 14 where we cover mineralocorticoids and electrolytes.

The fluid balance situation becomes extremely complex in those with adrenal insufficiency due to hypopituitarism, because of the potential compounding effect of the loss of arginine vasopressin action and a full discussion should take place on managing this situation with the patient's endocrinologist.

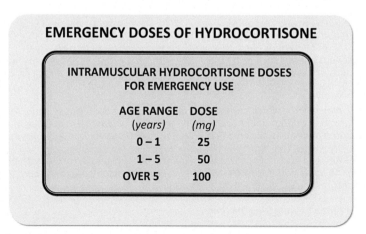

EMERGENCY DOSES OF HYDROCORTISONE

INTRAMUSCULAR HYDROCORTISONE DOSES FOR EMERGENCY USE

AGE RANGE (years)	DOSE (mg)
0 – 1	25
1 – 5	50
OVER 5	100

Figure 12.14 *Intramuscular hydrocortisone doses for emergency use for different age groups. Children over the age of 5 years have the same dose as adolescents and adults, 100 milligrams.*

An intravenous hydrocortisone infusion can be extremely helpful rather than intermittent intravenous boluses of hydrocortisone, as the latter can lead to swings in blood pressure and elevated plasma glucose concentrations. Hydrocortisone is the preferred drug for treatment of an adrenal crisis because of its physiological glucocorticoid pharmacokinetics, plasma protein binding, tissue distribution and balanced glucocorticoid as well as mineralocorticoid effects. If hydrocortisone is unavailable, then dexamethasone (4 mg every 4 hours) or methylprednisolone (40 mg every 24 hours) can be used.

Monitoring of heart rate, blood pressure and plasma sodium, as well as blood glucose should be undertaken over the next 12 to 24 hours. If blood glucose is < 2.5 mmol/l a bolus of 2 ml/kg of 10% glucose should be given. In extreme situations where the patient is drowsy, hypotensive, peripherally shut down with poor capillary return and has very low plasma sodium concentration (less than 120 mmol/l) then an intravenous bolus injection of 1 ml/kg of 3% saline, is helpful. This should only be carried out in a high dependency setting.

More details on managing a low plasma sodium are provided in Chapter 14.

SURGERY IN PATIENTS RECEIVING GLUCOCORTICOIDS

Hopefully, surgery will not be a common place event although at the end of this chapter we do cover dental surgery! There are times when surgery or some intervention is needed and this is usually done in a planned way known as an elective procedure. The other type of surgery is emergency surgery, for example, when you have appendicitis. The ways in which we advise glucocorticoid cover for these two types of surgery differ slightly, but the basic principle is the same — more glucocorticoid is needed.

For all surgical procedures including tests where anaesthesia is required e.g., MRI scanning, we use hydrocortisone as the preferred glucocorticoid.

Elective Surgery

There are a number of useful points to remember for planning elective surgery. Elective surgery is pre planned, so it is a good idea to know what the medical team are planning so you are aware of what to expect and can ensure relevant procedures are put in place. For example, dosing schedules for pre and after the operation/procedure, ensuring that hydrocortisone is prescribed and available on the day, as well as if any testing is required, such as monitoring blood glucose levels, if any pre/after treatment is needed such as a dextrose and saline drip, are known to all the team involved.

1. The doctor in charge, usually the surgeon, should always let the anaesthetist know beforehand so they can plan for the operation, for example, ordering and ensuring intravenous hydrocortisone is available.

2. It is best if patients with adrenal insufficiency are placed first on the surgical list in the morning. This is not always possible because lists are arranged in terms of complexity and whether the case is infective or noninfective, but the principle should be where possible, patients with adrenal insufficiency first.

   Fasting from food and fluid intake is often required prior to surgical procedures. The length of time for food and fluids does vary with age and the type of procedure undertaken. It is always best to discuss this with the surgical and anaesthetic teams particularly if hydrocortisone doses would normally be taken during this time period. If this occurs during the period when starved, this should be discussed with the endocrine team and anaesthetist.

If on the morning surgical list and an inpatient, the normal evening dose of hydrocortisone should be taken the night before. The ward staff should start monitoring blood glucose concentrations from 6 am (06:00) and hourly thereafter until arriving at the operating theatre. At the same time a dextrose and saline (sugar and salt mixture) intravenous drip should be commenced at 6 am (06:00) and maintained until tolerating oral fluids.

These blood glucose checks should be continued at 2 hourly intervals after the operation until the patient is taking food and drinking normally.

3. If on an afternoon list, double the usual morning dose of hydrocortisone and standard dose of fludrocortisone should be taken.

4. Before surgery, an intravenous dose of hydrocortisone (2 mg/kg body weight), should be given on arrival at the operating theatre. Extra bolus injections should be given if the operation is expected to exceed 4 hours. Alternatively, for prolonged procedures and when after surgery recovery is likely to be slow a hydrocortisone infusion using a standard intravenous infusion pump should be set up.

Minor Surgery

Minor Surgery can be defined as a procedure that lasts less than 90 minutes in total and this includes dental work needing a general anaesthetic.

At induction: Hydrocortisone IV 2 mg/kg and repeated if the procedure unexpectedly exceeds 4 hours.

After surgery: Can use repeat IV regimen of hydrocortisone (2 mg/kg) in lieu of routine medication until tolerating oral fluids. Then return to oral therapy which must include that day's fludrocortisone dose. Note that after short procedures, particularly an MRI or CT scan where an anaesthetic is needed (mainly children), an increased need for cortisol is required (see Figure 12.3) so a bolus intravenous hydrocortisone dose the same as that given pre procedure should be given and then continue rest of the day on usual therapy.

Major Surgery

Major Surgery is defined as a procedure which lasts more than 90 minutes for example chest or abdominal operation.

At induction: Hydrocortisone IV 2 mg/kg.

During operation: Repeat IV hydrocortisone on 4 hourly basis or use a hydrocortisone infusion.

After surgery: Can use repeat IV bolus regimen of hydrocortisone or when after surgery recovery is likely to be slow, it is better to use a hydrocortisone infusion. The IV administration of hydrocortisone should be continued until tolerating fluids. The patient should then return to oral therapy at twice normal dose for 24 hours, although this will be determined by the extent of the surgical procedure and will be decided in conjunction with the endocrine team. Extra hydrocortisone as part of More@4 AM should be given until back on normal dosing schedule. Once tolerating food and fluids then return to normal daily requirements. As soon as on oral therapy, the fludrocortisone dose is reintroduced.

Fluid therapy is based on body size and should be the following:

Fluids: 100 ml/kg/day if weight less than 10 kg

   80 ml/kg/day if weight 10 - 30 kg

   60 ml/kg/day if weight greater than 30 kg

In individuals with salt-wasting CAH or other forms of salt-wasting adrenal insufficiency, we would use 5% glucose with 0.45% sodium chloride, whereas for other cases use 4% glucose with 0.18% sodium chloride. Higher volumes are needed in younger children due to higher blood volumes per kilogram of body weight as well as different metabolic rates.

Fludrocortisone is not required until taking fluids orally as the sodium balance can be maintained with intravenous fluids and additional hydrocortisone. Regular daily checks of electrolytes should be undertaken whilst on intravenous fluid treatment.

For patients receiving DDAVP this should be given as normal before the operation. Once on intravenous fluids the rate of infusion can be matched with the urine loss. When surgery is complete, then arginine vasopressin can be given as an intravenous infusion after surgery until drinking fluids when a switch can be made back to oral dosing. This may need to be adjusted carefully by the endocrine team, as the dose of glucocorticoids may be higher than usual which will require careful titration of the DDAVP doses to the measurements of plasma and urine osmolalities, as well as urine output.

The intravenous infusion rate to achieve the average serum cortisol concentration achieved on intensive care during sepsis for example of 1000 nmol/l, is shown in Figure 12.15. The infusion rate is designed to attain a steady state plasma cortisol concentration and depicts an average cortisol clearance rate which influences the infusion rate required.

This will vary between individuals and can be checked by measuring the plasma cortisol concentrations attained. In order to achieve this quickly, a loading intravenous bolus dose of 10 mg for pre pubertal children and 15 mg for pubertal adolescents and adults is required.

HYDROCORTISONE INFUSION RATES

SITUATION	INFUSION RATE (mg/24 hr)
Pre pubertal <10 kg 10 kg — 20 kg >20 kg	25 50 100
Pubertal	155
Post pubertal	105
Infusion Rate (mg/24hrs) = clearance (ml/24hr) x steady state cortisol concentration (mg/ml) ©PCHindmarsh	

Figure 12.15 *Infusion Rate to achieve the average serum cortisol concentration encountered on intensive care during sepsis of 1000 nmol/l. These rates are based on average clearance rates which will vary from person to person and can be adjusted based on measurement of plasma cortisol concentrations attained.*

Emergency Surgery

If emergency surgery is required, then hydrocortisone will be given intravenously, either as a bolus or infusion following the protocol for major surgery. Blood glucose should be checked prior to and at the end of surgery as this is a very stressful situation. In individuals, without adrenal insufficiency adrenaline release will contribute to potentially raising blood glucose. However in patients with adrenal insufficiency this action is compromised so there is a risk that blood glucose may go low.

Fludrocortisone is not needed until the patient is switched back to oral therapy.

Plasma sodium can be maintained by altering the intravenous fluid therapy with varying concentrations of sodium to maintain a normal plasma sodium concentration.

Regular checks of plasma electrolytes and blood glucose should be undertaken whilst on intravenous fluid treatment.

Events can happen rapidly in emergency situations, so it is particularly important the staff know that the patient is taking glucocorticoids and this is why it is so crucial to carry an 'Adrenal Insufficiency' card and to wear a medic alert bracelet with the words '**Adrenal Insufficiency**' stamped on it and any other relevant information.

Dental Surgery

By dental surgery we mean fillings and root canal work that can be undertaken with a local anaesthetic. If a general anaesthetic is needed then the Minor Surgery routine above will need to be followed. Extra hydrocortisone is not needed for a routine dental appointment even though people feel very stressed about visiting the dentist!! However, it is important to ensure there is a reasonable concentration of cortisol in the system prior to any procedure. For example, if the morning hydrocortisone dose was taken at 6 am (06:00) and the appointment is at 11 am (11:00), cortisol levels will be low, so an extra dose, equal to the early morning dose should be taken 30 minutes prior to fillings etc., particularly if it is a deep filling, or preparation for a crown.

We have put our thinking on a variety of dental procedures in Figure 12.16 as a general guide for patients. This covers most areas but it is important for the patient to liaise with their dentist to ensure what dental work is planned and any concerns discussed with the endocrine team.

All general anaesthetics should be given in a hospital.

Vaccinations

The full vaccination programme is recommended for children and adults with adrenal insufficiency (see Chapter 16 for more detail). There are rules about giving some vaccines to people receiving glucocorticoids. These rules are specifically for those receiving high doses of glucocorticoids for inflammatory conditions and do not apply to the replacement doses used in adrenal insufficiency. The way a person reacts to a vaccination varies:

- If there is a rise in temperature, then double dosing with hydrocortisone should be started and the Sick Day Rules outlined above, followed.

- If you are unsure about how the person is reacting to the vaccine then it is always best to get medical advice either from the endocrine team, general practice or accident and emergency.

DENTAL PROCEDURES – GENERAL ADVICE

Something to consider when going to the dentist for treatment is when you took your last dose of hydrocortisone. For example, if you took your dose at 6 am (06:00) with your next dose due at noon (12:00) and your appointment time is 11 am (11:00), due to the half-life of hydrocortisone which results in hydrocortisone lasting at most 6 hours in the system as cortisol, your cortisol levels may have dropped very low. As a double dose doesn't last longer, only peaks higher, even doubling the morning dose may still leave you with a lower cortisol level. So, to ensure you have a good concentration of cortisol, it is best to take an extra dose (the amount dependent on the procedure) at least 30 minutes before your appointment as this will ensure you have a good amount of cortisol in the bloodstream. Depending on treatment you can then take your next dose an hour later than usual and the dose after at the usual time.

GENERAL CHECK UPS
These often cause great anxiety, however you should not need to increase the dose as this is an adrenaline effect not cortisol.

FILLINGS WITH A LOCAL ANAESTHETIC
Take an extra dose, equal to the last dose taken approximately 30 minutes before the procedure. Depending on how close the next dose is due then if less than an hour, take your next dose (usual amount) an hour later than the usual dosing time. Then return to normal doses and times.

ROOT CANAL TREATMENT
Take an extra dose, double the last dose taken approximately 30 minutes before the procedure. Depending on how close the next dose is due then if less than an hour, take your next dose (double amount) an hour later than the usual dosing time. Continue with double dose for rest of day then return to normal doses the next day. You will also need an extra dose at 4am (More@4 AM).

CROWN PREPARATION
Take an extra dose, equal to the last dose taken approximately 30 minutes before the procedure. Depending on how close the next dose is due then if less than an hour, take your next dose (usual amount) an hour later than the usual dosing time. Then return to normal doses and times.

EXTRACTIONS WITH A LOCAL ANAESTHETIC
Take an extra dose, double the last dose taken approximately 30 minutes before the procedure. Depending on how close the next dose is due then if less than an hour, take your next dose (double amount) an hour later than the usual dosing time and continue with double dose for rest of day then return to normal doses the next day.

COMPACTED AND DIFFICULT EXTRACTIONS UNDER GENERAL ANAESTHETIC
This should always be carried out in a hospital and not in the dentist's chair. A bolus of IV hydrocortisone should always be given before and after a general anaesthetic. This needs to be planned between your endocrinologist, the dental team and anaesthetist.

If you have any concerns contact your endocrine team.   ©PCHindmarsh

Figure 12.16 *General advice for patients with adrenal insufficiency attending for dental procedures.*

SUMMARY GENERAL DOSING GUIDE

We have covered a lot of information in the previous sections and have compiled a table for easy reference for illness and stress Figure 12.17.

Note this is a general guide and advice should always be sought from the endocrine team. It is always safer to give a dose, than not to as an occasional extra dose will not do any harm and then discuss the situation with the specialist at the next appointment.

ILLNESS – GENERAL DOSING GUIDE

ISSUE/CIRCUMSTANCE	AMOUNT OF EXTRA HYDROCORTISONE NEEDED	COMMENTS
RAISED TEMPERATURE >38ºC	Double dose	*Extra double dose at 4 am (04:00) equal to double morning dose. See GP for diagnosis of cause of raised temperature*
RAISED TEMPERATURE >39ºC	Triple dose	*Extra triple dose at 4 am (04:00) equal to triple morning dose. See GP for diagnosis of cause of raised temperature*
BROKEN BONE	IM injection (see dose schedule)	*Give IM injection (appropriate dose) call for ambulance*
UNCONSCIOUS	IM injection (see dose schedule)	*Give IM injection (appropriate dose) call for ambulance*
SERIOUS BURNS	IM injection (see dose schedule)	*Give IM injection (appropriate dose) call for ambulance*
SEVERE SCALDING	IM injection (see dose schedule)	*Give IM injection (appropriate dose) call for ambulance*
MINOR BURNS	Double dose	*Extra double dose at 4 am (04:00) equal to double morning dose. See GP or A & E for assessment of burn area*
HEAD INJURY WITH LOSS OF CONSCIOUSNESS	IM injection (see schedule)	*Give IM injection (appropriate dose) call for ambulance*
SERIOUS INJURY	IM injection (see schedule)	*Give IM injection (appropriate dose) call for ambulance*
MINOR INJURY (GRAZES AND BRUISES)	None needed	
SURGERY WITH GENERAL ANAESTHETIC	Bolus pre surgery and bolus after surgery	*See surgery guidelines*
MINOR SURGERY WITH LOCAL ANAESTHETIC	Depending on surgery extra dose 30 minute pre surgery	*This will ensure there is adequate cortisol at time of procedure*
DENTAL WORK WITH GENERAL ANAESTHETIC	Bolus pre surgery and bolus after surgery	*See surgery guidelines must always be carried out in hospital not in dentist chair*
DENTAL WORK WITH LOCAL ANAESTHETIC	Depending on surgery extra dose 30 minute pre surgery	*This will ensure there is adequate cortisol at time of procedure*
COMMON COLD WITH NO TEMPERATURE	None needed	*An extra dose equal to the usual morning dose can be taken at 4 am (04:00) if feeling very unwell*
VACCINATIONS	None needed unless a fever develops	*If fever develops include extra dose at 4 am (04:00) (More @4 AM)*

©PCHindmarsh

STRESS – GENERAL DOSING GUIDE

OCCASION	AMOUNT OF EXTRA HYDROCORTISONE NEEDED	COMMENTS
EXAMS	Small extra dose 30 minutes pre exam start time	*Too much cortisol can cause short term memory problems. If dose was taken more than 2 hours prior to exam, take half the previous dose 30 minutes pre exam*
BIRTHDAY PARTIES	None needed	
SHOCK FROM BEREAVEMENT	If needed an extra dose equal to double the last dose taken can be taken	
SPORT	None needed	*Some people may need extra if exercise is done before next dose is due*

©PCHindmarsh

Figure 12.17 *Summary guide of what to do with hydrocortisone dosing in various situations.*

MEDIC ALERT

We recommend that everyone with adrenal insufficiency should wear a medic alert. These should be inscribed with 'Adrenal Insufficiency' although additional information can be added, such as 'Hydrocortisone treatment,' (Figure 12.18).

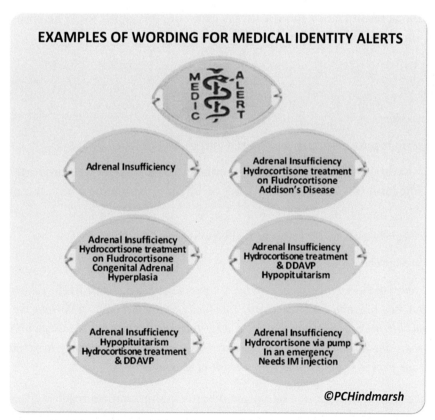

Figure 12.18 *Illustration of suggested engravings on a Medic Alert bracelet, with the key phrase 'Adrenal Insufficiency' with additional information below.*

The medic alert must be worn by the person that has the condition.

It should not be attached to seat belts or school bags as the person may have moved seats or the bag is in another part of the building or car. The emergency services do not have time when in attendance, to search vehicles or the building and they are not allowed to go through bags and personal belongings. The only item they recognise and act on is the medic alert worn by the person. Signs in cars though well intentioned, are not helpful as it does not identify the person and the person may for some reason not be in the car, which can cause confusion and delay. This is also relevant for seatbelt insignias, as for some reason someone else may be in the identified seat!

Remember, in an emergency situation, it might be that the patient is unconscious, so it is very important to wear a medic alert in order to alert all emergency staff that they have adrenal insufficiency. This is also important for children, although parents may feel they are always with their children, the parent could be unconscious in the event of an accident and therefore medic alerts should always be worn by everyone irrespective of age. Other medical identity brands can also be used but must include the wording 'Adrenal Insufficiency' and other relevant information as suggested by the patient's endocrinologist.

We do not recommend an identifiable tattoo in children, as they may not appreciate the permanent identification when older and again a tattoo is not what the paramedics are trained to look for.

It is important that children understand the importance of wearing a medic alert and that it is specifically for them.

EMERGENCY KIT

All patients with adrenal insufficiency should always carry an emergency kit. This should include several vials of hydrocortisone with diluent, syringes, as well as needles.

- Cotton wool ball
- Alcohol wipe
- Syringe and needle
- AmpSnap (plastic top to help snap open glass ampoules safely)
- Ampoules of hydrocortisone for injection either : Solu-Cortef (Hydrocortisone Powder for Solution for Injection or Infusion in the UK) or Hydrocortisone Sodium Phosphate or ACT-O-VIAL®
- Tube of Glucogel® (used to be known as (HypoStop).
- Emergency care letter.

Glucogel® should be only used when the patient is showing signs of low blood glucose levels. Glucogel® should be used AFTER the hydrocortisone injection has been given. Gradually squirt the Glucogel® into the side of the mouth, between the gums and the cheek. Up to one third of a 25 g tube may be needed. Massage into the cheek to allow the gel to be absorbed, this should raise blood glucose levels within 10 minutes. It is not recommended to administer glucogel if the patient is unconscious due the risk of choking.

The emergency pack should be kept in a safe place where children cannot reach it. It needs to be kept at room temperature, out of direct sunlight or heat. The injection ampoules do not need to be kept in the fridge. Injections should not be made up and kept in the fridge. It is also very helpful to keep a copy of an emergency letter with all relevant information and up to date phone numbers which will be helpful to the emergency services. (See Figure 11.20 for a hydrocortisone pump example and Figure 12.19 for a generic adrenal insufficiency example).

EMERGENCY CARE FOR ADRENAL INSUFFICIENCY

PATIENT NAME:

HOME ADDRESS:

POST CODE:

DATE OF BIRTH:

HOSPITAL NUMBER:

NEXT OF KIN CONTACT NUMBER:

HOSPITAL LETTERHEAD WITH RELEVANT TELEPHONE CONTACT NUMBERS

The above person has adrenal insufficiency and must be seen by a medical physician IMMEDIATELY. Time in a waiting room or triage situation is INAPPROPRIATE.

…………………………………………… is on **replacement glucocorticoid steroids** *and is at risk of a life-threatening adrenal crisis if not treated quickly. A crisis will occur when there is an electrolyte imbalance with febrile illness, fluid depletion from vomiting and diarrhoea, burns, serious illness and injury. Signs of an impending crisis can include, weakness, dizziness, failure to respond, nausea and vomiting, hypotension, hypoglycaemia, pallor, and clammy sweating.*

1. INSERT IV CANNULA

2. URGENT BLOOD TESTS REQUIRED
  - *Basic metabolic panel including urea and electrolytes, glucose and calcium.*
  - *Cortisol and 17OHP to get idea of current status.*
  - *Check capillary blood glucose level and perform any other appropriate tests (e.g. urine culture).*

3. TREATMENT

STAT: Hydrocortisone injection IV or IM if NOT already administered

Dose: *Standard emergency hydrocortisone injection dosing schedule should be used:*
    0 – 1 year 25 mg, 1 to 5 years 50 mg and over 5 years including adults 100 mg

4. IV FLUIDS:
  1. *Commence IV fluids. Infusion of sodium chloride and glucose to replace deficit. Add potassium depending on electrolyte balance.*
  2. *Commence hydrocortisone infusion (50 mg hydrocortisone in 50 ml 0.9% sodium chloride) via syringe pump.*
  3. *Monitor for at least twelve hours before discharge.*
  4. *IMPORTANT If blood glucose is <2.5 mmol/l give bolus of 2 ml/kg of 10% glucose.*
  5. *If patient is drowsy, hypotensive and peripherally shut down with poor capillary return give 20 ml/kg of 0.9% sodium chloride stat. Otherwise once sodium is at 120 mmol/l raise it slowly at a rate of no more than 0.3 mmol/l/hour.*

Contact Dr …………………………………… on ………………………………………… for further information.

©PCHindmarsh

Figure 12.19 *Example of an emergency letter for adrenal insufficiency. Further detail can be added for the individual conditions causing adrenal insufficiency such as congenital adrenal hyperplasia.*

HYDROCORTISONE FOR INTRAVENOUS AND INJECTION USE

Solu-Cortef - Hydrocortisone Powder for Solution in the UK (Sodium Succinate)

Solu-Cortef now known as Hydrocortisone Powder for Solution for Injection or Infusion in the UK, is a freeze dried powder (hydrocortisone sodium succinate) which comes with a separate vial of water for injections. For the quick safe opening of the glass vial, we also recommend the use of an Ampsnap. Solu-Cortef has a shelf life of approximately 60 months. The sterile water for injection is made specifically for this purpose and dissolves the powder very quickly. Once mixed the hydrocortisone can then be given as a bolus, an intravenous infusion or as an emergency injection. In other parts of the world, Solu-Cortef also comes as ACT-O-VIAL® which is an automated solution generator using a self-mixing system.

Hydrocortisone Sodium Phosphate 100 mg/1 ml and 500 mg/5 ml solution for Injection

Hydrocortisone Sodium Phosphate is a ready prepared liquid preparation that has a shelf life of 24 months. Hydrocortisone Sodium Phosphate is popular as an emergency injection although it is a thick liquid which makes it harder to inject. Several of our patients have had reactions to Hydrocortisone Sodium Phosphate with one patient being severely allergic to one of the excipients. However, it is convenient and sometimes the glass vials are difficult to snap open. We suggest using an Ampsnap which is a plastic cap that fits over the glass top of the ampoule allowing it to be snapped open easily and safely (Figure 12.20).

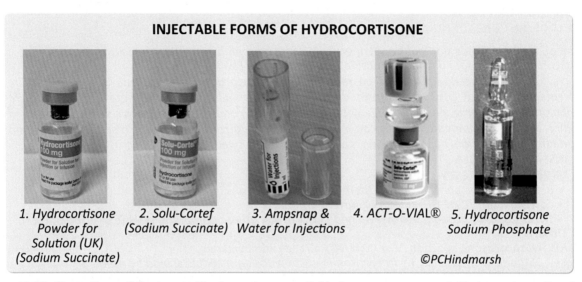

INJECTABLE FORMS OF HYDROCORTISONE

1. Hydrocortisone Powder for Solution (UK) (Sodium Succinate)
2. Solu-Cortef (Sodium Succinate)
3. Ampsnap & Water for Injections
4. ACT-O-VIAL®
5. Hydrocortisone Sodium Phosphate

©PCHindmarsh

Figure 12.20 *Illustrations of the types of hydrocortisone available for emergency use. 1. Hydrocortisone Powder for Solution (UK). 2. Solu-Cortef (Hydrocortisone Sodium Succinate). 3. Water for injections with the plastic Ampsnap which fits over the glass ampoule top, allowing for easy and safe snapping of the top. 4. Act-O-Vial® system. 5. Hydrocortisone Sodium Phosphate.*

Solu-Cortef contains less excipients than Hydrocortisone Sodium Phosphate (Figure 12.21) and all our studies and clearance work is done using Solu-Cortef. For pump use, we recommend using Solu-Cortef only, as Hydrocortisone Sodium Phosphate due to its consistency, can pool under the skin causing lumps and skin irritation.

EXCIPIENTS OF INJECTABLE HYDROCORTISONE

SOLU-CORTEF	HYDROCORTISONE SODIUM PHOSPHATE
Sodium Biphosphate	Disodium Edetate
Sodium Phosphate	Disodium Hydrogen Phosphate
PLEASE NOTE: In the UK Solu-Cortef is now known as Hydrocortisone Powder for Solution for Injection or Infusion (Hydrocortisone Sodium Succinate) No change to the excipients	Anhydrous Sodium Acid Phosphate
	Sodium Formaldehyde Bisulphite Monohydrate
	Phosphoric Acid (10% solution)
	Water for injections
Medicines Information MHRA Government UK	

Figure 12.21 *List of excipients (additional components) in Solu-Cortef compared with Hydrocortisone Sodium Phosphate preparations for intramuscular use.*

Needles

The following information is a general guide to help parents and patients with which needle to use but as always, it is best to discuss fully with the team caring for the patient:

- The size of needle needed is important because if the needle used is too short, the injection will not only go into fat tissue, but it will hurt and not be absorbed as well as it should be.

- Fixed needles need to be considered carefully as the they might be too short.

- If the needle is too fine or narrow, it will make giving the injection difficult.

- The thickness and width of the needle tube is known as the Gauge of the needle.

- Longer needles hurt less and cause less of a local reaction. It is important to dispose of the needle safely once used.

- The Gauge varies so for children less than 12 months of age a Gauge 25 needle can be used. This is coloured orange. However, this is probably a bit too small for the premixed solution of hydrocortisone (UK), Hydrocortisone Sodium Phosphate, (formerly known as Efcortesol) as it is a relatively thick liquid, so it is better to use a needle with a wider bore, this being a Gauge 23 or blue needle.

- When using Hydrocortisone Sodium Phosphate, due to the viscosity of the solution, when administering the injection, it needs to be given slowly.

- For children, young people and adults the blue Gauge 23 works well, but again if using Hydrocortisone Sodium Phosphate (UK), it is better to use the wider Gauge 21 needle (Figure 12.22).

- Our recommendation on the length of the needle for all ages from infants to adults is 1 inch or 2.5 cm.

- In an emergency pack it is always best to have several needles, particularly if mixing Solu-Cortef, as drawing up and pushing the needle through the rubber stopper can on occasions cause it to bend.

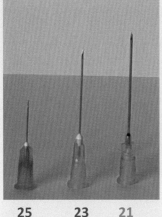

NEEDLE SIZES FOR INTRAMUSCULAR INJECTION OF HYDROCORTISONE

AGE (years)	HYDROCORTISONE dose (mg)	Needle Gauge and Colour	
		Solu-Cortef * (Sodium Succinate)	Hydrocortisone Sodium Phosphate
0 - 1	25	25	23
1 - 5	50	23	21
Over 5	100	23	21

Renamed in UK to Hydrocortisone Powder for Solution for Injection or Infusion

25 Gauge   23 Gauge   21 Gauge

©PCHindmarsh

Figure 12.22 *Picture on the left illustrates the difference between the various gauge needles and on the right an advisory summary of the type and gauge of needles (colour coded to match the needle colours in the picture on the left) which can be used with the different preparations at different ages.*

CONCLUSION

It is very important for patients and carers to understand the reasons why extra medication is required in illness, when it is appropriate to increase doses, when it should be administered, and how the increase should be given such as increasing orally or by an emergency injection of hydrocortisone. Most importantly if in a situation where it is felt an emergency injection might be needed but the patient or carer is unsure, then it should be given as it is safer to do so than not to and will do no harm. Once an emergency injection has been given, the patient needs to be examined in accident and emergency to establish the cause as to why the injection was needed. This is not wasting the staff's time as no one should mind checking a patient with adrenal insufficiency even if all is well. Understanding the reasons for increasing medication in illness is important as it will help to enforce the sick day rules. The cortisol binding globulin alters shape so the glucocorticoids will go straight to the target site to dampen down the infection/inflammation and extra cortisol is then needed to keep the levels in the bloodstream to travel to the body's organs at the normal expected level.

Emergency injection training should be given to parents, carers, and/or where appropriate, to patients. General Practitioners should also be given relevant information regarding dosing in illness and emergency care. Oral hydrocortisone should be used as it absorbs and peaks more quickly than other glucocorticoids. We recommend an extra double dose based on the morning dose of hydrocortisone should be given at around 4 am (04:00) (More@4 AM) as cortisol concentrations from the evening dose will have dropped very low or become depleted. The doubled morning dose should be taken at the usual time. This action of giving an extra dose at 4 am (04:00) is backed up by studies that have shown there is a natural surge of ACTH around 4 am (04:00) to drive the adrenal glands to increase cortisol production. In this chapter, we have considered the initial response in illness which is activation of the hypothalamo-pituitary-adrenal axis. In critical illness this is followed by cortisol metabolic adaptations; a reduction in cortisol binding globulin and increased free cortisol and glucocorticoid receptor activity. The increased cortisol exerts negative feedback at the pituitary, reducing ACTH production. Care needs to be exercised when stress dosing with hydrocortisone as circulating concentrations in prolonged illness can be already high. Careful monitoring of cortisol levels is required and further research is needed in this area.

FURTHER READING

Bolli, G.B., Gerich, J.E., 1984. The "Dawn-Phenomenon" — a common occurrence in both non-insulin-dependent and insulin-dependent diabetes mellitus. N Engl J Med 310, 746—750.

Costello, H.M., Gumz, M.L., 2021. Circadian rhythm, clock genes, and hypertension: recent advances in hypertension. Hypertension 78, 1185—1196.

Dagogo-Jack, S., Rattarasarn, C., Cryer, P.E., 1994. Reversal of hypoglycemia unawareness, but not defective glucose counterregulation, in IDDM. Diabetes 43, 1426—1434.

Hahner, S., Burger-Stritt, S., Allolio, B., 2013. Subcutaneous hydrocortisone administration for emergency use in adrenal insufficiency. Eur J Endocrinol 169, 147—154.

Hsu, C.Y., Rivkees, S.A., 2005. Chapter 9 Stress Dosing. In: Hsu, C.Y., Rivkees, S.A. (Eds.), Congenital Adrenal Hyperplasia: A Parents' Guide. Author_House, Indianna.

Langouche, L., Téblick, A., Gunst, J., Van den Berghe, G., 2023. The Hypothalamus-pituitary-adrenocortical response to critical illness: a concept in need of revision. Endocrine Rev 44, 1096—1106. https://doi.org/10.1210/endrev/bnad021.

Mushtaq, T., Ali, S.R., Boulos, N., et al., 2023. Emergency and perioperative management of adrenal insufficiency in children and young people: British Society for Paediatric Endocrinology and Diabetes consensus guidance. Arch Dis Child Epub ahead of print. https://doi.org/10.1136/archdischild-2022-325156.

Plumpton, F.S., Besser, G.M., 1969. The adrenocortical response to surgery and insulin-induced hypoglycaemia in corticosteroid-treated and normal subjects. Br J Surg 56, 216—219.

Rushworth, R.L., Torpy, D.J., Falhammar, H., 2019. Adrenal crisis. N Engl J Med 381, 852—861.

Tsigos C, Kyrou I, Kassi E, et al. Stress: Endocrine Physiology and Pathophysiology. [Updated 2020 Oct 17]. In: Feingold KR, Anawalt B, Boyce A, et al., editors. Endotext [Internet]. South Dartmouth (MA): MDText.com, Inc.; 2000-. Available from: https://www.ncbi.nlm.nih.gov/books/NBK278995/

Weise, M., Drinkard, B., Mehlinger, S.L., et al., 2004. Stress dose of hydrocortisone is not beneficial in patients with classic congenital adrenal hyperplasia undergoing short term, high-intensity exercise. J Clin Endocrinol Metab 89, 3679—3684.

Wilson, G.R., Dorrington, K.L., 2017. Starvation before surgery: is our practice based on evidence? BJA Education 17, 275—282. https://doi.org/10.1093/bjaed/mkx009.

CHAPTER 13

Glucocorticoid Replacement — Interaction With Other Hormones

GLOSSARY

Cortisol binding globulin A protein made by the liver which attaches itself to cortisol and carries it around the bloodstream. This is known as bound cortisol. 90% to 95% of cortisol is bound in this way with 5% in the free state.

Cortisol-cortisone shuttle A system that uses the isoenzyme 11beta-hydroxysteroid dehydrogenase type 1 to convert inactive cortisone to cortisol mainly in the liver and the isoenzyme 11beta-hydroxysteroid dehydrogenase type 2 to inactivate cortisol to cortisone mainly in the kidney and salivary glands.

DDAVP 1-desamino-8-d-arginine vasopressin. Synthetic form of arginine vasopressin where the first amino acid has been deaminated and the arginine at position 8 is in the right (dextro) rather than the left (levo) form.

Diabetes insipidus The passing of a dilute urine in the face of a reduced blood volume. This can arise due to lack of arginine vasopressin formation in the hypothalamus and storage in the posterior pituitary gland (cranial diabetes insipidus) or to lack of action of arginine vasopressin in the kidney tubules (nephrogenic diabetes insipidus).

Osmosis The movement of water molecules from a solution with a high concentration of water molecules to a solution with a lower concentration of water molecules, through the partially permeable cell membrane.

Peptide Peptides, like proteins are made up of strings of amino acids. The differences between a peptide and a protein are size and structure. Peptides are smaller than proteins and are defined as molecules that consist of between 2 and 50 amino acids, whereas proteins are made up of 50 or more amino acids. Proteins, because they are bigger can adopt complex conformations known as secondary, tertiary, and quaternary structures.

Tonicity The tonicity of a solution refers to its solute concentration relative to that of another solution on the opposite side of the cell membrane. A solution outside of a cell is called hypertonic if it has a greater concentration of solutes than inside the cell. When a cell is immersed in a hypertonic solution, osmosis tends to force water to flow out of the cell in order to balance the concentrations of the solutes on either side of the cell membrane. A solution outside of a cell is called hypotonic if it has a lower concentration of solutes than inside the cell. Isotonic is where the solute balance is the same across the cell membrane.

Transdermal Across the skin.

GENERAL

In the previous chapters we have considered drug interactions between hydrocortisone and other commonly used drugs. The hallmark of these drugs is they largely alter liver metabolism and because the glucocorticoids use similar enzyme systems to other drugs, there are often generic effects of these drugs on metabolism which incidentally impact on glucocorticoid replacement therapy. We have tabulated many of these in Chapter 6 (Figure 6.8). Many utilise the enzyme Cytochrome P450 3A4 system which can also increase hydrocortisone clearance.

Replacement Therapies in Adrenal Insufficiency. https://doi.org/10.1016/B978-0-12-824548-4.00013-9

Cytochrome P450 3A4 (CYP3A4) is an important enzyme in the body which is mostly found in the liver and intestine. It oxidizes small foreign organic molecules known as xenobiotics. These are chemical substances found within an organism which are not naturally produced or expected to be present, such as toxins or drugs. The cytochrome system is very efficient at removing toxins from the body, but CYP3A4 if switched on strongly by xenobiotics, can lead to an increase in hydrocortisone clearance. A good example of this is the anti-tuberculosis drug rifampicin which increases CYP3A4 activity and increases hydrocortisone clearance which means that if on replacement hydrocortisone treatment, extra hydrocortisone will be needed. The cytochrome system can be switched off as well by things such as grapefruit juice and other drugs and this can lead to the inhibition of cortisol metabolism, leading to increasing cortisol levels.

These drug interactions can lead to side effects themselves and we have considered many of the side effects we associate with over and under treatment with glucocorticoids in previous chapters. In this chapter, we are going to review some of the medications which are used specifically in association with glucocorticoids for the management of patients with adrenal insufficiency.

In adrenal insufficiency particularly associated with hypopituitarism, there is the potential for the glucocorticoid, particularly hydrocortisone, to either be affected by the other medications which are necessary for hormone replacement, or the glucocorticoids themselves impact on the metabolism of the other hormones which are being substituted. In this chapter we will consider a number of these, especially the most commonly encountered medication, the oral contraceptive pill.

It is also worth mentioning other ways in which glucocorticoid action can be modified through natural genetic variance in either cortisol binding globulin or the glucocorticoid receptor. Although there have been a number of reports of these in the literature, it is surprising that the natural variance which results from these changes, does not seem to produce much of an overall impact on cortisol binding globulin concentrations or binding to the glucocorticoid receptor. As such we will not consider further these particular issues and will concentrate more on the impact of associated hormonal therapies.

GLUCOCORTICOIDS AND MINERALOCORTICOIDS

We are used to the idea of glucocorticoid (cortisol) and mineralocorticoid (aldosterone) replacement therapy with hydrocortisone and 9 alpha-fludrocortisone respectively. In general, there isn't much in the way of interaction between these two. However, because 9 alpha-fludrocortisone has dexamethasone like activity, it does need to be factored into the total daily dose of glucocorticoid when calculating appropriate replacement regimens. This is particularly important because often when hyponatremia (low sodium) presents in the newborn, there is a tendency to increase the dose of 9 alpha-fludrocortisone without altering the sodium intake.

Despite such a dose increase if the intake of sodium is limited to a certain amount per day, then increasing the dose will not cause any further sodium retention. You can only retain what you have available and no more than that. The sodium content of milk, particularly breast milk, is low and sodium loss in the urine is naturally quite low suggesting that there is maximum resorption of sodium in the kidneys. The side effect of increasing the 9 alpha-fludrocortisone dose is that we will get an increased glucocorticoid like effect, so inadvertently over treatment from a glucocorticoid standpoint might result from the increase in 9 alpha-fludrocortisone. High doses of 9 alpha-fludrocortisone will not necessarily lead to hypertension unless there is freely available sodium in the diet which for the neonate and newborn, is not the case.

This is not the situation in older individuals on a normal western diet, because the sodium content of the western diet even though sodium has been reduced in it, is still very high and higher doses of 9 alpha-fludrocortisone would lead to a rise in blood pressure and ultimately hypertension. High doses of hydrocortisone can in themselves lead to a rise in blood pressure so we need to think of both hydrocortisone and 9 alpha-fludrocortisone doses when we encounter high blood pressure or hypertension in a patient with adrenal insufficiency who is also deficient in aldosterone.

Cortisol is present in the circulation in nanomolar amounts (nmol/l - nanomoles per litre), whereas aldosterone is present in picomolar amounts (pmol/l - picomoles per litre). In other words, there is 1000 times as much cortisol present than aldosterone. Cortisol in this amount would attach to the mineralocorticoid receptor (or docking station) in the kidneys leading to sodium retention and with that water, which will raise blood pressure. This is because the receptors for the glucocorticoids and the mineralocorticoids are structurally similar with 15% shared similarity at one end of the receptor and 57% at the other (please see Chapter 3, Figure 3.13 for receptor structural comparisons). To prevent this, the body has devised a protective mechanism called the cortisol shuttle (Figure 13.1). The enzyme 11beta-hydroxysteroid dehydrogenase type 2 is found in similar places to where the mineralocorticoid receptor is, such as the kidneys. This enzyme converts active cortisol to inactive cortisone, thereby protecting the receptor from the large amount of cortisol which is present and allowing aldosterone to gain access and work. The other half of the shuttle is 11beta-hydroxysteroid dehydrogenase type 1 which is found in the liver and converts inactive cortisone to cortisol. The enzyme system is easily saturated once cortisol levels get over 550 - 600 nmol/l.

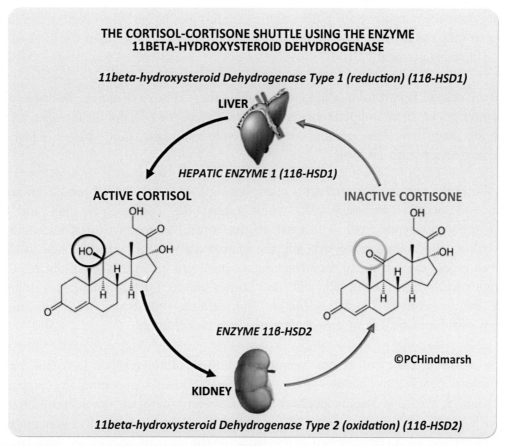

Figure 13.1 *Illustration of the cortisol shuttle where cortisone is converted to cortisol mainly in the liver and adipose tissue by the enzyme 11beta-hydroxysteroid dehydrogenase type 1 (11β-HSD1) and cortisol is converted to cortisone mainly in the kidneys and salivary glands by the enzyme 11beta-hydroxysteroid dehydrogenase type 2 (11β-HSD2).*

ESTROGENS AND CORTISOL

The main effect of estrogens are on the cortisol binding globulin in the circulation. Estrogens are known to stimulate liver protein production and this includes the production of cortisol binding globulin. There is a difference between the way estrogen is presented to the liver. When estrogen or rather estradiol is produced by the ovaries, it goes into the inferior vena cava, the large vein returning blood to the heart. The heart then passes the blood on to the lungs for oxygenation and this returns to the left side of the heart to be sent out into the main arteries. Estradiol can then act on its various target tissues, whilst some will reach the liver where it will be metabolised. The amount of estradiol which the liver is exposed to is a lot less than produced by the ovaries.

In hypopituitarism where estrogen replacement is undertaken because of gonadotropin deficiency, or in other situations where the oral contraceptive pill is used for contraception, the oral administration of estrogen leads to a far higher local concentration of estrogen in the portal circulation from the gut to the liver, compared to the same dose administered via the transdermal (across the skin using a patch) route. This may help explain why oral estrogen replacement more consistently elevates total cortisol concentrations compared to the transdermal route.

All routine laboratory measures of cortisol measure both the free cortisol and the cortisol which is bound to cortisol binding globulin and this is called the total cortisol concentration. In fact, we do not actually call it this and simply refer to the plasma cortisol concentration whereas we should really call it the plasma total cortisol concentration.

This means when we are interpreting cortisol levels, we have to remember that some is free and some is bound. Under normal circumstances this does not matter too much, but when cortisol binding globulin levels change, as they can do with oral contraceptive pill use (Figure 13.2), then the total concentration we measure will change as well.

The effect of the change in cortisol binding globulin takes some time to disappear. In our experience the oral contraceptive pill has to be stopped some 6 to 8 weeks before the effect of the estrogen on the cortisol binding globulin disappears. This explains why adult endocrinologists stop estrogen replacement well before measuring total plasma cortisol.

Figure 13.2 shows the cortisol measurements taken during a 24 hour cortisol profiles of an individual before taking an oral contraceptive pill, whilst taking the contraceptive pill and then after discontinuing the contraceptive pill. The total plasma cortisol concentration is increased when the individual is taking the oral contraceptive pill, the plasma cortisol then returns back to the previous values achieved before the individual took the contraceptive pill when it is discontinued. Overall, this means the individual whilst on the pill, will have higher plasma total cortisol concentrations due to the increase in the cortisol binding globulin. Side effects will occur from the high cortisol concentrations and the cortisol replacement dose needs to be adjusted.

The situation is not as clear cut as oral versus transdermal administration. It is true oral estrogen replacement more consistently elevates the plasma total cortisol concentration compared to the transdermal route as we have already pointed out. However, there are other components to these treatments such as the inclusion of progestins in the preparation. Incidentally, you might hear the term progestogens also used. Progestogen is the name of the class of hormones, while progestin is a synthetic progestogen and progesterone is a natural progestogen. The effects of progesterone on cortisol binding globulin production is less well established than that for the estrogens.

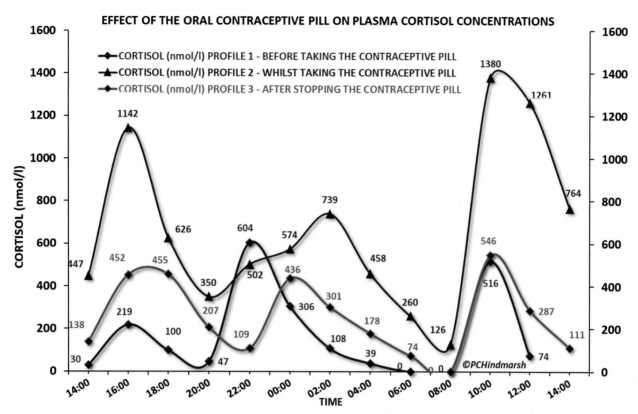

Figure 13.2 *Effect of introducing and then stopping the oral contraceptive pill on plasma cortisol levels in a single individual with adrenal insufficiency. The pill markedly increases the total cortisol measures (red line) compared to values pre (purple line) and post (blue line) taking the oral contraceptive pill. No change to the doses taken was made during these profiles apart from moving the last dose of the day from 20:00 (8 pm) (Profiles 1 and 2) to 22:00 (10 pm) (Profile 3). Note sampling start time is at 14:00 (2 pm) in these studies.*

It has been reported that high concentrations of progesterone can suppress cortisol binding globulin formation. If there is a progestin in the oral contraceptive pill, this would then lead to high local concentrations of progestin in the portal circulation which we also noted for estrogen. There then becomes a balance between how much estrogen is delivered from the oral replacement therapy compared to the amount of progestin. If this is constant, the effect of the increase in cortisol binding globulin by the estrogen will be offset to a certain degree by the suppression of cortisol binding globulin production by the progestin.

Eventually a new equilibrium will be established between the two. However, should there be any situation where the proportions change, then major changes will then take place in the balance between the estrogen and progestogen effects on cortisol binding globulin, leading to changes which would impact on the total cortisol measured and the free cortisol available for action. It should be pointed out that there is very little information of what is happening to free cortisol in many of the published studies. Some studies have demonstrated that low dose oral contraceptive therapy can increase free cortisol levels from 18 nmol/l to 28 nmol/l. This seems a small increase but is actually a 56% change and has been associated in some studies with an increase in triglyceride levels (triglycerides are molecules made up of fatty acids which help store and move fats around the body). Each person's response will be variable and we have observed similar effects in a number of patients. Further research is required to confirm and detail these findings.

This then leaves a very complex potential picture for those embarking on estrogen replacement therapy. For a variety of other reasons, transdermal estrogen is probably to be preferred to oral administration of estrogen as a form of hormone replacement therapy. These reasons relate mainly to alteration in the clotting factors and an increased tendency to formation of blood clots in the circulation, reflecting the high exposure in the liver to estrogen via the oral route.

This means in the consideration of the use of estrogen replacement therapy there is a choice which has to be made between oral and transdermal applications. In addition, consideration needs to be given to the dosage and ratio of estrogens and progestins which are administered as part of the hormone replacement therapy. These will alter the effects on plasma total cortisol concentrations in particular. Although we have painted a very broad picture with respect to oral versus transdermal estrogen delivery, there is even more detail which needs to be considered when looking at the contribution of dose and estrogen/progestin ratio in the various products available.

Like many things in endocrinology and particularly in adrenal insufficiency, careful attention to the effects of these medications on our hydrocortisone replacement therapy is essential and detailed biochemical studies, including 24 hour cortisol profiles are required to aid our understanding of the effect of these products on circulating cortisol concentrations, as well as overall efficacy of the hydrocortisone we are administering. In particular, it is common practice to stop hormone replacement therapy prior to cortisol day curves, but this does not tell us what is happening on a day to day basis and what is needed is all medication to be taken as usual when profiles are done, so we can see any effect on cortisol levels.

ARGININE VASOPRESSIN AND CORTISOL

Arginine vasopressin (AVP) is the natural peptide which is produced by the posterior pituitary gland and is involved in regulating water balance, in particular increasing water uptake in the kidneys. Figure 13.3 shows where AVP sits in the regulation of blood volume and blood pressure. A reduction in blood volume is detected by pressure (baroreceptors) receptors in the large blood vessels coming from the heart, the aorta and the carotid arteries and by the osmoreceptors in the hypothalamus, resulting in the development of a more concentrated blood (osmolality).

The baroreceptors sense pressure changes by responding to a change in the tension of the arterial wall. They respond very quickly to changes in blood pressure. A sudden increase in blood pressure stretches the baroreceptors and results in a switch off of the sympathetic nervous system input to the heart and increase in the parasympathetic input, which leads to a slowing of the heart rate in order to correct the increase in pressure. When a person has a sudden drop in blood pressure, for example standing up, the decreased blood pressure is sensed by the baroreceptors and the changes in the sympathetic and parasympathetic nervous systems increase the heart rate.

These are very quick changes compared to the mechanisms set in play by the osmoreceptors as they are mediated by the nervous system, but the baroreceptors also alter AVP production particularly if blood pressure falls.

The osmolality of the blood is detected by osmoreceptors in the hypothalamus. Activity in both these areas (osmoreceptors and baroreceptors) increases the feeling of thirst as well as promoting the release of AVP from the posterior pituitary. Arginine vasopressin via its V1 receptor, constricts blood vessels leading to a rise in blood pressure and action via the V2 receptors in the kidney leads to increased retention of water, thereby increasing blood volume and blood pressure.

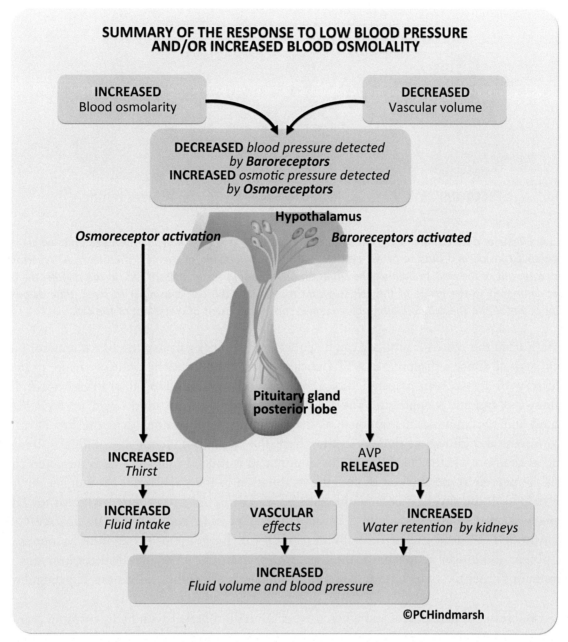

Figure 13.3 *Arginine vasopressin (AVP) release results from a reduction in blood volume and/or an increase in blood osmolality. This leads to constriction of the blood vessels increasing blood pressure along with an increase in water retention by the kidney which increases blood volume and blood pressure.*

Arginine vasopressin release is closely related to the osmolality of the blood. In fact, we are really talking about the tonicity of fluids and tonicity is the effect blood has on cells. When blood is hypotonic (blood contains a lot of water compared to the cells) cells swell as water moves from blood into the cell. When blood is hypertonic (blood contains less water than the cells) water moves from cells into the blood and the cells shrink (Figure 13.4). Osmolality is the way we measure this. These are important points we will return to when we look at how to treat low sodium levels in Chapter 14. Arginine vasopressin is not secreted when the blood osmolality is below 285 mOsmol/kg. If blood osmolality starts to rise as in the example in Figure 13.3, then the amount of AVP increases. Once the blood osmolality reaches 295 mOsmol/kg AVP production is maximal and the thirst mechanism is switched on. This leads to maximum water retention from the kidneys and prevents the blood becoming hypertonic.

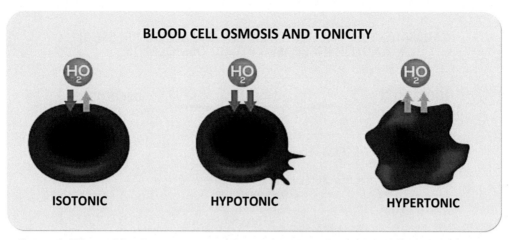

BLOOD CELL OSMOSIS AND TONICITY

ISOTONIC   HYPOTONIC   HYPERTONIC

Figure 13.4 *Effects of different blood tonicity on a cell. On the left is the normal situation (isotonic) where water is equally balanced inside and outside of the cell. On the right the outside of the cell, the blood, is hypertonic and this pulls water out of the cells to balance the situation and in doing so the cell shrinks. In the middle, the blood is hypotonic compared to the inside of the cell so water moves into the cell causing it to swell. Blue arrows show movement of water into the cell and lighter blue arrows show movement of water out of the cell.*

Loss of AVP from the posterior pituitary can be either isolated or as part of a loss of the anterior pituitary hormones as well. Once a diagnosis of AVP deficiency (cranial diabetes insipidus) is made, treatment is commenced with the synthetic preparation of AVP which is known as DDAVP, or to give it its full name, 1-desamino-8-d-arginine vasopressin. The full name tells us the first amino acid in AVP has been deaminated and the arginine at position 8 is in the right (dextro) rather than the left (levo) form. These forms are also known as isomers so they have the same components but different strengths of action depending on whether in this case, the amino acid is rotated right or left, as this alters the way in which the peptide is metabolised prolonging its duration in the circulation. Prolonging duration of action is helpful in this situation because the half-life of AVP is only 10 minutes, whereas for DDAVP the changes increase this to 3.5 hours. Because it is a peptide and quite small, DDAVP can be absorbed through the nasal passage or orally in tablet form. 1-desamino-8-d-arginine vasopressin itself is more potent and longer acting and is the mainstay of treatment of cranial diabetes insipidus. There are a number of other uses which it can be used for such as bed wetting and various bleeding disorders.

Arginine vasopressin is quite potent and when used as DDAVP together with hydrocortisone, care needs to be exercised because it may increase the risk of developing low plasma sodium concentrations (hyponatremia). Symptoms of hyponatremia may include nausea, vomiting, lethargy, muscle cramps, confusion seizures and if not noticed and treated can lead to death because of prolonged seizure activity and coma.

The exact mechanism of this glucocorticoid-AVP interaction is unclear. Glucocorticoid deficiency is believed to impair free water excretion via mechanisms which are both dependent and independent of AVP. Cortisol induces a state of relative resistance to AVP at the level of the AVP receptors, leading to movement of the aquaporin water channels to the surface of the cells in the kidneys involved in water reabsorption. When cortisol is low, it is not easy to clear water from the body.

In patients with deficiency of AVP who are replaced with DDAVP, extreme caution needs to be taken in changing any associated glucocorticoid doses. This is most likely to occur when hydrocortisone doses are changed in illness.

Increasing the dose of hydrocortisone either doubling or tripling, is the correct procedure in terms of coping with stressful events and illness. However, this will lead to an increase in water clearance from the body which will make the plasma sodium rise (hypernatremia). To counteract this, the dose of DDAVP often needs to be increased and because this requires fine adjustments and measurement of the effect on plasma sodium concentrations, this is best done by specialists in hospital. We cover in more detail the effects of hyper and hypo natremia in Chapter 14. The main message is to carefully adjust glucocorticoid and DDAVP doses to avoid sudden and rapid changes in the plasma sodium concentration. If plasma sodium concentrations have been high for some time, usually more than 24 to 36 hours, changes start to take place in the brain and a sudden reduction in the plasma sodium concentration can lead to seizures.

Equally, when the reason for the increase in hydrocortisone dosing has resolved, e.g., post infection, careful adjustment of the DDAVP dose in light of reducing hydrocortisone doses is required to avoid over retention of water and subsequent hyponatremia. These changes in the dosing regimen, need to be undertaken with appropriate monitoring of plasma sodium and plasma osmolality levels and are made even worse in some situations of hypopituitarism, where the thirst mechanism may also have been lost. Careful assessment in hospital is essential.

It is also important to remember that all drugs have interactions with other drugs, or rather other drugs may modify the actions of our drug of interest. We have talked here about cortisol, but other agents that may be used in the management of hypopituitarism may be important. In congenital hypopituitary patients, epilepsy might be a problem and treatments such as carbamazepine, or the more modern drug lamotrigine, used. These appear to cause water retention due to an effect centrally on AVP release, so care needs to be exercised when these medications are introduced, particularly if a patient has partial diabetes insipidus as excess water retention can occur leading to hyponatraemia.

Finally, other drugs may alter AVP/DDAVP action. Lithium is used to treat bipolar disorders and also acts to inhibit AVP action on the kidney, producing a nephrogenic diabetes insipidus picture. This may mean that if already on DDAVP, a higher dose may be required if treatment with lithium is introduced. Careful monitoring of electrolytes is required.

GROWTH HORMONE AND CORTISOL

Growth hormone deficiency can occur in isolation or as part of hypopituitarism. In hypopituitarism, growth hormone deficiency is almost an inevitable component, whereas the loss of other anterior pituitary hormones can be more variable.

Figure 13.5 shows the normal profile of growth hormone over a 24 hour period. In contrast to the cortisol circadian rhythm, growth hormone appears in distinct bursts or pulses roughly every 3 hours. This is more obvious during night time when most growth hormone is produced — so perhaps we do grow as children when we go to bed early and sleep well!! Notice that the highest peak is seen immediately after sleep has commenced and is usually at a time when cortisol is at its lowest.

As growth hormone and cortisol both increase blood glucose, or rather prevent blood glucose going low, losing one or both of these hormones leaves the person at a high risk of developing hypoglycaemia at night, as these two hormones work together to maintain blood glucose when fasting occurs during sleep overnight.

24 HOUR PROFILE OF PLASMA GROWTH HORMONE

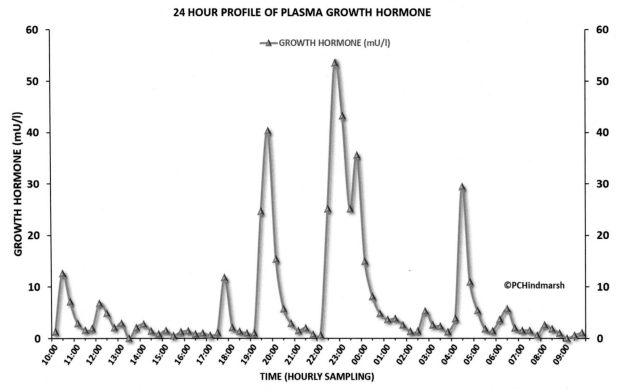

Figure 13.5 *24 hour plasma growth hormone profile in a person with short stature showing distinct normal bursts of growth hormone with the largest peak occurring at 23:00 (11 pm).*

In Figure 13.6 Chart A we see a profile from a patient with growth hormone deficiency where there is very little growth hormone measured over the 24 hour period. Figure 13.6 Chart B shows the profile after a subcutaneous injection of biosynthetic human growth hormone.

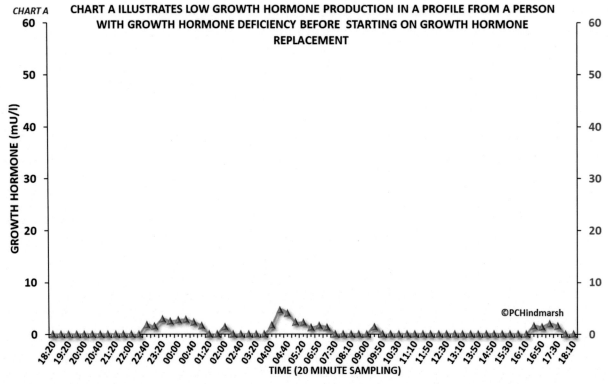

Figure 13.6 *Chart A illustrates the result of a 24 hour growth hormone profile in a person with growth hormone deficiency showing two pulses of growth hormone with very low peak values.*

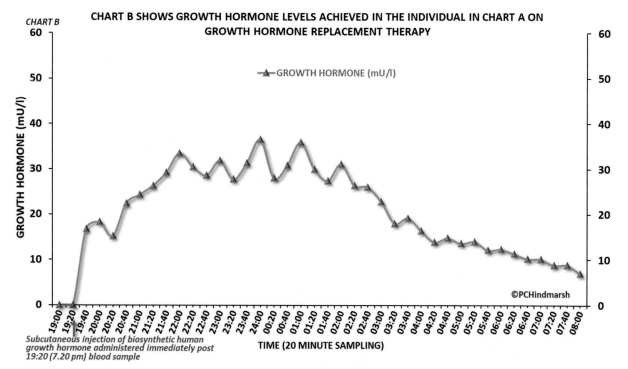

Figure 13.6 *Chart B illustrates an overnight profile in the same person studied in Figure 13.6 Chart A. Immediately following the blood sample drawn at 19:20 (7.20 pm) a subcutaneous injection of biosynthetic human growth hormone was given which attained a similar peak to that observed in Figure 13.5 but lacking the discrete bursts associated with normal growth hormone secretion.*

The replacement of growth hormone, in this case with a subcutaneous injection of biosynthetic human growth hormone, delivers a similar peak growth hormone concentration to that seen in Figure 13.5, but the profile lacks the distinct bursts of growth hormone that characterise normal growth hormone secretion. Despite this, this therapy does produce a normalisation of growth.

The prolonged exposure to growth hormone may alter how other endocrine pathways function. Examples are growth hormone, increasing insulin resistance (please see Chapter 8, Part 2) and as already mentioned in this chapter (Figure 13.1), growth hormone effects on the cortisol–cortisone shuttle.

Growth hormone therapy is used extensively in hypopituitarism in both children, to promote growth and in adults, to allay some of the metabolic consequences of growth hormone deficiency, such as adverse cardiovascular lipid profiles with high total cholesterol and very low-density lipoprotein cholesterol. Very low-density lipoprotein cholesterol is very damaging to the wall of the blood vessels, particularly those supplying the heart muscle. Growth hormone therapy reduces total cholesterol, as well as that present as very low-density lipoprotein cholesterol.

Growth hormone therapy appears to be associated with less circulating cortisol and an increase in cortisol concentration in the urine. This is likely to pose problems, particularly if the hydrocortisone replacement is suboptimal, because cortisol will be lost in the urine and as the dose of hydrocortisone is already inappropriately low, the person may develop symptoms of cortisol under replacement.

From the data available, it appears growth hormone may directly or indirectly modulate the activity of 11beta-hydroxysteroid dehydrogenase type 1 (Figure 13.1), by reducing enzyme activity so that cortisone cannot be converted as efficiently back into cortisol.

It is unclear whether the effect is a direct one of growth hormone, or is mediated indirectly via the production of insulin-like growth factor-1 (IGF-1) by growth hormone. What is clear is either growth hormone and/or IGF-1 are associated with inhibition of 11beta-hydroxysteroid dehydrogenase type 1, decreasing the conversion of cortisone to cortisol. Studies would suggest that *in vitro* it is IGF-1 which is responsible for this effect. These findings have important clinical implications.

1. Firstly, the growth hormone increase in cortisol metabolism might precipitate adrenal insufficiency in hypopituitary patients commencing on growth hormone therapy but who are only partially ACTH deficient, as they cannot compensate for the lower cortisol by increasing ACTH production.

2. Secondly, these changes mean there becomes an imbalance in the cortisol to cortisone shuttle. If dosing with hydrocortisone is fixed on a daily basis, then a deficiency or insufficiency in cortisol will result as there is now an inability to convert back from cortisone to cortisol in the liver. This would imply alterations to the dosing of the hydrocortisone would be required when growth hormone therapy is instituted in individuals already on hydrocortisone replacement. Prednisolone doses also have to be altered. Dexamethasone doses will also need some adjustment which is more difficult to get right due to the flattish profile of dexamethasone. Blood levels of both prednisolone and dexamethasone are hard to check as there are no commercial assays available.

Growth hormone has a similar effect on thyroxine metabolism. In this situation, long term GH replacement therapy decreases serum free thyroxine (FT4) and increases serum free triiodothyronine (FT3) levels. These changes result from increased peripheral conversion of T4 to T3. Generally, this does not constitute a problem unless FT4 was low to begin with. Careful monitoring of thyroid function during growth hormone treatment is required.

THYROXINE AND CORTISOL

Thyroxine, like cortisol plays an important role in many metabolic processes. We saw in Chapter 8 that cortisol has many effects on the cardiovascular system. Thyroxine does too. Too much thyroxine increases the heart rate, whereas too little has the opposite effect. In adrenal insufficiency, thyroxine deficiency can coexist with cortisol deficiency especially in autoimmune conditions such as Addison's disease or in secondary adrenal insufficiency due to hypopituitarism. If we diagnose both at the same time it is important to be careful with commencing replacement with hydrocortisone or any glucocorticoid. Although 9 alpha-fludrocortisone has glucocorticoid properties, it does not seem to cause problems, probably because it is usually introduced after the person has been established on glucocorticoid therapy.

If thyroxine is started before the patient has been established on cortisol replacement, then a rapid acceleration in heart rate, particularly in older people, can result. This can lead to heart failure or atrial fibrillation. Further, adrenal crises have been reported when thyroxine therapy has been started in patients with undiagnosed hypoadrenalism. Cortisol replacement should always be started first for 2 to 3 days before introducing thyroxine.

Glucocorticoids themselves can alter thyroxine production and metabolism. Thyroxine (T4) is produced in the thyroid gland and is converted to its active form T3. Doses of prednisolone used for their anti-inflammatory effect, may reduce plasma T4 and T3 levels due to suppression of thyrotropin-releasing hormone from the hypothalamus and thyroid-stimulating hormone from the anterior pituitary gland.

These high doses also increase T4 binding to thyroxine-binding globulin, which may contribute to lower T4 transfer rates from plasma to extravascular sites and decreased T3 production from T4.

Figure 13.7 shows the production of T4 and T3 under the control of the hypothalamus and pituitary. Most of the circulating T3 comes from conversion of T4 to T3 in tissues other than the thyroid. Conversion of FT4 to FT3 uses the deiodinase (D) enzyme system, which is present as the D1 isoenzyme in the liver, kidneys and thyroid and the D2 isoenzyme in the hypothalamus, pituitary, thyroid and heart. Notice that T4 feedback on the hypothalamus and pituitary is mediated by conversion to T3 in both structures via the D2 isoenzyme.

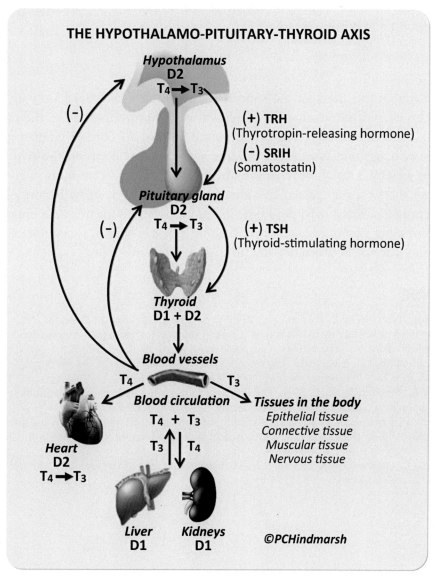

Figure 13.7 *The hypothalamo-pituitary-thyroid axis showing where thyroxine (T4) is converted to triiodothyronine (T3) in the body by the deiodinase isoenzymes D1 in the liver, kidneys and thyroid and D2 in the hypothalamus, pituitary, thyroid and heart. Thyrotropin-releasing hormone (TRH) stimulates thyroid-stimulating hormone (TSH) release from the pituitary and somatostatin (SRIH) switches off TSH release. Thyroid-stimulating hormone causes T4 and T3 to be synthesised and released from the thyroid.*

Finally, it is worth mentioning that thyroxine is influenced by similar drugs to those which affect cortisol. You will notice we have referred to thyroxine as T4 and FT4. Thyroxine, like cortisol, is carried around the bloodstream by carrier proteins, particularly thyroid binding globulin (TBG) which like cortisol binding globulin, is made in the liver. When we measure thyroxine in the blood, we can measure total thyroxine (T4) or free thyroxine (FT4). Most laboratory systems measure the latter these days. A similar situation pertains to T3 and FT3. Like our discussions on factors which influence cortisol binding globulin, there is a similar one for TBG. First and foremost are the oral contraceptive pill and also pregnancy, which alters the level of TBG, but unlike cortisol binding globulin, thyroid binding globulin is decreased by male hormones such as testosterone, so care needs to be taken when patients with hypopituitarism need replacement with both thyroxine and testosterone, thyroxine doses may need to be reduced. A person with intact thyroxine production taking testosterone, adjusts thyroxine production to normalise the FT4, but this cannot happen if on a fixed dose of thyroxine so the dose needs adjusting based on FT4 measurements. It is also important to be aware that absorption of thyroxine is decreased by oral iron therapies.

CONCLUSION

In endocrinology we tend to think of the various hormone systems as separate with little interaction between them. This chapter shows that the effects of some hormones such as the estrogens can alter cortisol by altering the balance between free and bound cortisol via cortisol binding globulin. In other situations, such as with arginine vasopressin the interaction occurs between the two hormones at the cellular level in the kidney. Finally, enzyme systems that modulate the amounts of cortisol in the body such as the cortisol shuttle are impacted by other hormones such as growth hormone which would alter how much cortisol is available to the body. These complex interactions are important to consider when we are determining dosing regimens and creating sick day rules for example. This is particularly the case in secondary adrenal insufficiency due to hypopituitarism.

FURTHER READING

Gelding, S.V., Taylor, N.F., Wood, P.J., et al., 1998. The effect of growth hormone replacement therapy on cortisol-cortisone interconversion in hypopituitary adults: evidence for growth hormone modulation of extrarenal 11beta-hydroxysteroid dehydrogenase activity. Clin Endocrinol (Oxf) 48, 153–162.

Hertel, J., König, J., Homuth, G., et al., 2017. Evidence for stress-like alterations in the HPA-axis in women taking oral contraceptives. Sci Rep 7, 14111. https://doi.org/10.1038/s41598-017-13927-7.

Qureshi, A.C., Bahri, A., Breen, L.A., et al., 2007. The influence of the route of oestrogen administration on serum levels of cortisol-binding globulin and total cortisol. Clin Endocrinol (Oxf). 66, 632–635.

Ufer, F., Diederich, S., Pedersen, E.B., et al., 2012. Arginine vasopressin-dependent and AVP-independent mechanisms of renal fluid absorption during thirsting despite glucocorticoid-mediated vasopressin suppression. Clin Endocrinol (Oxf) 78, 431–437.

White, P.C., Mune, T., Agarwal, A.K., 1997. 11β-Hydroxysteroid dehydrogenase and the syndrome of apparent mineralocorticoid excess. Endocr Rev 18, 135–156.

CHAPTER 14

Sodium and Water Balance

GLOSSARY

Cerebral oedema Swelling of the brain with water due to rapid correction of chronic hypernatraemia or to a sudden infusion of water into the circulation.

Fludrocortisone Cortisol modified with a fluorine atom which prolongs action on the mineralocorticoid receptor retaining salt and water.

Glucocorticoids A member of the steroid family similar to cortisol that are particularly involved in carbohydrate, protein and fat metabolism and have anti-inflammatory and immunomodulating properties.

Haematocrit An indirect measure of the circulating blood volume. When high this implies dehydration when low water overload. Haematocrit is a ratio of total red blood cell volume and the total blood volume. As total red blood cell volume does not change much haematocrit reflects changes in total blood volume.

Mineralocorticoid A member of the steroid family similar to aldosterone that is involved in sodium and water balance in the body.

Osmotic Demyelination Syndrome Destruction of the myelin sheath surrounding neurones resulting from too rapid correction of plasma sodium in chronic hyponatraemia. Can lead to severe neurological impairment.

Renin Protein made by the kidney that instructs the liver to make angiotensin which in turn is involved in making aldosterone (salt retaining hormone) in the adrenal glands.

Severe Hyponatraemia A plasma sodium concentration less than 120 mmol/l.

Severe Hypernatraemia A plasma sodium concentration greater than 150 mmol/l.

GENERAL

Sodium and water are critical for the functioning of all human cells. How well cells function depends on the ability of the body to regulate the sodium content of the fluid outside the cells, the extracellular fluid. Plasma sodium concentrations stay within a remarkably narrow range from 135 to 145 mmol/l despite large variations in salt (usually as sodium chloride) intake. There is tight regulation of this system together with water balance and failure of the system to regulate within this sodium range presents severe stresses to virtually all cells in the body, but particularly in the brain.

This is because the brain is contained in the skull so there is not much room for expansion (only 5%) and the cells are also very sensitive and easily damaged if they are forced to contract in size due to changes in sodium levels in the blood.

Water can move quickly into and out of brain cells, whereas sodium cannot, therefore imbalances between the blood and brain can establish rapidly. Figure 14.1 shows the distribution of fluids in the various body compartments in a 70 kilogram male where 60% of body weight is water. Notice that of the 42 litres of water in the body, only 3.5 litres are in the blood circulation (intravascular fluid).

Replacement Therapies in Adrenal Insufficiency. https://doi.org/10.1016/B978-0-12-824548-4.00005-X

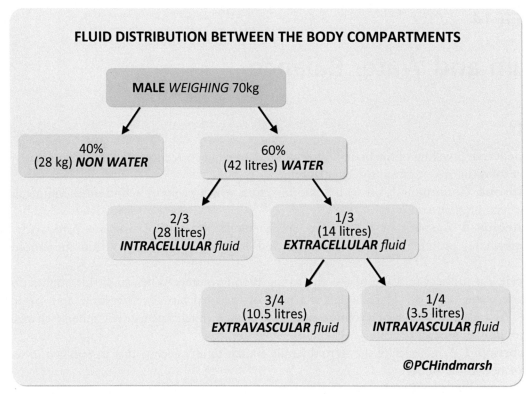

Figure 14.1 *The distribution of fluid in the various body compartments in a 70 kilogram adult male.*

This cellular stress arises because plasma sodium concentration affects cell volume. The term tonicity is used to describe the effect of plasma on cells.

Hypotonicity means there is either lower than normal amounts of sodium in the plasma or more water present than usual. This means there is more water outside the cell than inside (a gradient) and water will move into the cell causing it to swell.

Hypertonicity means there is more sodium outside the cell and/or less water, so the net gradient here means water will move out of the cell, causing the cells to shrink. Raised plasma sodium concentrations (hypernatremia) always indicates hypertonicity.

Usually hyponatraemia (low plasma sodium) indicates hypotonicity but there are some exceptions, such as hyponatraemia associated with hyperglycaemia. In this situation the glucose also contributes to the tonicity. We illustrate this concept of tonicity in Chapter 13, Figure 13.4.

If we now consider how sodium is distributed around the body, then we find that most of the sodium is in bone (45%), between cells (interstitial fluid) (30%) or in connective tissues (10%). Only 10% of sodium is present in the plasma of the blood (Figure 14.2). Glycosaminoglycans (GAGs) are important as places for sodium storage and those in connective tissues, particularly cartilage, are critical for maintaining cartilage structure and flexibility, as well as the ability of structures such as the vertebral discs in the spine to withstand the forces transmitted through the spine due to our standing posture.

Understanding sodium and water balance is important in primary adrenal insufficiency because of the loss of aldosterone formation, as well as the permissive effects of cortisol on the kidneys handling a water load. In hypopituitarism, loss of arginine vasopressin (AVP) as in cranial diabetes insipidus, leads to major problems in water retention particularly if associated with disorders of thirst (Chapter 13, Figure 13.3).

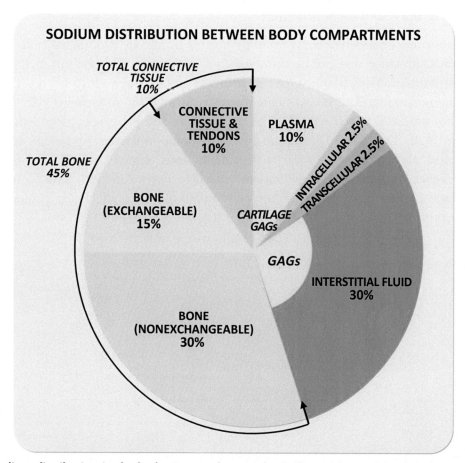

Figure 14.2 *Sodium distribution in the body. Most sodium in the body is in bone (45%), interstitial fluid (30%) and connective tissue (10%) whereas the amount in plasma which we measure in the laboratory only amounts to 10% of the total. Excess sodium is stored in cartilage and interstitial fluid (between cells) attached to glycosaminoglycans (GAG). (Redrawn from Ellison, D.H., Welling, P., 2021. Insights into salt handling and blood pressure. N Engl J Med 385, 1981—1993 with kind permission).*

PLASMA SODIUM AND WATER

The concentration of sodium is equal inside and outside of cells because water channels (aquaporins) makes cell membranes permeable to water. Within the membrane of the cell, there is a 'sodium pump' which functionally excludes sodium from cells and swaps it for potassium by means of an energy dependent process. It is potentially possible to create a situation where there is an imbalance of values across the cell membrane but any such gradient is quickly abolished by water movement across the cell membranes.

As a result, the concentration of sodium in plasma should equal the concentration of sodium plus potassium in total body water.

It is important to realise that a substantial amount of sodium is bound to large polyanionic macromolecules or proteoglycans which make up the substance of bone, connective tissue and cartilage. Proteoglycans in the skin, for example, serve as a sodium reservoir. Sodium concentration in cartilage is twice that of plasma. This is extremely important as it helps the cartilage tissue withstand high pressures when we stand up for long periods of time. A further example of the importance of sodium is in bone tissue.

It is well known through laboratory experimentation that chronic hyponatraemia is a more potent cause of osteopenia and fractures than vitamin D deficiency. Looking at Figure 14.2 this is not surprising given how much of the total body sodium is in bone (45%).

SODIUM AND THE BLOOD-BRAIN BARRIER

The blood-brain barrier is a highly selective semipermeable border of endothelial cells which prevents solutes (a solute is a substance that can be dissolved in a solution such as sodium in the blood) in the circulating blood from non-selectively crossing into the extracellular fluid of the central nervous system where neurons reside. The blood-brain barrier is formed by endothelial cells of the capillary wall, astrocyte foot processes which wrap around the capillary and pericytes embedded in the capillary wall itself (Figure 14.3). This system allows the passage of some molecules by passive diffusion, as well as the selective and active transport of various nutrients, ions, organic anions, and macromolecules such as glucose, water and amino acids which are crucial to nerve function. The blood-brain barrier restricts the passage of pathogens and immune cells and molecules, effectively protecting the brain from damage by these agents.

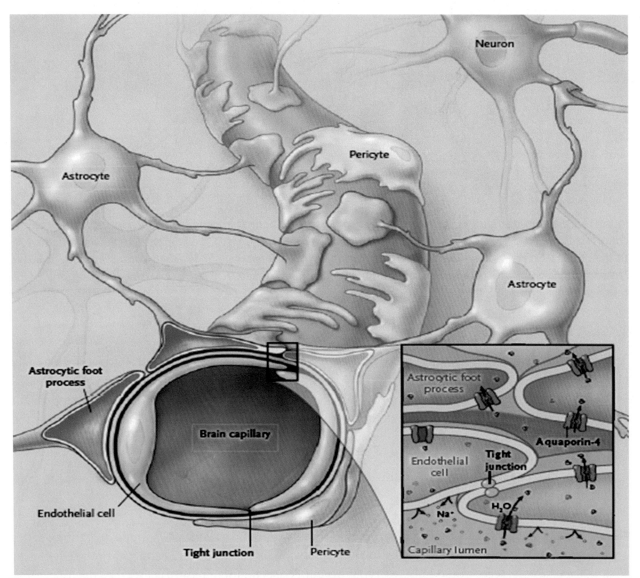

Figure 14.3 *The blood-brain barrier made up of the endothelial cells lining the capillary blood vessels of the brain, astrocyte supporting cells that are applied around the capillary and the pericytes sitting around the capillary. Both the endothelial cells and astrocyte foot processes have aquaporin-4 water channels that make them permeable to water but not to sodium (inset picture). (Reproduced with permission from Sterns, R.H., 2015. Disorders of plasma sodium - causes, consequences, and correction. N Engl J Med 372, 55—65).*

Sodium readily crosses permeable membranes through special clefts between endothelial cells. In most tissues therefore, the sodium concentrations of plasma and the fluid around the cells are nearly identical. However, this situation does not occur in the brain. Brain capillaries have the blood-brain barrier that sodium cannot cross. Both the endothelial cells and astrocyte foot processes have aquaporin-4 water channels which make them permeable to water but not to sodium.

In this situation, an abnormal plasma sodium concentration causes water to enter or leave the brain tissue. Because the brain is situated within the skull only a small degree of brain swelling (5%) or shrinkage is possible.

REGULATION OF THE PLASMA SODIUM CONCENTRATION

Two systems regulate the plasma sodium concentration. The first uses a series of cell volume receptors which are responsible for adjusting thirst and AVP secretion from the brain. These receptors are situated in the brain which is not too surprising given the effects the plasma sodium concentration can have on brain volume. Tight regulation is required.

The receptors are situated in the hypothalamus. In the day to day situation both thirst and AVP secretion are inhibited when the plasma sodium concentration falls below 135 mmol/l. As plasma sodium concentrations start to rise from 135 mmol/l, the levels of AVP increase linearly with the increasing sodium concentrations (Figure 14.4).

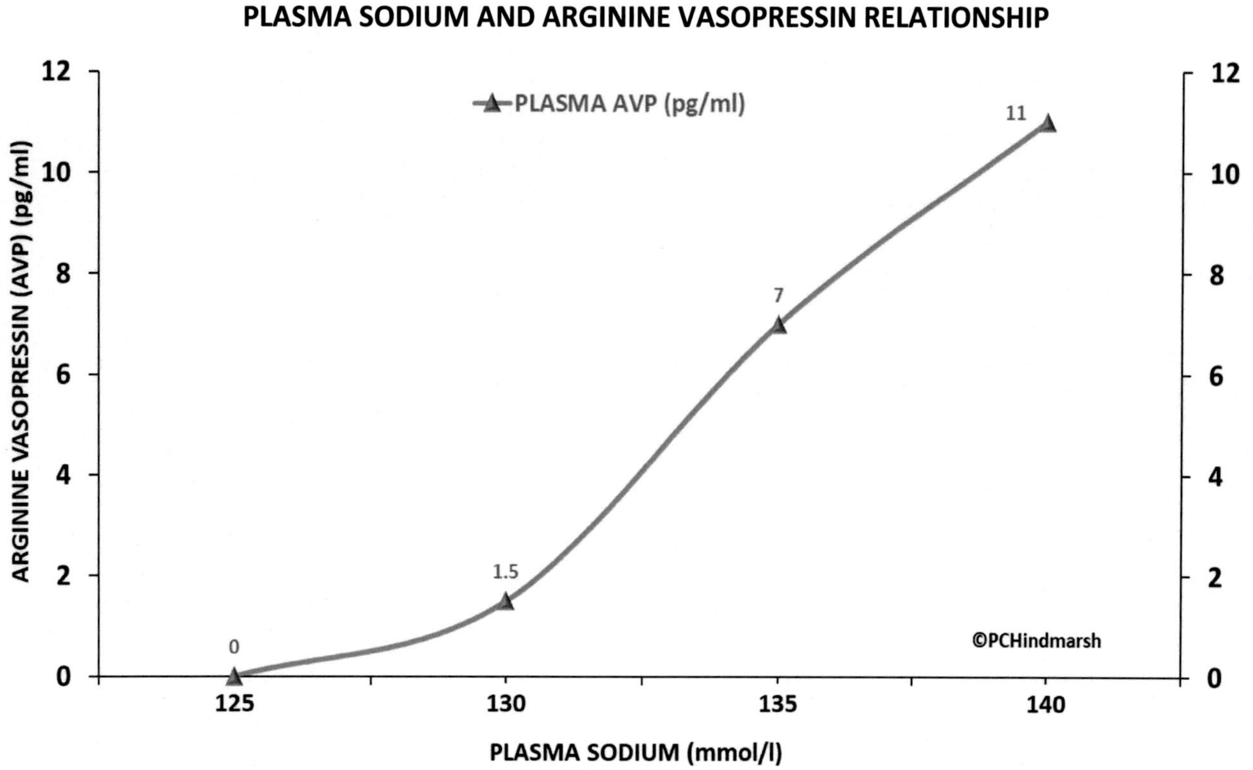

PLASMA SODIUM AND ARGININE VASOPRESSIN RELATIONSHIP

Figure 14.4 *As the plasma sodium concentration reaches 135 mmol/l arginine vasopressin (AVP) secretion increases linearly thereafter through the normal plasma sodium range.*

Arginine vasopressin binds to its V2 receptor in the cells lining the renal collecting duct and aquaporin (acquaporin-2) water channels are then inserted into the membrane facing the lumen, which allows water to flow from the lumen back into the kidney structure itself and into the bloodstream (Figure 14.5).

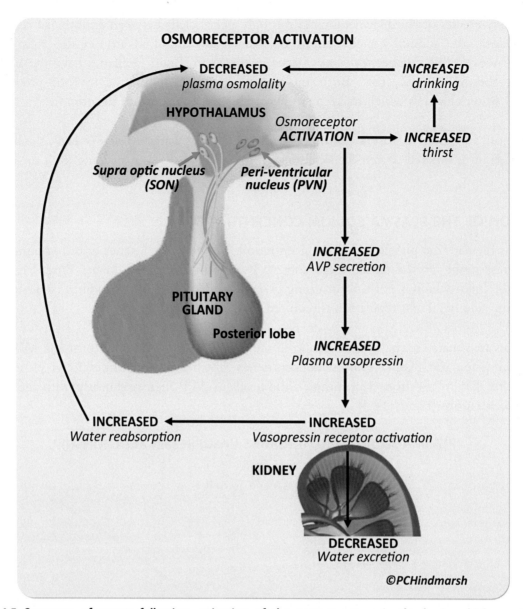

Figure 14.5 *Sequence of events following activation of the osmoreceptors in the brain which monitor blood concentration. In the situation shown the receptors are simulated by dehydration leading to arginine vasopressin release and water retention as well as simulating the sensation of thirst — SON is the supra optic nucleus and PVN the peri-ventricular nucleus where the AVP neurones originate.*

When the plasma sodium concentration increases to 145 mmol/l, AVP is high enough to result in a maximum concentrated urine of 1200 mOsmol/kg. If the urine is dilute when the plasma sodium concentration is above 145 mmol/l this implies either deficiency in AVP secretion (cranial diabetes insipidus) or a failure of the kidneys to respond to AVP (nephrogenic diabetes insipidus). Recent terminology suggests that in the future these two conditions will be referred to as AVP deficiency or AVP resistance respectively. It is important to realise that even complete diabetes insipidus with total absence of AVP, does not cause hypernatremia because the thirst mechanism prompts the person to drink to replace the urinary water loss. The thirst mechanism becomes active at a plasma sodium concentration of 145 mmol/l. The thirst mechanism can be damaged by the presence of some tumours in the hypothalamic area which damage both the AVP cells and the thirst centre. This produces a very dangerous situation because the individual cannot compensate for water loss by drinking more and can become seriously dehydrated. This dehydration can lead to thrombosis in the veins in the brain. Other situations which can be dangerous are if the patient is too young or old, or too sick to seek water themselves.

The second system that regulates the plasma sodium concentration is the renin-angiotensin-aldosterone system (Figure 14.6). This system senses changes in blood pressure and/or circulating blood volume in the kidneys. Cells in the juxtaglomerular area of the kidney synthesise, store and secrete the protein renin which acts on the liver to form angiotensin I. Angiotensin I is then converted into angiotensin II by angiotensin converting enzyme situated in the lungs.

Angiotensin II has two effects. First, it promotes vasoconstriction of the blood vessels and second, it regulates the production of aldosterone by the zona glomerulosa of the adrenal cortex. Aldosterone acts then on the kidney to retain sodium, and therefore water, in exchange for potassium. The net effect of these two actions of angiotensin II, direct and indirect, leads to an increase in circulating blood volume and restoration of blood pressure.

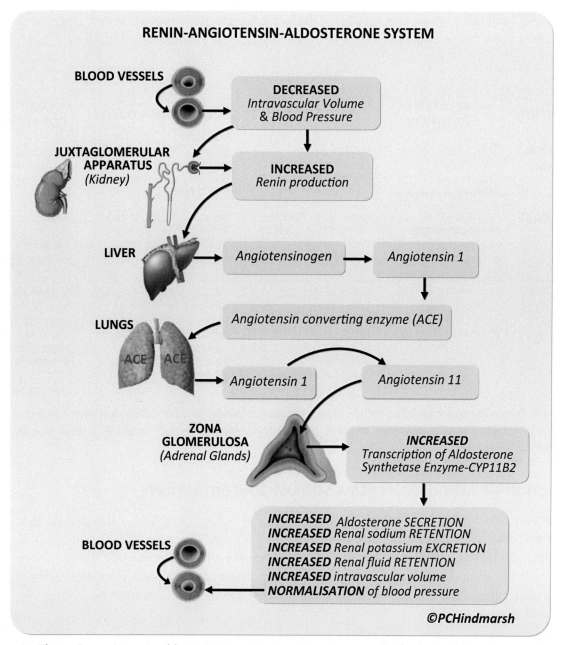

Figure 14.6 *The renin-angiotensin-aldosterone system responding to a reduction in intravascular volume and fall in blood pressure.*

CAUSES OF RAPID CHANGES IN PLASMA SODIUM CONCENTRATIONS

Plasma sodium concentrations will decrease rapidly if the amount of water ingested or infused intravenously exceeds the capacity of the kidneys to excrete free water. Plasma sodium concentration increases rapidly if large amounts of concentrated salt are ingested or infused, or if there are large unreplaced losses of electrolyte free water because of an osmotic diuresis as occurs in diabetes insipidus. A good guide is to note that loss or gain of approximately 3 ml of water per kilogram of body weight, will change the plasma sodium concentration by approximately 1 mmol/l. The results of abnormal plasma sodium concentrations and extremes of tonicity both damage cells. Hypotonicity ruptures cell membranes whereas extreme hypertonicity damages the cytoskeleton inside the cell and causes breaks in DNA, leading to cell death. Although these disturbances affect all cells, the clinical manifestation of hyponatraemia and hypernatremia are mainly neurological and rapid changes in plasma sodium concentrations in either direction can cause severe, permanent and sometimes lethal brain injury.

Figures 14.7 and 14.8 show the effects of hyponatraemia and hypernatraemia respectively while Figure 14.9 shows the consequences of rapid changes in plasma sodium concentrations.

HYPONATRAEMIA

DURATION	RELATED CONDITION	FEATURES	INITIAL TREATMENT	LIMIT OF CORRECTION
SEVERAL HOURS	*Self-induced water intoxication. Ecstasy use. Marathon running.*	*Seizures, coma, brain swelling and fatal brain herniation.*	*Bolus of 3% saline three times. Increase plasma sodium by 4 - 6 mmol/l in first 6 hours.*	*Excessive correction not known to be harmful.*
1 - 2 DAYS	*Postoperative hyponatraemia. Hyponatraemia associated with intracranial disease.*	*Headache, seizures, coma brain swelling and fatal brain herniation.*	*Bolus of 3% saline three times. Increase plasma sodium by 4 - 6 mmol/l in first 6 hours.*	*Maximum plasma sodium increase 10 mmol/l/day.*
UNKNOWN OR MORE THAN 2 DAYS	*High risk of osmotic demyelination syndrome with plasma sodium less than 105 mmol/l.*	*Malaise, fatigue, 10% risk of seizures if plasma sodium less than 110 mmol/l. Minimal risk of brain swelling. No risk of brain herniation.*	*3% bolus saline if having seizures. High risk of osmotic demyelination syndrome so increase in plasma sodium by 4 - 6 mmol/l in first 24 hours.*	*Maximum limit of sodium increase first day and thereafter 8 mmol/l/day.*

©PCHindmarsh

Figure 14.7 *Treatment and limits of correction of severe hyponatraemia (plasma sodium less than 120 mmol/l). If the duration of hyponatraemia is unknown or more than 2 days rapid correction results in a high risk of osmotic demyelination syndrome.*

CORRECTION OF ABNORMAL PLASMA SODIUM CONCENTRATIONS

Whilst prompt management of hyponatraemia and hypernatraemia is required, it is important to recognise the dangers posed by excessive corrections which can be potentially harmful. This is particularly important in patients with adrenal insufficiency due to primary adrenal problems because salt loss is an ever present concern and the salt loss either at presentation or during illness can take place over short or long periods of time, which alters how we deal with the subsequent replacement of sodium.

The hyponatraemia in primary adrenal insufficiency is usually associated with a reduced blood volume and increased kidney loss of sodium.

HYPERNATRAEMIA

DURATION	RELATED CONDITION	FEATURES	INITIAL TREATMENT	LIMIT OF CORRECTION
MINUTES TO HOURS	Acute salt poisoning. Use of hypertonic saline in IV fluids. Errors in dialysis.	Seizures, coma, brain thrombosis and intracranial haemorrhages.	Rapid infusion of 5% dextrose in water plus emergency haemodialysis.	Excessive correction is not known to be harmful.
1 - 2 DAYS	Unreplaced water from urine loss associated with diabetes mellitus or diabetes insipidus.	Coma and brain demyelination.	Decrease plasma sodium by 2 mmol/l/hr until reaching 145 mmol/l. Stop or replace water loss.	Excessive correction is not known to be harmful.
UNKNOWN OR MORE THAN 2 DAYS	Diarrhoea in children. Lack of drinking in adults.	Coma, rehydration associated seizures and cerebral oedema in children in particular.	Children decrease plasma sodium by 0.3 mmol/l/day. Adults reduce by 0.5 mmol/l/day. Replace water loss.	Children 0.5 mmol/l/hr 3% saline for seizures associated with rehydration.

©PCHindmarsh

Figure 14.8 *Treatment and limits of correction of severe hypernatraemia (plasma sodium more than 150 mmol/l). If the duration of hypernatraemia is unknown or more than 2 days a rapid reduction can result in a high risk of cerebral oedema.*

EFFECTS OF RAPID CHANGES IN PLASMA SODIUM CONCENTRATION

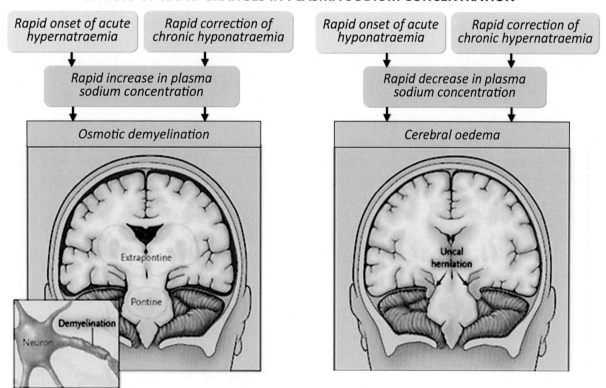

Figure 14.9 *Schematic representation of the effects of rapid increase in plasma sodium concentration on the brain (left panel) leading to osmotic demyelination of the brain neurones or a rapid decrease in plasma sodium concentration leading to (right panel) cerebral oedema and brain herniation. (Reproduced with kind permission from Sterns, R.H., 2015. Disorders of plasma sodium - causes, consequences, and correction. N Engl J Med 372, 55—65).*

Hyponatraemia can occur in secondary adrenal insufficiency particularly when cortisol is deficient or poorly replaced. This is because the kidneys cannot excrete a water load in the absence of cortisol, so water is retained and sodium levels in the blood fall. The increased water retained dilutes the amount of sodium in the blood lowering the concentration. This means the blood volume is normal or increased and these patients are rarely dehydrated, so fluid therapy is different. Large volumes of fluid are not needed as they are already replete, but care is needed when cortisol is replaced, as a sudden loss of water via the kidney (water diuresis) can occur.

This contrasts with primary adrenal insufficiency where sodium is lost through the kidney due to the lack of aldosterone. The sodium loss is accompanied by some water loss, so the net effect is a low plasma sodium concentration (hyponatraemia) along with a reduced blood volume. Treatment in this situation is to carefully replete the body with water and sodium.

In secondary adrenal insufficiency when there is also cortisol and AVP deficiencies, extreme care is needed when adjusting cortisol doses as the fine balance between the interaction of cortisol and DDAVP in the kidney can easily be upset with water loss and retention occurring.

Severe hyponatraemia is defined as a plasma sodium concentration of less than 120 mmol/l. It is important to determine the time over which the person is likely to have developed hyponatraemia as this influences how the patient is managed (Figure 14.7), because the length of time influences the way in which it should be treated/corrected. Brain swelling from an abrupt onset of hyponatraemia results in increased intracranial pressure, impaired cerebral blood flow and sometimes causes brain herniation (Figure 14.9). In this situation for severe symptoms such as seizures, a bolus of 3% saline can be given. A good rule of thumb is that 1ml of 3% saline/kg body weight (to a maximum of 100 ml) will raise the plasma sodium by 1 mmol/l. This can be repeated three times.

Because the sodium adaptation across the blood-brain barrier is slow, the acute situation can be managed as above. However, for chronic hyponatraemia a more cautious approach is required to avoid brain demyelination.

Fatal brain swelling is relatively rare in acute hyponatraemia and has only been reported in those with intracranial disease. Because the brain is contained within the rigid skull it cannot swell by much more than 5%, correction of hyponatraemia by this amount would be expected to prevent the most serious complications of acute water intoxication. In this situation where the hyponatraemia has come on rapidly, a simple increase in the plasma sodium concentration of 4 − 6 mmol/l is enough to reverse impending brain herniation or to stop active seizures. This can be easily achieved with a 1 ml of 3% saline/kg body weight (to a maximum of 100 ml). This is administered at 10 minute intervals to a total of three doses, if necessary, to control symptoms.

Brain injury after the rapid correction of chronic hyponatraemia manifests as a biphasic syndrome called the osmotic demyelination syndrome. In this situation an initial reduction of symptoms is followed by a gradual onset of new neurological problems. The clinical spectrum is quite broad and includes seizures, behavioural abnormalities and movement disorders.

The most severely affected patients become 'locked in.' They are unable to move, speak or swallow because of demyelination of the central pons (Figure 14.10). Similarly, acute hypernatremia may also cause brain demyelination but without this biphasic clinical course.

CENTRAL PONTINE MYELINOLYSIS

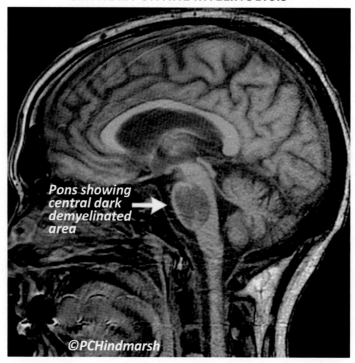

Figure 14.10 *Magnetic resonance image of central pontine myelinolysis showing the demyelination of the pons in the brain stem (white arrow).*

In practical terms, hyponatraemia is usually a chronic condition and it should be presumed to be chronic when the actual duration is unclear as this will reduce symptoms and improve potential outcomes. Chronic hyponatraemia should be corrected gradually with use of fluid restriction, salt supplementation, slow infusions of 3% saline, frusemide or vasopressin antagonists, or by treatment of the underlying cause. Severe symptoms of hyponatraemia may require more aggressive interventions, but there is no need to increase the plasma sodium concentration by more than 4 to 6 mmol/l/day.

Overcorrection can be dangerous. If the plasma sodium concentration is less than 120 mmol/l or if there are risk factors for osmotic demyelination, correction of the plasma sodium concentration by more than 8 mmol/l/day should be avoided through replacement of lost water or prevention of water loss with desmopressin.

If severe hypernatremia develops over a period of minutes or hours following a massive intake of salt, vascular injury created by a suddenly shrinking brain, causes intracranial haemorrhage. In the acute situation, prompt interventions are required as detailed in Figure 14.8.

Chronic hypernatremia like chronic hyponatraemia causes a reversible encephalopathy. This is particularly the case in infants and children and if rehydration is not undertaken with care, cerebral oedema and seizures can ensue. In the case of chronic hypernatremia, limiting the correction of the elevated plasma sodium concentration by decrements less than 0.5 mmol/l/hr reduces the risk of cerebral oedema and seizures associated with rehydration.

In both hyponatraemia and hypernatraemia a guide to the therapy comes from the frequent monitoring of the plasma sodium concentration and overreliance on formulas for sodium replacement is to be tempered.

FLUDROCORTISONE — 9 ALPHA-FLUDROCORTISONE

In this section, we will consider the drug 9 alpha-fludrocortisone and how its use can be monitored. At the end of the chapter, we will look at blood pressure itself and what can be done when problems develop.

What is 9 alpha-Fludrocortisone?

9 alpha-fludrocortisone which we will refer to from now on as fludrocortisone is a synthetic corticosteroid which has a structure very similar to cortisol. As we have previously mentioned, introducing a fluorine atom prolongs the action of a steroid and this has happened with the construction of fludrocortisone where fluorine has been introduced into the ring structure at position 9. The orientation of this is in the 'alpha' position and this gives the full name to the drug '9 alpha-Fludrocortisone'. Figure 14.11 shows the comparison between fludrocortisone and hydrocortisone.

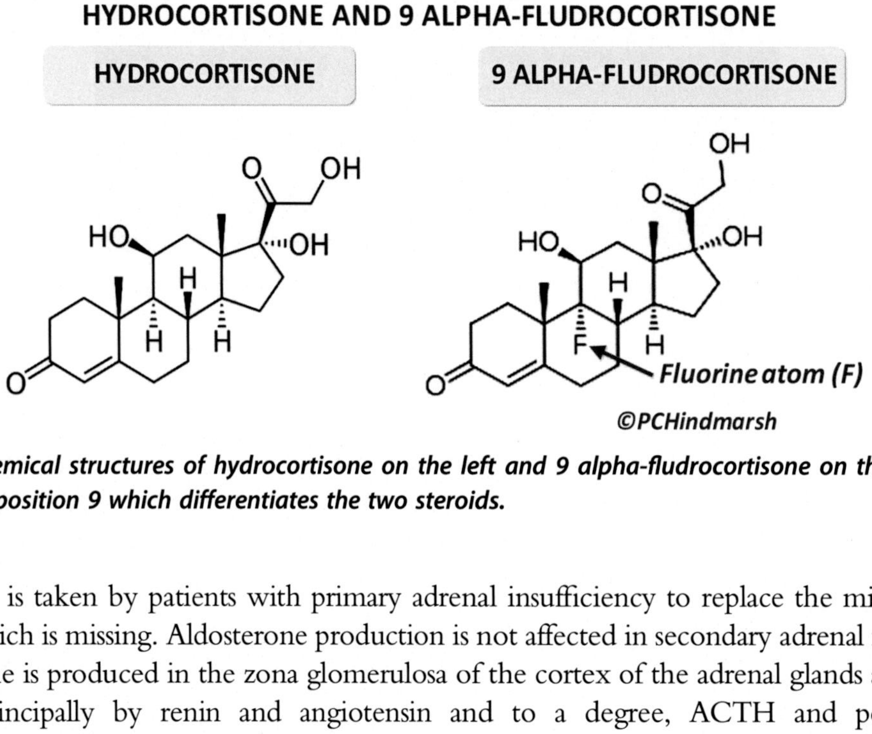

Figure 14.11 *Chemical structures of hydrocortisone on the left and 9 alpha-fludrocortisone on the right. Note the fluorine atom at position 9 which differentiates the two steroids.*

Fludrocortisone is taken by patients with primary adrenal insufficiency to replace the mineralocorticoid, aldosterone, which is missing. Aldosterone production is not affected in secondary adrenal insufficiency. In brief, aldosterone is produced in the zona glomerulosa of the cortex of the adrenal glands and its secretion is mediated principally by renin and angiotensin and to a degree, ACTH and potassium levels. Aldosterone retains sodium in the kidney as well as the large bowel and details of the control system are illustrated in Figure 14.6.

Fludrocortisone and hydrocortisone have salt retaining properties, whereas dexamethasone does not and prednisolone has some. Of interest is that fludrocortisone was the first synthetic corticosteroid to be marketed followed the introduction of cortisone in 1948 and hydrocortisone (cortisol) in 1951 and was also the first fluorine containing pharmaceutical drug.

How Does Fludrocortisone Work?

Fludrocortisone like hydrocortisone is rapidly and completely absorbed after oral administration and the blood levels are reached as a peak, between 4 and 8 hours. Like hydrocortisone, fludrocortisone is attached to various proteins in the blood which act as a pool for the drug and evens out the way that it is distributed throughout the 24 hours.

The half-life of fludrocortisone is approximately two to three hours and the fluorine molecule prolongs its duration of action.

The introduction of the fluorine atom means that fludrocortisone is no longer easily broken down by the enzyme 11β-hydroxysteroid dehydrogenase type 2 (HSD-2) (see Chapter 6). As you may recall, this is part of the cortisol shuttle and converts cortisol, which is the active glucocorticoid to cortisone, which is biologically inactive. The levels of HSD-2 are very high around the mineralocorticoid (salt retaining hormone) receptor in the kidney. This prevents cortisol from binding to the aldosterone receptor. This is important because the concentration of aldosterone in the blood is measured in picomoles (pmol/l) whereas cortisol is measured in nanomoles (nmol/l). In other words, there is a thousand times more cortisol around than aldosterone and if the HSD-2 was not operative, then cortisol would swamp the mineralocorticoid receptor leading to excessive salt and water retention which ultimately would raise blood pressure. This can be seen in situations where there is a genetic abnormality in the HSD-2 gene leading to an inactive enzyme and the clinical manifestation is severe hypertension. This clever manipulation of fludrocortisone allows for a prolonged duration of action and avoids conversion to an inert product.

As such, fludrocortisone has salt retaining properties, but it also has a dexamethasone like action because it is very similar in structure to dexamethasone.

Fludrocortisone Action

Fludrocortisone acts in the kidney to direct the absorption of sodium in exchange for potassium. Fludrocortisone not only retains sodium in the kidney but also in the large bowel. The amount of sodium which can be retained per day by the kidney or reabsorbed through the gut, is limited to the total amount of sodium taken in. In a western diet we normally take in at least 2 millimoles/kilogram body weight of salt/day.

If you become salt depleted, unless you increase the amount of sodium in the diet, you will never make up the deficiency because there is only a certain amount of salt fludrocortisone can retain per day, namely the normal daily intake.

This is particularly the case in the newborn. It is often common practice in situations where plasma sodium concentrations have been low, to continue to increase the amount of fludrocortisone to try and increase the plasma sodium. This is unlikely to achieve very much because the amount of sodium present in the diet and being absorbed is relatively limited and all that will happen, is the individual will suffer from the glucocorticoid effects of the fludrocortisone.

Other situations where salt balance can be quite important is during very hot days in the summer, but particularly when travelling to very hot countries near the equator. In such situations it is often important to have additional salt supplementation, particularly because of increased salt loss in sweat.

Dosing with Fludrocortisone

As with hydrocortisone, the dose of fludrocortisone is calculated initially in terms of the size of the body. The amount required varies with age. In the newborn, the dose is 150 micrograms/m^2 body surface area/day, whereas in childhood this decreases to 100 micrograms/m^2 body surface area/day and by adulthood may be as low as 50 micrograms/m^2 body surface area/day.

The reason for the changes is the newborn baby's kidneys are not as responsive to aldosterone as later in childhood due to reduced expression of the mineralocorticoid receptor (docking station). In the preterm baby the situation is even more complicated because not only is the mineralocorticoid receptor not adequately expressed in the kidney, but aldosterone formation is also compromised (Figure 14.12).

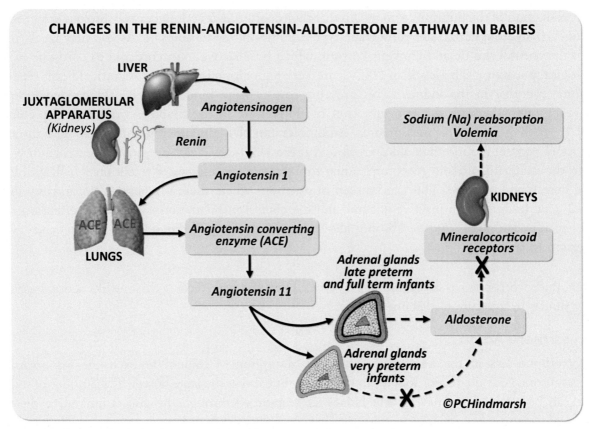

Figure 14.12 *Changes in the renin-angiotensin-aldosterone pathway in babies. In the preterm infant there is reduced aldosterone production and in both preterm and term babies there is also reduced mineralocorticoid receptor expression in the kidney so aldosterone action is impaired.*

Monitoring Fludrocortisone Replacement

Although it has been suggested fludrocortisone replacement can be evaluated clinically, in practice it is difficult to achieve. Salt cravings and/or lightheadedness might indicate a need for an increased dose and body swelling might indicate water overload.

Such an approach, however, only detects marked under or over replacement, so overall it is more accurate to use biochemical measures to determine how good the replacement is.

MEASURES AVAILABLE TO ASCERTAIN ADEQUACY OF FLUDROCORTISONE REPLACEMENT

1. Plasma sodium measurements. The amount of sodium in blood can be easily measured and is a very useful measure after a salt-wasting crisis but it does not give us a good overview of the total body sodium (Figure 14.2). Simply trying to measure total body sodium is complicated and what many people do, is to measure the plasma sodium coupled with an estimate of the plasma renin activity or actual plasma renin concentration.

   In situations where we are using fludrocortisone because of an absence of aldosterone, if the fludrocortisone dosing is correct and by that we mean that it is acting on the kidney to retain sodium, then the plasma renin activity, or plasma renin concentration, once the body sodium has been restored after a salt-wasting crisis, should be within the normal range.

   Not getting the plasma sodium correct leads to long term problems. Firstly, the total blood volume will be low and symptoms of this may be headaches or dizziness particularly when standing up quickly. This is known as postural hypotension. Secondly, in the long term low sodium concentrations (less than 135 mmol/l) lead to osteoporosis (Chapter 8, Part 1). Thirdly, sodium is present in many other tissues of the body, as mentioned it is present in cartilage and ligaments. The sodium in cartilage takes with it water, which is what makes cartilage, particularly in the vertebral discs of the spine, very strong and capable of resisting huge stress forces when we walk, run or jump. It is not clear what persistent low sodium concentrations means with respect to cartilage and ligaments, but it might mean the bones and joints are unable to withstand the usual wear and tear of daily activity.

In addition to measuring plasma sodium, we can also measure plasma potassium. These two tend to go in opposite directions, if the fludrocortisone dose is too low, sodium will be lost in the urine and the plasma potassium will be high and we see this in a salt-wasting crisis. High and for that matter low potassium levels, can lead the heart to beat irregularly and particularly if potassium is too high, the heart can stop beating altogether.

If the fludrocortisone dose is too high the sodium will move towards the upper end of the normal range but will not go over 145 mmol/l, as the body will always compensate by retaining water which will have the effect of increasing blood pressure. However, a high plasma sodium will be accompanied by a low plasma potassium which is not good for heart function or blood pressure. We know that a diet high in sodium and low in potassium, which is most western diets, can through the way the kidneys work, lead to high blood pressure. This is probably why a high fibre and potassium containing diet reduces blood pressure.

Salt intake should be minimised throughout the general population, which will reduce water retention, ankle swelling and high blood pressure. The American Heart Association recommends a sodium intake of no more than 1200 mg/day (2 to 2.5 mmol/kg/day) in children aged 4 to 8 years of age and 2300 mg/day (1.5 mmol/kg/day) in adults moving toward an ideal limit of no more than 1500 mg/day for most adults. In fact, the body needs only a small amount of sodium (less than 500 mg/day) to function properly. Note the guideline to reduce to 1500 mg may not apply to people who lose large amounts of sodium in sweat, like competitive athletes and workers exposed to major heat stress, such as foundry workers and firefighters.

Sodium replacement should be carefully considered for those who take fludrocortisone and guided by measurements of renin, plasma sodium and potassium levels, as well as side effects such as ankle swelling and raised blood pressure. It is important to remember that other factors might be responsible for high blood pressure, such as obesity, genetics and family history and physical inactivity.

Overall, however, using plasma sodium to monitor fludrocortisone replacement is not the best method. The amount of sodium in blood can be easily measured and is an extremely useful measure after a salt-wasting crisis, but it does not give us a good overview of the total body sodium.

A considerable amount of sodium can be lost before it shows in a blood test.

When contemplating fludrocortisone as replacement therapy in patients with adrenal insufficiency, there are two other problems/factors to consider:

i)   Firstly, the normal range of plasma sodium concentrations. If at the lower end (less than 135 mmol/l), then we do need to increase the fludrocortisone dose and some extra salt may be required. At the other end of the range (145 mmol/l) interpretation is difficult. If the fludrocortisone dose is too high, the sodium will move towards the upper end of the normal range but will not go over 145 mmol/l, as the body will always compensate by retaining water which will have the effect of increasing blood pressure. The problem is that we cannot be sure when sodium is at the upper end of the range, whether the fludrocortisone dose is adequate or too much. We can measure blood pressure which would be high if too much sodium and water are retained, but this is a late effect and if present for a long time may not be reversible. We do not want that to happen, so we need to be warned of any potential problem earlier before blood pressure increases.

ii)   Secondly, in adrenal insufficiency due to hypothalamus and pituitary problems, a low sodium is more likely to reflect low hydrocortisone dosing as when cortisol is low the kidneys are less able to excrete water, so water is retained in the body diluting body spaces and reducing the plasma sodium. Treatment here is to ensure both the hydrocortisone and DDAVP balance is optimal before thinking fludrocortisone is required. The latter is unlikely as the renin-angiotensin-aldosterone axis is not affected in secondary adrenal insufficiency.

2. Plasma renin activity (PRA) or plasma renin concentration. There is a slight difference between these two measurements. Plasma renin concentration is the measurement of the actual amount of renin in the blood. Plasma renin activity is a measure of the enzymatic effect of renin, so is more a measure of its biological activity. Plasma renin and PRA need to be measured carefully. We usually undertake this in the resting position after lying down for a period of 2 to 3 hours and then after standing or being active for 2 to 3 hours. This is easily done during a 24 hour cortisol profile. These measurements give us important information because plasma renin or PRA tends to increase slightly in the standing position, in order to cope with the change in blood volume resulting from the upright position. What we want in individuals where we are replacing with fludrocortisone, is to keep both the resting and the standing plasma renin or PRA within the normal range (less than 10 ng/ml/hr for PRA). A high value might indicate that we are under replacing with fludrocortisone and the blood volume is low.

This often leads to the phenomenon of postural hypotension (low blood pressure on standing upright quickly). This can be identified by measuring blood pressure in the lying and standing positions. A drop in systolic blood pressure of more than 20 mm Hg, or in diastolic blood pressure of more than 10 mm Hg, is considered abnormal.

In more detail we use the recumbent and standing plasma renin or PRA as follows. If taking fludrocortisone and the blood sample is taken after a period of rest and lying down and shows a high plasma renin or PRA, the dose needs increasing. If the lying down value is normal but the standing up value is high, then an increased dose is needed as well, as this indicates the blood volume is on the low side, as when standing up the blood pressure falls further. The low blood volume increases renin signaling to the renin-angiotensin system which tries to instruct the adrenal glands to make aldosterone.

In primary adrenal insufficiency, the adrenal glands are unable to produce aldosterone of course, but the rise in renin/PRA informs us the fludrocortisone dose needs to be adjusted and more fludrocortisone is needed to prevent the decrease in blood volume and blood pressure change. Lying and standing renin/PRA measures provide a more complete picture of what is happening and these results will be more accurate than a normal blood test, where the result could be raised by the activity (often rushed) prior to getting the blood test. The range of renin values is such that we can easily ascertain if we are giving too much or too little fludrocortisone and this occurs with plasma sodium values which are still within the normal range. So, renin/PRA is a much more sensitive indicator of sodium and water balance than just plasma sodium alone.

3. Blood pressure. This is more of a long term measure of how well the fludrocortisone has been dosed. As fludrocortisone retains sodium, water will also be retained with it. This increase in the retention of water in the body leads to an increase in blood pressure. As long as the renin is within normal range then blood pressure will also be within the normal range for height. However, what we do not want to occur is for blood pressure to start tracking upwards into the upper half of the normal range, because if this happens it could indicate that in the long term, we are giving too much fludrocortisone. Blood pressure changes with age and size particularly in children, so any measurement has to be plotted on a set of standards. Just as a high blood pressure (hypertension) can be a problem, low blood pressure (hypotension) can indicate that we are under dosing with fludrocortisone. We would see this in our measurement of lying and standing blood pressure.

4. Haematocrit. The final way of assessing fludrocortisone replacement is to measure the haematocrit. The haematocrit is the ratio of total red blood cell volume and the total blood volume. As the total red blood cell volume does not change much most of the time, haematocrit reflects a change in blood volume. This gives a guide to how the circulating blood volume is maintained. If the haematocrit is raised, this suggests that the circulating blood volume is reduced and often means that more fludrocortisone is needed.

Haematocrit is really useful for fine tuning as it can show changes before they manifest in terms of blood pressure or renin/PRA.

Another way we can check on the blood volume is to measure the urea level in the blood. Urea levels that are low may reflect too much water in the circulation whereas a high urea level might imply dehydration or a low blood volume. Unfortunately, urea is also influenced by other factors such as body nitrogen turnover, so it is not as specific as the other measures we have talked about.

Side Effects, Contra Indications and Drug Interactions

As fludrocortisone resembles cortisol, the side-effects, drug interactions and contra indications are exactly the same as those we have described in Chapter 6. The most important difference from hydrocortisone is the effect on blood pressure.

There are some specific drugs which need to be considered as they also interface with fludrocortisone. Diuretics and drugs that affect blood pressure and electrolytes might interact with fludrocortisone and may require dose adjustments. This is because it is quite easy to produce hypokalemia (low plasma potassium) which as we have already said can be problematic in terms of heart function. Liquorice and grapefruit juice potentiate the mineralocorticoid effect of hydrocortisone, in particular by reducing the conversion of cortisol to cortisone in the case of the former and inhibition of cytochrome P450 3A4 which helps metabolise cortisol in the case of the latter, so this may enhance the overall effect of fludrocortisone and they should be avoided.

An important aspect of fludrocortisone use is the effect on the eyes.

Both glucocorticoids and fludrocortisone can produce cataracts (opacification in the lens of the eye). However, the increase in water retention which can occur with high doses of fludrocortisone may increase the pressure within the eye and lead to glaucoma, or if the person already has glaucoma this may worsen. (Chapter 8, Part 6). The increase in water retention in the eye, may also lead to blurred vision and dosing with fludrocortisone should only be increased in small increments of 25 micrograms and checks undertaken with respect to the effect on plasma sodium, renin/PRA and blood pressure.

Extreme care needs to be undertaken with fludrocortisone because of this sodium and water retention effect.

We have mentioned above the effects on the eye, but it is also important to note that if the doses are kept high for long periods of time, not only will hypertension and peripheral swelling occur, but cardiac enlargement can follow along with congestive heart failure. The ongoing potassium loss can lead to total body potassium depletion which may place a person at particular risk of cardiac rhythm abnormalities.

High doses will also draw water from the large bowel into the circulation leading to harder stools and constipation.

Do I need to double dose with Fludrocortisone when unwell?

This is a good question. **The answer is *NO*.**

The reason that extra dosing is not needed is that you will only generate more problems by doing this. If you take extra fludrocortisone, it will retain slightly more sodium and therefore water which will expand the blood volume and may even lead to high blood pressure. Although this might be thought of as a good idea, the major problem is that fludrocortisone will retain sodium and lose potassium.

Potassium loss leads to low blood potassium levels which are really dangerous as this leads to heart rate problems and can lead, if they get too low, to the heart stopping working.

The right treatment if unwell is to double the hydrocortisone and also ensure a good intake of fluids. Clear fluids are ideal especially with some additional glucose. Sports Drinks contain extra sodium and can lead to protein breakdown, whereas extra salt in food during illness does not, so is preferred.

If you have an adrenal crisis and the sodium is low, then intravenous fluids are the way to rectify the problem, as the total body sodium will have fallen and no matter how much fludrocortisone is given, it will not raise the sodium. The only way to do that is to give more as fluid.

Finally, if unwell you will be increasing the hydrocortisone which has a salt retaining effect which will also ensure that plasma sodium is maintained in the normal range.

SALT AND WATER BALANCE AND BLOOD PRESSURE

Raised blood pressure is a major health risk for cardiovascular disease. The ideal blood pressure has been harder to define and still remains controversial in some circles. Rather than try to determine the normal range for blood pressure as we would for other biological measures, a more pragmatic approach has been undertaken to determine at what levels of blood pressure are problems likely to be encountered in the future.

Figure 14.13 shows the risk of cardiovascular disease related to blood pressure with risk standardised to a value of 1 for the lowest blood pressure of 115 mm Hg systolic and 75 mm Hg diastolic.

Increases in both systolic and diastolic pressure are associated with an increase in cardiovascular risk.

From these data, in adults, it is generally viewed that blood pressure values of 135 mm Hg systolic and 85 mm Hg diastolic (135/85 mm Hg systolic/diastolic) and over should be treated, with a target to reduce the systolic below 130 mm Hg and closer to 120 mm Hg and the diastolic down to 70 mm Hg.

In children, blood pressure changes with age and body size so both of these need to be adjusted for in order to interpret the recorded value. Blood pressure measures can be plotted on centile charts (Figure 14.14) or recorded using an app that adjusts for age and body size (National Institutes of Health Peds CV Guidelines version 2.0.6.20150407).

An annual review should include measurement of blood pressure in children and in adults and we use measurements overnight to allow us to identify blood pressure problems sooner. The first sign of problems emerging is the loss of the normal 10% drop in blood pressure which takes place overnight.

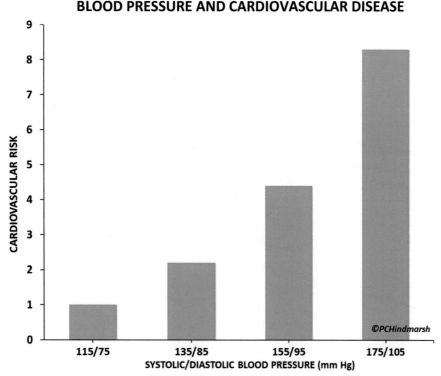

Figure 14.13 *Risk of developing cardiovascular disease at different levels of blood pressure standardised against risk with a blood pressure of 115 mm Hg systolic and 75 mm Hg diastolic.*

High Blood Pressure

We have already mentioned how high blood pressure can be defined on the risk of developing cardiovascular disease. In paediatrics, high blood pressure is defined as blood pressure values between the 90th and 95th centile on the blood pressure charts (Figure 14.14). Hypertension is defined as a blood pressure value over the 95th centile. Recording both systolic or diastolic blood pressures is important because they tell us a lot of about how the heart and circulation is responding. You can have high or low blood pressure in either the systolic or diastolic components but the one that is really important is high systolic blood pressure.

High blood pressure nearly always responds to reconsideration of the dose of glucocorticoids and in particular the dose of the mineralocorticoid fludrocortisone. For example, in rheumatoid arthritis, prednisolone doses greater than 7.5 mg/day are associated with a 17% increased risk of hypertension. Simply reducing the dose based on careful biochemical work is often all that is needed. However, aldosterone induced hypertension is mediated initially by an increase in blood volume, but after 8 weeks the volume falls back towards normal and the raised blood pressure is maintained by changes in the blood vessels themselves. This is when the high blood pressure or hypertension persists and it may then be necessary to use the various drugs which block angiotensin formation or action. Treating raised blood pressure can be difficult and despite the availability of several medications and lifestyle measures to treat hypertension, approximately 20% of patients have resistant hypertension. Interestingly, there is a promising new medication (Baxdrostat) being developed to tackle untreatable high blood pressure, which decreases aldosterone production by blocking the enzyme CYP11B2 (see Chapter 2, Figure 2.3). It is only by careful testing of the renin axis along with measuring blood pressure and sodium that careful adjustments can be made to the fludrocortisone dose. Increasing the fludrocortisone dose without careful checks, can lead to major problems because it is not only blood pressure that may be affected but the pressure in other organs such as the eye.

BLOOD PRESSURE CENTILES

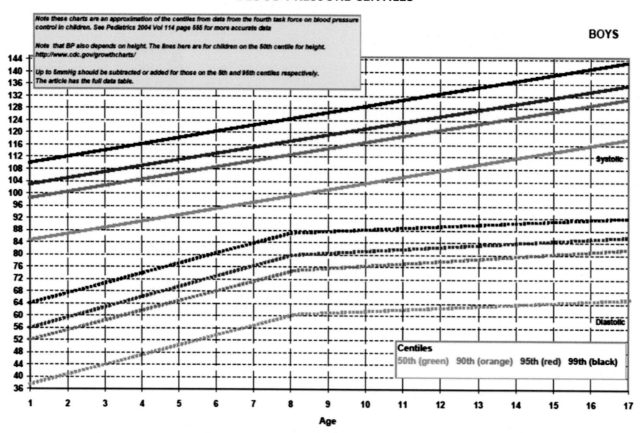

Figure 14.14A *Blood pressure centile chart for boys with systolic blood pressures in solid lines and diastolic blood pressures in dashed lines. (With permission from International Paediatric Task Force).*

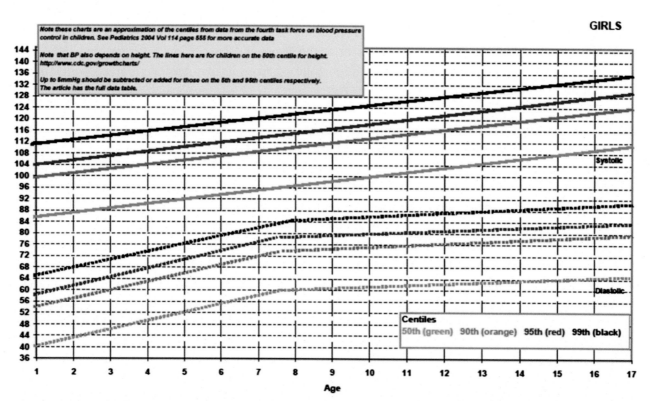

Figure 14.14B *Blood pressure centile chart for girls with systolic blood pressures in solid lines and diastolic blood pressures in dashed lines. (With permission from International Paediatric Task Force).*

Dose increases of fludrocortisone need to be undertaken carefully to avoid causing high blood pressure and if an increase is necessary based upon the findings of all the carefully conducted testing mentioned in this chapter, the dose should be increased by 25 mcg increments and the impact checked by biochemical testing.

Low Blood Pressure

Low blood pressure in the population is quite common. When we see it in adrenal insufficiency however, we are always concerned the low blood pressure might indicate either under replacement with glucocorticoid or mineralocorticoid. The glucocorticoids and mineralocorticoids interact in the generation of blood pressure because glucocorticoids are involved in maintaining the tone of the muscles in the walls of the main arteries. When cortisol is low, the walls of the arteries are quite lax and can easily distend. This generates low blood pressure.

If the dose of fludrocortisone is too low, then the person will have low blood pressure and the symptoms of this are dizziness on standing from the sitting position. People often crave salt and will switch to or crave salty foods. If this happens, then a check of plasma renin/PRA and sodium levels in the blood is important. Glucocorticoids have several roles in maintaining blood pressure. They act directly on blood vessels and are also important for the effect adrenaline has on the blood vessels. Adrenaline itself acts to increase blood pressure, so if you are under dosed with glucocorticoids you might also end up in a very similar situation with low blood pressure. Figure 14.15 shows the interaction of changes in blood pressure on the renin-angiotensin-aldosterone system

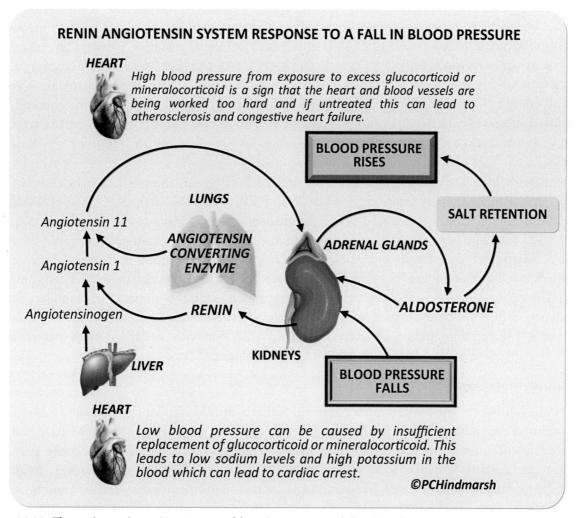

Figure 14.15 *The renin angiotensin system and how it reacts to a fall in blood pressure.*

In high blood pressure situations, we block angiotensin converting enzyme, so the body stops making angiotensin II, which allows the blood vessels to dilate and stops the kidney absorbing water and salt both of which bring down blood pressure. Careful adjustment of the mineralocorticoid and glucocorticoid doses is warranted to maintain blood pressure within the normal range.

One additional point is with respect to sodium. In the Western diet even with everyone trying to reduce salt, intake is still high (see page 393 for recommendations on daily sodium intake). The exception to this is in the newborn who are dependent initially on either breast or infant formula milk. In newborn babies with primary adrenal insufficiency, such as CAH or adrenal hypoplasia congenita, salt supplementation is often required to replace the salt lost up to the point they present. This is because as we have mentioned already the newborn kidneys are less responsive to aldosterone than later in life. Newborn babies need around 2 mmol sodium/kg body weight/day and breast milk or infant formula milk only just delivers that amount. So, if salt has been lost, additional salt supplements will be required to stabilise blood pressure, plasma sodium and renin/PRA.

ARGININE VASOPRESSIN AND DESMOPRESSIN

One further factor is involved in regulation of blood volume and blood pressure and that is arginine vasopressin (AVP). It is important to mention this at this stage because there are important effects of AVP that we need to consider, particularly the interaction with cortisol.

Arginine vasopressin regulates the tonicity of body fluids. Tonicity is the balance of solutes inside and outside of cells which determines the flow of water between and into cells. An indirect measure of this is osmolality. As noted previously, AVP is released from the posterior pituitary in response to hypertonicity or hyperosmolality and causes the kidneys to reabsorb water and return it to the circulation, returning the tonicity of the body fluids toward normal. This is what happens if you do not drink enough water. A consequence of this kidney reabsorption of water is a concentrated urine and reduced urine volume. High amounts of AVP also raise blood pressure by causing the arteries to narrow or vasoconstrict.

In patients with hypopituitarism and are ACTH and AVP deficient, there is a fine balance between cortisol replacement therapy and replacement of AVP with the synthetic form DDAVP or desmopressin (actual name 1-deamino-8-D-arginine vasopressin). Day to day variations in plasma cortisol leads to suppression of AVP secretion into the bloodstream. Arginine vasopressin levels are highest between (00:00) midnight and 02:00 (2 am) at a time when cortisol is at its nadir and starting to rise towards its peak in the morning. Cortisol feeds back on hypothalamic AVP synthesis and release. The action of AVP is also dependent on how much cortisol is present. In secondary adrenal insufficiency with AVP deficiency, if we double dose with hydrocortisone for illness, we may find that water loss through the kidneys increases so extra DDAVP may be needed. This is quite complex and any changes need to be discussed with your endocrinologist.

Desmopressin (DDAVP)

DDAVP is available for the management of cranial diabetes insipidus in liquid, spray and tablet forms. The dose used depends on which method of delivery is used. Care needs to be exercised when used with other medications that lead to water loss such as the diuretics. The main side effect is water retention and hyponatraemia so careful monitoring is required when starting treatment. Anti-epileptic drugs may accentuate hyponatraemia so as with all medications it is best to check with your endocrinologist for any potential drug interaction.

EXERCISE AND SODIUM AND WATER BALANCE

So far in this book, we have not discussed glucocorticoid or mineralocorticoid dosing with respect to exercise. We know from studies of exercise that additional glucocorticoid is not required for short bursts of exercise. Hypoglycaemia can occur, but this is due to a blunted adrenaline response and should be manged by pre-exercise loading with readily available and complex carbohydrate. Extreme high intensity exercise may require some extra glucocorticoid one hour beforehand and repeated depending on the duration of the exercise. This needs to be carefully worked out with an endocrinologist and an expert in sports medicine.

Fludrocortisone dosing does not need to change for most exercise. Care needs to be taken with intense forms of exercise such as marathon running where hyponatraemia can develop - Exercise Associated Hyponatraemia (EAH). The causes of EAH include sweat loss, excessive intake of (low-sodium or hypotonic) fluids and possible hormonal imbalances (some athletes increase AVP production). Cases of hyponatremia can occur outside extreme sports, for example, in team sports and rowing. Involvement of an endocrinologist and sports medicine specialist is needed to advise on drinking rates and pre-race increases in salt intake as well as in hypopituitarism in formulating what dose changes to DDAVP are required.

CONCLUSION

Salt and water balance is extremely important as cell size and function is dependent on it. The regulation of plasma sodium is kept within a tight range and requires interaction between the renin-angiotensin-aldosterone system and AVP production. The blood-brain barrier is relatively impermeable to sodium and sodium therefore equilibrates slowly across it. This leads to problems when correcting situations where the plasma sodium is high or low. Fludrocortisone is a synthetic modification of cortisol which allows it to retain sodium. Careful dosing is required as the dose changes with age. Higher doses when expressed per metre squared body surface area are needed in the first 2 years of life compared to late adolescence and adulthood. This is because the number of mineralocorticoid receptors in the kidney is less in the neonate and infant, so more fludrocortisone is required to retain sodium via this route. The aim of therapy is to maintain a normal plasma renin/PRA and blood pressure and at the same time ensuring that under treatment does not lead to troubling effects such as headaches and dizzy spells. We also want to avoid over treatment which will lead to hypertension, the potential for heart rhythm abnormalities due to a low potassium and increased water retention leading to glaucoma.

FURTHER READING

Adrogue, H.J., Madias, N.E., 2023. The syndrome of inappropriate antidiuresis. N Engl J Med 389, 1499–1509. https://doi.org/10.1056/NEJMcp2210411.

Carey, R.M., 2010. Aldosterone and cardiovascular disease. Curr Opin Endocrinol Diabetes Obes 17, 194–198.

Ellison, D.H., Welling, P., 2021. Insights into salt handling and blood pressure. N Engl J Med 385, 1981–1993.

Flynn, J.T., Ingelfinger, J.R., Redwine, K.M. (Eds.), 2018. Pediatric Hypertension, 4th edition. Springer, New York.

Freeman, M.W., Halvorsen, Y-D., Marshall, W., et al., 2023. Phase 2 Trial of baxdrostat for treatment-resistant hypertension. N Engl J Med 388, 395–405. https://doi.org/10.1056/NEJMoa2213169.

Green-Golan, L., Yates, C., Drinkard, B., et al., 2007. Patients with classic congenital adrenal hyperplasia have decreased epinephrine reserve and defective glycemic control during prolonged moderate-intensity exercise. J Clin Endocrinol Metab 92, 3019–3024.

Klingert, M., Nikolaidis, P.T., Weiss, K., et al., 2022. Exercise-associated hyponatremia in marathon runners. J Clin Med 11, 6775. https://doi.org/10.3390/jcm11226775.

Krone, N., Webb, E.A., Hindmarsh, P.C., 2015. Keeping the pressure on mineralocorticoid replacement in congenital adrenal hyperplasia. Clin Endocrinol (Oxf) 82, 478–480.

Lloyd-Jones, D.M., Hong, Y., Labarthe, D., on behalf of the American Heart Association Strategic Planning Force and Statistics Committee, et al., 2010. Defining and setting national goals for cardiovascular health promotion and disease reduction: the American Heart Association's Strategic Impact Goal through 2020 and beyond. Circulation 121, 586—613.

Sterns, R.H., 2015. Disorders of plasma sodium - causes, consequences, and correction. N Engl J Med 372, 55—65.

CHAPTER 15

Weaning Glucocorticoids

GLOSSARY

Adrenal suppression A general term to describe loss of cortisol production due to the exogenous administration of glucocorticoids.

Adrenocorticotropin Hormone produced by the pituitary gland that regulates cortisol synthesis and secretion from the adrenal glands.

Corticotropin-releasing hormone Hormone produced by the hypothalamus that regulates adrenocorticotropin synthesis and secretion from the pituitary gland.

Cortisol profile Measurement of cortisol in the blood at one hourly intervals to build up a profile of what levels are achieved from treatment with hydrocortisone.

Synacthen test A means of making the adrenal gland produce and release cortisol, synacthen is the name given to a synthetic form of andrenocorticotropin (ACTH).

Weaning glucocorticoids The process of reducing exogenous doses of glucocorticoids balancing the amount and speed of reduction against the activity of the disease being treated. The aim is to take the patient off all exogenous glucocorticoids in a safe manner without reactivating the disease being treated.

GENERAL

Glucocorticoids are used in many areas of medicine predominately for their anti-inflammatory and immunosuppressive effects. It has been estimated that glucocorticoids are used in 10% of inpatients with the majority used for respiratory problems and 2% to 3% of the general population receive systemic or topical glucocorticoid treatment. Prednisolone and dexamethasone were developed as synthetic glucocorticoids with a high anti-inflammatory potency and lower salt retaining effects than hydrocortisone, (20% lower in the case of prednisolone and no salt retaining effect in the case of dexamethasone).

The dosing used for an anti-inflammatory or immunosuppressant effect, is much higher than that used in replacement hydrocortisone therapy. As such, it is quite easy to supress the hypothalamo-pituitary-adrenal axis (HPA) when prednisolone or dexamethasone are used as anti-inflammatory or immunosuppressant agents.

For example, oral prednisolone given for giant cell arteritis (inflammation of the blood vessels) at a dose of 0.7 mg/kg/day for 1 week and then reduced to 0.35 mg/kg/day for 4 to 6 weeks, was associated with 50% of individuals adrenal glands not responding to a synacthen test one week after therapy was discontinued. More concerning was the time to recovery which took 14 months and 5% of those involved in the study, never showed any recovery of the HPA axis. Several aspects need to be considered when a person is receiving glucocorticoid therapy for any situation other than adrenal replacement therapy. Many people say that they have developed Cushing's Syndrome because of high dose glucocorticoid therapies. We will look at this before we think through the issues of HPA suppression and how to wean down the high glucocorticoid doses.

Replacement Therapies in Adrenal Insufficiency. https://doi.org/10.1016/B978-0-12-824548-4.00017-6

CUSHING'S DISEASE AND CUSHING'S SYNDROME

In Chapter 8 we looked at many of the problems which occur as a result from over and under replacement with glucocorticoids. Over treatment is often referred to as Cushing's syndrome or developing a Cushingoid appearance. Cushing's syndrome occurs when the body is exposed to too much cortisol over time. It is important to note the statement 'over time', which means that double dosing for illness over say 5 to 7 days will not lead to Cushing's syndrome unless it happens frequently. Cushing's syndrome are the signs and symptoms which result from an increase in the amount of cortisol produced, with a reduction in or loss of the normal circadian rhythm of cortisol.

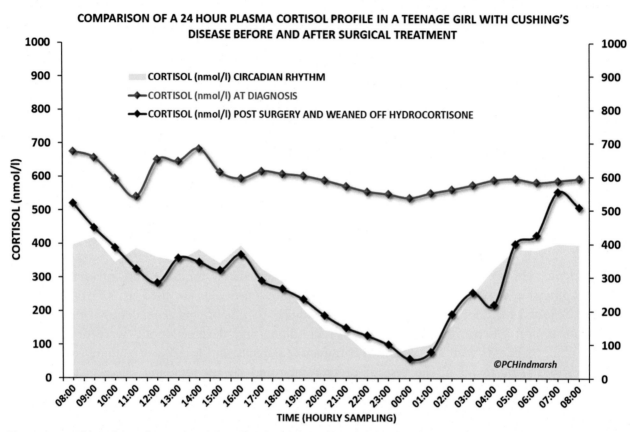

COMPARISON OF A 24 HOUR PLASMA CORTISOL PROFILE IN A TEENAGE GIRL WITH CUSHING'S DISEASE BEFORE AND AFTER SURGICAL TREATMENT

Figure 15.1 *The 24 hour plasma cortisol profile of a teenage girl with Cushing's disease prior to (light blue line) and after transsphenoidal surgery when all hydrocortisone replacement therapy was weaned (dark blue line). Note the return of the normal cortisol circadian rhythm after surgery. The average circadian rhythm of cortisol is shown in the blue shaded area.*

This book is about adrenal insufficiency, but it is worth briefly reviewing Cushing's disease and syndrome as there are important learning points for weaning exogenous glucocorticoids. The syndrome takes its name from a Boston neurosurgeon Harvey Cushing who at the beginning of the last century, described the signs and symptoms (as listed in this section) in association with the presence of a pituitary tumour. Figure 15.1 shows the 24 hour plasma cortisol in a teenage girl with Cushing's disease at diagnosis and after surgery once weaned off replacement hydrocortisone compared with the normal circadian rhythm of cortisol. The term Cushing's disease refers to an ACTH cause for the raised cortisol usually due to a problem in the pituitary gland. Cushing's syndrome refers to adrenal autonomatous cortisol production or high dose exogenous glucocorticoid administration.

The striking features are the elevation of plasma cortisol (light blue line at diagnosis) throughout the 24 hour period with a near loss of the circadian rhythm. In this case the excess cortisol production arises from excess adrenocorticotropin hormone (ACTH) production from a microadenoma within the pituitary gland (Figure 15.2).

PITUITARY MICROADENOMA

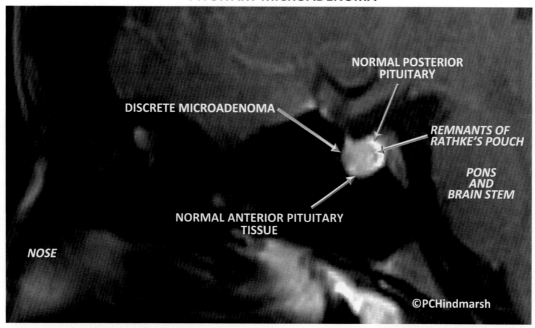

Figure 15.2 *Sagittal section from an MRI scan of the pituitary region in a teenage girl showing a discrete pituitary microadenoma causing Cushing's disease. The microadenoma was removed in its entirety by transsphenoidal surgery.*

Cushing's syndrome can arise from over secretion of cortisol by the adrenal glands alone, secondary to an adrenal tumour. Cushing's disease is a specific cause of Cushing's syndrome due to an ACTH secreting tumour of the pituitary gland which is what Harvey Cushing described.

Excess ACTH secretion can also result from ectopic production in the lungs due to an oat cell also known as a small cell carcinoma. Ectopic ACTH production also informs us that exogenous ACTH (as used for the treatment of infantile spasms in children), will have a similar effect in that cortisol will be high from the exogenous ACTH stimulation of the adrenal glands, while hypothalamic corticotropin-releasing hormone (CRH) and pituitary ACTH will be suppressed by the elevated cortisol. This means once exogenous ACTH is stopped, the patient will be at risk of adrenal insufficiency and crises until the CRH and ACTH function of the axis recovers. Replacement hydrocortisone will be required to cover this period and this will need to be weaned down in due course. Adrenal androgens can be normal or increased depending on how long the adrenal glands are stimulated by the ectopic/exogenous ACTH.

BIOCHEMISTRY OF CUSHING'S DISEASE AND SYNDROME

BIOCHEMISTRY	CUSHING'S SYNDROME *Due to Adrenal Tumour*	CUSHING'S SYNDROME *Due to Exogenous Glucocorticoid*	CUSHING'S DISEASE *Due to Pituitary Tumour*	CUSHING'S DISEASE *Due to Ectopic ACTH e.g. Lung Cancer*
ACTH	↓/UD	↓/UD	↑↑	↑↑↑
CORTISOL	↑↑	↓/UD	↑↑	↑↑↑
(UD - *undetectable* ↓ - *low* ↑- *high*)				©PCHindmarsh

Figure 15.3 *Plasma ACTH and cortisol measurements in Cushing's syndrome and Cushing's disease. Plasma cortisol is suppressed by exogenous glucocorticoid administration and the level of exogenous glucocorticoids cannot be measured in routine laboratories.*

Finally, the commonest cause of Cushing's syndrome is exogenous administration of glucocorticoids. Figure 15.3 summarises the biochemical findings in these situations and Figure 15.4 gives a pictorial representation of changes in the HPA axis for these causes.

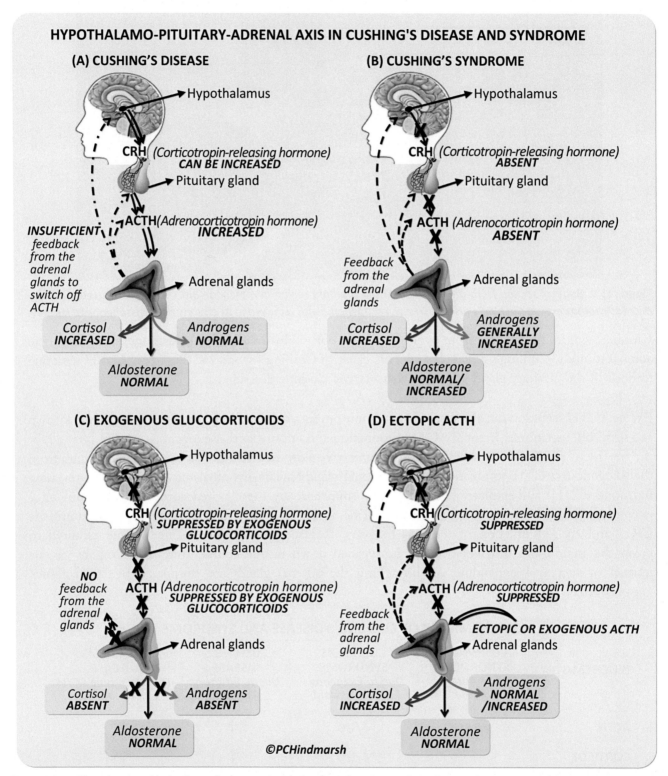

Figure 15.4 *The changes in the hypothalamo-pituitary-adrenal axis in (A) Cushing's disease, (B) Cushing's syndrome, (C) Cushing's syndrome resulting from exogenous glucocorticoid administration and (D) Cushing's syndrome due to ectopic ACTH production. Note in Cushing's disease CRH may be increased if problem is in the hypothalamus or suppressed if ACTH production in the pituitary is from an autonomous tumour.*

A Cushingoid appearance can also be seen in obesity, chronic alcoholism and depression and is sometimes referred to as Pseudo-Cushing's syndrome. Careful testing to diagnose these needs to be undertaken.

We covered many of the effects of over treatment in Chapter 8, but it is worth a recap of them again with respect to Cushing's syndrome and the Cushingoid appearance. The hallmark signs of Cushing's syndrome are:

- Fatty tissue deposits particularly between the shoulders (buffalo hump), a rounded face (moon face), and around the midriff but sparing the limbs
- Weight gain
- Pink or purple stretch marks (striae) on the skin of the abdomen, thighs, breasts and arms
- Thinning, fragile skin that bruises easily
- Slow healing of cuts and infections
- Acne
- High blood pressure, osteoporosis and type 2 diabetes mellitus

An important fact we learnt from the patient with Cushing's disease is the length of time which it takes to wean down from high amounts of cortisol or other glucocorticoids. The microadenoma was removed surgically in its entirety. Afterwards, as normal CRH and ACTH production had been switched off by the high cortisol produced because of the microadenoma producing ACTH autonomously, we had to cover her with hydrocortisone replacement. Initially, this needed to be at a higher amount than normal replacement because she was so accustomed to high levels. This weaning process took some 2 years for the normal pituitary ACTH cells to recover and to generate normal cortisol production from the adrenal glands and a normal circadian rhythm illustrated in Figure 15.1 (dark blue line).

As we shall see with recovery of the axis from exogenous glucocorticoids this can take a long period of time. This reflects firstly, the need for the hypothalamo-pituitary-adrenal axis to reactivate after being switched off by the exogenous glucocorticoid. The recovery of the axis takes place in a hierarchical order starting with CRH, then ACTH and finally cortisol. Cortisol production from the adrenal glands can take longer to recover than CRH and ACTH, as often due to the exogenous glucocorticoid administration, the adrenal glands will have shrunk in size so the glands need to increase in size first before cortisol is generated. Secondly, consideration also has to be given to the potential for relapse of the condition for which the glucocorticoids were prescribed in the first instance.

HYPOTHALAMO-PITUITARY-ADRENAL SUPPRESSION

Effect of dose and timing

Suppression of the HPA axis is dose dependent.

Most glucocorticoid use is for less than 5 days but 22% is for 6 months or more and 4% for periods of 5 years or more.

A prednisolone dose of 0.2 mg/kg/day is unlikely to suppress the axis even if given for a long period of time. Even a dose of prednisolone of 0.3 to 0.5 mg/kg/day given for a period of 3 weeks is unlikely to cause suppression. Doses higher than this and certainly if given for periods of time greater than 2 to 3 weeks, are likely to lead to suppression of the axis.

In childhood leukaemia, where high doses of prednisolone and dexamethasone are used, 28 days of treatment was associated with recovery of the adrenal axis over a 4 to 10 week period, although some patients (13%), still had adrenal insufficiency 20 weeks after the therapy was discontinued. In adults receiving prednisolone 40 mg (approximately 0.5 mg/kg/day for 14 days) for acute exacerbation of their asthma, 89% showed a blunted response to synacthen testing at the end of the 14 days treatment and 33% still had a blunted response 21 days later. Frequent oral courses of glucocorticoids act in a dose dependent manner with an increased risk of adrenal insufficiency for every course of treatment per year.

When considering these time frames, it is important to remember that following the acute loss of ACTH production from the pituitary due to trauma, adrenal atrophy results in 6 weeks. There is a window therefore, during which recovery can take place speedily, but once beyond this window of 4 to 10 weeks adrenal atrophy is likely to have occurred and recovery will be much slower.

How and when the glucocorticoid is taken, are also important factors. There is literature suggesting if the medication is given on alternate days, treatment is less likely to suppress the axis. This at face value can seem reassuring, but it is important to also remember on the day the individual is not receiving the glucocorticoid, the response of the axis may still be blunted or impaired. As we shall discuss later in this chapter, recovery of the stress response occurs later than the return of the circadian rhythm, so although the individual may appear to be cortisol replete on a day to day basis, they may lack the increase of cortisol production required during illness or the stress associated with trauma or surgery.

The timing of the anti-inflammatory glucocorticoid dose is also important. Doses given in the evening are more likely to cause suppression. In addition, doses given during the day are more likely to raise blood glucose because of food intake. There is no easy way to resolve this but the majority of anti-inflammatory glucocorticoid treatments use daytime dosing.

Potency of the Glucocorticoid

The potency of the glucocorticoid used varies. Figure 15.5 shows the growth retarding and anti-inflammatory effects of hydrocortisone, prednisolone and dexamethasone. We looked at this earlier in the book but it is worth another review here. In all instances, hydrocortisone has been ascribed an effect of 1 for comparison. Note that prednisolone is approximately 4 to 5 times more potent than hydrocortisone, whereas dexamethasone is the most potent glucocorticoid used in the management of inflammatory conditions.

PROPERTIES OF COMMONLY USED GLUCOCORTICOIDS

GLUCOCORTICOID	HYDROCORTISONE	PREDNISOLONE	DEXAMETHASONE
Half-Life in Blood (hours)	1.5	2 – 3	3.5 – 4.5
Duration as Glucocorticoid (hours)	~ 6	~ 8	~ 12
Duration of Inflammatory Action (hours)	~ 8	~ 12	~ 36
Time to Peak Level (hours)	1 – 2	3 – 4	Rather flat profile
Growth Suppressing Effect	1	5	80
Dosing Effect on Growth (mg)	30	6	0.35 – 0.45

©PCHindmarsh

Figure 15.5 *Table comparing the duration and peak of action of the three glucocorticoids hydrocortisone, prednisolone and dexamethasone along with effects in dosing terms on growth. Hydrocortisone is ascribed a growth suppressing effect of 1. The symbol ~ is short for approximately.*

Not surprisingly, the potency of a glucocorticoid in terms of anti-inflammation and growth suppression also applies to the degree of suppression which is likely to be encountered within the HPA axis. Suppression occurs with a total daily hydrocortisone dose of 12 to 15 mg/m^2 body surface area. As the body surface area of an adult male is 1.73 m^2 this equates to 20 to 25 mg of hydrocortisone per day, 5 to 6.25 mg of prednisolone per day, or 0.4 to 0.5 mg of dexamethasone per day. These are guides to what might happen but will vary from person to person, depending on how they metabolise glucocorticoids and how sensitive their glucocorticoid receptors are. Note that based on these doses, adrenal suppression is likely to occur before growth suppression.

Method of Administration

In the vast majority of individuals receiving anti-inflammatory therapy, the glucocorticoid will be administered orally. Figure 15.5 is based on oral administration with respect to the growth affect. There are other ways of administering glucocorticoids, for example, both prednisolone and dexamethasone can be administered into joints for the management of arthritis, as can hydrocortisone. Once in the joint, the glucocorticoid can be absorbed into the circulation and it has been noted that some 52% of individuals having intra-articular steroid injections have adrenal suppression. This occurs with frequent injections but can be observed after a single dose. Inhaled glucocorticoids are used in the management of asthma and also for allergic rhinitis. In asthma the dose of the inhaled glucocorticoids, budesonide and beclomethasone which leads to adrenal suppression, is somewhere in the region of 40 mcg/kg body weight/day. Figure 15.6 shows the dose response relationship between overnight cortisol and the total daily dose of inhaled glucocorticoid (beclomethasone). Inhaled fluticasone is more potent at suppressing the hypothalamo-pituitary-adrenal axis. The ratio is roughly 1:2 for beclomethasone to fluticasone. Budesonide, beclomethasone and fluticasone are structurally very similar to dexamethasone.

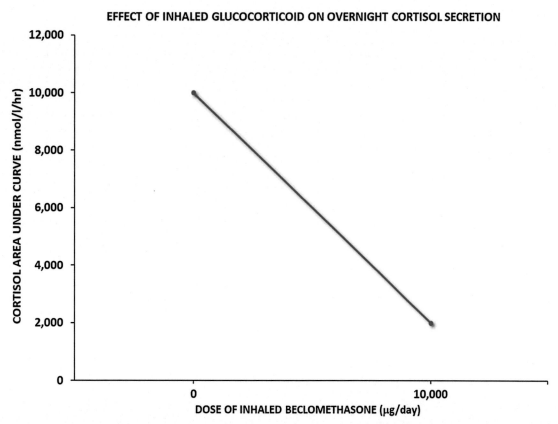

Figure 15.6 *Dose response relationship between the total daily dose of inhaled beclomethasone and overnight cortisol. (Figure redrawn from the data of Law, C.M., Marchant, J.L., Honour, J.W., Preece, M.A., 1986. Nocturnal adrenal suppression in asthmatic children taking inhaled beclomethasone dipropionate. Lancet 26, 942—944.)*

Figure 15.7 shows inhaled glucocorticoid doses commonly used in asthma based on the licensing system. For people who need prolonged treatment with high dose inhaled glucocorticoids, steroid treatment cards should be provided. The exact dose which will supress the adrenal glands when using intranasal administration is less clear, but it has been reported that 4.2% of individuals receiving intranasal steroid therapy for allergic rhinitis will experience adrenal suppression.

GLUCOCORTICOID DOSING FOR ASTHMA - ADULTS (AGED 17 YEARS AND ABOVE)

DRUG	LOW DOSE	MODERATE DOSE	HIGH DOSE
Beclomethasone standard particle	200 - 500 micrograms per day in 2 divided doses	600 - 1000 micrograms per day in 2 divided doses	1200 - 2000 micrograms per day in 2 divided doses
Beclomethasone extra-fine particles	100 - 200 micrograms per day in 2 divided doses	300 - 400 micrograms per day in 2 divided doses	500 - 800 micrograms per day in 2 divided doses
Fluticasone propionate	100 - 250 micrograms per day in 2 divided doses	300 - 500 micrograms per day in 2 divided doses	600 - 1000 micrograms per day in 2 divided doses

©PCHindmarsh

Figure 15.7(A) *Inhaled glucocorticoid dosages for adults aged 17 years and above. (Table derived from Asthma Guidelines produced by the United Kingdom National Institute for Health and Care Excellence (NICE) 2018.)*

GLUCOCORTICOID DOSING FOR ASTHMA - CHILDREN (AGED 16 YEARS AND BELOW)

DRUG	LOW DOSE	MODERATE DOSE	HIGH DOSE
Beclomethasone standard particle	100 - 200 micrograms per day in 2 divided doses	300 - 400 micrograms per day in 2 divided doses	500 - 800 micrograms per day in 2 divided doses
Beclomethasone extra-fine particles	100 micrograms per day in 2 divided doses	150 - 200 micrograms per day in 2 divided doses	300 - 400 micrograms per day in 2 divided doses
Fluticasone propionate	100 micrograms per day in 2 divided doses	150 - 200 micrograms per day in 2 divided doses	250 - 400 micrograms per day in 2 divided doses

©PCHindmarsh

Figure 15.7 (B) *Inhaled glucocorticoid dosages for children. (Table derived from Asthma Guidelines produced by the United Kingdom National Institute for Health and Care Excellence (NICE) 2018.)*

A difficulty in understanding many of the studies arises as they have been conducted in individuals who are relatively well from their asthma or allergic rhinitis standpoint. It is likely that absorption of the glucocorticoid is even greater when there are exacerbations of allergic rhinitis or asthma, because absorption of the glucocorticoid occurs more easily across inflamed surfaces. Not only does the inflammation allow the steroid easier access to the circulation, the increased blood flow to the area also enhances absorption.

Again, the inhaled preparations vary in their potency. If patients are receiving doses above 40 mcg/kg body weight/day of inhaled glucocorticoid, assessment of adrenal function should be undertaken (20 mcg/kg body weight/day for fluticasone preparations). More general recommendations focus on monitoring high risk patients for adrenal insufficiency which includes:

- Those using moderate to high dose of high potency inhaled glucocorticoids (particularly fluticasone) for longer than 6 months.

- The concurrent use of inhaled or topical glucocorticoids.

- Frequent medication with oral glucocorticoids and a low body mass index.

Finally, it is important to be aware of other sources of glucocorticoids. Some unbranded skin whitening creams contain glucocorticoids and use the glucocorticoids to produce thinning of the skin which gives it a whiter appearance. Not only may this damage the skin but it could also lead to adrenal suppression.

Extreme care is needed with the use of topical creams for eczema because like nasal glucocorticoids, when there is a large, inflamed area of skin this allows easier absorption into the circulation than if the skin surface was normal.

FACTORS INFLUENCING GLUCOCORTICOID WITHDRAWAL

The adrenal suppression which follows treatment with exogenous glucocorticoids is classified as secondary adrenal insufficiency. This is because the exogenous glucocorticoid feeds back on to the hypothalamus and pituitary gland to switch off the production of corticotropin-releasing hormone from the hypothalamus. This reduces production of adrenocorticotropin (ACTH) from the pituitary gland, which in turn switches off cortisol formation and release from the adrenal cortex (Figure 15.8).

The upper part of the panel in Figure 15.8 shows the normal relationship and feedback of cortisol on the hypothalamus and pituitary gland. Primary adrenal insufficiency is associated with loss of cortisol production from the adrenal glands, so the negative feedback loop back to the hypothalamus and pituitary is broken and ACTH is raised. In secondary adrenal insufficiency, the problem lies at either the hypothalamus and/or pituitary, so ACTH is low and does not stimulate cortisol release from the adrenal glands.

There is no negative feedback, but this does not alter ACTH production because this is damaged.

When exogenous glucocorticoids are administered to a person with a normal HPA axis, they will act like cortisol and switch off CRH and ACTH production from the hypothalamus and pituitary respectively, leading to low cortisol secretion by the adrenal glands and if the exogenous glucocorticoids are administered for a long period, they will lead to adrenal atrophy.

The biochemical hallmark of secondary adrenal insufficiency is absence of cortisol and ACTH. This is in contrast to the situation in primary adrenal insufficiency where there is loss of cortisol, but because the feedback system is intact, ACTH rises in an attempt to normalise cortisol. Because of the damage to the adrenal glands this cannot be achieved, so in primary adrenal insufficiency cortisol is low and ACTH very high.

This means in secondary adrenal insufficiency the production of aldosterone, the mineralocorticoid from the adrenal glands, is unaffected as this system is not influenced to any significant degree by ACTH. This is why replacement therapy with fludrocortisone is not usually required in secondary adrenal insufficiency from whatever cause. In the short term if ACTH is low, cortisol production will be switched off. If suppression of ACTH continues for 6 weeks or more, then the adrenal glands shrink in size due to the lack of the growth maintaining effect of ACTH on adrenal cortex cell size. This poses a considerable problem when considering weaning of glucocorticoids, as it means not only has ACTH production to recover, but also the adrenal glands have to grow back to their normal size so their normal function can resume.

The process of weaning takes time and is often slowed down due to a relapse of the underlying condition being treated, which necessitates temporary higher doses of exogenous glucocorticoids.

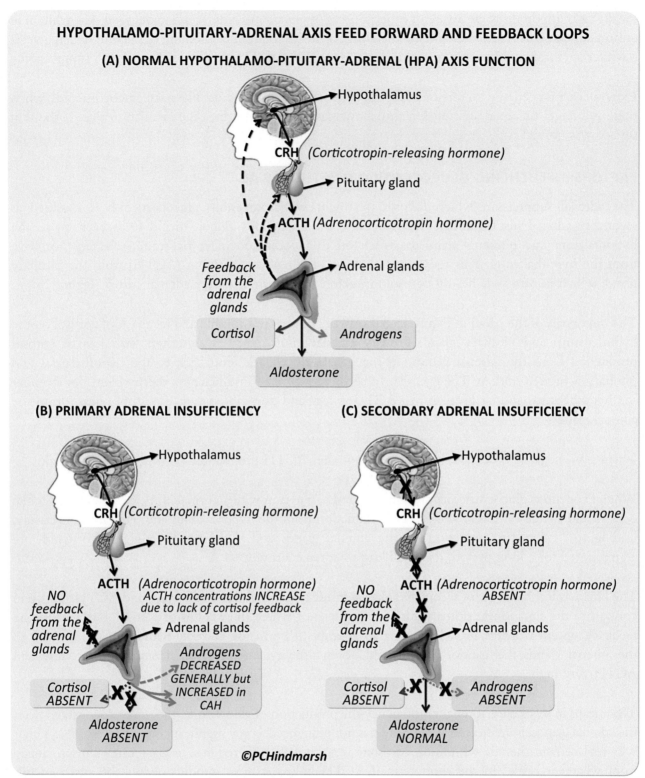

HYPOTHALAMO-PITUITARY-ADRENAL AXIS FEED FORWARD AND FEEDBACK LOOPS

(A) NORMAL HYPOTHALAMO-PITUITARY-ADRENAL (HPA) AXIS FUNCTION

Hypothalamus

CRH *(Corticotropin-releasing hormone)*

Pituitary gland

ACTH *(Adrenocorticotropin hormone)*

Adrenal glands

Feedback from the adrenal glands

Cortisol

Androgens

Aldosterone

(B) PRIMARY ADRENAL INSUFFICIENCY

Hypothalamus

CRH *(Corticotropin-releasing hormone)*

Pituitary gland

ACTH *(Adrenocorticotropin hormone)*
ACTH concentrations INCREASE due to lack of cortisol feedback

NO feedback from the adrenal glands

Adrenal glands

Androgens *DECREASED GENERALLY but INCREASED in CAH*

Cortisol ABSENT

Aldosterone ABSENT

(C) SECONDARY ADRENAL INSUFFICIENCY

Hypothalamus

CRH *(Corticotropin-releasing hormone)*

Pituitary gland

ACTH *(Adrenocorticotropin hormone)*
ABSENT

NO feedback from the adrenal glands

Adrenal glands

Cortisol ABSENT

Androgens ABSENT

Aldosterone NORMAL

©PCHindmarsh

Figure 15.8 *In the top panel (A) is a representation of the Hypothalamo-Pituitary-Adrenal (HPA) axis generating cortisol and the adrenal androgens. CRH = corticotropin-releasing hormone. ACTH = adrenocorticotropin. High levels of ACTH will generate aldosterone but the main regulator is the renin-angiotensin-aldosterone system. Primary adrenal insufficiency (B) (lower left panel) leads to loss of cortisol production with loss of cortisol feedback and consequently elevated ACTH. Note androgens are low in primary adrenal insufficiency except when congenital adrenal hyperplasia is the cause where they are elevated. In secondary adrenal insufficiency (C) (lower right panel) ACTH is not produced so cortisol is low due to the loss of ACTH stimulation of the adrenal glands. There is no cortisol feedback because the adrenal glands are not producing cortisol. In glucocorticoid induced secondary adrenal insufficiency, the glucocorticoid given switches off CRH and ACTH production and release from the pituitary, which in turn leads to low or no cortisol production.*

Two factors influence the speed of weaning from glucocorticoid use:

1. The first and most important, is the disease activity for which the glucocorticoid is administered. A rapid reduction in glucocorticoid dose could lead to a resurgence of the disease activity for which the glucocorticoid was prescribed. Several attempts at weaning are often required because of relapse of the condition for which the glucocorticoids have been prescribed for. This means the weaning process has to be done in conjunction with the physician involved in managing the inflammatory condition. This may be a gastroenterologist in conditions such as Crohn's disease, or a kidney specialist in the various conditions which lead to inflammatory disease of the kidney.

2. The second factor which influences the rate of glucocorticoid withdrawal is how fast the HPA axis recovers.

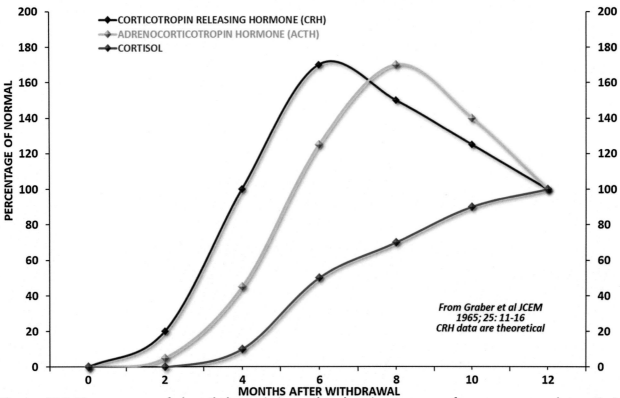

RECOVERY OF THE HYPOTHALAMO-PITUITARY-ADRENAL AXIS AFTER EXOGENOUS GLUCOCORTICOID USE

Figure 15.9 *Time course of hypothalamo-pituitary-adrenal axis recovery after exogenous glucocorticoid administration. CRH = corticotropin-releasing hormone (purple line). ACTH = adrenocorticotropin (yellow line). Cortisol is the blue line. CRH is stated as theoretical as it had not been identified in 1965.*

Figure 15.9 shows the hierarchy of recovery:

1. Corticotropin-releasing hormone (CRH)

2. Adrenocorticotropin hormone (ACTH)

3. Cortisol

The data has been set with 100% being normal function. Of note, both CRH and ACTH start to recover within 4 months of withdrawal from the glucocorticoids and there follows a period of some 6 to 8 months where they are being produced in greater amounts than normal. This probably reflects the need for cortisol generation which is slower in recovery than CRH and ACTH and also reflects the need for the adrenal glands to return to their normal size.

The data from an individual when weaned off hydrocortisone is shown in Figure 15.10 where Chart A shows the cortisol profiles and Charts B and C synacthen tests.

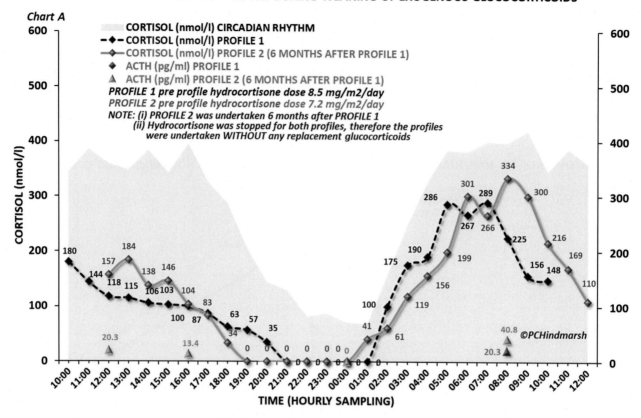

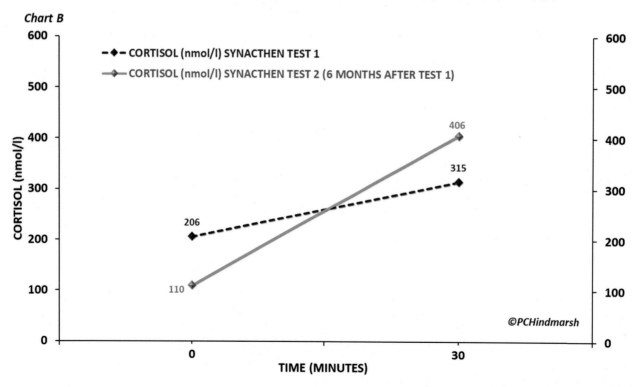

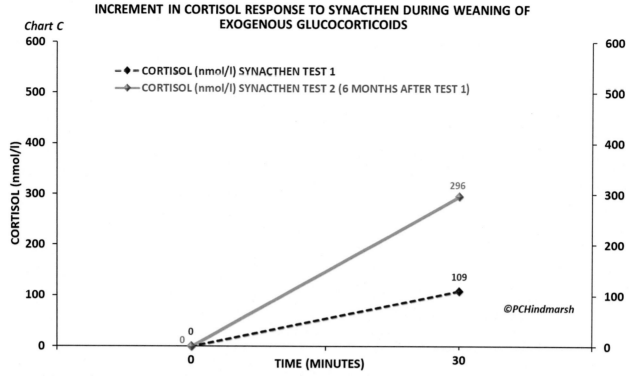

INCREMENT IN CORTISOL RESPONSE TO SYNACTHEN DURING WEANING OF EXOGENOUS GLUCOCORTICOIDS

Chart C

Legend:
- – ♦ – CORTISOL (nmol/l) SYNACTHEN TEST 1
- —♦— CORTISOL (nmol/l) SYNACTHEN TEST 2 (6 MONTHS AFTER TEST 1)

Y-axis: CORTISOL (nmol/l)
X-axis: TIME (MINUTES)

Data points: 0, 0, 296, 109

©PCHindmarsh

Figure 15.10 *The 24 hour profile in Chart A was undertaken during the process of weaning the individual off hydrocortisone and no hydrocortisone was taken over the 24 hours, therefore the cortisol measured was naturally produced by the adrenal glands. The normal average circadian rhythm is shown as the pale blue shaded zone with spontaneous cortisol secretion on two occasions at the start of weaning (dark blue line) when the daily hydrocortisone dose was 8.5 mg/m²/day and 6 months later (light blue line) when the daily hydrocortisone dose was 7.2 mg/m²/day. The profiles and ACTH measures are similar. In contrast Chart B shows that the cortisol response to synacthen stimulation is blunted initially (dark blue line) and improved after 6 months (light blue line). This is shown more clearly when we look at the increment in cortisol during the synacthen test in Chart C.*

The recovery of cortisol production over a 24 hour period is shown in Figure 15.10. In this situation the patient has been on hydrocortisone and this has been weaned down to below the normal cortisol production rate of 8 mg/m²/day. The profile was performed when off replacement hydrocortisone. Overall, there was recovery of the 24 hour cortisol production at both time points, whereas the cortisol response to synacthen was blunted initially but showed recovery 6 months later.

This is a key point illustrating that the circadian rhythm of cortisol recovers first and the stress response later. This means that even when the 24 hour cortisol profile looks normal, an emergency care plan will still be required for sick days or trauma situations.

Figures 15.11 and 15.12 show the pre synacthen ACTH measurements along with the results of synacthen testing in two further patients. The hydrocortisone weaning doses are shown on each line.

In Figure 15.11, there is a progressive improvement in the pre synacthen plasma cortisol concentrations, along with recovery of the peak cortisol response to synacthen stimulation over a 2 year period as the replacement hydrocortisone dose was gradually reduced and discontinued. The ACTH measures show an initial increase to 82 pg/ml even when the cortisol is low indicating that the ACTH had recovered and was now trying to wake up the suppressed adrenals as illustrated also in Figure 15.9.

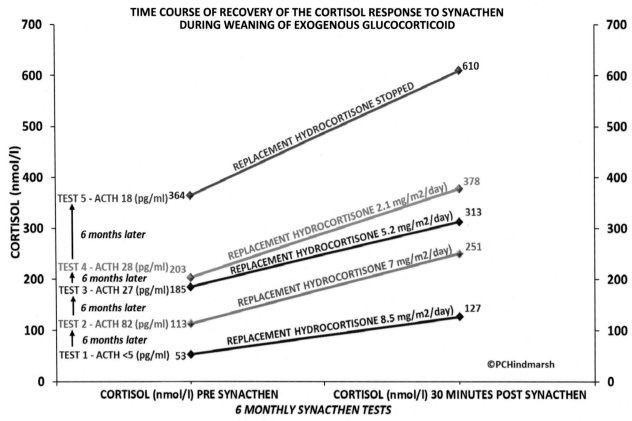

Figure 15.11 *Cortisol response to 6 monthly synacthen testing showing gradual recovery of the pre synacthen cortisol concentration along with the post synacthen cortisol response during the weaning period and normal values once hydrocortisone replacement was discontinued. Pre synacthen adrenocorticotropin (ACTH) measures are shown on the left.*

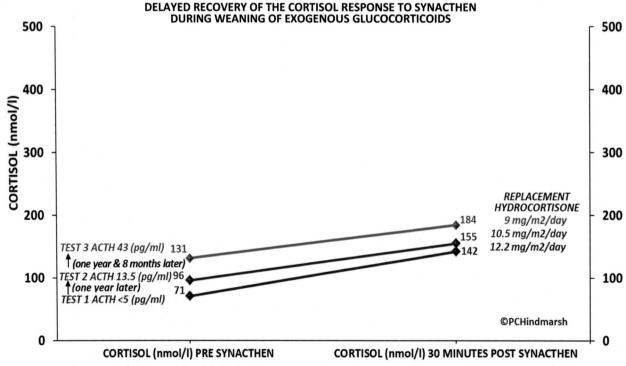

Figure 15.12 *Cortisol response to yearly synacthen testing showing slow recovery of the pre synacthen cortisol concentration along with the post synacthen cortisol response during the weaning period which has not gone below the normal cortisol production rate of 8 mg/m²/day. Pre synacthen adrenocorticotropin (ACTH) measures are shown on the left with a suggestion of recovery in ACTH on Test 3.*

In Figure 15.12 even after nearly three years, the weaning dose is only down to the lower end of the normal cortisol production rate and despite a steady increase in the pre synacthen cortisol, the response is still attenuated. Weaning has been slow due to constant exacerbations of asthma over the winter periods. Note the improvement in ACTH again reflecting the changes seen in Figure 15.9. The doses calculated for weaning are carefully calculated based on the individual as everyone will not only need different doses based on their absorption and clearance, but also depending on the disease activity that the glucocorticoid was given for initially.

RULES FOR WEANING EXOGENOUS GLUCOCORTICOID THERAPY

We can now put all this information together to create several guidance rules to implement when stopping glucocorticoid therapy.

DISCONTINUATION RULES FOR SHORT COURSE OF GLUCOCORTICOID THERAPY

STATUS OF DISEASE AND THERAPY	SUGGESTED WITHDRAWAL PATTERN
Disease unlikely to relapse and less than 3 weeks of treatment and: - No recent repeated courses - No previous long term therapy - No other causes of adrenal suppression - Dosing no greater than 0.3 – 0.5 mg/kg daily prednisolone or equivalent - No evening dosing	Abrupt stop **but** for stress (infection, trauma, surgery) 1 week after stopping therapy then systemic glucocorticoid cover is still needed ©PCHindmarsh

Figure 15.13 *Glucocorticoid therapy stopping rules if the disease is unlikely to relapse and treatment has been for less than 3 weeks. (From National Institute for Health and Care Excellence British National Formulary (Accessed 2023).)*

Figure 15.13 shows the withdrawal plan for disease unlikely to relapse and for which there has been less than three weeks of treatment. There are a number of additional caveats such as, no recent repeated courses of anti–inflammatory glucocorticoid therapy, no previous long term therapy with glucocorticoids and no other causes of adrenal suppression. The table also shows the dosing requirements and makes a note that the anti–inflammatory dosing has not been given in the evening. If all of this is fulfilled, then glucocorticoid therapy can be stopped without any weaning taking place, but it is advised that additional glucocorticoid cover is still needed if the individual becomes unwell or suffers trauma one week after stopping the glucocorticoid therapy.

DISCONTINUATION RULES FOR PROLONGED COURSES OF GLUCOCORTICOID THERAPY

STATUS OF DISEASE AND THERAPY	SUGGESTED WITHDRAWAL PATTERN
Disease unlikely to relapse and more than 3 weeks of treatment or less than 3 weeks therapy but: - Repeated courses recently - Previous long term therapy - Other causes for adrenal suppression - Dose greater than 0.3 - 0.5 mg/kg daily prednisolone or equivalent - Evening dosing	Gradual withdrawal of systemic glucocorticoids ©PCHindmarsh

Figure 15.14 *Glucocorticoid therapy stopping rules if the disease is unlikely to relapse and treatment for 3 weeks or more along with less than 3 weeks of treatment with additional caveats. (From National Institute for Health and Care Excellence British National Formulary (Accessed 2023).)*

In contrast, Figure 15.14 shows the situation when treatment has been given for more than 3 weeks or less than 3 weeks with caveats. In this situation a gradual withdrawal of the glucocorticoid is suggested. This can be done by reducing the anti-inflammatory dose of glucocorticoids to the normal glucocorticoid replacement dose. This should be done by reducing the total dose by 25% on a 1 to 2 week basis. As mentioned above, the rate of reduction will depend on disease progress/activity. When the dose is weaned down to a physiological dose, we would then advise to switch to an equivalent dose of hydrocortisone of 10 mg/m^2/day in four divided doses.

The advantage of switching to hydrocortisone at this stage is that we are dealing with normal cortisol production rates and hydrocortisone, which is synthetic cortisol, is the preferred glucocorticoid replacement. It is also easy to measure in the circulation. Hydrocortisone doses can then be reduced by 2.5 mg per week until a total daily dose is reached which is at the lower end of the normal daily requirement of approximately 7 to 8 mg/m^2/day. This part of the weaning process may take some time as the closer the dose gets to the lower end of the normal daily requirement the more likely there may be symptoms of cortisol deficiency. In which case a lower weaning programme of 1.25 mg per week may be required. Once on this dose, the HPA axis can be assessed. Throughout this time on hydrocortisone, it is important the patient is aware of sick day rules, what to do during trauma and stressful procedures and that the patient receives More at 4 am. All these aspects are covered in detail in Chapter 12.

Specific weaning plan in congenital adrenal hyperplasia

One final situation where weaning down high doses of glucocorticoids is necessary, is in congenital adrenal hyperplasia when high doses of glucocorticoids are used to shrink the adrenal glands, which have increased in size due to the glucocorticoid replacement therapy not been optimised and ACTH has been elevated for a long period of time. It is often very difficult with conventional glucocorticoid replacement dosing, to reduce the ACTH, 17-hydroxyprogesterone (17OHP) and androstenedione concentrations to acceptable levels without over suppressing the adrenal glands which can happen when treatment is based solely on 17OHP levels. Enlarged adrenal glands arise from increased ACTH production. This can occur despite cortisol replacement assessed on 24 hour profiles seemingly looking like appropriate replacement therapy. This happens if sampling intervals are too long or the time when below 50 - 100 nmol/l is too long, so although the peaks may look acceptable the actual exposure to cortisol is reduced. This can also occur simply because the cortisol from the dosing schedule is incorrectly distributed from incorrect dose timings, fast metabolism of glucocorticoids, in some cases poor compliance or just simply under treatment.

In this situation higher doses of glucocorticoid are often required. This is because high levels of androstenedione and 17OHP in particular, compete for the glucocorticoid receptor impairing the feedback effect of cortisol on ACTH production at the level of the pituitary gland. Before increasing the glucocorticoid dose, it is important to consider whether there are adrenal rests present and not to rely on elevated 17OHP levels only. Both androstenedione and 17OHP are raised indicating the adrenal glands are enlarged. In both the following cases, the patients had a sonogram to check for adrenal rests. Both showed normal testicular structures, and CT scans of the adrenal glands showed enlargement, which concurred with the biochemical findings. The high doses can be weaned down once ACTH levels have been suppressed and the size of the adrenal glands reduced which can take anything from 6 to 12 weeks. Once this has been achieved, the glucocorticoid doses can be weaned down to standard replacement doses based on ACTH measurements returning to within the normal range. 24 hour cortisol profiles as in Figure 15.10 with measurements of ACTH, 17OHP and androstenedione are useful in determining the adequacy of the hydrocortisone replacement in these situations.

Shrinking the adrenal glands in congenital adrenal hyperplasia using the continuous hydrocortisone subcutaneous pump method and the Peter Hindmarsh formula

A successful example of weaning down doses to shrink the adrenal glands in a patient with congenital adrenal hyperplasia, whose adrenal glands were enlarged due to a problem with the cortisol shuttle (Chapter 11, Figure 11.7 Charts A and B), with replacement treatment via the continuous subcutaneous hydrocortisone infusion pump using the Peter Hindmarsh formula has been already mentioned.

The starting dose was high at 80 mg per day with the basal hydrocortisone infusion rates calculated to mimic the circadian rhythm. This resulted in the normalisation of androstenedione (Chapter 11, Figure 11.10) and 17OHP (Chapter 11, Figure 11.5), both of which remained stable as the pump rates were carefully reduced over time towards a final total daily dose of 32 mg per day. This also resulted in the normalisation of testosterone, LH and FSH (Chapter 11, Figure 11.24).

Interestingly, it was documented that this individual needed to take high doses of hydrocortisone since diagnosis. The pump delivery system overcame the problem with the cortisol shuttle, which had resulted in a cortisol half-life of 40 minutes and by mimicking the circadian rhythm using the Peter Hindmarsh formula, the adrenal glands were reduced to normal size. It is often thought the daily hydrocortisone dose of 32 mg is high, but this is needed in an individual who has a fast clearance and is not excessive as evidenced by the normal circadian plasma cortisol profiles.

The overall daily dose required using the pump was less than the oral hydrocortisone daily dose previously taken, with the continuous delivery on the lower dose resulting with no periods of over and under treatment which had occurred daily formerly when on oral therapy using 6 high doses per day, due to the very rapid clearance of hydrocortisone.

Further, for many years because of the problem with the cortisol shuttle, the patient was underweight which normalised and remained stable after this shrink and wean approach.

Shrinking the glands in congenital adrenal hyperplasia using oral hydrocortisone medication

Figure 15.15 Charts A, B and C illustrate a situation in a teenage boy with congenital adrenal hyperplasia where 17OHP and androstenedione were elevated despite seemingly good cortisol replacement. A CT of the adrenal glands showed bilateral enlargement (adrenal hyperplasia). Each chart shows the three profiles undertaken, in the process of shrinking the glands as well as the weaning process. In this case the patient remained on oral hydrocortisone. However, several adjustments were made to both doses and dose timings.

Chart A compares the plasma cortisol, Chart B the plasma 17OHP and Chart C the plasma androstenedione profiles.

Chart A Profile 1, the initial profile was undertaken with a long sampling interval (2 hourly) and does not give as clear a picture over the 24 hours when compared to the hourly sampling taken both in Profile 2 and Profile 3.

- Profile 1 was undertaken on 35 mg of hydrocortisone per day.
- Profile 2 was undertaken six months after the dose was increased to 45 mg per day with dose times adjusted.
- Profile 3 was undertaken six months after the daily dose was reduced back to 35 mg with adjusted dose timings (same dose times as Profile 2).

MANAGING AN INADEQUATE REPLACEMENT SCHEDULE (PROFILE 1) BY INCREASING THE HYDROCORTISONE DOSES (PROFILE 2). THEN AS THE ADRENAL GLANDS NORMALISED IN SIZE, WEANING THE HYDROCORTISONE DOSING SCHEDULE BACK TO A MORE PHYSIOLOGICAL CORTISOL REPLACEMENT (PROFILE 3)

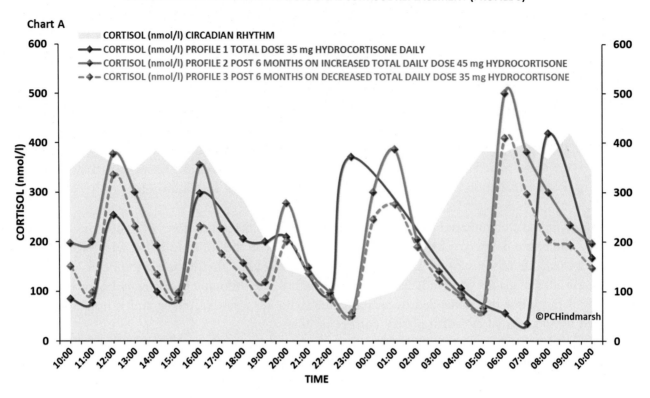

EFFECT ON 17-HYDROXYPROGESTERONE MANAGING AN INADEQUATE REPLACEMENT SCHEDULE (PROFILE 1) BY INCREASING THE HYDROCORTISONE DOSE (PROFILE 2) THEN WEANING THE HYDROCORTISONE DOSE BACK TO A MORE PHYSIOLOGICAL REPLACEMENT SCHEDULE (PROFILE 3)

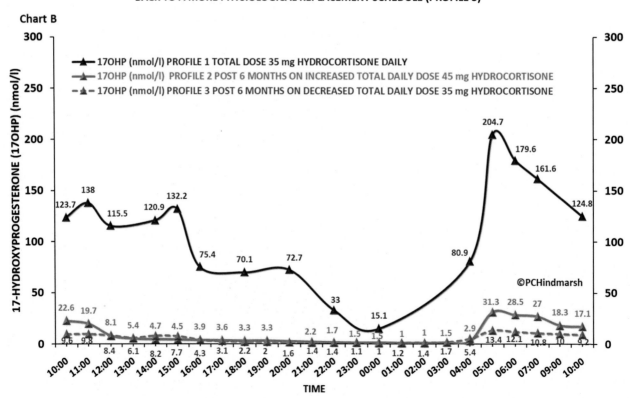

EFFECT ON ANDROSTENEDIONE WHEN MANAGING AN INADEQUATE CORTISOL REPLACEMENT SCHEDULE (PROFILE 1) BY INCREASING THE HYDROCORTISONE DOSE (PROFILE 2) THEN WEANING THE HYDROCORTISONE DOSE BACK TO A MORE PHYSIOLOGICAL REPLACEMENT SCHEDULE (PROFILE 3)

Figure 15.15 *Effect of increasing and then weaning total daily oral hydrocortisone dose in a teenage boy with congenital adrenal hyperplasia with elevated 17-hydroxyprogesterone and androstenedione levels due to unsatisfactory replacement therapy. The charts show the adrenal steroids cortisol (Chart A), 17-hydroxyprogesterone (Chart B) and androstenedione (Chart C). Cortisol half-life was 73 minutes so fast clearance was not the explanation for lack of treatment efficacy (Profile 1). The 45 mg per day hydrocortisone dose (Profile 2) allowed shrinkage of the enlarged adrenal glands and a return to the original daily dose of 35 mg per day of hydrocortisone but redistributed to avoid periods of time when plasma cortisol was very low (Profile 3). Note the doses used are specific to this individual and will be different for different people. Patient became an early riser taking first dose at 05:00 (5 am) to help improve cortisol profile.*

When we compare the Profile 1 data in Chart A, B and C, the cortisol (Chart A solid blue line) showed seemingly good values on the initial 35 mg per day. However, the 17 OHP (Chart B solid purple line) and androstenedione levels (Chart C solid green line) were elevated reflecting an increased ACTH drive. What appears to be happening here, is the raised androstenedione competing against cortisol for access to the glucocorticoid receptor at the level of the hypothalamus and pituitary, blocking cortisol feedback on ACTH resulting in an increased ACTH drive to the adrenal glands.

The morning plasma cortisol peak is reasonable at 419 nmol/l (Figure 15.15), however the time spent within and below the critical plasma cortisol concentration of 50 – 100 nmol/l, which brings the plasma 17OHP (unless the patient has adrenal rests) into the normal range, was approximately 5 hours on Profile 1. This is probably an underestimate as the sampling interval was long which will have missed times of low plasma cortisol concentrations. Further, the androstenedione levels were high for many hours through the profile. The raised 17OHP and androstenedione indicate enlargement of the adrenal glands and to regain control of the situation, higher doses of hydrocortisone are required to reduce the ACTH drive to the adrenal glands and to reduce/shrink them in size. To achieve this without producing side effects from very high doses, the dose was increased to 45 mg of hydrocortisone per day with the dosing times carefully calculated and adjusted on the results of a clearance test (half-life 73 minutes).

All results on the increased dose (Profile 2 undertaken after six months on this higher dose) are represented by an orange solid line in all three charts. The increased dose raised the cortisol peak to 501 nmol/l as well as provided more appropriate cortisol concentrations between 06:00 (6 am) and 09:00 (9 am) and more importantly, reduced the time cortisol levels were in the 50 - 100 nmol/l range to approximately 2 hours. This would shift the competition at the glucocorticoid receptor in favour of cortisol. As can be seen in Profile 2, the 17OHP (Chart B) and androstenedione (Chart C) levels reduced as the higher dose decreased the size of the adrenal glands, but even after 6 months of the increased dose the 17OHP was still elevated during the night period.

Even with this slight elevation in 17OHP after 6 months on the higher dose, a repeat CT scan showed normal sized adrenal glands. The daily dose was then reduced to the original dose of 35 mg, with the adjusted dosing times remaining and after 6 months a further 24 hour profile (Profile 3) was undertaken. Chart A Profile 3 (light blue dashed line) shows the dosing regimen better approximated the normal circadian rhythm of cortisol, with a lower peak cortisol of 410 nmol/l and only 3 hours spent between 50 - 100 nmol/l. These changes can be attributed to adjusted dosing taking into account the biological half-life of oral hydrocortisone. Further, Charts B and C Profile 3 show both the 17OHP and androstenedione were now within the normal range which would be expected as the adrenal gland size had been returned to normal. The increased dose simply reduced the ACTH drive which led to a reduction in size of the adrenal glands and normalisation of 17OHP and androstenedione without over exposure to cortisol. As everyone absorbs and clears hydrocortisone differently, we have not added in the actual cortisol values to Chart A but have shown values for 17OHP (Chart B) and androstenedione (Chart C) to illustrate how the hypothalamo–pituitary–adrenal feedback loops have been brought into range.

In CAH, although short term high glucocorticoid doses can bring 17OHP and androstenedione levels down, as soon as the dose is reduced the adrenal glands will become active as they are still enlarged, because it takes some time for them to reduce back to normal size. Slow reduction using an increased dose, dependent on the size of the adrenal glands and with the distribution calculated using the individual's clearance and half-life, will over time normalise 17OHP and androstenedione. This example illustrates another very important point particularly in the variation in the androstenedione concentrations over the 24 hours in Figure 15.15 Chart C Profile 1, because if a single measurement had been taken at 10:00 (10 am) the result of 9.9 nmol/l would have been within the normal range, however the sample taken an hour later was high at 28.2 nmol/l. This example also highlights the important information more frequent sampling i.e., hourly over a 24 hour period provides which aids interpretation and medication adjustment more accurately.

USING SYNACTHEN TO STIMULATE SUPPRESSED ADRENAL GLANDS

One final comment is regarding the use of the prolonged synacthen test to stimulate recovery of switched off adrenal glands. In this test a fixed dose synacthen subcutaneous depot is used which releases ACTH slowly over a 2 to 3 day period. This stimulates the adrenal glands to produce cortisol and may well waken up the adrenal glands to start to produce some cortisol. This approach has not been tested formally and will probably only work if there is already some endogenous ACTH to continue adrenal stimulation once the depot synacthen (synthetic ACTH) wears off.

ASSESSING THE RECOVERY OF THE HYPOTHALAMO-PITUITARY-ADRENAL AXIS

There are two questions which need to be asked when considering recovery of the axis. The first, is whether the day to day cortisol production is normal and the second, is whether the system can respond to stressful situations. These two questions require two different approaches. The physiological question whether cortisol is being produced normally can only be really answered by undertaking a 24 hour cortisol profile.

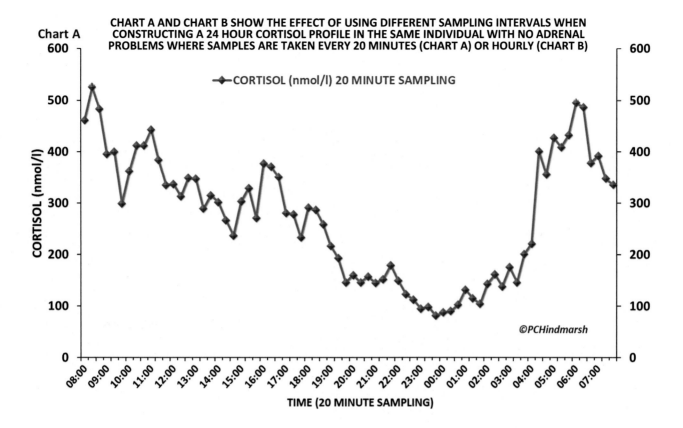

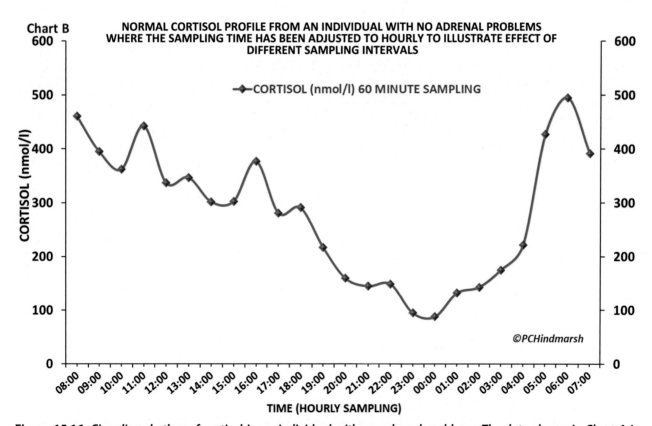

Figure 15.16 *Circadian rhythm of cortisol in an individual with no adrenal problems. The data shown in Chart A is constructed using a 20 minute sampling interval. Chart B is the same data set but with a 60 minute sampling interval. Note the loss of detailed description of the peaks but the overall rhythm is maintained Please remember it is the circadian pattern of cortisol over the 24 hours which is important. The actual cortisol values will vary between individuals.*

The profile data gives a considerable amount of information regarding the attainment of a normal circadian rhythm as shown in Figure 15.16 Charts A and B. The Figure also illustrates the importance of the sampling interval with hourly sampling losing detail compared to 20 minute sampling. In assessing adequacy of recovery, consideration needs to be given to the peak concentrations attained in the morning as well as how closely the cortisol production matches the normal circadian profile.

The use of a 24 hour urinary free cortisol or urinary steroid profile to assess total cortisol excretion is different to using a blood profile. The reason for this is the urinary free cortisol measurement requires a reasonable amount of cortisol to be filtered by the kidney and this will only occur when cortisol concentrations are high and the saturation of the cortisol binding globulin is 100%. As saturation only takes place around a plasma cortisol concentration of 500 nmol/l, the urinary measure is not a good measurement of adequacy of cortisol production. The urinary steroid profile can give a better approximation of cortisol production if all the metabolites in the urine from cortisol are considered. However, it does not describe whether the circadian rhythm has been attained or not.

Salivary cortisol suffers the same drawbacks as urinary free cortisol.

Whenever we are assessing cortisol in these situations, we need to be very careful that the assay used does not cross react with some of the glucocorticoids used as anti-inflammatory agents. If there is cross-reactivity with some of these drugs with prolonged durations of action, then falsely normal cortisol levels may be obtained during testing.

The stress response is usually assessed by using the synacthen test. This involves the administration of synthetic ACTH and measuring the adrenal response in terms of cortisol produced over a 30 or 60 minute period. A variety of doses of synacthen have been proposed and in general a peak response of greater than 500 nmol/l is generally presumed an adequate stress response. In addition to the absolute cortisol value attained, it has been proposed that a doubling of the baseline unstimulated plasma cortisol concentration be included in the definition of adequacy of response. The problem with this is if the initial unstimulated plasma cortisol concentration is low, for example 150 nmol/l then doubling only achieves 300 nmol/l which would still be viewed as an inadequate stress response to synacthen stimulation. A full discussion of synacthen testing is provided in Chapter 4 and illustrated in Figure 4.15.

CONCLUSION

The anti-inflammatory effects of glucocorticoids has revolutionised modern medicine allowing many conditions to be treated and transplanted organ rejection prevented. Such success comes with the price of potential adrenal suppression. Care needs to be taken with other sources of glucocorticoids such as inhaled steroids for asthma which vary in potency. It may not be obvious that a glucocorticoid is present in the inhaler simply from the brand name. For example, Fostair or Luforbec contain a long acting beta receptor agonist to open the airways and beclomethasone (glucocorticoid) which prevents relapse. Glucocorticoid withdrawal needs to be carefully planned and related to disease activity, duration of therapy, type of glucocorticoid used and the dosing regimen. Short term exposure for less than 3 weeks can be simply managed by stopping the therapy (with a set of caveats outlined in Figure 15.13), but exposure greater than 3 weeks needs careful dose reduction. There is a hierarchy of recovery with ACTH first along with the circadian rhythm. The stress response recovers last. Recovery of physiological cortisol secretion can be assessed with 24 hour plasma cortisol profiles, however if not possible, then to undertake a day curve with hourly sampling. The stress response is evaluated using the short synacthen test. Emergency regimens and sick day rules need to be in place until the stress response has fully returned. Although in most patients full recovery of the hypothalamo-pituitary-adrenal axis occurs, a small proportion do not and they will require long term glucocorticoid replacement therapy.

FURTHER READING

Aronson, J.K., 2006. Meyler's Side Effects of Drugs. Volume 1: A-B, 15th edn. Elsevier, Amsterdam.

Burki, T., 2021. Skin-whitening creams: Worth the risk? Lancet 9, 10.

Iliopoulou, A., Abbas, A., Murray, R., 2013. How to manage withdrawal of glucocorticoid therapy. Prescriber 19 May, 23–29.

Mayer, M., Rosen, F., 1975. Interaction of anabolic steroids with glucocorticoid receptor sites in rat muscle cytosol. Am J Physiol 229, 1381–1386.

National Institute for Health and Care Excellence, 2018. Inhaled corticosteroid doses for NICE's asthma guideline.

National Institute for Health and Care Excellence, 2020. Clinical knowledge summaries. Corticosteroids – oral. https://cks.nice.org.uk/topics/corticosteroids-oral/.

National Institute for Health and Care Excellence. British National Formulary, Hydrocortisone. https://bnf.nice.org.uk/drugs/hydrocortisone, https://bnfc.nice.org.uk/drugs/hydrocortisone. (Accessed 2023).

Pijnenburg-Kleizen, K.J., Engels, M., Mooij, C.F., et al., 2015. Adrenal Steroid Metabolites Accumulating in Congenital Adrenal Hyperplasia Lead to Transactivation of the Glucocorticoid Receptor. Endocrinology 156, 3504–3510.

Pofi, R., Caratti, G., Ray, D.W., Tomlinson, J.W., 2023. Treating the side effects of exogenous glucocorticoids; can we separate the good from the bad? Endocrine Rev 44, 975–101. https://doi.org/10.1210/endrev/bnad016.

Rensen, N., Gemke, R.J.B.J., van Dalen, E.C., Rotteveel, J, Kaspers, G.J.L., 2017. Hypothalamic-pituitary-adrenal (HPA) axis suppression after treatment with glucocorticoid therapy for childhood acute lymphoblastic leukaemia. Cochrane Database Syst Rev 11, CD008727. https://doi.org/10.1002/14651858.CD008727.pub4.

Younes, A.K., Younes, N.K., 2017. Recovery of steroid induced adrenal insufficiency. Transl Pediatr 6, 269–273.

CHAPTER 16

Chronic Health Care and Adrenal Insufficiency

GLOSSARY

Stages of reaction Various steps in the process from diagnosis to acceptance. The original five were denial, anger, bargaining, depression and acceptance.

Selective serotonin reuptake inhibitors Selective serotonin reuptake inhibitors are antidepressants that stop nerve cells in the brain from reabsorbing serotonin, which plays a key role in mood regulation.

GENERAL

Chronic health conditions are generally associated with poorer quality of life compared to the general population and the more health problems there are, then the worse the person usually feels. This is true in adrenal insufficiency where a number of studies including our own surveys, point to the poor subjective and objective health status of patients with various forms of adrenal insufficiency. There are likely to be many causes for these observations. The causes of adrenal insufficiency are varied and the factors causing the condition may play a role in the health outcomes themselves. In Addison's disease it is recognised that the disease itself seems to be an important factor and one cannot exclude what the impact of going from having a normal cortisol circadian rhythm to cortisol replacement, will have on someone.

Treatment regimens must also play a role in health outcomes and a number of these have been explored in Chapter 8. Weight gain and obesity reflect over treatment as do changes in cardiovascular risk factors and bone mineral density. Under treatment is associated with lack of energy as well as increasing the risk of episodes of adrenal crises.

LIVING WITH A CHRONIC ILLNESS

For the patient, attending clinics and meeting health care professionals can be daunting. Just dealing on a day to day basis with adrenal insufficiency is demanding. Tablets to take at set times of the day, checks to be made as to whether that headache is a sign that cortisol might be low, or is it just the odd headache that we all get from time to time. How well am I today and do I need to double my dose. And of course, how do I deal with the dentist!!?

Two problems present themselves immediately and are related. The numbers with the various forms of adrenal insufficiency are low when we look at the total population of a country. The number of new cases of Congenital Adrenal Hyperplasia (CAH) is estimated to be 40 per year in the United Kingdom which means that there are approximately 600 under 20 years of age with the condition and some 2000 adults. If we say there are some 250 to 300 adult endocrinology units in the United Kingdom, then each will see 6 to 8 cases each. This means that expertise in managing adrenal insufficiency will not be high. Even if we look to the Greater London area, we are only taking into account about 400 adult patients with CAH, a number we can double for other forms of primary adrenal insufficiency so that if we include all causes of adrenal insufficiency, this will only total some 1600 adults. Distribute those numbers between the 8 major

Replacement Therapies in Adrenal Insufficiency. https://doi.org/10.1016/B978-0-12-824548-4.00016-4

centres, then we have 200 per centre which is reasonable size as long as they are all seen by the same person in each centre. This means that for adequate expertise to be developed, then larger centres are the way to achieve this. Not only does this improve expertise, but it also provides a patient base which allows for interactions to develop between patients, especially if care is delivered in dedicated adrenal insufficiency clinics which provide consultations and annual checks (Chapter 7) as a 'one stop shop'.

The second problem for the person with adrenal insufficiency in addition to the day to day routine, is the isolation which can be felt as there are so few with the actual condition that the person can interact with. Social media can be advantageous, but unregulated sites without sound medical support can be dangerous and should be avoided.

As Franklyn D Roosevelt famously said, 'We have nothing to fear but fear itself.' This is true for chronic conditions, especially those where the person has to rely on life-saving medications such as cortisol where day to day judgements are important. The seriousness of the condition is rightly impressed upon patients, but this can lead to fear and paralysis in undertaking day to day activities. If I do such and such a thing, how will that affect me with this condition? Many patients experience this feeling and it is perfectly natural. It is part of a natural and normal reaction to a diagnosis or life event of which adrenal insufficiency is one.

Figure 16.1 puts these feelings into a series of events which have been identified from careful studies of how people react to serious events. The various steps in the cycle have been expanded over time from the original five described by Elisabeth Kubler-Ross. The original five were denial, anger, bargaining, depression and acceptance. It is important to stress that they do not all have to happen, or happen in the order outlined, although it is more than likely that the original five will happen.

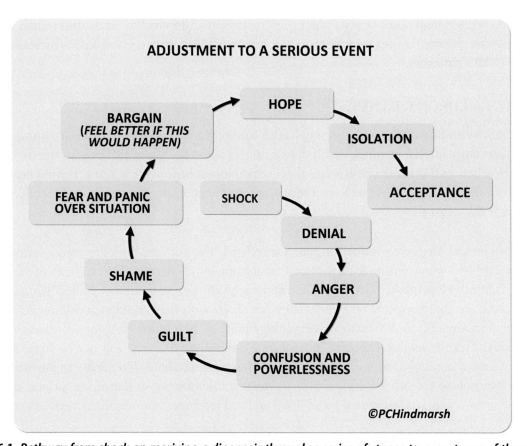

Figure 16.1 *Pathway from shock on receiving a diagnosis through a series of stages to acceptance of the condition.*

What is important, is that the person does not get 'stuck' at one particular stage and this requires skilful practice by all care providers to recognise if this is happening and to involve psychologists early to assist in helping the patient move to the next stage. For example, being stuck at the stage of denial makes it hard to get the replacement therapy adequately tailored and taken.

It is important to realise that these stages do not just apply to the person with the condition but also to other family members, particularly when the patient is a child i.e., the parents. Many of the causes of primary adrenal insufficiency arise from inheritance of a faulty gene from one or both parents. This certainly influences the guilt component and this component needs careful handling by the clinical team who need to be aware of this broader context and help the family through this difficult set of stages. Time spent at these stages is time well spent.

We now look at the five steps.

Denial

Denial is a natural stage which helps cope with the news of the diagnosis. This can present itself with reactions such as, life makes no sense, has no meaning and everything is too overwhelming. It is common to think —how will I live with this condition, everything has changed? You might think — is the diagnosis correct? It must be a mistake!

The denial stage is important as it helps in spacing out feelings about the diagnosis, so instead of becoming completely overwhelmed with grief, it is spread out. It can be likened to a natural defence mechanism. The brain is buying time to process the information and to work out how this will all impact on day to day life.

Over time, the denial and shock start to fade. This is good news as this is the start of the recovery phase. This is all to the good but in making this progress, the feelings which have been suppressed during the denial stage come to the surface and will have to be acknowledged and dealt with, as one goes through the whole process to reach the point of acceptance.

Anger

This is a common stage and can best be summarised as the thinking 'why me?' and 'life's not fair!' It is hard to think how something like adrenal insufficiency could happen to you. This is a very uncomfortable stage but studies show the anger step is extremely important to reach and to go through. It is the stage many people get stuck at. It is important to feel angry and it does resolve. The quicker you get through this stage, the quicker you get to acceptance.

Directing anger at someone or something is really important, as it means connections with other people are starting again, which is a critical step. It can be difficult for the other person as well, so when thinking about seeking help it is important to also involve others who may be involved in your life. This may be partners, siblings, parents, or close friends. They may find it hard too, especially as they will have noticed how you have changed in reaction to the diagnosis.

Bargaining

This is something that we do within our minds. We make deals saying things such as, if someone can change this, I'll do the following... This is a natural reaction as it is hope which we are trying to grasp, although because of the actual bargaining we go through, the hope can be false. This uses the 'what if' situation. It can be quite irrational at times. For example, what if I had not thought such and such or not eaten that food, I would not have developed Addison's disease. It can be a really difficult stage especially when we know very little about what triggers the autoimmune process in Addison's disease.

It may have a more concrete base say in a person with hypopituitarism following a pituitary tumour, where the 'what if' might be what if I had gone to see a doctor six months ago, it would have been picked up sooner and I might not have needed such extensive treatment.

We also see this in secondary adrenal insufficiency because of exogenous glucocorticoids used for treating inflammatory conditions. Here not only the underlying inflammatory condition has to be accepted and managed, but also the unintended consequence of the glucocorticoid therapy which helps with the inflammation, but at the cost of producing adrenal insufficiency. This can lead to anger at both conditions and a question of if I had known I might have explored other treatment options before accepting the glucocorticoid therapy.

It may seem that these thought processes are not helpful as what has happened is reality. In fact, having thoughts such as these are extremely important as they are part of the process of adapting and accommodating to the diagnosis. They may not seem rational to the observer as they are about what might have been, however should not be dismissed but carefully discussed allowing the patient to fully explore the thoughts and to come to terms with the situation.

Depression

Depression is the feeling which is most associated with this whole process. You can definitely feel depression. In adrenal insufficiency it is quite common and may be long standing and associated sometimes with the treatment, particularly if high dose and potent glucocorticoids such as prednisolone are used. Depression represents the feeling of realising that you have this condition and it is not possible to go back to what things were like beforehand. This is especially the case in adrenal insufficiency which has an onset outside of childhood where the person knows what it is like to have a life with normal cortisol production but has to adapt to replacement therapy.

In this stage several things can happen. You might withdraw from life, feel numb, live in a fog with the outside world seeming overwhelming and experience feelings of hopelessness. You might even experience suicidal thoughts. This stage may need a lot of involvement from psychology and even occasionally medication with antidepressants.

Acceptance

This stage is not just about it is alright that I have adrenal insufficiency, but rather I have adrenal insufficiency but I'm going to be alright. In this stage, emotions stabilise. The 'new' reality is that adrenal insufficiency is not going to go away. It is not great to have it — but it's something you can live with. There will be good and bad days and with time the good days outnumber the bad. In this stage, the fog lifts and you start to engage with friends again.

This stage really puts the onus on health care professionals to get the replacement therapy right. Before this stage is reached, it can be very difficult to determine whether the symptoms are due to the reaction and accommodation to the diagnosis, or to how optimal the replacement therapy is. Once at the acceptance stage, then the focus is more on getting the replacement therapy right if symptoms persist.

Figure 16.2 lists the symptoms which may manifest during these stages.

COMMON EMOTIONS AND SYMPTOMS WHEN ADJUSTING TO A NEW DIAGNOSIS

- Crying
- Headaches
- Difficulty Sleeping
- Questioning the Purpose of Life
- Feelings of Detachment
- Isolation from Friends and Family
- Worry and anxiety
- Frustration
- Guilt
- Fatigue
- Anger
- Loss of Appetite
- Aches and Pains
- Stress
- Fear of the future
- Hopelessness
- Depression

©PCHindmarsh

Figure 16.2 *List of symptoms which may manifest in adjusting to a new diagnosis.*

Treatment of the Grief Reaction

The prescribing of medication and engagement in counselling are the mainstays of helping people through the stages. Medications may include the use of sedatives, antidepressants, or anti-anxiety medicines. There is a fine line to be walked between the use of these treatments, as it is easy to become dependent on them and some doctors would argue that they slow down the process towards acceptance. Nonetheless in the short term they can be helpful.

As with any medication, it is worth checking how they might interact with the medications that you are on and many of these might do just that. Chapter 6, Figure 6.8 contains a useful table that looks at potential drug interactions.

The medications available range from antidepressants and anti-anxiety agents such as the selective serotonin reuptake inhibitors (SSRI), to the more symptomatic treatments such as propranolol.

Although SSRIs are a type of antidepressant, they are considered also by some as the first-line drug treatment for anxiety. Selective serotonin reuptake inhibitors stop nerve cells in the brain from reabsorbing serotonin, which plays a key role in mood regulation.

Benzodiazepines are a type of sedative drug that reduce the physical symptoms of anxiety, such as tense muscles. These drugs also encourage relaxation and their effects take place within a few minutes. They are however prone to make the person sleepy so are not good for use during the day especially in the workplace. They are also known to promote dependence on them in the person so need to be used for short periods of time and reduced slowly when coming off them.

Finally, beta blockers which are usually used to reduce high blood pressure, reduce the effects of noradrenaline which gives many of the feelings of anxiety.

Counselling is the more commonly used approach. This may be individual or in the group setting usually with a psychologist or psychotherapist. The counsellor needs to be knowledgeable about the adrenal condition that the patient has. This would include not just the cause of the adrenal insufficiency, but also the replacement therapy used as well as understanding the life-threatening issues associated with the condition and its treatment. The latter is extremely important as so many patients and their families are scared of illness and feel that they live their lives on a knife-edge. Counselling is very good when your reaction to the diagnosis is creating obstacles in your everyday life. None of these approaches offers a 'cure,' but they do provide coping strategies to help you deal with all this in an effective way.

The important point to remember in all of this is that these are normal reactions to the situation. There is nothing to be ashamed of in having or admitting to these types of feelings. Recognising them is a key step and getting appropriate help will lead to a quicker resolution. More work needs to be done also with health care professionals particularly. Family Practitioners who often have a better grasp of the situation the person finds themselves in, are likely to be in better touch with local services which can help, than more remote endocrine clinics. The role of the family doctor can be enhanced with good communication between the endocrinologist and the practice. Simple leaflets explaining the condition, which is rarely encountered in family practice, are helpful. So too are treatment plans, these are useful especially when they state that treatment is lifelong, extra medication needs to be prescribed for extra cover in illness and hydrocortisone for injections prescribed for emergency kits. These prescriptions are life long and should never be stopped. This is a constant worry for many patients.

Above all it is too easy to take judgemental positions. This has no place. We all should be there to listen and help.

HAVING A CHILD WITH A LONG TERM CONDITION

Having any child can be immensely rewarding but at times stressful. This is especially so when the child or young person has a chronic medical condition. When they are babies and also at junior school, parents have control over what they do and in terms of adrenal insufficiency, with how the medication is given. In adolescence, this control is gradually handed over to the young person. It is done however, on the developmental background of understanding causation. Something you might do today might have an impact in the future. That future might be weeks, months or years ahead. The realisation of causation and the fact that what you do today might have an impact on something tomorrow, develops slowly during adolescence and isn't fully in place until about 16 to 18 years of age. This can make taking medications regularly challenging, because telling an adolescent that they will become ill tomorrow if they do not take medications regularly today, is difficult for them to grasp. They will probably understand over a short period of time, but over longer periods they are less likely to. A more common problem is not that doses are missed, but are taken at the wrong time, which is a problem with our treatments that rely on timing to replace correctly and avoid side effects. Although annoying, this behaviour lasts for a very short duration.

This is part of a broader issue in adolescents of being in control. The young person may want to be in control, for example, taking their tablets but social activities, for example sports and lunchtime may mean medicines are forgotten. This is rarely wilful and more a 'I forgot because there was so much going on' event. The standoff arguments which can arise at home are unhelpful. Rather, gentle persuasion and questions such as 'what might you do to remind yourself' are better approaches. The idea is to promote responsibility, which is what they want, but in a way which is safe and achievable.

The 'you must' approach is counterproductive; people, as always, are more likely to do something if it is their own idea, even if it isn't!

Parents should encourage children to believe they are normal and can live a normal life but need to take tablets and the key is to get the replacement correct. They will not die suddenly if they get overexcited as has appeared in some newspaper reports. If that were the case no one would survive as emotional challenges are faced all the time at home, in school and when out with friends. Only a lack of cortisol will cause an adrenal crisis, and/or in the case of those who are salt losers, a fall in sodium, which can be due to the imbalance of electrolytes. The condition needs to be put into perspective. It is serious but manageable within the framework of normal day to day activities. With the correct individualised replacement regimen, there is no reason for patients not to live a normal life and normal life span. It is important to keep reinforcing this positive aspect.

Long term side effects should be understood because noncompliance can cause long term health problems. Early education and understanding can prevent noncompliance too. Being too protective, a natural parental response can cause resentment. Again, it is 'the being different' that we mentioned above.

We explored how to talk to a child and young person about congenital adrenal hyperplasia (CAH) in Chapter 35 of our book Congenital Adrenal Hyperplasia: A Comprehensive Guide by Peter Hindmarsh and Kathy Geertsma. Here we looked at the various child ages and what could be said at the various stages to help the person understand their condition. It is not just down to the parents although they can seize on moments which crop up to explain the situation. Situations such as when the child asks 'why do I take this medicine and my friend does not' should be seized as great opportunities to raise the topic. Parents can also benefit from skilled health care professionals to guide them on the journey. Health care professionals need to be non-judgemental, open, and easily accessible.

Parents and carers often turn to social media groups for support, where they find they can share experiences, feelings, and concerns. Emotional support is great as members can relate to the condition. However, it is extremely important to discuss any medical concerns with your endocrinologist and not on social media, because as we have seen throughout this book, adrenal insufficiency is an individual disorder and each and every patient who has this will have different needs regarding replacement therapy.

Medical advice and suggestions on doses and dosing times should never be discussed even if well meaning. This could be libellous to the person giving advice if something untoward happens. Also be very aware, that experiences shared may sometimes not be completely accurate and written at a time when the person is feeling very emotional. The details shared may not be completely true or give the complete picture and may be exaggerated in order to create a dramatic story in an attempt to seek compassion from other parents. This is understandable but the incorrect facts may colour other families reactions and cause unnecessary worry and stress.

Opinions on blood results should not be sought or shared, again these can be misinterpreted, erroneously presented and shared without important factors the person may choose to omit or not even understand. Different assays are often used to measure the various hormones in the blood which result in various normal range parameters. Any concerns regarding tests and treatments should be shared with your consultant, not in social media groups. Exaggerated stories lead to unnecessary fear.

The connection between consultant and patient/parent is based on trust. The patient/parent trusts the consultant to use their knowledge to do the best for them/their child and the consultant trusts the patient/parents to follow the treatment plan set out for the individual. The treatment plan is based on clinical findings and experience and by acting on interpretations or suggestions other patients/parents make, even if the person is medically trained, it is not advisable without discussion with their consultant. This is becoming a serious problem and it might occur in the future that consultants will refuse to see patients if this trust is broken or make patients/parents sign an agreement. Problems should be discussed with endocrinologists or specially trained endocrine nurses and should be welcomed. A second opinion should be sought if the patient/parent has lost faith in the consultant, but it is important to discuss the problem with the consultant first without social media influence.

Parents should be extremely careful in sharing photographs of their children on social media stating their condition. Although this is well meaning, it is important to appreciate that children when they are older, may not wish to have their medical condition known for obvious reasons. If fundraising, a relevant logo could be used. On social media, even in private groups, there are usually many participants and it can never be certain of what these participants might share.

IMPACT OF THE CAUSE OF ADRENAL INSUFFICIENCY

Adrenal insufficiency is a collection of conditions that cause problems with cortisol production from the adrenal glands, either primarily or due to problems at the hypothalamus and/or pituitary level. In addition, we also need to add the effect of our replacement therapy and how close we come to mimic the circadian rhythm. We have covered some of this in Chapter 8 where we consider the side effects of replacement therapy. It also has to be remembered that when we have an established complication such as hypertension, then we have additional therapies which are needed to treat the side effects and these additional treatments bring with them their own side effects. Multiple drug therapies are common in chronic health problems, increasing the chance of drug interactions as well as adverse effects on mood and day to day activities. There is also a relationship between the number of medications taken and the person's compliance with the treatment. Finally, the greater the number of medications taken the lower the quality of life.

It is worth reiterating that the underlying condition causing adrenal insufficiency can also impact on a person's mental health. In CAH, both genders are often very self-conscious about their bodies when side effects from over and under treatment cause obvious signs such as precocious puberty and/or weight gain. Addison's disease, which is an autoimmune condition affecting the adrenal glands, also appears to impact on mood and this effect is not to do with any replacement therapy but appears to be a direct effect of the disease process. This may reflect the loss of the normal cortisol circadian rhythm which the person has had until developing the condition and despite our best endeavours with replacement with glucocorticoid therapy, we do not exactly reproduce the rhythm.

Similarly, in X-linked adrenoleukodystrophy we have effects of both the condition and its impact on brain function, as well as loss of cortisol and aldosterone from adrenal involvement. In addition, unless the deterioration in brain cognitive and motor function is not treated with bone marrow transplantation (which brings its own problems), this will lead to early death, so the young person also has to cope with this knowledge.

With respect to the secondary causes, hypopituitarism again has problems due to early deficiency of key hormones involved in brain development such as thyroxine along with the effects of hypoglycaemia on the developing brain, either due to the lack of counterregulatory hormones or inadequate replacement of them so coverage with cortisol may be poor, leading to periods of increased risk of developing low blood glucose.

As mentioned in Chapter 1, the genes involved in pituitary development are also important in other parts of brain development, so intellectual impairment can be quite complex to disentangle with the genetic effects, intermingled with hormone deficiencies and the problems with hormone replacement which we have noted in Chapters 8 and 13.

Finally, acquired hypopituitarism can have associated problems in terms of neurological function, cognition and emotions. Intracranial brain tumours can be successfully dealt with using a combination of neurosurgery, chemotherapy and radiotherapy. Radiotherapy can have profound effects on cognition in children, but both surgery and chemotherapy also have long term effects. This is in addition to the impact of having a diagnosis of cancer and the trauma of undergoing the intensive treatments required.

Managing all these aspects patients face, need to be factored into any follow up programme so that the individual and their problems is seen as a whole rather than a simple focus on the hormone missing.

CHRONIC HEALTH CONCEPTS

We now need to look at what is required in a health system that delivers chronic health care. As medical science and technology have advanced at a rapid pace, the healthcare delivery systems for chronic care have struggled to provide consistent high-quality care. Adrenal insufficiency is no exception and perhaps has fared worse than several other chronic conditions. This may well reflect the fact that there are very few hard end points to measure and surrogate markers, for example 17-hydroxprogesterone in CAH, do not necessarily reflect the problems which can be encountered with respect to side effects or drug interactions. Perhaps, in the past there has been an over emphasis on markers such as these, without much development in other important components on how adrenal insufficiency impacts on the life and family of the young person with adrenal insufficiency, or for that matter any environment in which the person with adrenal insufficiency finds themselves.

Adrenal insufficiency is a chronic disease which requires continuous monitoring and input which often involves different specialities along with a high level of patient/family involvement. Although the complexity is acknowledged, in practice there is little evidence that healthcare systems really understand these complexities and they tend to go on providing the same type of care which was delivered 10 to 20 years ago without the benefit of a more holistic approach to the patient's condition. This is largely because the models which were devised are based on acute medicine which uses as its base, the handling of infectious diseases in the 1950's and 1960's.

These approaches work along the lines that an individual presents with a problem, a diagnosis is made and then treatment instigated – the person either gets better or does not. For the infectious disease approach this worked well, particularly with antibiotic use.

Generally speaking, the acute medical model worked well also for other conditions such as heart attacks. The model is not good at dealing with chronic health problems. Endocrinology is essentially about managing chronic health because none of the interventions cure the condition as you might a sore throat with antibiotic treatment for 5 to 7 days.

We have seen throughout this book that adrenal insufficiency needs to be viewed from a chronic health standpoint, because the underlying physiology and treatment modalities force the clinician and the patient/carers to embark on a more equal interrelationship rather than the hierarchical model previously employed. The pharmacology of glucocorticoid replacement requires that medication is administered 3, 4 or more times per day, with adjustments made according to overall assessment of replacement therapy and changes made acutely to adjust for events such as illness.

This approach places the emphasis more on the patient/carers as the centre for decision making albeit in conjunction with their healthcare professionals, who act as a resource for advice and ongoing support.

Healthcare professionals have a very specific role in addition as they provide input into events such as planned surgery or the management of additional problems, such as excessive weight gain or those we outline in Chapter 8. There have also been further changes in the way in which individuals view making decisions about themselves. Healthcare in the early part of the 21st Century should now recognise the autonomy of the patient. This switch necessitates, however, a rethinking in the education and training programs provided for health care professionals and delivered to families and carers.

Education and training become an absolute necessity rather than a desirable part of the healthcare provision and this is best exemplified in helping patients and families with adrenal insufficiency, to understand their treatment regimens and the importance of 'sick day rules' for example. In fact, the purpose of this book was based on broadening the exposure of patients and their family/carers to understanding the condition they have and how this is managed with various treatments and the problems which can be associated with either the condition itself, or the treatment regimens employed.

In chronic health care, the challenge is to provide the patient with easy access to the information they require for executing their daily tasks, plus a background feedback system of how well they are doing with respect to their overall targets they have set themselves and agreed with their health care practitioners.

Sometimes this is not immediately obvious and partly reflects the fact that healthcare professionals have probably not identified the type of outcomes which are to be expected with the various conditions which fall under the category of adrenal insufficiency. We have outlined some of these in Chapter 7 where we looked at outcomes at different ages. The outcomes can be medical in nature or biochemical measures but whatever they are they have to be of value to the patient/family/carer themselves.

This is a particularly important concept because what may be a desirable outcome measure to a healthcare professional, for example, a normal 17-hydroxyprogesterone concentration, may be less important to a young person deciding on their A level course, or what job to pursue.

Striking this balance between all these potential outcomes is the task for all involved in chronic healthcare.

Switching the thinking from a hierarchical, 'you must do' approach to one of negotiation in the light of what is important to the individual has benefits in a number of areas. The clinician still has a duty to point out practices which are dangerous, but setting such information in the context of the patients' beliefs is more likely to be successful than a confrontational style.

If of course, what is being proposed to the clinician is frankly dangerous, then they must adopt a 'you must do,' for obvious safety reasons. This shift in perceptive is not a laissez-faire approach to a serious condition but a more collaborative approach to get the best for the patient and their carers and families. This transforms the occasional clinic meeting into a process of care, rather than a one-off single entity.

Too often, medical consultations consist of the patient attending and being seen by someone not necessarily the same person each time with a lot of time wasted in reiterating and going over the past. If these attendances are infrequent, then the worthiness of them becomes less and if the concerns and worries of the patient are not addressed, it is very easy for the patient to disengage from these as they cannot see any benefit of attendance.

THE ROLE OF FAMILY PRACTICE

In chronic health care, family doctors play an important role as they are very good at dealing with common problems and have a good understanding of how the patient and family are coping with the demands of a chronic health problem. However, they are unlikely to know a lot about adrenal insufficiency.

That said, there is a lot they can do and we outline this below. What the family doctor can do is to make sure that all the normal things which occur in children and adulthood such as immunisation and flu vaccinations, happen.

There is no reason why a child with adrenal insufficiency should not have all their immunisations including for Covid-19 and everyone should have the annual flu vaccine.

What is important is that responsibility for care is clearly defined between the hospital and the family doctor, so everybody knows what is expected of them. This is particularly important during illness when rapid review by the family doctor can prevent an admission to hospital.

Hospital Responsibilities

Hospitals take charge of monitoring the condition and in particular:

- Height and weight.

- Blood pressure monitoring.

- Medication dose changes.

- Arrangement of specialist hospital appointments.

- Annual review assessments and 24 hour profiles.

It is important that this information is supplied regularly to the family doctor to keep them up to date.

General Health

This can be provided as is usual for any person without adrenal insufficiency, by the family doctor. It is also important that everyone is aware of potential drug interactions with the glucocorticoids and Chapter 6 (Figure 6.8) contains a useful table of these.

Included under this heading are the full range of immunisations, developmental checks, health monitoring and screening for conditions.

Emergency Care

There are several aspects that a family doctor can help with:

1. Arranging and ensuring the continuation of 'Open Access' to avoid unnecessary delays in accident and emergency.

2. Have a copy of the emergency letter for all health care professionals at hand along with a copy of the hospital emergency guidelines plan.

3. Allow priority appointments when unwell.

4. Ensure that practice nurses and out of hours services are aware of the emergency protocol and are familiar with the importance of increasing steroids when ill, as well as the correct dose of hydrocortisone which should be administered intramuscularly.

5. Ensure the patient's condition is flagged on the practice GP system, so locum doctors, practice nurses are alerted that the patient has adrenal insufficiency.

6. Reinforce the need to wear a medic alert with the wording 'Adrenal Insufficiency.'

VACCINATIONS

Another area that Family Practices can get involved is with vaccination programmes. Every person with adrenal insufficiency, child or adult, should receive the full immunisation schedule.

Having adrenal insufficiency and receiving replacement glucocorticoids is not a reason not to be vaccinated.

It is true that patients receiving high dose glucocorticoids for anti-inflammatory conditions need to be careful when having vaccinations and they should not be undertaken until there has been a discussion between the clinician dealing with the inflammatory condition and the family practice.

People can have reactions to vaccines such as headaches, joint pains and a raised temperature. These should be dealt with symptomatically with analgesics and paracetamol to reduce the temperature and introduce the usual sick day rules outlined in Chapter 12. These reactions are short term lasting no more than 24 to 48 hours.

In addition to the vaccine programme for children, additional vaccines should be given to patients with adrenal insufficiency particularly the yearly influenza vaccine. For Covid-19 all with adrenal insufficiency should have the two initial doses followed by a booster dose 6 months after the second vaccine. Whether further yearly boosters will be needed is unclear at present. Figure 16.3 illustrates the current 2020 vaccination programme within the United Kingdom National Health Service.

The routine immunisation schedule   from June 2020

Age due	Diseases protected against	Vaccine given and trade name		Usual site
Eight weeks old	Diphtheria, tetanus, pertussis (whooping cough), polio, *Haemophilus influenzae* type b (Hib) and hepatitis B	DTaP/IPV/Hib/HepB	Infanrix hexa	Thigh
	Meningococcal group B (MenB)	MenB	Bexsero	Left thigh
	Rotavirus gastroenteritis	Rotavirus	Rotarix	By mouth
Twelve weeks old	Diphtheria, tetanus, pertussis, polio, Hib and hepatitis B	DTaP/IPV/Hib/HepB	Infanrix hexa	Thigh
	Pneumococcal (13 serotypes)	Pneumococcal conjugate vaccine (PCV)	Prevenar 13	Thigh
	Rotavirus	Rotavirus	Rotarix	By mouth
Sixteen weeks old	Diphtheria, tetanus, pertussis, polio, Hib and hepatitis B	DTaP/IPV/Hib/HepB	Infanrix hexa	Thigh
	MenB	MenB	Bexsero	Left thigh
One year old (on or after the child's first birthday)	Hib and MenC	Hib/MenC	Menitorix	Upper arm/thigh
	Pneumococcal	PCV booster	Prevenar 13	Upper arm/thigh
	Measles, mumps and rubella (German measles)	MMR	MMR VaxPRO[2] or Priorix	Upper arm/thigh
	MenB	MenB booster	Bexsero	Left thigh
Eligible paediatric age groups[1]	Influenza (each year from September)	Live attenuated influenza vaccine LAIV[2, 3]	Fluenz Tetra[2, 3]	Both nostrils
Three years four months old or soon after	Diphtheria, tetanus, pertussis and polio	dTaP/IPV	Repevax or Boostrix-IPV	Upper arm
	Measles, mumps and rubella	MMR (check first dose given)	MMR VaxPRO[2] or Priorix	Upper arm
Boys and girls aged twelve to thirteen years	Cancers caused by human papillomavirus (HPV) types 16 and 18 (and genital warts caused by types 6 and 11)	HPV (two doses 6-24 months apart)	Gardasil	Upper arm
Fourteen years old (school year 9)	Tetanus, diphtheria and polio	Td/IPV (check MMR status)	Revaxis	Upper arm
	Meningococcal groups A, C, W and Y disease	MenACWY	Nimenrix or Menveo	Upper arm
65 years old	Pneumococcal (23 serotypes)	Pneumococcal Polysaccharide Vaccine (PPV)	Pneumococcal Polysaccharide Vaccine	Upper arm
65 years of age and older	Influenza (each year from September)	Inactivated influenza vaccine	Multiple	Upper arm
70 years old	Shingles	Shingles	Zostavax[2]	Upper arm

1. See Green book chapter 19 or visit www.gov.uk/government/publications/influenza-the-green-book-chapter-19 or www.nhs.uk/conditions/vaccinations/child-flu-vaccine/
2. Contains porcine gelatine.
3. If LAIV (live attenuated influenza vaccine) is contraindicated and child is in a clinical risk group, use inactivated flu vaccine.

For vaccine supply information for the routine immunisation schedule please visit www.immform.dh.gov.uk and check vaccine update for all other vaccine supply information.

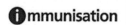 **mmunisation** | The safest way to protect children and adults   **NHS**

Selective immunisation programmes

Target group	Age and schedule	Disease	Vaccines required
Babies born to hepatitis B infected mothers	At birth, four weeks and 12 months old[1,2]	Hepatitis B	Hepatitis B (Engerix B/HBvaxPRO)
Infants in areas of the country with TB incidence >= 40/100,000	At birth	Tuberculosis	BCG
Infants with a parent or grandparent born in a high incidence country[3]	At birth	Tuberculosis	BCG
At risk children	From 6 months to 17 years of age	Influenza	LAIV or inactivated flu vaccine if contraindicated to LAIV or under 2 years of age
Pregnant women	During flu season At any stage of pregnancy	Influenza	Inactivated flu vaccine
Pregnant women	From 16 weeks gestation	Pertussis	dTaP/IPV (Boostrix-IPV or Repevax)

1. Take blood for HBsAg at 12 months to exclude infection.
2. In addition hexavalent vaccine (Infanrix hexa) is given at 8, 12 and 16 weeks.
3. Where the annual incidence of TB is >= 40/100,000 – see www.gov.uk/government/publications/tuberculosis-tb-by-country-rates-per-100000-people

Additional vaccines for individuals with underlying medical conditions

Medical condition	Diseases protected against	Vaccines required[1]
Asplenia or splenic dysfunction (including due to sickle cell and coeliac disease)	Meningococcal groups A, B, C, W and Y Pneumococcal Influenza	MenACWY MenB PCV13 (up to ten years of age)[2] PPV (from two years of age) Annual flu vaccine
Cochlear implants	Pneumococcal	PCV13 (up to ten years of age)[2] PPV (from two years of age)
Chronic respiratory and heart conditions (such as severe asthma, chronic pulmonary disease, and heart failure)	Pneumococcal Influenza	PCV13 (up to ten years of age)[2] PPV (from two years of age) Annual flu vaccine
Chronic neurological conditions (such as Parkinson's or motor neurone disease, or learning disability)	Pneumococcal Influenza	PCV13 (up to ten years of age)[2] PPV (from two years of age) Annual flu vaccine
Diabetes	Pneumococcal Influenza	PCV13 (up to ten years of age)[2] PPV (from two years of age) Annual flu vaccine
Chronic kidney disease (CKD) (including haemodialysis)	Pneumococcal (stage 4 and 5 CKD) Influenza (stage 3, 4 and 5 CKD) Hepatitis B (stage 4 and 5 CKD)	PCV13 (up to ten years of age)[2] PPV (from two years of age) Annual flu vaccine Hepatitis B
Chronic liver conditions	Pneumococcal Influenza Hepatitis A Hepatitis B	PCV13 (up to ten years of age)[2] PPV (from two years of age) Annual flu vaccine Hepatitis A Hepatitis B
Haemophilia	Hepatitis A Hepatitis B	Hepatitis A Hepatitis B
Immunosuppression due to disease or treatment[4]	Pneumococcal Influenza	PCV13 (up to ten years of age)[2,3] PPV (from two years of age) Annual flu vaccine
Complement disorders (including those receiving complement inhibitor therapy)	Meningococcal groups A, B, C, W and Y Pneumococcal Influenza	MenACWY MenB PCV13 (up to ten years of age)[2] PPV (from two years of age) Annual flu vaccine

1. Check relevant chapter of green book for specific schedule.
2. If aged two years to under ten years of age and unimmunised or partially immunised against pneumococcal infection, give one PCV13 dose.
3. To any age in severely immunocompromised.
4. Consider annual influenza vaccination for household members and those who care for people with these conditions.

immunisation | The safest way to protect children and adults

Figure 16.3 *Routine, selective and additional immunisations schedules in the United Kingdom for the year 2020.*

TRAVEL AND TIME ZONES

We have put this section in here because it is important that we do all the things that we want to do in life and having adrenal insufficiency should not stop you from doing so. A common request we get is for advice on travel and what to do with medications during travel and at what times should they be given. Holidays and trips away are exciting and there is no reason why a person with adrenal insufficiency cannot go where they want. It just needs some forward planning. This is best discussed early on with your endocrinologist. Other good sources are specialist travel clinics for advice on additional vaccinations or tablets. Many family practices run a specialised 'Travel Clinic' as do many hospitals.

Before you go

- Wear your medic alert bracelet or equivalent at all times.

- Ensure you have a copy of your emergency letter, and it is always a good idea to get it translated into the local language.

- Take your steroid or treatment card or recent clinic letter detailing dosing with you and make sure it is up to date.

- Carry your supply of tablets and the hydrocortisone for emergency use (make sure it is in date) in your hand luggage. It is always a good idea to get a customs letter from your consultant to explain this and the fact that you are carrying medications.

- Ensure you have enough supplies of everything for the length of your holiday. Then double the amount as getting medicines abroad can sometimes be difficult and the formulations are not always the same. Hydrocortisone is not available in some countries.

- For travel to the United States of America make sure that all your medications are carried in the boxes that were issued by your pharmacist. They need to show the name of the drug and that they were dispensed by the pharmacist. Most pharmacies place their label on the drug package which is all that is needed. Do not carry loose medications.

- Ensure you have your hospital contact number in your phone.

- For patients who take fludrocortisone. Some brands of fludrocortisone need to be refrigerated. For those that do it is perfectly safe to keep them out of a fridge for a 2 week holiday as only the backup supply needs to be kept cool. Putting them in and out of a fridge for short periods will do no harm.

- If you are going to a really hot country where the temperature will be above $35°C$ it is a good idea to take extra salt with you or make sure that snacks are savoury foods such as crisps.

- It is always best to keep medication in their labelled boxes along with a copy of your repeat prescription.

On your way

- If you are flying, all medication needs to be carried in your hand luggage as it is then accessible during the flight. If it goes in the baggage in the hold and the baggage goes missing, you could be left short!

- Also, the hold on an aircraft gets very cold, so the intense cold might alter how the medication works.

- You will need a letter from your endocrinologist to enable you to carry your emergency kit through customs (Figure 16.4). The letter should give flight details and which medications you are carrying.

On arrival

Increasing air travel means that many patients receiving oral hydrocortisone treatment have to face changes to their dosing schedule. For those on hydrocortisone pumps it is much easier to handle changes across time zones. You simply adjust the clock on the pump to the local time on arrival.

TRAVEL LETTERS

EXAMPLE A *(Oral Medication)*

Hospital letterheaded paper
(with relevant contact telephone numbers)

Name of patient:

Date of Birth: **Hospital Number:**

Medical Condition: *(Cause of Adrenal Insufficiency e.g. Addison's Disease)*

To Whom it May Concern

_____ has the above medical condition and receives treatment with hydrocortisone and fludrocortisone. This is lifesaving medication as is the emergency injections of hydrocortisone that he/she is also carrying. He/she needs to have this medication with them in the cabin of the plane and not in the luggage in the hold, to avoid freeze damage to the medications. He/she will also need to carry syringes and needles for the emergency intramuscular injection.

He/she will be flying to: _____ (full details of all flights including dates and times for both outgoing and return journeys should be provided).

I trust this letter will facilitate his/her safe passage through customs. Should there be any questions please contact _____ on the above telephone number.

Signature

(of either an endocrinologist, endocrine specialist nurse or member of the endocrine team)

EXAMPLE B *(Hydrocortisone Pump Therapy)*

Name of patient:

Date of Birth: **Hospital Number:**

Medical Condition: *(Cause of Adrenal Insufficiency e.g. Addison's Disease)*

To Whom it May Concern

_____ has the above medical condition and receives treatment with hydrocortisone and fludrocortisone. The hydrocortisone is delivered through a pump system which he/she wears and the pump must not be disconnected. He/she will be travelling with spare equipment for the pump, needles and an injection device, which will be used in emergency situations as well as the oral medications needed for the medical condition. He/she needs to have this medication with them in the cabin of the plane and not in the luggage in the hold, to avoid freeze damage to the medications.

He/she will be flying to _____ (full details of all flights including dates and times for both outgoing and return journeys should be provided).

I trust this letter will facilitate his/her safe passage through customs. Should there be any questions please contact _____ on the above telephone number.

Signature
(of either an endocrinologist, endocrine specialist nurse or member of the endocrine team)

©PCHindmarsh

Figure 16.4 *Example of a letter for customs for oral medications (Example A) and for a hydrocortisone pump (Example B).*

For oral medications, travel within Europe is not a problem but longer journey times may need some adjustment to the timings of doses (Figure 16.5). The times relate to travel from and to the UK.

TIME ZONE DOSE CHANGES

AFRICA   (Including South Africa)
Journey to and from Africa
No change required as within a 1 to 3 hour time shift.

EUROPE
Journey to and from Europe
No change required as within a 1 to 3 hour time shift.

EAST ASIA, AUSTRALIA OR NEW ZEALAND
Journey to and from East Asia, Australia or New Zealand
No significant changes as dose schedule is already 6 to 8 hourly.
Simply take tablets as normal until arrival then switch to local time
and dose as normal at usual times.

MIDDLE EAST OR INDIA
*Journey **to** Middle East or India*
   ➢ Evening dose as usual.
   ➢ Half morning dose on arrival.
   ➢ Normal dose schedule from the morning of arrival day including the morning dose as normal.

*Journey **from** Middle East or India*
   ➢ Repeat evening dose on boarding plane.
   ➢ Usual morning dose on arrival in UK.
   ➢ Second dose late afternoon.
   ➢ Late afternoon dose at 20:00 (8pm).
   ➢ Normal late evening dose.
   ➢ Normal dose schedule the following day.

UNITED STATES OF AMERICA
*Journey **to** USA*
   ➢ Morning dose as usual.
   ➢ Normal UK dosing until arrival.
   ➢ Half morning dose on arrival.
   ➢ Evening dose before going to bed.
   ➢ Normal dose schedule the following day.

*Journey **from** USA*
   ➢ Evening dose as usual.
   ➢ Normal dose schedule the following day.

©PCHindmarsh

Figure 16.5 *Changes to dosing times for different time zone travel. The travel times are based on travel from and to the UK.*

Fludrocortisone

No change to fludrocortisone is required as it is taken on a once daily basis and this should be continued. In those travelling to hot climates an increase in salt intake may be required.

When you are there

Most people do not get ill on holiday or become involved in accidents, however in the event these problems arise, they need to be dealt with in the same way that they would be at home (see Chapter 12).

However in illness always:

- When unwell, double or triple the hydrocortisone dose.
- If there is associated vomiting intramuscular hydrocortisone should be administered.
- If you have used the intramuscular injection of hydrocortisone, go to the nearest Accident and Emergency department as soon as possible and inform the doctors of the condition and that emergency hydrocortisone has already been given.
- The doctors need to check with blood tests for salt balance and blood glucose, so do not leave until this has been done.
- In any situation of doubt insist on admission for glucose, electrolyte and blood pressure monitoring. Particularly so if the patient is a child.
- Give an additional double dose of hydrocortisone at 04:00 (4 am). This extra dose should be equal to double the usual morning dose, which must also be a double dose and given at the usual time the morning dose is given.
- Diarrhoea is the major problem because of the fluid loss. This is the same whether the person has adrenal insufficiency or not. If it is associated with vomiting, you are best to get medical help quickly as you cannot be sure that any of the medication has either stayed down or been absorbed.
- When visiting some countries it is wise to use only bottled water for drinking, even when cleaning teeth and avoid ice in drinks.

Key points related to diarrhoea are:

- Diarrhoea is a particular problem due to the fluid losses.
- Oral rehydration solutions such as Dioralyte should be used.
- Make sure urine is passed regularly (see colour guide in Chapter 12).

Seek medical advice early especially:

- If there is a fever.
- Blood in the diarrhoea.
- The person becomes confused.
- The diarrhoea does not stop after 24 hours.
- There is associated vomiting.
- Do not use antidiarrhoeal drugs.

Antidiarrhoeal Drugs

Antidiarrhoeal drugs should always be used with caution.

In most cases of diarrhoea, taking an antidiarrhoeal medication will not treat the underlying cause (such as an infection or inflammation), but they may help with the discomfort that comes from having repeated watery bowel movements.

However, antidiarrhoeal drugs should not be taken when diarrhoea is accompanied by fever, severe illness, abdominal pain, or if there is blood or pus (mucus) in the stool. This can make the condition worse. These findings mean a medical opinion is needed urgently as taking antidiarrhoeal medication can lead to problems with the gut and the development of dilated pieces of bowel which can be dangerous.

SCHOOLS, COLLEGES AND THE WORKPLACE

With chronic health conditions it is important to determine how to fit the demands of the condition into everyday activities. It is best to think of it that way round rather than trying to fit day to day demands to the needs of the condition. In adrenal insufficiency, this means thinking about the daily dosing schedule and the need to be alert for situations where extra dosing may be required, for example illness.

Schools, nurseries, colleges and the workplace need to know exactly what to do as they will need to give doses during the day and also double doses if the person has an accident or becomes unwell. This is extremely important, not just from a safety perspective, but as we shall see later informing these bodies is an essential part of your rights under the Equality Act 2010. This applies to England and Wales and other countries have similar legislation.

In the European Union this is contained in Chapter 3 of the European Union Charter of Fundamental Rights 2012 and in the United States of America the Equality Act of 1974 which has undergone several amendments since.

Schools, colleges and the workplace need to make it possible to take medications on site so this means that glucocorticoid dosing can take place during the day or during shift work. Shift work is a difficult area, because the timing of the doses may need to be readjusted to work with the sleep wake cycle that has changed as a result of the shift work. This needs to be carefully worked out with the endocrine team.

Schools, colleges and the workplace are not obliged to give the emergency injections but many will if shown how to. Figure 16.6 is an outline school/nursery/college plan for the administration of hydrocortisone and a plan of how to handle illness and trauma at school/nursery/college. It is important to ensure the school, colleges and the workplace have the contact numbers for both parents/carers and are updated if those contacts change.

Children and young people do not like to be excluded from normal activities and there is no reason why any child or young person with adrenal insufficiency cannot be included on school trips and activities. What is important, is to ensure that medication is taken along as well as the emergency kit and that the staff understand if a dose needs to be taken, that it needs to be given on time and what needs to happen if the child becomes unwell. A drink should always be taken too, so the individual is able to take medication.

MEDICAL MANAGEMENT PLAN FOR SCHOOLS, NURSERY OR COLLEGE

NAME:

DATE OF BIRTH:

EMERGENCY CONTACT DETAILS:

STEROIDS TAKEN

Type of steroid: hydrocortisone

Dose of steroid to be administered at school: ....mg

Time of administration: ....hr

ILLNESS
In adrenal insufficiency extra medication is needed if the individual becomes unwell or has a serious injury to prevent a life-threatening adrenal crisis occurring. For minor falls, scratches, bumps and bruises no extra hydrocortisone is needed if they recover immediately and are able continue what they were doing before their accident.

Always notify the designated guardian or emergency contact of any illness or injury.

SERIOUS INJURIES
An intramuscular injection of hydrocortisone is needed immediately for the following:
* *Broken limb.*
* *Bump on the head leading to unconsciousness.*
* *Burn injury.*
* *If for any reason the individual is found in a condition where they are pale, clammy, drowsy and unresponsive (do not respond as they would normally do).*

After administering the hydrocortisone injection, dial 999 (UK) ask for an ambulance.

Advise ambulance control the individual has **Adrenal Insufficiency** *and must be taken to hospital to be monitored.*

Note: Even if the individual did not necessarily need the IM hydrocortisone injection, it will do no harm and it is always better they have the injection as more serious problems may occur if it is not given when needed.

GENERAL ILLNESSES
* *If an individual becomes unwell extra medication will be needed as soon as possible:*
* *High temperature (38°C degrees centigrade and over).*
* *If the individual faints.*
* *Stomach upset severe enough to prevent normal activities.*

A double dose of hydrocortisone should be given, whether the dose is due or not.

VOMITING
It takes 60 minutes for an oral hydrocortisone dose to be absorbed so if the individual vomits up their last administered dose within 60 minutes of taking it:
* *Repeat oral dose but double the amount.*
* *Contact parent/or their designated contact.*
* *If the second dose is vomited up, then give intramuscular hydrocortisone.*
* *Call ambulance on 999 and the individual should be taken by ambulance to nearest Accident and Emergency department.*

If vomiting occurs 60 minutes after a dose of hydrocortisone, then the medication is likely to have been absorbed and no repeat dose is needed. However, if vomiting occurs within 60 minutes, then the dose should be repeated.

If vomiting occurs again, then an intramuscular injection of hydrocortisone is needed and the person should go straight to Accident and Emergency. If the individual starts to vomit before medication is due, parents or their designated contact should be contacted immediately and seek medical advice. Closely monitor the individual's level of consciousness and if they become drowsy give an intramuscular hydrocortisone injection and call an ambulance.

©PCHindmarsh

Figure 16.6 *General guidelines for a medical care plan for a patient with adrenal insufficiency which can be adapted for use for those attending nursery, school or college.*

For schools, it is important that all staff are aware the student has adrenal insufficiency and problems can arise if there are new members of staff. To overcome this, the medical plan should have a photo of the child on it and a brief set of instructions of what to do in illness/injury placed on the staffroom or office information board. This needs to be updated at the start of every year with a new injection kit supplied. A note should be made of the expiry date of the hydrocortisone injection kit, so it is kept in date.

A new supply of tablets should be given to the school/nursery/college each term and the medical management plan renewed if a relevant dose is changed.

For college and universities, the general assumption is that students are responsible for administering their own medication. However, the University should be made aware of the student's medical condition and needs in illness and emergency situations. This is particularly important for participation in sporting activities and also the recognition that the student will be on their own so may have no support if unwell. In addition, places for the safe storage of medications (including fridges) in Halls of Residence should be provided for students using that type of accommodation.

This brings us to the Equality Act 2010. The Equality Act 2010 covers employment, provision of services and schools and higher education, the workplace and their premises. This defines conditions such as adrenal insufficiency as a disability because the condition has a long term adverse effect on the person. It does not matter that treatment seeks to prevent adverse effects, it is that without treatment adverse events would happen.

The Act protects the individual from direct (e.g. less favourable treatment because of the disability – exclusion from school activities would be an example) and indirect (e.g., a sickness policy that does not take into account the condition or need to attend clinic appointments) discrimination. It is important therefore, that all people involved with the person know about the condition because the Act does not apply if say the employer did not know that the person had adrenal insufficiency.

You do not have to declare a disability before interview only after acceptance of the job or place in school or college. Further, you should not be asked to declare a disability in the lead up application either.

There is also within the Act, a duty for the organisation/employer to make reasonable adjustments for the person. This might, in the case of adrenal insufficiency, mean places to store medications and emergency kits, awareness for all associated with the person of the needs of a person with adrenal insufficiency and patterns of working which allow for time to be taken off for medical appointments.

In England and Wales all components of the Act are enforced through Employment Tribunals or in the case of schools and colleges, Educational First Tier Tribunals.

CONCLUSION

Patients need to feel safe in the knowledge that their problems and concerns are taken seriously and addressed. This has to be done in the setting where experts work closely with patients and their carers to maximise their wellbeing. Patients must not give up on seeking answers, their issues may not be caused by adrenal problems but something else, but endocrinologists should strive to ensure cortisol replacement is correct first, so that it can be removed from the equation and teams should work together. This should not stop at childhood, or teenage years but for life as these conditions are incurable.

It is important that patients feel able to talk about what they face either with their endocrinologist or others such as psychologists. We need to remove the fear of talking about feelings after having gone through all the things that they face. Listening is key.

Adrenal insufficiency qualifies as a disability and there is legislation in countries to ensure equality of opportunity and the prevention of discrimination. In England and Wales this is enshrined in the Equality Act 2010. Patients need to be aware of this to ensure that their rights are respected and the patient has the right to seek redress if there are problems that cannot be resolved at school, college or in the workplace.

FURTHER READING

Buning, J.W., Brummelman, P., Koerts, J., et al., 2016. Hydrocortisone dose influences pain, depressive symptoms and perceived health in adrenal insufficiency: A randomized controlled trial. Neuroendocrinol 103, 771—778.

Equality and Human Rights Commission. www.equalityhumanrights.com.

Hindmarsh, P., Geertsma, K., 2017. Congenital Adrenal Hyperplasia: A Comprehensive Guide. Elsevier, New York.

Kubler-Ross, E., 2014. On Grief and Grieving. Simon and Schuster.

Lee, T.H., 2012. Care redesign—a path forward for providers. N Engl J Med 367, 466—472.

Rubin, R.T., Phillips, J.J., Sadow, T.F., McCracken, J.T., 1995. Adrenal gland volume in major depression. Increase during the depressive episode and decrease with successful treatment. Arch Gen Psychiatry 52, 213—218.

Vreeburg, S.A., Hoogendijk, W.J.G., van Pelt, J., et al., 2009. Major depressive disorder and hypothalamic-pituitary-adrenal axis activity: results from a large cohort study. Arch Gen Psychiatry 66, 617—626.

APPENDIX 1

Converting System International (Si) Blood Measures Into North American Values or Conventional Units

In this book, we have used the units of measurement used in Europe named the System International (SI). If you are from North America and some other parts of the world where this system is not commonly used, the blood results will be presented in different units. To help make the graphs easier to understand, the SI measures can be converted to North American measures by using the following table:

MEASURE	SI Units	Conversion	North American Units
Cortisol	nmol/l	*divide by 27.6*	mcg/dl
17-hydroxyprogesterone	nmol/l	*divide by 0.03*	ng/dl
Androstenedione	nmol/l	*divide by 0.035*	ng/dl
Testosterone	nmol/l	*divide by 0.035*	ng/dl
ACTH	pg/ml	*no difference*	pg/ml
LH	U/l	*no difference*	U/l
FSH	U/l	*no difference*	U/l
Estradiol	pmol/l	*divide by 3.67*	pg/ml
Blood glucose	mmol/l	*multiply by 18*	mg/dl
Growth Hormone	mcg/l	*no difference*	ng/ml

APPENDIX 2

List of Abbreviations

Common Abbreviations	
11beta-HSD1	11beta-hydroxysteroid dehydrogenase type 1
11beta-HSD2	11beta-hydroxysteroid dehydrogenase type 2
17OHP	17-hydroxyprogesterone
α	Alpha
ACTH	Adrenocorticotropin Hormone
AHC	Adrenal Hypoplasia Congenita
AVP	Arginine Vasopressin
β or b	Beta
BG	Blood Glucose
BMI	Body Mass Index
CBG	Cortisol Binding Globulin
C_{max}	Maximum peak concentration
CRH	Corticotropin-Releasing Hormone
CYP	Cytochrome P450 enzyme systems
CYP11B1	11beta-hydroxylase
CYP21	21-hydroxylase
DDAVP	1-Deamino-8-D-Arginine Vasopressin
DHEA	Dehydroepiandrosterone
DI	Diabetes Insipidus
E2	Estradiol
FSH	Follicle-Stimulating Hormone
FT4	Free Thyroxine
GH	Growth Hormone
GnRH	Gonadotropin-Releasing Hormone
hCG	Human Chorionic Gonadotropin
HPA	Hypothalamo-Pituitary-Adrenal Axis
IC_{50}	Concentration that inhibits an effect by 50%
IIHT	Insulin Induced Hypoglycaemia Test
LH	Luteinising Hormone

LOCAH	Late-onset Congenital Adrenal Hyperplasia
PTH	Parathyroid Hormone
PRA	Plasma Renin Activity
SRD5A1	Steroid 5-alpha reductase
StAR	Steroidogenic Acute Regulatory Protein
SULT2A1	Sulphotransferase family 2A member 1
SVCAH	Simple Virilising Congenital Adrenal Hyperplasia
SWCAH	Salt-wasting Congenital Adrenal Hyperplasia
T_{max}	Time to maximum peak concentration
TSH	Thyroid Stimulating Hormone

nmol/l	Nanomoles per litre
mmol/l	Millimoles per litre
mU/l	Milli Units per litre
pmol/l	Picomoles per litre
pg/ml	Picograms per millilitre
U/l	Units per litre

INDEX

'*Note:* Page numbers followed by "f" indicate figures.'

Printed in the United States
by Baker & Taylor Publisher Services